Y0-BQA-757

RISK ANALYSIS

Prospects and Opportunities

ADVANCES IN RISK ANALYSIS

This series is edited by the Society for Risk Analysis.

Volume 1 — **THE ANALYSIS OF ACTUAL VERSUS PERCEIVED RISKS**
Edited by Vincent T. Covello, W. Gary Flamm, Joseph V. Rodricks, and Robert G. Tardiff

Volume 2 — **LOW-PROBABILITY/HIGH-CONSEQUENCE RISK ANALYSIS**
Issues, Methods, and Case Studies
Edited by Ray A. Waller and Vincent T. Covello

Volume 3 — **RISK ANALYSIS IN THE PRIVATE SECTOR**
Edited by Chris Whipple and Vincent T. Covello

Volume 4 — **UNCERTAINTY IN RISK ASSESSMENT, RISK MANAGEMENT, AND DECISION MAKING**
Edited by Vincent T. Covello, Lester B. Lave, Alan Moghissi, and V. R. R. Uppuluri

Volume 5 — **RISK ASSESSMENT AND MANAGEMENT**
Edited by Lester B. Lave

Volume 6 — **NEW RISKS**
Issues and Management
Edited by Louis A. Cox, Jr., and Paolo F. Ricci

Volume 7 — **RISK ASSESSMENT IN SETTING NATIONAL PRIORITIES**
Edited by James J. Bonin and Donald E. Stevenson

Volume 8 — **RISK ANALYSIS**
Prospects and Opportunities
Edited by Constantine Zervos
Contributing Editors: Kathleen Knox, Lee Abramson, and Rob Coppock

Volume 9 — **THE ANALYSIS, COMMUNICATION, AND PERCEPTION OF RISK**
Edited by B. John Garrick and Willard C. Gekler
Contributing Editors: Caron Chess, Roger Kasperson, and Curtis Travis

A Continuation Order Plan is available for this series. A continuation order will bring delivery of each new volume immediately upon publication. Volumes are billed only upon actual shipment. For further information please contact the publisher.

RISK ANALYSIS
Prospects and Opportunities

Edited by
Constantine Zervos
Food and Drug Administration
Washington, D.C.

Contributing Editors
Kathleen Knox
U.S. Environmental Protection Agency
Washington, D.C.

Lee Abramson
Nuclear Regulatory Commission
Washington, D.C.

and
Rob Coppock
National Academy of Sciences
Washington, D.C.

PLENUM PRESS • NEW YORK AND LONDON

Library of Congress Cataloging-in-Publication Data

Society for Risk Analysis. Meeting (1988 : Washington, D.C.)
Risk analysis : prospects and opportunities / edited by Constantine Zervos.
p. cm. -- (Advances in risk analysis ; v. 8)
"Proceedings of the Annual Meeting of the Society for Risk Analysis, held October 30-November 2, 1988, in Washington, D.C."--CIP galley.
Includes bibliographical references and index.
ISBN 0-306-44113-6
1. Health risk assessment--Congresses. 2. Risk assessment--Congresses. 3. Cancer--Risk factors--Congresses. 4. Environmental health--Congresses. I. Zervos, Constantine. II. Series.
RB152.S63 1988
363.1--dc20 91-39959
CIP

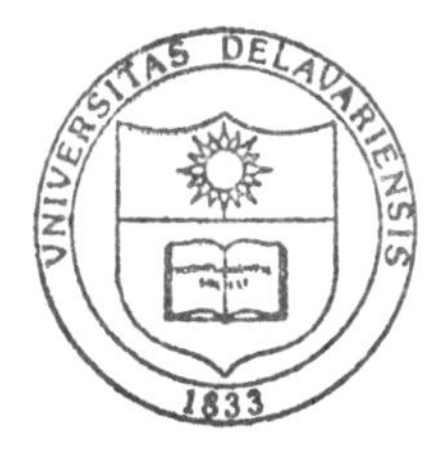

Proceedings of the annual meeting of the Society for Risk Analysis,
held October 30–November 2, 1988, in Washington, D.C.

ISBN 0-306-44113-6

A Division of Plenum Publishing Corporation
233 Spring Street, New York, N.Y. 10013

Printed in the United States of America

Preface

This volume of the series *Advances in Risk Analysis* consists of papers presented at the 1988 Annual Meeting of the Society for Risk Analysis, which was held October 30 through November 2 at the Mayflower Hotel in Washington, DC. The papers span the gamut of the increasing number of risk assessment topics addressed by the Society since it held its first annual meeting in June 1981, also in Washington DC. Organized to promote interdisciplinary analyses, the Society approaches risks from three broad perspectives: (1) the impact of various risks on the health of the world's populations and on the environment; (2) the social and political implications of specific risks, and (3) the management and reduction of risks through the development of a risk analysis methodology and corresponding data bases.

The papers included in this volume typify these three approaches and illustrate their interdependence. For example, both cancer and noncancer health risks are examined for a variety of situations that exist within society. The public's perception of risks and the correlation between that perception and the acceptance or nonacceptance of certain risks is also addressed. In addition, the progress to date on predicting and quantifying specific risks, including the risks associated with the construction and use of large engineered systems, is reported. Included among the papers are several dealing with recent current issues, such as the impact of California's Proposition 65, hazardous waste disposal, and chemical accidents.

As is usually the case in a compilation of this size, the cooperation of a number of individuals and organizations has made the publication of this volume possible. Particular thanks for paper reviews are extended to Kathleen Knox of the Environmental Protection Agency, to Lee Abramson of the Nuclear Regulatory Commission, and to Rob Coppock of the National Academy of Sciences. Appreciation is also expressed for the support received from the Division of Drug Research and Testing, Center of Drug Evaluation and Research of the U.S. Food and Drug Administration, both during the planning of the 1988 SRA meeting and during the editing of the papers submitted for these proceedings

Finally, gratitude is expressed to Katie Ingersoll of Tec-Com, Inc., for her diligence and patience in producing the camera-ready pages of this book for the publisher.

Constantine Zervos

Contents

Plenary: Twenty Year Retrospective on 1969 *Science* Paper of C. Starr, "Social Benefit vs. Technological Risk"

Chauncey Starr
Electric Power Research Institute
Palo Alto, CA

ABSTRACT

Those of us who believe that human welfare is significantly aided by technological progress have a clear motivation to accentuate the positive and to mitigate the negative consequences of technology. We thus share a common objective to allocate our limited societal resources effectively so as to improve public health and safety by minimizing real risks, both present and future.

Health and safety have no absolute measures—they are perceived as the absence of harm and risks. In a world in which zero risk is impossible and safety has no absolute measure, the question then arises as to how to determine "how safe is safe enough." This question specifically applied to large technological systems was the stimulus for the study which I published in *Science* in 1969. In the two following decades this subject has blossomed into a major field of study, as best symbolized by the membership of the Society for Risk Analysis. My talk is a short scan of the several approaches to this subject which have developed in the past two decades.

KEYWORDS: Revealed preferences, involuntary risk, acceptable risk

INTRODUCTION

The 1969 paper was based on two assumptions:

1. The performance criteria for a mature technological system is a balanced trade-off of societal benefits and societal costs, indirect as well as direct. The history of motor vehicle safety illustrates this point (Fig. 1). This societally accepted balance is a measure of "How safe is safe enough."

2. Historical data are adequate for revealing the acceptable balance of social preferences and costs, and show that these change only very slowly. Implicitly, this indicates a much greater faith in the validity of a demonstrated balance rather than in the publicly voiced attitudes and preferences.

Risk Analysis, Edited by C. Zervos
Plenum Press, New York, 1991

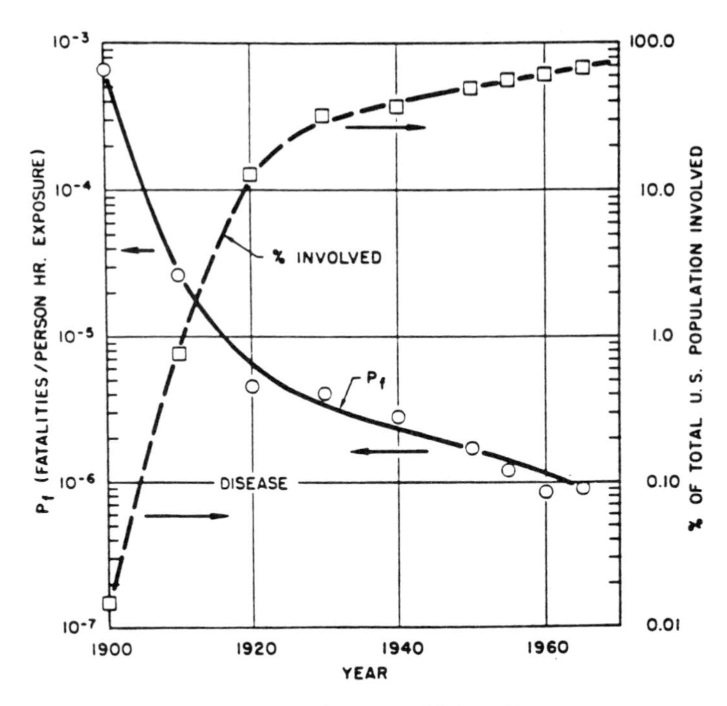

Fig. 1. History of motor vehicle safety.

Starting with these assumptions and the historical data available from many sources, I examined the risks of mining, motor vehicles, air carriers, general aviation, railroads, skiing, hunting, smoking, the Vietnam war, electric power, natural disasters and several other activities. The minimal benefits of each activity were based on the costs the public was willing to pay and the estimated value of time savings, etc. Other intangible benefits were not estimated. The result was condensed into Fig. 2, and subsequently proposed as a generalized hypothesis in Fig. 3. A very evident result was the separation of voluntary risk taking from involuntary exposure. Subsequent studies of recreational boating and commercial vessels verified this separation.

The publication of the 1969 paper provoked considerable interest and criticism. The paper suggested that simple monetary cost/benefit analysis was not an adequate acceptability criterion, but that a spectrum of social values should be included.

However, the paper also suggested that rough quantification of such social values could be based on the historically revealed preferences sufficiently well to permit a risk/benefit analysis useful for societal decision making. The principal point was that the revealed preference study suggested that societal safety targets were based on an societally acceptable level rather than on economic factors, although the economics was one of the elements in determining acceptability.

For those seeking the risk management comfort of a defined objective, the revealed preference approach offered a reasonable path to establishing a socially acceptable risk level. It opened the door to comparative risk assessments to guide resource allocations. It established an analytic basis for evaluating the consequences of risk transference between technologies when regulatory or public constraints shifted choices among alternatives. To a technologist, it appeared to be a logical approach to societal decisions.

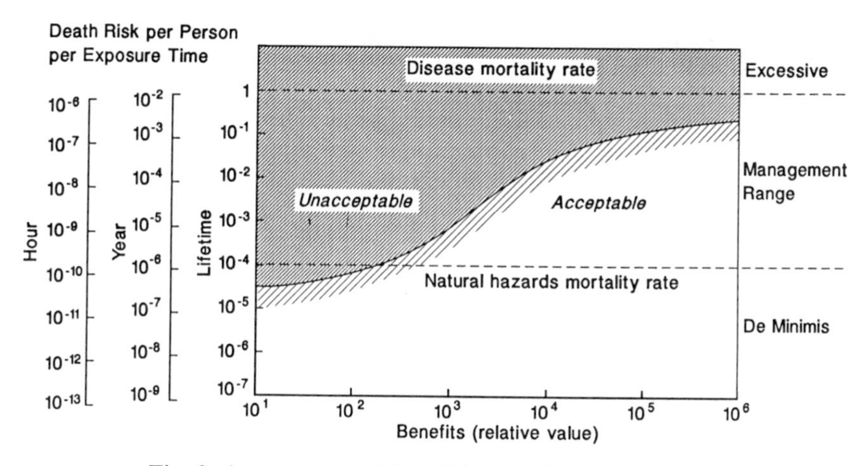

Fig. 2. Average annual benefit/person involved (dollars).

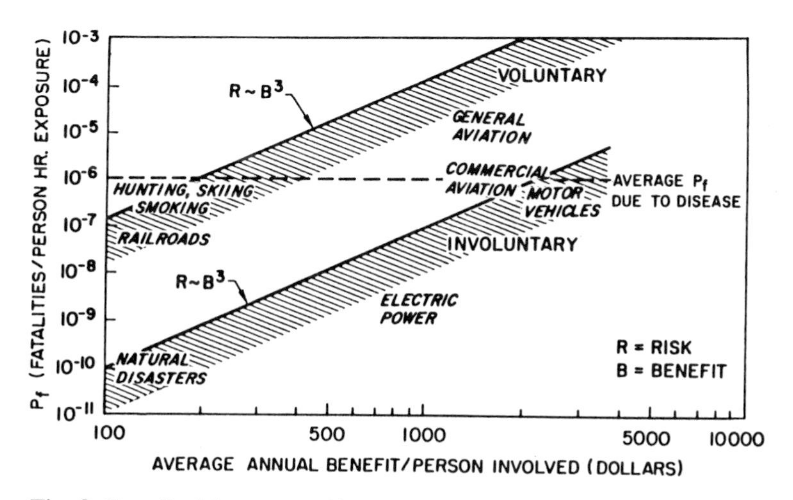

Fig. 3. Benefit-risk pattern of involuntary exposure to technical systems.

However, there were many non-technologists who were deeply concerned with the apparent power of such quantification to influence decisions while neglecting the social intangibles which might be involved with a fuller public participation. Quantification is very persuasive to a decision maker when all else is vague. Further, there was a concern among some that the interlocking of technical systems with our changing social and political structures would not be considered in the revealed preference analysis. While it was generally recognized that the reality of risks was primarily technology based, the acceptability of risk was considered primarily a social and political determination which could be changed at any time by the political process.

The several criticisms of the quantified revealed preference approach arose from the differing philosophies for arriving at societal decisions on public health and safety, particularly with regard to low level risks. With an almost mystical faith of the public in the power of science and technology, the public view of low level risks has slowly shifted from fatalism (e.g. acts of God) to an expectation that societal risk management will ameliorate such risks. This gave rise to a central theme that pervades the flourishing literature on risk analysis that followed the 1969 paper. In its simplest form, this central theme is embodied in the question: "how do we analyze and predict what determines the societal acceptability of a risky technology?" In studying this question, a new and very broad spectrum of participants became involved, whose work has constructively illuminated many facets of our public decision making processes. I will briefly list some of these diverse approaches.

DESCRIPTIVE REVEALED PREFERENCES

This is a continuation and expansion of the revealed preference study presented in the 1969 paper. A few of the contributors are Rowe, Wilson, Cohen, Litai and, of course, Whipple and Starr. These concepts are inherent in such regulatory actions as the safety goals of the Nuclear Regulatory Commission, the criteria of EPA, and the precedent setting vinyl chloride decision which will be discussed later at this meeting. Most notably, the nuclear industries development of Probabilistic Risk Assessment (PRA), which is now commonly used for nuclear power plants, assumes quantitative goals established by the NRC as the target of nuclear engineering and risk management.

PUBLIC PERCEPTION PATTERNS

The public perception of the quality of risks clearly plays a role in societal acceptability. The quantitative calculation of projected probabilities and harm, which is central to the revealed preference approach, apparently is secondary in determining public attitudes. The study of public perceptions includes such participants as Slovic, Fischhoff, Lichtenstein, Keeney, Hohenemser, Kates. The Clark University group has studied the topology of social responses to risk. This body of work has shown the importance of risk perception at the individual level, as contrasted with the quantitative societal balance of the revealed preference approach.

CULTURAL ROOTS

It has been suggested by Clark, Douglas, Wildavsky, Thompson, that our cultural heritages have developed a diversity of values and constraints on the social acceptability of risk. Thus the acceptability of risk is sensitive to the culture of the groups involved.

REGULATORY PRACTICE

The studies of the past actions of regulatory agencies by Travis, Milvy, Bird, and Lave have suggested patterns for regulatory decisions. Travis has shown that federal regulatory decisions on environmental carcinogens follow a probabilistic distribution around an acceptable low level risk.

POLITICAL PROCESSES

Several political analysts, such as Nelkin and Ruckelshaus, have studied the role of our political processes in risk decisions. Of course, this is closely related to the influence of communication to the public, particularly through the journalistic media. The infamous Delaney Amendment is a historic remnant of the political process functioning in the absence of risk analysis, but certainly with public and media support.

PUBLIC RISK MANAGEMENT

It should be particularly noted that during the past several decades the role of public bodies in organizing to ameliorate risk consequences through management has been emphasized by Gil White and the Natural Hazards Center that he nurtured. This acceptance both of the probability of harm and of the societal capability to prepare in advance to mitigate the consequences is a key contribution to dealing with all public risk exposure.

CONCLUSION

It is clear from the wide scope of the current participants in risk analysis work that my 1969 paper presented only one part of a very complex problem. The basic issue we all face is how to reconcile the reality of risk with both the political processes and public perceptions. Unfortunately, only in a limited number of public risks does an actuarial fact base exist, as with motor vehicles. Usually, we are faced with rough judgmental estimates or projections of effects on health, environment, social structure, and a variety of secondary individual consequences. However, these are the common characteristics of almost all societal issues, and we should not be dismayed that they exist in risk analysis. I am very encouraged by the broad progress in this field. In a deep fog, the dim glow of a street light provides some guidance. Our collective efforts are certainly making a constructive contribution to the development of sound and more sophisticated public policies on risks.

Proposition 65: Risk Communication and Regulatory Policy

Brenda Nordenstam
University of California
Irvine, CA

ABSTRACT

Regulatory guidelines for the provision of information to the public regarding environmental hazards are expanding at the federal, state, and local levels. Most of the effort to develop and implement these regulations has focused primarily on scientific and legal aspects, despite the psychological implications of such legislation. Little effort has been made to address the impact and effectiveness of these regulations on the risk perception and behavior of those individuals whom the information is intended to protect. The rapid increase in such right-to-know regulations, combined with the lack of attention to social and behavioral considerations, has generated problems in developing effective risk communication programs. This paper discusses these issues by first presenting a brief background on both the history and information disclosure requirements of California's Proposition 65. Next, a model for a hierarchical system of public warning requirements utilizing the knowledge derived from risk communication research is presented. Lastly, consideration is given to issues raised by the social policy aspects of regulating the communication of risk.

KEYWORDS: Proposition 65, right-to-know, risk communication, warning message, regulatory policy

INTRODUCTION

Proposition 65 is one of the most recent in a series of "right-to-know" laws that have been passed at the federal, state, or local level. Despite the psychological implications of regulatory action of this type, most of the efforts to develop right-to-know regulations have been focused primarily on scientific questions pertaining to accurate risk assessment, and on legal analysis of such legislation. Little effort has been made to address the impact and effectiveness of these laws in producing changes in the knowledge, perception, and behavior of the individuals whom the information is intended to protect.[1] As a result, legal guidelines outlining the adequacy of warnings have led to the development of legally sufficient but ineffective and in some cases perhaps even counterproductive warnings.[2]

Right-to-know communication guidelines of this type have become a kind of ritualistic activity, in which the formal action of conveying risk information has taken precedence over the actual impact of the information in reducing health risks.[3]

Making the information available is a necessary but not sufficient step in decreasing health risks. The information at some level must be able to stimulate the individual to make changes that lead to a reduction in risk.[3] Although a great deal of research has been carried out that would serve to increase the efficacy of risk communication programs, government agencies have rarely used these principles in developing regulations for information disclosure requirements.[4] However, in order to implement risk information programs successfully, an understanding of the strengths and weaknesses of risk communication techniques should be developed and utilized by public policymakers.

These issues are examined below first by presenting a brief background on both the history and the information disclosure requirements of California's Proposition 65. Next, a model utilizing a hierarchical system for the presentation of risk warnings as required by Proposition 65 is presented. This hierarchical system is based upon principles derived from risk communication and information processing theories. Lastly, consideration is given to issues raised by the social policy aspects of regulating the communication of risk.

PROPOSITION 65

Proposition 65, officially known as The Safe Drinking Water and Toxic Enforcement Act of 1986, began as a citizen-sponsored initiative which was overwhelmingly approved by the people of California. As such, it represents a signal from the public indicating a perceived need to be better informed and protected against potential environmental risks. Indeed, the citizens of California felt the need for greater protection and information in regard to the increasing number of hazards present in their environment despite the existing state and federal laws designed to protect the public from exposure to environmental hazards.[5] Proposition 65 represents the outcome of this desire for more effective right-to-know laws and more adequate protection of drinking water supplies. It is a statutory initiative which was placed directly on the general election ballot by the process of citizen petition. On November 4, 1986, 63% of the citizens of California voted to approve Proposition 65.[6]

Proposition 65 represents a new trend in citizen initiated right-to-know legislation. Its implementation and success is being closely watched by other states considering the development of similar laws. With the passage of Proposition 65 the burden of proving that a chemical is not a health risk has been shifted to the business using the chemical, and the responsibility for informing the public, the workforce, or the consumer of possible exposure also falls upon the business. This type of innovative "preventive strategy" approach taken by Proposition 65 has created a new concept in environmental hazard management. Although at the present time this strategy exists only within California, it may eventually become the model for other states to follow.[7]

Proposition 65 contains two major objectives. The first objective is to prohibit the release of detectable amounts of toxic chemicals which have been determined by the state of California to cause cancer or reproductive harm into any source of drinking water. The second objective (and the primary focus of this paper) is to require the makers and sellers of toxic chemicals to give the public a "clear and reasonable warning" of possible exposure to such chemicals when they are released into the environment, used in the workplace, or present in consumer products. To ensure enforcement of the two major objectives of Proposition 65, several new and innovative provisions were included within the language of the Initiative Measure. These major provisions of Proposition 65 are listed in Fig. 1.[8]

1. The governor must publish a list of chemicals known to the state to cause cancer or reproductive toxic effects.

2. Twelve months following the listing of a chemical, the public may not knowingly be exposed to a significant level of this chemical without first receiving a clear and reasonable warning.

3. Twenty months following the listing of a chemical, the chemical may not knowingly be discharged at a significant level into any source of drinking water.

4. If the business can show that the listed carcinogen does not pose a significant risk, or that the reproductive toxicant has no observable effect at 1000 times the exposure level, the business will be exempt from the warning requirement.

5. Civil penalties of up to $2,500 per day per violation of these requirements are imposed.

6. A citizen may bring suit against a business that violates any of these requirements after notifying the proper authorities and allowing 60 days for them to prosecute. If the suit is successful, 25% of the penalties may be collected by the citizen.

7. The burden of proof from the potential victims of exposure is shifted onto the companies that make and sell products containing hazardous substances by requiring the defendant to show that the exposure or discharge was lawful.

Fig. 1. Major provisions of Proposition 65.

WARNING REQUIREMENTS OF PROPOSITION 65

When passed, Proposition 65 did not contain a clear definition of key terms or phrases used in the measure. This resulted in some controversy as opponents sought a minimal interpretation of the Initiative language while public interest groups sought to interpret it to the fullest extent possible. The regulations covering the methods used to determine if a chemical should be listed, the types of businesses that are exempt, and the types of warnings that are acceptable were all developed following the passage of Proposition 65.[6]

Proposition 65 defines warnings as general communications to the public, including labels on consumer products, notices in mailings to water customers and notices in public places. Warnings are required to be clear and reasonable but need not be provided separately to each exposed individual.[8]

The regulations developed to implement Proposition 65 establish three types of exposure categories and require specific language to be used in the warning method chosen by the business. The three types of categories are (1) environmental exposure, (2) occupational exposure, and (3) consumer product exposure.[9]

Regarding environmental exposure, the regulations implementing the warning requirement of Proposition 65 allow companies to meet the community notification requirements by printing occasional notices in local newspapers stating that chemicals known to the state of California to cause cancer are used by the company. To comply with the employee notification provision, companies are required only to post a warning notice on company property. The posted notice must contain the following language: **"Warning: This area contains a chemical known to the state of California to cause cancer."** If the chemical has been identified as a reproductive toxin the following language is required: **"Warning: This area contains a chemical known to the state of California to cause birth defects or other reproductive harm."**[9]

Proposition 65 regulations do not require stores selling consumer products to identify individually products containing toxic chemicals (except for tobacco products). For example, grocery stores have complied with the warning requirements by posting a single notice at the store entrance stating that some products are sold in the store which contain chemicals known to the state of California to cause cancer. Additionally, a toll-free number is provided for consumers to call if they wish to find out which products within the store contain chemicals known to cause cancer or reproductive harm (see Fig. 2).

This method makes it difficult for the average consumer to obtain information on a specific product. The consumer must correctly identify the item by the exact brand name or he will be informed that there is no listing for that particular product. Even a variation in package size may cause the caller to be told that the product is not listed. If the caller is persistent, he may be given a number to call the manufacturer. However, the manufacturer will not always return a consumer's call.[10]

Although these warning methods fulfill the legal requirements to provide individuals with a clear and reasonable warning of possible exposure to toxic chemicals, it is questionable whether they fulfill the intent of Proposition 65 to effectively inform individuals of the potential risks from toxic chemicals. In fact, the State Attorney General has stated that the regulations meant only to make it clear that a toll-free information number could be used as part of an overall system of warnings, but that it was never meant to be used alone. The State Attorney General further stated that an adequate warning system should provide the required information to all consumers, not just to those who are willing to invest unusual amounts of time and effort to obtain the facts.[11]

In the following section a proposed model for a hierarchical warning system based upon principals of risk communication and information processing research will be presented. The implementation of a warning system of this type into the overall design of a risk information program should serve to increase the efficacy of the warning methods currently required by Proposition 65 regulations.

HIERARCHICAL WARNING SYSTEM

An often overlooked consideration in the development of risk communication programs is that only about 10% to 20% of consumers are information seekers. Information seekers tend to have high incomes, high education levels, high media use, and high confidence in scientific test data.[12] Many information programs are used almost exclusively by these information seekers and not by the majority of consumers. This may be because designers of risk communication programs are themselves information seekers and fail to consider that the information needs of their target audience may differ from their own.[13] A risk communication program which requires active information seeking by the individual will reach only a small minority of the intended audience. Therefore, the use of a warning system that requires an 800 number effectively excludes the majority of the public from

1. For exposure to a chemical known to the state of California to cause cancer: "Warning: This area contains a chemical known to the state of California to cause cancer."
2. For exposure to a chemical known to the state of California to cause reproductive toxicity: "Warning: This area contains a chemical known to the state of California to cause birth defects or other reproductive harm."
3. Pre-recorded warning message available through the 800-number: "The state of California requires that the following statement be given to you. Warning: This product contains chemicals known to the state of California to cause cancer, birth defects, or other reproductive harm. For further information about this product, please stay on the line and an operator will assist you."

Fig. 2. Warning messages required by Proposition 65.

ever receiving the information they need to make an informed decision concerning their risk.

To reach a larger segment of the population, steps should be taken to ensure the availability of risk information for each product within the store. However, in designing information provision programs policymakers must distinguish between the availability and the processability of risk information. Processability refers to the ease with which information can be comprehended and used. To be effectively utilized, information must be both available and easily processable. Presenting information that is well-organized and in formats that facilitate processing can increase the processability.[14] In developing risk communication programs, policymakers must consider the limitations and complexities of human judgment and decision making. Individuals have a finite ability to process information and find it difficult to understand complex information about risks.

In making decisions about risks, people tend to use judgmental heuristics (mental strategies that help to reduce complex judgments to simpler and more manageable forms).[15] In some cases, the use of mental strategies can lead to serious errors in overestimating or underestimating risk. For example, a strategy used to judge the frequency or likelihood of an event, known as the availability heuristic,[16] is especially important to consider when informing people about risk. People will tend to judge a risk according to how easy it is to imagine other relevant examples of that risk. However, the ease of recall may be influenced by factors unrelated to the actual probability of the risk, such as sensational events heavily reported in the news media. This research illustrates the need to increase the vividness and relevance of the warning message currently utilized to convey the risk associated with some toxic chemicals.

Research studies in human information processing indicate that a hierarchical warning system would be more effective than the current indiscriminate type of message now being utilized for Proposition 65 warnings. This approach involves the regulation and standardization of warning labels to minimize the effects of overloading the public with the

Tier One: Symbol on product

Tier Two: Warning label on product

Tier Three: Information booklet available in store

Tier Four: Computerized information available through 800 number

Fig. 3. Hierarchy of warning messages.

sheer volume and complexity of risk information. This model is based upon similar models used in product labeling and consumer marketing research.[4,14,17,18]

An effective way to increase an individual's ability to process risk information is to arrange the warning on the label so that increasing tiers of detail are provided on the warning label itself. A hierarchy of information formatted on the label would reference additional information available within the store in the form of information booklets. Finally, the highest tier of detail would be available via an 800 number linked to a computer information system (See Fig. 3).

In any information warning system a signal word or symbol should serve as the first tier of risk information.[19] Symbols representing a cancer causing or reproductive toxin would be placed on the product. If feasible, color coding or a number system could be utilized to indicate the degree of risk. It should be noted that this symbolic level of warning does not require translation into another language to be understood. This symbol system would serve to reduce information overload by allowing consumers to quickly determine whether they needed to seek additional information and also by making the most important information more salient to the consumer.[14]

After being alerted by the symbol, the consumer would proceed to the second warning tier provided on the product—the actual warning label. Providing risk information to consumers via a product label does not involve introducing a new concept for consumers to master. Research indicates that consumers already use nutritional labels as a means of obtaining risk information for certain ingredients that they wish to avoid, such as sugar, salt, or preservatives.[20] The warning label could simply consist of the warning message presently required by Proposition 65, or it could also reference more detailed information, available from other tiers of the hierarchy. For example, the warning message specific to lung cancer that cigarette packages now carry could be placed on other tobacco products also known to cause lung cancer. In the case of alcoholic beverages, a description of fetal alcohol syndrome could be provided. The addition of such information would serve to increase the personal relevance of the message for the intended audience, a risk communication process known to heighten attention to risk information.[21]

Of course care must be taken to insure that the degree and type of information provided does not err on the opposite side of the spectrum and induce a fear response from those reading the message. If an individual feels vulnerable to a threat, then psychological resistances may be aroused. Studies have shown that if warning messages are made too threatening, without providing effective methods of avoiding the danger, the individual may respond by ignoring the threatening message or actually taking steps that increase the risk.[22]

Subtle changes in the format of the message can have a marked change in the reception and response of the intended audience.[23] Research indicates the need for surveys of the targeted audience in order to measure their perceptions and responses to the warning message. The needs of subpopulations of the community should be assessed. For example, evidence clearly reveals that those with lower income and education are less likely to seek out and use information than are those with high income and education. This points to the need for warning messages targeted to these audiences.[12,24]

The next tier of warning messages would consist of the information available within the store itself. This could take the form of booklets containing more detailed information on the health risks of the chemicals. Comparisons of different products could also be provided so that consumers would feel that they had some choices and control over their possible exposure. Research in risk communication and public health campaigns indicates that one effective method of inducing behavioral change is to furnish positive coping strategies for the individual to implement. Simply supplying information without furnishing any means of avoiding the hazard may create feelings of lack of control over exposure to the risk and help induce denial that the risk even exists.[3,22,23] In fact, it may be that an inadvertent result of the overuse of generic warning messages is the general perception that everything causes cancer.

Although it would be necessary to conduct comprehensive studies in order to assess accurately the perceptions and reactions of the public, it appears that the reaction of a large number of people to the warning messages has not been panic and cancer-phobia, as predicted by opponents of Proposition 65, but rather apathy and lack of interest. This is consistent with research studies in risk perception which indicate that when exposed to multiple warnings, those at risk reach a saturation point: so many risks appear to be present that they feel overloaded and stop responding to the messages.[3] In fact, in terms of the health impact, it may be that widespread underreaction to risk messages represents a more serious problem than overreaction to risk information.

The final tier of warning messages to be provided in this hierarchical warning system would be the 800 number for those individuals who wish to obtain further information concerning the health risks of certain products or chemicals. Those particularly benefited by this level of information would include hypersusceptible individuals or those who make frequent use of a certain product. This 800 number could be tied into a computer or library system to supply the additional information.

The utility of a computerized information bank for consumers has long been suggested by researchers in marketing psychology.[12] The development of data bases such as the Environmental Protection Agency's Integrated Risk Information System[26] points to the feasibility of eventually providing a service which describes health risks from chemical exposure in a format accessible to the general public. This approach could be modeled to meet the needs of those companies required by right-to-know laws to provide risk information to the public.

The use of computerized data bases available in libraries would require the standardization of risk information now required by various agencies.[18] This leads to the final suggestion for the implementation of a successful risk communication system — the development of a consistent method of risk communication for the different agencies now involved in regulating risk information. The increasing amount of duplicate effort required in reporting potential risks points to the need for a uniform risk communication system.[18,27] In addition, a uniform method of risk communication for all right-to-know laws would increase the confidence of the public in risk management programs. The large and inconsistent amount of information now available tends to confuse and overwhelm the public. Research indicates that inconsistent risk information can make scientific evidence seem uncertain, leading to such possible public reactions as hypervigilance or panic.[28,29]

In conclusion, the passage of Proposition 65 represents the needs of the citizens of California to receive more information about the possible health risks in their environments. The fact that the scientific data is both difficult to interpret and to present should not frustrate this desire to be better informed, but rather should serve to encourage those responsible for implementing the warning provisions of the initiative to provide the best risk communication program possible, given reasonable cost and feasibility considerations.

REFERENCES

1. B. J. Nordenstam and J. F. DiMento, Right-To-Know: Risk Communication and Regulatory Policy, *U.C. Davis Law Review* (1990).
2. V. E. Schwartz and R. W. Driver, Warnings in the Workplace: The Need for a Synthesis of Law and Communication Theory, *Cincinnati Law Review* **38**:83 (1983).
3. C. Needleman, Ritualism in Communicating Risk Information, *Science, Technology, and Human Values* **12**:20-25 (1987).
4. M. B. Mazis and R. Staelin, Using Information-Processing Principles in Public Policymaking, *Journal of Public Policy and Marketing* **1**:3-14 (1982).
5. J. A. DeFranco, California's Toxics Initiative: Making It Work, *The Hastings Law Journal* **39**:1195-1128 (1988).
6. Orange County Register, Feb. 17, 1988, A3, Col. 5.
7. K. W. Kizer, T. E. Warriner, and S. A. Book, Sound Science in the Implementation of Public Policy: A Case Report on California's Proposition 65, *JAMA* **260(7)**:951-955 (1988).
8. California Health and Safety Code, Chp. 6.6, Safe Drinking Water and Toxic Enforcement Act of 1986, Section 25249.5 - 25249.13.
9. California Administrative Code, Title 22, Chp. 3, Safe Drinking Water and Toxic Act of 1986, Section 12601.
10. Environmental Defense Fund, Letter to the State Attorney General, Aug. 22, 1988.
11. J. K. Van de Kamp, State Attorney General, and A. S. Ordin, Assistant Attorney General, Letter addressed to Assemblyman Lloyd G. Connelly, California State Capitol, 3/18/88.
12. H. B. Thorelli and J. L. Engledow, Information Seekers and Information Systems: A Policy Perspective, *Journal of Marketing* **44**:9-27 (1980).
13. T. C. Earle and G. T. Cvetkovich, Risk Communication: A Marketing Approach, NSF/EPA Workshop on Risk Perception and Risk Communication, Long Beach, CA, December, 1984.
14. J. R. Bettman, J. W. Payne, and R. Staelin, Cognitive Considerations in Designing Effective Labels for Presenting Risk Information, *J. of Public Policy and Marketing* **5**:1-28 (1986).
15. A. Tversky and Kahnerman, Judgment Under Uncertainty: Heuristics and Biases, *Science* **185**:1124-1131 (1974).
16. P. Slovic, B. Fischhoff, and S. Lichtenstein, Facts and Fears: Understanding Perceived Risk, in *Societal Risk Assessment: How Safe is Safe Enough?* pp. 273-285, R. C. Schwing and A. A. Albers, eds., Plenum Press, New York (1980).
17. P. Slovic, B. Fischhoff, and S. Lichtenstein, Informing People About Risk, in *Product Labeling and Health Risks*, Banbury Report 6, L. Morris, M. Mazis, and B. Barofsky, eds., Cold Spring Harbor, New York (1980).
18. S. G. Hadden, *Read the Label: Reducing Risk by Providing Information*, Westview Press, Boulder, Colorado (1986).
19. M. S. Wogalter, S. S. Godfrey, G. A. Fontenelle, D. R. Desaulniers, P. R. Rothstein, and K. R. Laughery, Effectiveness of Warnings, *Human Factors* **29(5)**:599-612 (1987).
20. R. B. Smith, J. A. Brown, and J. P. Weimer, Consumer Attitudes Toward Food Labeling and Other Shopping Aids, U.S. Dept. of Agric., Report #439 (1979).

21. E. Vaughan, Some Factors Influencing the Nonexpert's Perception and Evaluation of Environmental Risks, Doctoral Dissertation, Stanford, CA (1986).
22. R. W. Rogers and C. R. Mewborn, Fear Appeals and Attitude Change: Effects of a Threat's Noxiousness, Probability of Occurrence, and the Efficacy of Coping Responses, *Journal of Personality and Social Psychology* **34(1)**:54-61 (1976).
23. W. A. Magat, J. W. Payne, and P. F. Brucato, How Important Is Information Format? An Experimental Study of Home Energy Audit Programs, *Policy Analysis and Management* **6**:20-34 (1986).
24. D. P. Robin, The Need for a New Class of Information to Aid Public Policy Decision-Makers, *Journal of Public Policy and Marketing* **5**:58-75 (1986).
25. R. F. Soames, Effective and Ineffective Use of Fear in Health Promotion Campaigns, *American Journal of Public Health* **78(2)**:163-167 (1988).
26. IRIS User Support, Environmental Criteria and Assessment Office, Environmental Protection Agency, Cincinnati, OH.
27. P. L. Stenzil, The Need for a National Risk Assessment Communication Policy, *Harvard Environmental Law Review* **11**:381-413 (1987).
28. I. L. Janis and L. Mann, Coping with Decisional Conflict: An Analysis of How Stress Affects Decision-Making Suggests Interventions to Improve the Process, *American Scientist* **64**:657-666 (1976).
29. V. T. Covello, D. V. Winterfeldt, and P. Slovic, Risk Communication: An Assessment of the Literature on Communication Information about Health, Safety and Environmental Risks, Environmental Protection Agency (1986).

Societal Acceptance of Controversial Facilities: The Role of Two Public Participation Strategies—Negotiation and Risk Communication

Amy K. Wolfe
Oak Ridge National Laboratory
Oak Ridge, TN

ABSTRACT

Public participation in decision making about the siting of controversial facilities is viewed in contradictory ways by different groups of people. Some see public participation as an impediment, while others think it is an important mechanism in gaining societal acceptance for eventual siting. This paper discusses two strategies for obtaining societal acceptance — negotiation and risk communication — in light of the extent to which they (1) involve members of the public; (2) focus on risk-related issues; and (3) contribute to decisions to site controversial facilities. The paper presents an integrated conceptual model for public participation in siting decisions that incorporates risk as well as social, political, and historical contexts.

KEYWORDS: Risk communication, negotiation, public participation, technology acceptance, facility siting

INTRODUCTION

In recent years, much attention has been focused on ways in which to obtain public acceptance for the siting of controversial facilities. Two approaches to technology acceptance that have been gaining favor are dispute resolution and risk communication. Dispute resolution processes are intended to resolve conflicts before they escalate to the point of requiring litigation. Methods used to resolve conflicts include consensus-building, negotiation, and policy dialogue. Risk communication, on the other hand, often is viewed as a means by which experts or proposers of particular technologies educate members of the public about the 'true' (i.e., quantitatively determined) risks associated with those technologies. In the case of some technologies, risk communication is intended to convince different publics that certain technologies are (relatively) safe. Implicit in the literature on risk communication is the idea that effective communication will increase societal acceptance of these technologies.

In their efforts either to educate or to include members of the public, both dispute resolution and risk communication require forms of public participation. The role of public participation in decision making about the siting of controversial facilities is viewed in conflicting ways by different groups of people. For example, some members of the public, such as people involved in some civic or environmental associations, may think that it is their right to be involved in siting decisions. From the point of view of some sponsors of technological facilities, such participation is seen as a form of delay and disruption that can be caused by public protest. Still other sponsors consider public participation as an important mechanism for gaining societal acceptance for eventual siting.

In this paper, I compare two strategies for obtaining societal acceptance of controversial facilities — negotiation and risk communication. Discussion focuses on the goals of negotiation and risk communication and comparisons of the extent to which they (1) involve members of the public; (2) focus on risk-related issues; and (3) contribute to decisions to site controversial facilities. Finally, I present and discuss a preliminary integrated conceptual model for public participation in siting decisions that incorporates risk as well as social, political, and historical contexts.

NEGOTIATION

Within the category of dispute resolution techniques, negotiation and mediation sometimes are separated.[1] Thus, for example, the latter employs the use of an independent mediator or facilitator, while negotiations involve face-to-face discussions among affected parties in the absence of an independent party. However, they are similar because of the way participants are selected and topics discussed, and in their links to technology acceptance. For the purposes of this paper, therefore, negotiation and mediation will be discussed together and the terms used interchangeably.

Negotiation, like other dispute resolution techniques, has grown in use in recent years. It has been used both for policy and site-specific issues. According to Bingham,[1] implementation of agreements reached through negotiation has been more successful for site-specific than for policy matters. In some cases, negotiation has become an institutionalized part of decision making processes. Statutes enacted in Massachusetts, Rhode Island, Texas, Virginia, and Wisconsin, for instance, require negotiated siting agreements for solid or hazardous waste facilities. On a site-specific basis, the format of negotiations has differed with regard to timing, participants, procedures, and goals. While negotiation has been applied to a wide variety of issues, of interest here are those cases that deal with site-specific technology acceptance — facility siting.

Objectives for negotiations generally fall into two categories. The first pertains to those aimed directly at facility or technology acceptance. Involved parties try to reach consensus or agreement regarding the conditions for acceptance. The second pertains to the establishment or enhancement of communication channels between affected parties. The idea here is to reduce adversarial relationships, increase trust, and establish a dialogue where information and alternatives can be discussed and generated. Often these processes are intended to pave the way for more informed and less highly charged traditional decision making.

Determining the affected parties in a particular dispute is of critical importance for the eventual success of negotiations. Non-participants may not agree either with the decisions or recommendations made by negotiating parties or with the negotiation process. They will consider the process unfair because it neglected them. Non-participants also may be moved to try to stop the implementation of negotiators' agreements or recommendations. When mediators are involved, usually they are given the task of identifying affected parties.[1] Reports on negotiations sometimes fail to discuss specifically how participants were selected, saying only that affected parties were contacted and invited to participate.[2] Direct citizen involvement in negotiations tends to be minimal. Citizens generally are represented either by citizens groups or by public agencies.

Further, because many negotiations are voluntary, not every identified party decides to become involved. Some groups intentionally avoid becoming parties to negotiations to retain their distance and assure their power to halt the implementation of agreements. Other groups decline involvement because they do not see enough incentives for them to become involved; their stakes are not high enough. Once the participants are selected, successful negotiation depends partially on the communication both among large interest groups and within the groups themselves (i.e., between representatives and the groups they represent, whether citizen, corporate, government, etc.).

Among the first decisions that must be made during negotiations is the scope of issues to be addressed. Some researchers/negotiators look upon compensation as the primary condition for acceptance.[3] For them, negotiations may center on the nature and amount of compensation. In the case of potentially hazardous facilities, some researchers believe that risk spreading or risk reduction also is critical to the acceptance of a controversial facility.[4,5,6]

Another topic of negotiation recommended by the National Governors' Association Subcommittee on the Environment[7] is the encouragement of people at the local level to participate within the decision making system rather than outside the system. Further, the National Governors' Association suggested that negotiations regarding hazardous waste facilities should center on mitigation packages that stipulate the conditions under which a facility siting would be acceptable and reduce risks as well as tangible and intangible community costs such as stigma. More specific issues for mediation reported in case studies presented by Bingham[1] include the following: accident cleanup; emergency preparedness; air and water quality monitoring; waste reduction; enforcement of regulations; establishment of a continuing citizen role in planning; restrictions in hours of construction and operation; and facility design. In summary, negotiations can include a range of topics. Although many of these topics are risk-related, communications apparently do not center on quantitative assessments of risk.

RISK COMMUNICATION

Fundamentally, formal risk communication is a method used to gain public acceptance of technologies. This may be an implicit rather than explicit goal of risk communication. More often, risk communication is viewed as a formal process in which experts or officials inform members of the public about probabilistic risk assessments. Insofar as risk communicators develop messages to deliver to certain audiences, they are involved in a version of participatory dispute resolution. The problem is that, too often, such participation involves members of the public only as targets of change, not as participants in an interactive risk communication process. Professional risk communicators tend to frame the terms of the dispute and try to resolve the dispute on behalf of the public without eliciting from affected people what concerns they truly have. Thus, one reason why risk communication efforts so often fail to convince people of the safety of particular technologies is that they are slanted toward selling risk acceptance, like advertisements for consumer products.

In this regard, risk communication differs from negotiation. Negotiation is a process that involves reciprocal dialogue between representatives of participating affected parties. As has been discussed, the roles such participants play and the acceptability of settlements to the larger groups represented therefore vary from case to case. Formal risk communication campaigns, however, tend to limit the role of members of the public to passive receptors of expert wisdom.

Historically, one reason for this risk communication approach derives from the emergence of risk communication from the field of risk perceptions. Among the questions asked by path-breaking researchers in this field was why the public (frequently conceived of as a single, homogeneous group) failed to see nuclear power as safe when the probabilities of morbidity or mortality were so remote.[8-14] The framing of this type of question led researchers to focus their attention on perceptions of probabilities and uncertainties, to the virtual exclusion of other factors that influence perceptions of the technology in question.

In seeking to understand why people perceive a technology somewhere along the continuum of safe to deadly, it would be more fruitful to ask a wider question about perceptions of the whole technology rather than about perceptions of its risk. Expanding the research question in this fashion allows investigation of social, cultural, economic, and historic factors that influence the perceptions and acceptability of a technology.[15-19] Emphasizing probabilistic assessments of risk may define inaccurately the boundaries of conflicts over technologies because they are overly restrictive. Probabilistic risk assessments may be neither the primary nor the sole determinant of people's confidence in the safety or acceptability of a technology.

This is recognized in the negotiation literature, which basically ignores the question of the accuracy of public perceptions of quantitative risk estimates. Instead, a host of issues are brought to the fore. Some of these issues indeed are risk-related and some even center on probabilistic risk assessments.[2] Thus, in negotiation risk-related concerns address in a straightforward manner how to reduce potential hazards and how to handle potential accident situations, not how to convince members of the public that the risk is small.

Within or outside of the negotiation setting, while communication undoubtedly is an essential component of conflict resolution, that communication may need to involve a number of aspects of a technology instead of just probabilities of risk. In this context, risk communication is a continuing, interactive process, a fact not well recognized in the risk communication literature. Although researchers involved in risk communication tend to acknowledge its interactive nature, two-way risk communication is not incorporated substantively in their studies or recommendations. Even when researchers suggest that learning about the target audience and its concerns may improve risk communication, they restrict their inquiry to short-term techniques for packaging the risk messages better.[20]

Because conventional risk communication literature fails to study the knowledge and perceptions of the participants, two additional issues are disregarded. First, researchers do not formalize the effect which risk communication (or miscommunication) has on each of the parties involved.[21] Second, much of the risk communication literature does not recognize that communication takes place both formally or intentionally and informally, as a by-product of continuing interactions. Day-to-day informal interactions between sponsors of a technology, managers and operators of facilities, and members of the public may do more to determine if (or what sort of) conflict arises over a particular facility than formalized communication efforts. An industry that generally has open channels of communication with its host community, for example, may be viewed as well-intentioned and trustworthy should a crisis occur. In contrast, an industry that has been viewed with suspicion may be the target of public outrage in the event of an accident, regardless of its culpability.

Conventional risk communication and conventional negotiation processes thus frequently are in conflict. Public policy makers appear, so far, to have kept the two endeavors separate, having assumed that the conflict is irreconcilable. Irreconcilability, however, is not intrinsic to the two approaches, and resolution is possible by making more formal the often non-formal negotiation and mediation processes. The following is a model that formalizes both reciprocal negotiation and one-way communication processes at the community level.

PRELIMINARY MODEL FOR PUBLIC ACCEPTANCE OF CONTROVERSIAL FACILITIES

Both negotiation and risk communication influence the degree to which proposed technological facilities are deemed acceptable by members of the public. However, in these cases, technology acceptance is not dichotomous; i.e., it is not simply a matter of acceptance or rejection. There are a range of public responses that fall under the category of technology acceptance. These responses include (1) active support for the facility; (2) passive acceptance; (3) apathy; (4) reluctant acceptance (i.e., feeling that matters are beyond individual or community control and that, in effect, there is no choice but to accept the technology); (5) optimizing reluctant acceptance through negotiation, compensation, and the like (i.e., making the most of a bad situation by attempting to derive some benefits for having to accept the facility); and (6) active opposition to the facility at any cost. Over time within a community, the nature of the responses to a particular facility may change. Further, different segments of one community may respond differently to the same proposed facility.

The preliminary model proposed here (see Figs. 1 and 2) depicts the range of TECHNOLOGY/FACILITY ACCEPTANCE responses as an eventual outcome of a particular FACILITY OR TECHNOLOGY. Figure 1 depicts interactions that occur at any point in time. Figure 2 lists historical stages that influence the nature of interactions during particular slices of time.

If regarded as an input/output model, the FACILITY or TECHNOLOGY is the primary input and levels of TECHNOLOGY/FACILITY ACCEPTANCE are the output of most concern. The facility or technology includes its operators and operations; managers and sponsors or owners; tangible and intangible costs and benefits to a community; local versus regional effects of the facility, its operations, by-products, and emissions; and the state of the art of the technology.

A particular community is affected by factors external to that community (although sometimes it is difficult to define the boundaries between internal and external). EXTERNAL FACTORS that may be of special importance in influencing technology acceptance in a particular community include: economic and social characteristics of the surrounding region; state and federal government; national or regional social organizations (e.g., Sierra Club); regulations; news media (the nature and extent of coverage); and scientific or expert analysts of the facility/technology. Interactions between these external factors and a community take place continually, shifting on occasion. They help to shape the community of interest.

This preliminary model focuses particularly on the community level. Thus, LOCAL CONTEXT is of utmost interest. Local context is the filter through which information about a facility is interpreted and given MEANING. The meanings attached to a technology/facility (and its owners, operators, etc.) determine levels of technology acceptance. Levels of acceptance, in turn, feed back directly into the other components of the model, except meaning. Indirectly, through social context, levels of acceptance feed back into the meaning component of the model. This model states that meaning does not exist outside of social context; it is through the filter of local context that meaning is derived.

Local context includes a number of components. "Physical/natural environment" refers to the built and natural environmental setting of the community. "Industrial/economic environment" denotes the extent of industrialization, the types of industries, and the economic status of the community currently and in the past. "Individuals" include the people residing or working within the community, their past experiences (especially with regard to the technology/facility of interest or similar

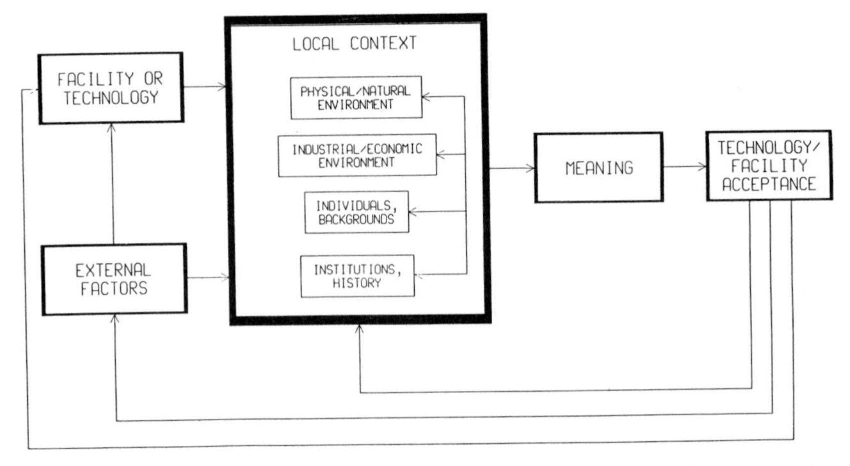

Fig. 1. Preliminary conceptual model for acceptance of technologies: interactions.

1. DETERMINATION OF NEED FOR FACILITY OR TECHNOLOGY

2. DECISION ON WHERE TO LOCATE FACILITY

3. FACILITY SITING

4. FACILITY CONSTRUCTION

5. FACILITY OPERATION

6. PERHAPS, FACILITY CLOSURE

Fig. 2. Preliminary conceptual model for acceptance of technologies: historical stages.

technologies), their power within and outside the community, and their psychology (e.g., risk-averse versus risk-taking). Finally, "institutions" include the past and present social structure of the community, and links and power established within and outside the community.

The model has historical depth, recognizing that current responses to facilities depend on past interactions and events. Thus, the HISTORICAL STAGES of the model (see Fig. 2) represent phases in the lifespan of a particular technology/facility. These stages are as follows:

- *Determination of the need for a technology or facility.* The circumstances of the development of the technology and the way a decision was made to site a facility are among the factors of concern in this historical phase.

- *Decision on where to locate the facility.* This decision can involve alternative locations. In this phase, what is of importance is not only where facilities may be sited, but on what bases such decisions were made.

- *Facility siting.* This phase includes preparing documents, obtaining permits, meeting regulations and requirements, designing and planning the facility, and any other preparations for the next phase.

- *Facility construction.* Among the factors of importance here are the quality of workmanship and oversight by managers and regulators.

- *Facility operation.* Again, quality of workmanship and oversight are important factors during this phase. Any accidents or incidents also can affect technology acceptance, as can the nature of the relationships between the owners of the facility and the community.

- *Facility closure.* In some cases, facility closure is a matter of concern in earlier phases. This phase may be neither planned nor relevant for particular cases.

This preliminary model predicts that both the interactions and the levels of technology acceptance within a community at any point in time are built upon past interactions. That is why historical stages are stated explicitly.

The preliminary model is predicated on the notion that informal technology communication takes place continually and that both formal risk communication and negotiations take place within that context. Whether formally or not, controversial facilities involve public participation. In deciding what form or forms of public participation to adopt, first a diagnosis must be made of the important factors operating in the community in question, as well as its surrounding area and state (external factors). Suppose, for example, it is clear that one reason people are wary of a facility is that channels of communication are blocked between facility sponsors, state government officials, and the local community. Negotiations aimed at improving communications may be one way to improve this state of affairs. Formal risk communication, as traditionally practiced, likely will not be of much use. However, cognizance that informal day-to-day technology communication influences technology acceptance may lead sponsors of technologies to use more adaptive behaviors. These behaviors, like those exhibited in a case of successful hazardous waste facility siting in North Carolina,[2] include eliciting from people their concerns and responding in meaningful ways to those concerns. This is an example of public participation in siting decisions that can span boundaries between formal and informal procedures and that can combine such techniques as negotiation and risk communication.

ACKNOWLEDGMENTS

I wish to thank Bruce Tonn, Martin Schweitzer, and Mark Schoepfle for their comments on this paper.

REFERENCES

1. G. Bingham, Resolving Environmental Disputes: A Decade of Experience, The Conservation Foundation, Washington, DC (1986).
2. Frances M. Lynn, Citizen Involvement in Hazardous Waste Sites: Two North Carolina Success Stories, *Environmental Impact Assessment Review* **7:347-361** (1987).
3. Michael O'Hare, Lawrence Bacow, and Debra Sanderson, *Facility Siting and Public Opposition*, Van Nostrand Reinhold, New York (1983).
4. R. Kasperson, Hazardous Waste Facility Siting: Community, Firm, and Governmental Perspectives, in *National Academy of Engineering, Series on*

Technology and Social Priorities, Hazards: Technology and Fairness, pp. 118-144, National Academy Press, Washington, DC (1986).
5. Lawrence E. Susskind, The Siting Puzzle: Balancing Economic and Environmental Gains and Losses, *Environmental Impact Assessment Review* **5**:157-163 (1985).
6. D. Swartzman, K. Croke, and S. Swibel, Reducing Aversion to Living Near Hazardous Waste Facilities Through Compensation and Risk Reduction, *Journal of Environmental Management* **20**:43-50 (1985).
7. National Governors' Association Subcommittee on the Environment, Siting Hazardous Waste Facilities, Final Report of the National Governors' Association Subcommittee on the Environment, Energy and Natural Resources Program, National Governors' Association, Washington, DC (1981).
8. B. Fischhoff, P. Slovic, and S. Lichtenstein, Which Risks Are Acceptable? *Environment* **21(4)**:17-20 and 32-38 (1979).
9. C. Starr, Social Benefit Versus Technological Risk: What Is Society Willing to Pay for Safety? *Science* **165**:1232-1238 (1969).
10. P. Slovic, Rating the Risks, *Environment* **21(3)**:1420+ (1979a).
11. P. Slovic, S. Lichtenstein, and B. Fischhoff, Images of Disaster: Perception and Acceptance of Risks from Nuclear Power, in *Energy Risk Management*, pp. 223-245, G. Goodman and W. Rowe, eds., Academic, London (1979b).
12. P. Slovic, B. Fischhoff, and S. Lichtenstein, Facts and Fears: Understanding Perceived Risks, in *Societal Risk Assessment: How Safe Is Safe Enough?* pp. 181-214, R. C. Schwing and W. A. Albers, Jr., eds., Plenum Press, New York (1980).
13. P. Slovic, Informing the Public About the Risks from Ionizing Radiation, *Health Physics* **41(4)**:589-598 (1981).
14. P. Slovic, B. Fischhoff, and S. Lichtenstein, Why Study Risk Perception? *Risk Analysis* **2(2)**:83-93 (1982).
15. Branden B. Johnson and Vincent T. Covello, eds., *The Social and Cultural Construction of Risk: Essays on Risk Selection and Perception*, D. Reidel, Dordrecht (1987).
16. Harry Otway, Experts, Risk Communication, and Democracy, *Risk Analysis* **7(2)**:125-129 (1987).
17. Steve Rayner and Robin Cantor, How Fair Is Safe Enough? The Cultural Approach to Societal Technology Choice, *Risk Analysis* **7(1)**:3-9 (1987).
18. A. K. Wolfe, Risk and Confidence in Industrial Communities: A Comparative History of Perceptions of Industrial Pollution in Oak Ridge and Rockwood, Tennessee, PhD Dissertation, University of Pennsylvania, University Microfilms International, Ann Arbor, MI (1986).
19. A. K. Wolfe, Risk Communication: Who's Educating Whom? *Practicing Anthropology* **10(3-4)**:13-14 (1988).
20. Vincent Covello *et al.*, Risk Communication, *Proceedings of the National Conference on Risk Communication*, Washington, DC, January 29-31, 1986, The Conservation Foundation, Washington, DC (1987).
21. Steve Rayner, Muddling Through Metaphors to Maturity: A Commentary on Kasperson *et al.*, The Social Amplification of Risk, *Risk Analysis* **8(2)**:201-204 (1988).

Liability and the Economic Risks of Genetically Engineered Microbial Agents in Agriculture

Beverly Fleisher
Office of Science and Technology Policy
Washington, DC

ABSTRACT

Decisions regarding the manufacture, sale, and use of genetically engineered microbial agents designed for deliberate release in agricultural settings are particularly complex because of the uncertainty surrounding the products' environmental impacts, the regulatory standards of safety that will be established and the incidence of liability for unintended adverse effects that may be created. The Office of Technology Assessment has encouraged approval of field testing of genetically engineered microbial agents, stating that there is reason for caution but no cause for alarm. At the same time, biotechnology firms engaged in research on deliberate release organisms often find it difficult to obtain liability insurance coverage. The risk of, and liability for, economic damage from the deliberate release of organisms in agriculture are discussed, and the implications of the likelihood of high probability/low consequence events versus low probability/high consequence events on regulation, liability, and insurability are explored. Particular attention is given to the problems of assessing the economic risk of genetically engineered microbial agents and determining the appropriate institutional division of labor between ex ante (regulatory) and ex post (legal) mechanisms for ensuring an optimal level of risk.

KEYWORDS: Genetically engineered microbial agents (GEMs), risks (associated with GEMs), Bt toxin, legal liability (associated with GEMs), regulatory approval

INTRODUCTION

Decisions regarding the manufacture, sale, and use of genetically engineered microbial agents designed for deliberate release in agricultural settings (hereafter referred to as GEMs) are particularly complex because of the uncertainty surrounding the products' environmental impacts, the regulatory standards of safety that will be established, and the incidence of liability for unintended adverse effects that maybe created. Uncertainty exists in the scientific community about the possibility of migration, mutation, and possible environmental, health, and crop damage from GEMs. However, there is an emerging consensus that these products present low probability/high consequence risks.[1,2,3] The effect of this risk profile on GEMs introduction and adoption in agriculture will be

Risk Analysis, Edited by C. Zervos
Plenum Press, New York, 1991

determined in two stages. The first is the standard of acceptable risk set by regulators before allowing a products' testing or release into the marketplace. Since regulatory approval is unlikely to require that there be absolutely no risk involved, input manufacturers and agricultural producers will be faced with assessing the financial risk posed by liability for externalities created by GEMs.

Because of biotechnology's ability to foster the next technological revolution in agriculture, economists are anxious to be able to perform ex ante analysis of its effects on the farm sector. Historical experience with the externalities generated by the chemical revolution in agriculture have made economists concerned with determining the socially optimal level of risk and mix of institutions for regulating any adverse effects of the new technologies.

Economists have at their disposal several models and methods for conducting both ex ante studies of the impact of a new technology on agriculture and for determining the socially optimal mix of ex ante (regulatory) and ex post (tort action) mechanisms for controlling externalities. Prediction of a new technology's adoption and effect on the agricultural sector is most commonly conducted in an uncertainty framework where uncertainty is introduced through yield risk. Optimal strategies for control of externalities is usually determined within a certainty framework with the implicit assumption that actors have at their disposal the means for controlling the level of adverse effects resulting from their actions. But fundamental scientific, legal, and institutional uncertainties prevent these models and methods from being adequate for conducting similar analyses with respect to GEMs. The extent and effect of these uncertainties on the economic risks faced by manufacturers and users of GEMs will be explored. Particular emphasis will be placed on the effect of the economic risk introduced by the possibility of tort action on the manufacture and adoption of GEMs in agriculture.

RISKS ASSOCIATED WITH GEMS

Since its inception, recombinant DNA technology has been surrounded by concerns over its safety. Initially this concern focussed on the accidental release of genetically engineered organisms from the laboratory. Now the primary concern is with the safety of organisms designed for deliberate release into the environment. Unlike organisms intended solely for use in confined situations, microorganisms used in deliberate release applications are selected specifically for their ability to function and survive in the open environment. Questions have been raised about microorganisms' ability to multiply and spread into environments other than those into which they are released and to exchange genetic information with other, related microorganisms. Subtle changes in host range or virulence could have deleterious ecological, property, and human health effects.[4]

The risks associated with deliberate release of GEMs are often described as being analogous to those associated with two other classes of environmental introductions: toxic chemicals, including pesticides, and exotic species. The analogy to toxic chemicals arises from concerns about how chemicals are altered by the environment, their migration through ecosystems, and the hazards associated with human exposure and effects on the environment. The possibilities of uncontrolled reproduction and mutation and profligation of GEMs also raise many of the concerns associated with the introduction of exotic species.[5] In spite of the principles and caveats they reveal, particular case histories of problems caused by exotic species or toxic chemicals may be of little direct value in assessing the effects of GEMs and their treatment in the courts. Furthermore, like other phenomena that involve a degree of risk, the hazards presented by the introduction of GEMs cover a continuum of severity, starting at zero and ending with the catastrophic outliers.[1]

The scientific community has by no means reached a consensus on the degree of concern which should be associated with deliberate release of GEMs. Proponents of a "business as usual" approach argue that recombinant DNA technology is simply an extension of previous genetic manipulation technologies such as cross-breeding and hybridization. It is argued that the precision offered by the new technologies leads to a more predictable product[6,7] and that concern should be diminished rather than enhanced by the use of recombinant DNA. Opponents of the "business as usual" approach argue that recombinant DNA leads to the mixing of genetic materials that would not be possible using traditional techniques and that this manipulation may lead to organisms that are, genetically, less stable. The idea that small genetic changes necessarily yield small ecological changes is not supportable, even though likely to be true in many cases.[1] More specifically, the genetic manipulations have the aim of increasing virulence, shifting host ranges, and expanding the ecological range of organisms.[3] These types of ecological shifts, if successful, may have at least three important effects. First, they release the engineered genotype from the potential for head-to-head competition. Second, they put the new genotype into contact with an expanded or altered range of other species, some of which may never have encountered the parent genotype.[1] Third, such shifts may have direct or indirect effects on the habitat itself. All three phenomena are cause for close scrutiny of unanticipated risks to human health and property as well as to the ecosystem.[8]

In comments on application to EPA for permits for field testing of engineered organisms incorporating the toxin found in *Bacillus thuringienesis*, often referred to as Bt, Toll[9] and Toll and McRae[10] acknowledge both the increased precision made possible by recombinant DNA technology and the argument that this increased precision does not eliminate the need for concern. They note that in at least two cases, the gene being used to confer toxicity through the use of a delta-endotoxin (the part of Bt that is toxic to certain pests) is not a complete delta-endotoxin gene. Instead of producing delta-endotoxin, these genes produce only the toxic portion of the protein. This production mechanism eliminates the unique environmental conditions in the target pests' gut that are required to activate the delta-endotoxin. So instead of being confined to the gut of the target insect, these products could introduce the Bt toxin into plant tissue, thus bypassing the chemical containment mechanism that limits exposure to the toxin to a narrow range of species. Many new species may be exposed to the Bt toxin for the first time. Toll and McRae question how increased persistence of the toxin will affect pest tolerance to the Bt toxin, given evidence that pests do develop resistance to such toxins over long periods of exposure. In addition, if weed species accidentally incorporate the toxin, they too may become insect resistant, thus increasing weed pressure. Some scientific evidence has shown that the toxin in Bt can also cause adverse human health effects.

The problems in assessing risks from biotechnology stem from difficulty in ascertaining the likelihood of and the means of handling the presence of outliers. The average risk to the environment from the products of traditional biotechnology and from the products of genetic engineering may prove to be about equal for any given kind of product (see Fig. 1). On the other hand, the variability in risk among successive individual cases may be higher for genetically engineered organisms, producing a broader risk profile.[11] In addition, the absolute number of outliers in any distribution depends not only on the variance of the distribution but on the sample size. As the pace of development of experimental genotypes accelerates, the "sampling rate" of possibilities will also increase. Although "risk outliers" represent a minuscule proportion of the total number of GEM introductions, they are serious, both economically and in terms of public perception.[1]

LEGAL LIABILITY FOR GEM-INDUCED DAMAGES

The potential for legal liability of manufacturers and agricultural producers for damages that may be caused by GEMs will affect decisions regarding their production and

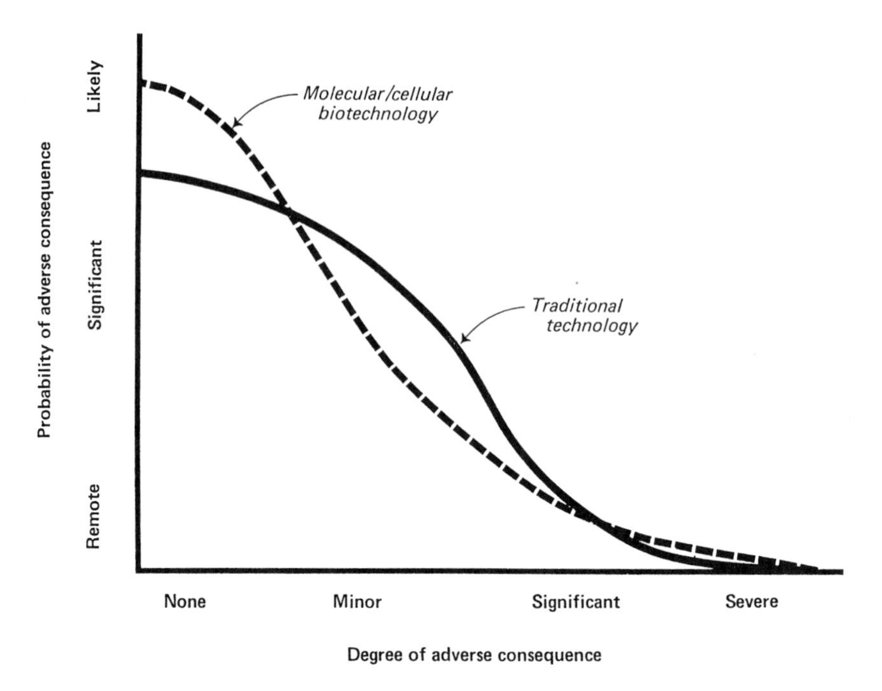

Fig. 1. A hypothetical ecological risk profile for the products of traditional biotechnology versus comparable products of modern molecular and cellular biotechnology intended for environmental use (adapted from Fiksel and Covello[11]).

use. Courts' treatment of liability cases for GEM-induced damages has not yet been determined because actual case law in this area has not been developed. Because of similarities in their function and use, the legal environment surrounding liability for GEMs would, at first glance, seem analogous to that for pesticides, particularly pesticide drift. However, there are three important differences. First, the technology is new, and there is debate over whether the courts will treat it as abnormally dangerous. Second, there are questions as to what manufacturers and users can do to demonstrate due care in the use of the technology. Third, it is not clear whether the courts will use the legal theory of negligence or strict liability in adjudicating cases that may be brought to court. The appropriate theory for examination of biotechnology in tort actions is the subject of heated debate in the legal profession.[12,13,14,15] The regulatory standards and legal theories used in court cases involving pesticide drift do provide a useful baseline for discussion.

While the basic concepts of the regulation of pesticides are derived from the Federal Insecticide, Fungicide and Rodenticide Act, most of the legislative initiative to control drift has evolved within the states and shows an impressive variety of approaches.[16] Many state statutes refer explicitly to drift or to concepts that indicate a concern with damage from drift. In some states, drift is expressly prohibited. At the other end of the spectrum are states that have statutes that do not directly regulate drift but imply the granting of authority for its regulation by repeated reference to environmental concerns. A wide variety of legal theories have been used to recover damages for injuries caused by the use of pesticides. The most common basis of recovery in pesticide cases has been negligence.[17] At the same time, most states have adopted some form of strict liability. Private nuisance and trespass are less used legal bases for private recovery. The application of strict liability and negligence rules poses problems in the treatment of GEMs because both rules imply some standard of action, usually based on precedent or best available techniques. The defendant in negligence cases must show use of "due care" in the application, use, or operation of the technology. In strict liability cases, the focus is on a standard of unreasonable danger in the design or working of the product and not on the subjective intention or fault of the user.

The rapid evolution of new techniques and products in biotechnology means, however, that courts will have difficulty in defining an appropriate level of due care and in assessing the user's true level of care under the negligence theory. The courts will also face difficulty in determining the standard of acceptable safety or use of state of the art in the development of products under a strict liability theory. The case law of each state determines whether strict liability is recognized and then whether the state of the art is to be defined by industry practice or by technological feasibility.

It is not clear whether courts will employ a strict liability or a negligence standard in adjudicating GEM cases. There are several arguments under which strict liability suits can be brought. O'Reilly notes that if genetic engineering is "abnormally dangerous," then courts could apply a standard of strict liability. Others, however, predict that courts will instead employ a standard of negligence, because as experience with recombinant DNA and associated technologies grows, they will no longer be considered abnormally dangerous.

Courts may still impose strict liability under the "escaping things" doctrine of Rylands v. Fletcher, or on the theory that genetically engineered microorganisms can be deemed "animals with known vicious or dangerous propensities." The Rylands rule states that "(i)f a person brings, or accumulates, on his land anything which, if it should escape, may cause damage to his neighbor, he does so at his peril."[16] Application of the Rylands rule to GEMs would be a reversal of the trend in pesticide cases where, according to Chiarella,[17] the Rylands precedent has been largely abandoned.

Strict liability could also be charged under the defect concept which ties the acceptability of a product to the relative risks presented by feasible alternatives. Courts often use a risk-utility analysis to decide whether a product's utility for its intended use exceeds the risks of its use. If the risk was undiscoverable by the designer and the product met the state of the art when designed, courts in some states would not regard it as unreasonably dangerous and therefore would not treat the product as being defective. But defining the actual state of the art is not simple. The term has at least two meanings: compliance with industry customs of design or compliance with the safest feasible alternative design standard. A defendant who poses a state of the art defense can assert that the product design was no worse than other products' designs at the time of manufacture. This criterion is tied to industry custom and current marketplace products. Alternatively, it could be argued that the design was at the leading edge of safe designs which this type of product could use and still remain functional. In at least one case,[18] however, the court refused to rule that a manufacturers' liability can be measured by the risks known at the time of the trial, but stated that "some products, though manufactured as designed and intended, are so dangerous in fact that the manufacturer should be liable for resulting harm though he did not know and could not have known of the danger at the time of marketing."

The legal uncertainty surrounding suits over biotechnology products arises, in part, from the conscious substitution of a pioneering technology of production for a well understood conventional alternative technology. If recombinant DNA is the only possible means of manufacture of a product, then the producer or user is less likely to be held liable if damages occur. (Consider, for example, the development of a new vaccine.) But if it is simply more economical, the producer or user is likely to be held liable [Restatement (Second) of Torts, at 402A, comment k, 1965]. At this point, use of biotechnology products will most likely occur because greater quantities, lower cost, or purer formulations (rather than a new function) can be achieved. The substitution leaves both manufacturer and user open to suit under strict liability.

Users of GEMs also have cause for concern if negligence theory is used as the basis for suit, since they have limited means of asserting due care once the decision to adopt is made. The plaintiff's use of liability or negligence arguments in bringing suit will determine whether the end user, the agricultural producer, can shift liability back to the manufacturer of the product. In traditional pesticide cases, manufacturers have been afforded some protection from this shift of liability by following appropriate labelling and warning practices, without which the product would be deemed defective [Restatement (Second) of Torts, at 402A, comment h, 1965]. In the recombinant DNA context, however, even a warning of the danger may not protect those likely to suffer harm[14] such as an agricultural producer whose fields are adjacent to those to which the GEM was applied.

LIABILITY AND THE MANUFACTURE OF GEMS

The risk of tort action from unintended adverse effects of GEMs will affect both the structure of the agricultural input industry and the types of products that are developed. The effect of uncertainty about the likelihood of cause for, and treatment of, tort actions is reflected in biotechnology firms' difficulty in obtaining liability insurance.

Although liability insurance is not required for the testing, manufacturing, or commercializing of biotechnologically-derived products, operating without insurance exposes both manufacturers and users of the technology to the potential for financial devastation. Biotechnology products are so new that many of the small companies that pioneered them cannot get product liability insurance. According to Bruce Mackler, of the Association of Biotechnology Companies, many firms will be forced to abandon promising new technology as a result.[19] Others will have to test products without coverage and run the risk of suits for amounts larger than their total assets should a product have unintended effects. The lack of insurance for many small firms raises questions about their ability or obligation to offer compensation for unintended side effects of their operations. Larger companies involved in agricultural biotechnology have not been affected as much as smaller companies because they have the size and safety record to give them clout with insurers, they offer a diversified set of products across which premiums and potential claim risks can be spread, and they can often afford to insure themselves.

Changes in liability concepts in the courts have also affected the insurance industry's willingness to offer product liability insurance to biotechnology firms. Insurers are concerned about the proliferation of punitive damages awarded and the trend towards shared liability in cases where any maker of a product deemed hazardous may be sued when an injured party does not know which one made the actual product that caused the injury, and where some companies have been held responsible for making a product even though the product met state-of-the-art standards at the time it was made.[20]

These changes have made assessing risk a new game for insurers. The actuarial risk that an adverse event will occur is becoming less important. Insurers are interested in knowing what the likelihood of a suit will be and the amount that has been awarded by jury or out-of-court settlements for certain types of products. What insurance executives say concerns them the most is the lack of predictability: the loss of ability to project with reasonable certainty the relations between losses and premiums paid.[21]

Although biotechnology firms are not required to have product liability insurance, its unavailability to small firms is likely to affect their role in the evolving biotechnology industry. For many small agricultural biotechnology firms, alliance with major agrichemical firms through licensing agreements may, in the short run, be the only feasible route towards protection from suit. However, this alliance will not come without cost to the smaller firms. In return for providing protection from possible liability claims, major agrichemical firms are likely to require lower licensing fees or other concessions.[22]

Table 1. Risks Associated with GEMs That Are of Direct Concern to Government Regulators and Agricultural Producers

Risk	Decisionmaker	
	Agricultural Producer	Government Regulator
Applicator health	X[a]	X
Food safety/residues		X
Ecosystem disruption		X
Liability	X	
Technology failure	X	

[a]Government regulation, through its focus on health and safety, provides some assurance of safety in this area.

LIABILITY AND THE ADOPTION OF GEMS

Most studies of the adoption and diffusion of new technologies in agriculture have been ex post.[23] Although economists have developed models that explicitly recognize the effect of uncertainty and risk aversion in ex ante prediction of adoption of new technology, their focus has been exclusively on yield risk.[24,25,26] Because of their focus on yield risk, the results of these models are of limited applicability in predicting the outcome of adoption decisions for GEMS or other technologies with a broader set of risks of concern to the producer.

Table 1 lists the types of risks associated with the release and use of GEMs. These include human health risks to the applicator and to consumers through residues, ecosystem disruption or pollution, and financial risk through liability to the farmer for damage to neighboring property, damage to his own property, or technological failure. The risks of direct concern to government regulators charged with approving the technology for use and the risks faced by farmers are almost mutually exclusive. However, they are not independent. The most obvious link is between regulatory standards for applicator health and safety and the consequent risk of this type faced by the producer. A less obvious but perhaps more important link for producer adoption exists between the regulatory standards set for effects external to the firm, specifically environmental disruption, and producer liability. As has been frequently demonstrated in pesticide drift liability cases, regulatory approval of a product is not an adequate defense in tort actions.[13,16]

To predict producer adoption of GEMs, we need to be able to establish appropriate probability distributions for yield and for tort action against the producer. In its simplest sense, tort action can be characterized by a Bernoullian or binomial distribution; you either get sued or you don't. However, development of a means of accurately determining the probability of suit and the damages awarded if such a suit is brought is hampered by scientific uncertainty about the probabilities associated with the factors that would lead to suit and uncertainty about how the courts will respond to such a suit.

Yassour *et al.*[24] demonstrate the importance of using the right specification for the probability distribution function of yield in ex ante prediction of the adoption of new technology and note that the importance of the correct specification increases with the decisionmaker's risk aversion. With the current state of knowledge on the probability of migration, mutation, and consequent property (crop) damage caused by GEMs, it is not possible to develop a probability distribution for the phenomena that would lead to tort action and subsequent liability for the producer using a GEM. At this point, the only information available to characterize such a distribution is that it is likely to be highly negatively skewed. But the probability associated with effective suit and the amount of damages awarded also depends on how the courts handle liability for damages from biotechnology.

ACCEPTABLE SAFETY IN REGULATION AND LEGAL LIABILITY

Although regulatory approval of a product is not a defense in tort actions for pesticides, the level of safety required before a product is approved for commercial release will affect the likelihood that producers will face tort actions. Therefore, we will examine the current standards for safety used by the Environmental Protection Agency in the approval of pesticides and GEMs, and the economic efficiency of controlling the possibility of adverse effects through the use of ex ante (regulation) and ex post (tort action) instruments.

GEMs, like chemical and biological pesticides, are regulated by the EPA under the Federal Insecticide, Fungicide, and Rodenticide Act (FIFRA). EPA balances the adverse effects of pesticides against their benefits to the economy, society, and the environment. FIFRA requires that EPA must conclude that a pesticide's use "will not generally cause unreasonable adverse effects in the environment."[27] Registration does not require that pesticides be proven absolutely safe to humans or to the environment. Such a requirement would effectively bar the use of pesticides because chemicals that are intended to kill pest organisms are often dangerous to other forms of life as well.

Both manufacturers and farmers may be caught in the bind that regulatory agencies and the courts use significantly different definitions of risk in determining the acceptability of a product and its use. Thompson's[28] distinction between the event-based concept of risk and the action-based concept of risk is useful in analyzing this difference. An action-based concept of risk presupposes that risk is a direct result of an individual's actions and can be distinguished from freak accidents or normal background risk. Action risk is therefore limited to behavior that is unreasonable or otherwise extraordinary by traditional precedents. In contrast, event risk is ubiquitous. The event-based concept of risk forms the basis for quantitative risk analysis and is based on the determination of probabilities and utilities. The definition of an acceptable risk depends, in large part, on how catastrophic risks are entered into the utility function. Individuals' responsibility for adverse events has little to do with defining an acceptable level of event risk.

Much of the controversy over how GEMs and other products of biotechnology should be regulated revolves around the question of whether an action-based or an event-based definition of risk should be used. The arguments for the use of an action or an event based concept of risk relate directly to the question of the relative importance of expectations and outliers. A key point of tension between the use of event and action risk arises over the type of inferences used to establish questions of fact. Since action-risk evaluation involves classifying of the action as to its "reasonableness" or its "exceptional" character, analogies between the act in question and other acts are crucial. Event-risk, on the other hand, requires probabilistic anticipation of all possible outcomes. Both perspectives rely upon facts, but each presupposes a different procedure for determining which facts are relevant.[28]

Many proponents of agricultural biotechnology advocate an action-based standard of risk in regulation. They portray agricultural genetic engineering as thoroughly mundane and consistent with reasonable actions. Under action-risk thinking, a risk is acceptable as soon as the act is judged to be analogous to accepted precedents. Any harmful effects that do occur would have to be considered to be so unexpected that they are freak accidents, the sort of outcomes for which no one can be held accountable.[28] Such a basis for regulation would free research and commercialization of GEMs and other agricultural biotechnologies. But at the same time it would increase liability concerns for their users where in the courts a different level of "abnormally dangerous" may be used as a standard for judgment.

Others argue that the event-based definition of risk should be used to determine acceptability. A risk becomes acceptable under event-risk thinking only when reliable quantification and comparison has been completed, not only for the planned action but for its principal alternatives. The meanings of responsibility, of acceptability, and even the type of factual information required all change as one shifts from an emphasis upon judging responsibility for actions to one of anticipating, then accepting or rejecting, a pattern of events.[28]

The selection of an action- or event-based risk standard also has implications for the institutional division of labor between the regulators and the courts in preventing or compensating individuals for exposure to adverse events. This leads to questions about the socially optimal means of controlling risk. Work in this area is exemplified by papers by Cooter,[29] Johnson and Ulen,[30] Segerson,[31] and Shavell.[32] All of the authors discuss a socially optimal mix of ex ante (regulatory) and ex post (tort) control of hazardous activities. Implicit in their analysis is the assumption that users of the technology or causers of externalities can choose the level of hazard or safety that they wish to promulgate. In other words, it is not an all or none situation. This situation can be contrasted with that of a user of a GEM who has, to date, limited economical means of control after adoption. A rule that may be socially optimal where actors have means for controlling the level of safety may not be an optimal rule for the producer who relies on a regulatory standard to indicate acceptability of use. Similarly, manufacturers may be unaware of the long term ecological impacts of their products at the time they are released after regulatory approval.

Economists, regulators, and scientists working in biotechnology are not the only ones perplexed by this problem. Legal scholars are in conflict about the efficacy of a strengthened regulatory regime[12,33] or a strengthened tort regime[14] for ensuring a socially optimal level of risk from biotechnology.

The stricter the regulatory standard imposed, the less likely it is that producers will be faced with suit because it will be less likely that the GEMs released for commercial use will have adverse effects. However, even a strict regime for regulatory approval does not completely protect producers from suit: regulatory approval does not protect producers from tort action and state courts may set different standards for what is an appropriate level of due care in negligence actions or what they deem to be abnormally dangerous products under strict liability. Neither a "utility greater than risk" or *de minimus* standard provides consequent insurance against suit because, at this point, GEMs will serve, in large part, as substitutes for existing products rather than serve new functions. A regulatory standard that would promulgate less risk for both manufacturers and farmers is one based on relative risk — approval of GEMs only if they are deemed to be less risky than the products for which they may serve as substitutes. However, at this point, EPA procedures emphasize a product-by-product standard of acceptable risk, rather than a comparison among products. Furthermore, there is little evidence that regulators and the courts evaluate expectations and outliers in the same manner.

CONCLUSIONS

Liability for unintended adverse effects of genetically engineered microbial agents designed for free release in agricultural settings and the consequent economic risk faced by both manufacturers and users of these products will play a crucial role in the technology's introduction and adoption in agriculture. Ex ante prediction of the impacts of possible liability is hindered by uncertainty about the probability of adverse environmental impacts of GEMs, unresolved debate about the appropriate regulatory standard of acceptable risk, and questions about how courts will treat manufacturers' and users' liability under either strict liability or negligence theories. The importance of higher moments of distributions of outcomes is highlighted by the skewed probability distributions associated with different biotechnology-related risks and the differing weights that courts and regulatory agencies attach to outliers.

Economists' repertoire of models and methods for predicting the introduction and adoption of technology and determining the socially optimal institutional division of labor for risk management cannot be applied, given the existing scientific, legal, and institutional uncertainty surrounding GEMs. GEMs may be a uniquely troublesome product within the broad range of biotechnologies anticipated to come on line in the near future because of their direct release into the environment. However, the case of GEMs does bring up points that will be important in the consideration of many new technologies in agriculture. One of the most important is that yield risk is not the only risk of concern to the agricultural producer. The regulatory standard of safety and individual state court decisions will shape new technologies' impact on the sector through their effect on manufacturers' and agricultural producers' liability.

REFERENCES

1. R. Colwell, Ecology and Biotechnology: Expectations and Outliers, in *Risk Analysis Approaches for Environmental Releases of Genetically Engineered Organisms*, Joseph Fiksel and Vincent Covello, eds., Springer-Verlag, Berlin (1990).
2. R. Harlow, The EPA and Biotechnology Regulation: Coping with Scientific Uncertainty, *The Yale Law Journal* **95**:555-576 (1986).
3. P. Regal, Models of Genetically Engineered Organisms and Their Ecological Impact, *Recombinant DNA Technical Bulletin* **10**:67-85 (1987).
4. F. Betz, M. Levin, and M. Rogul, Safety Aspects of Genetically-Engineered Microbial Pesticides, *Recombinant DNA Technical Bulletin* **6(4)**:135-141 (1983).
5. S. Offutt and F. Kuchler, Issues and Developments in Biotechnology: What's an Economist to Do? *Journal of Agricultural Economics Research* **39**:25-33 (1987).
6. W. Brill, Safety Concerns and Genetic Engineering in Agriculture, *Science* **227**:381-384 (1985).
7. B. Davis, Bacterial Domestication: Underlying Assumptions, *Science* **235**:1329,1332-1335 (1987).
8. F. Sharples, Regulation of Products from Biotechnology, *Science* **235**:1329-1332 (1987).
9. J. Toll, Will Biotechnology Improve Biological Controls? *Bio-Science* **38**:588 (1987).
10. J. Toll and G. McRae, Comments on Crop Genetics International's Experimental Use Permit Application OPP-50675 for Clavibacter xyll Cynodontis Containing a Segment of the Delta-Endotoxin Gene from Bacillus Thuringiensis var. Durstaki, *Federal Register* **53**:2641-2642, January 26, 1988.
11. J. Fiksel and V. Covello, The Suitability and Applicability of Risk Assessment Methods for Environmental Applications of Biotechnology, in *Biotechnology Risk*

Assessment: Issues and Methods for Environmental Introductions, pp. 1-34, Joseph Fiksel and Vincent Covello, eds., Pergamon Press, New York (1986).
12. R. Pierce, Encouraging Safety: The Limits of Tort Law and Government Regulation, *Vanderbilt Law Review* **33**:1281-1332 (1980).
13. J. O'Reilly, Biotechnology Meets Product Liability: Problems Beyond the State of the Art, *Houston Law Review* **24**:451-489 (1987).
14. D. Dahl, Strict Product Liability for Injuries Caused by Recombinant DNA Bacteria, *Santa Clara Law Review* **22**:117-149 (1982).
15. Designer Genes that Don't Fit: A Tort Regime for Commercial Releases of Genetic Engineering Products, *Harvard Law Review* **100**:1086-1105 (1987).
16. S. Redfield, Chemical Trespass? — An Overview of Statutory and Regulatory Efforts to Control Pesticide Drift, *Kentucky Law Journal* **73**:855-918 (1985).
17. M. Chiarella, Pesticide Spraying: Theories for Private Recovery, *New Hampshire Bar Journal* **26**:26-38 (1984).
18. Crocker vs. Winthrop Laboratories, 514 S.W.2d 432 (Texas, 1974).
19. K. Day, Biotechnology Companies Meet Insurer Reluctance, *Los Angeles Times*, May 28:IV.1, IV.14 (1985).
20. T. Lewin, The Liability Insurance Spiral, *The New York Times*, March 8:35,37 (1986).
21. N. Nash, Calculating Risk is a Riskier Business Now, *The New York Times*, p. D1, May 25, 1986.
22. B. Fleisher, The Evolving Biotechnology Industry and Its Effects on Production Agriculture, U.S Agricultural Policy in a Changing World, AFPR-6, U.S. Department of Agriculture Economic Research Service, Washington, DC (1989).
23. Z. Griliches, Hybrid Corn: An Exploration in the Economics of Technical Change, *Econometrica* **25**:501-522 (1957).
24. J. Yassour, D. Zilberman, and G. Rausser, Optimal Choices among Alternative Technologies with Stochastic Yield, *American Journal of Agricultural Economics* **63**:718-723 (1981).
25. G. Feder, Adoption of Interrelated Agricultural Innovations: Complementarity and the Impacts of Risk, Scale, and Credit, *American Journal of Agricultural Economics* **64**:94-101 (1982).
26. W. Lesser, W. Magrath, and R. Kalter, Projecting Adoption Rates: Application of an Ex Ante Procedure to Biotechnology Products, *North Central Journal of Agricultural Economics* **8**:159-173 (1986).
27. M. Mellon, Biotechnology, in *Law of Environmental Protection*, Sheldon Novick, Donald Stever, and Margaret Mellon, eds., pp. 18.1-18.64, Vol. 2, Clark Boardman Company, Ltd., New York (1987).
28. P. Thompson, Agricultural Biotechnology and the Rhetoric of Risk: Some Conceptual Issues, Resources for the Future National Center for Food and Agricultural Policy Discussion Paper FAP87-01 (1987).
29. R. Cooter, Liability Rules and Risk Sharing in Environmental and Resource Policy: Discussion, *American Journal of Agricultural Economics* **68**:1276-1278 (1986).
30. G. Johnson and T. Ulen, Designing Public Policy Towards Hazardous Waste: The Role of Administrative Regulations and Legal Liability Rules, *American Journal of Agricultural Economics* **68**:1266-1271 (1986).
31. K. Segerson, Risk Sharing in the Design of Environmental Policy, *American Journal of Agricultural Economics* **68**:1261-1265 (1986).
32. S. Shavell, A Model of the Optimal Use of Liability and Safety Regulation, *Rand Journal of Economics* **15**:271-280 (1984).
33. K. Viscusi, Product Liability and Regulation: Establishing the Appropriate Institutional Division of Labor, *American Economic Review* **78**:300-304 (1988).

A Method for Ranking the Severity of Foodborne Illnesses

Josephine Mauskopf and A. Scott Ross
Research Triangle Institute
Research Triangle Park, NC

ABSTRACT

Foods that violate the Food, Drug, and Cosmetic Act can cause a wide variety of illnesses when consumed. In this paper we present a method for ranking the severity of these foodborne illnesses. Such a ranking, in conjunction with information on the likelihood of experiencing each illness, might be useful to the Food and Drug Administration when determining compliance monitoring priorities. To develop the severity ranking, we describe the impact on patients of different levels of severity of illnesses likely to be associated with food products. This impact is described in terms of symptoms, duration of illness, impact on functional status, and fatality rates. These impacts are translated into changes in the time spent in a set of health states developed by Rosser and Kind. Relative utility weights, estimated for each of the health states, are used to convert these changes into estimates of losses in utility, measured as quality adjusted life years (QALY's) lost. Finally, severe botulism is defined as the reference illness with an index value of one. The index values for all other illnesses can then be computed as the ratio of the QALY's lost to the QALY's lost from severe botulism.

KEYWORDS: Severity index, foodborne illness, quality adjusted life years (QALYs)

INTRODUCTION

All foods produced for human consumption in the United States are regulated for composition, quality, safety, and labeling under the Food, Drug, and Cosmetic (FD&C) Act of 1938 and its subsequent amendments. The Food and Drug Administration (FDA) has only limited resources available for ensuring compliance of imported foods with these laws. These resources can be allocated among several compliance monitoring options, including memoranda of understanding (MOU) with the country of origin, wharf examinations, sample collections, and inspections of foreign plants. The resources divided to each compliance monitoring option must then be allocated among the wide variety of imported products, each of which might violate the FD&C Act in many different ways.

Compliance monitoring reduces the probability that any given imported food product that reaches the U.S. consumer violates the FD&C Act. Such monitoring reduces the probability that imported food is in violation of the FD&C Act, both directly because of inspections of foreign food processors or MOU's with foreign governments and indirectly because of the fear of detection by wharf exams or sample collection and subsequent penalty to the producer if the violation is detected. Wharf exams and sample collection also prevent foods that are in violation of the FD&C Act from reaching the U.S. consumer.

FDA's resource allocation problem is similar to that of EPA's Superfund. Potential Superfund sites are ranked in order of their seriousness so that the limited resources available to clean up such sites can be allocated as efficiently as possible. Several hazard ranking schemes have been developed. These hazard rankings depend on the probability of different levels of human or other exposure to the toxic substances found at the site, the potency of these toxic substances, and the severity of the adverse effects associated with such exposures. The hazard rankings help to identify the most hazardous sites, and subsequent cost-effectiveness analysis for these sites determines whether remedial action is feasible.

Similarly, FDA might find it efficient to develop a hazard ranking for imported foods as a first step for allocating scarce compliance monitoring resources. One key input for such a hazards ranking is a relative severity index for all the many different foodborne illnesses that can be caused by violations of the FD&C Act. Such a severity index is necessary if FDA is to be able to compare, for example, the overall hazards to the U.S. consumer from two imported products. The first imported food product has a high probability of being in violation of the FD&C Act, and the violation, if undetected, has a high probability of causing a generally non-serious foodborne illness, for example staphylococcal gastroenteritis. The second imported food product has a very low probability of being in violation of the FD&C Act, and the violation, if undetected, has a low probability of causing a very serious foodborne illness, for example botulism. In this case, the relative value to the consumer of preventing the different foodborne illnesses is an important component of the determination of the relative hazards from the two products.

In this paper, we describe a method that we have used to develop a severity ranking for a large number of foodborne illnesses. This method consists of the following five steps:

1. Identify the foodborne illnesses associated with each violation of the FD&C Act.
2. Describe the impacts of each foodborne illness on an individual consumer.
3. Translate these impacts into time spent in specific health states.
4. Estimate the losses in quality adjusted life years associated with each foodborne illness.
5. Use the estimated losses in quality adjusted life years to compute a relative severity index.

We will illustrate the proposed method for botulism only.

IDENTIFY FOODBORNE ILLNESSES

The first step is to use available human or nonhuman data to identify illnesses likely to be associated with violations of the FD&C Act.[1] In some cases the existence of a cause and effect relationship between a violation and an illness is well established, such as that between botulinum toxin and botulism. In other cases this relationship may be less well established, such as that between pesticide residues and excess risk of cancer. These differences should be factored into a complete hazards ranking but have not been considered when developing the severity ranking for the illnesses themselves.

In order to facilitate the later steps in the estimation procedure, the foodborne illnesses were subdivided into the following three categories:

1. Acute illnesses that occur with no latency period after exposure, have a well defined duration and end in either death or complete cure.
2. Chronic illnesses that have no or a short latency period after exposure, have a prolonged duration, and end in death.
3. Cancers that have a prolonged latency period, short or prolonged duration and end in either death or complete cure.

Most foodborne illnesses can be assigned to one or more of these categories. Table 1 presents some examples of violations of the FD&C Act and their associated foodborne illnesses. Botulism is caused by the presence of botulinum toxin in a food product and is classified as an acute illness. Survivors of a severe case of botulism might also suffer from residual chronic illness, but this was not included in our analysis.

DESCRIBE THE IMPACT ON CONSUMER

Most foodborne illnesses can manifest themselves at a variety of levels of severity, each of which impacts the consumer to a different degree. In order to simplify the analysis, three levels of severity were chosen for each illness: mild, moderate, and severe (local, regional, and distant at diagnosis for the cancers), and the impacts of the illnesses at each of these levels of severity determined. The definitions of mild, moderate, or severe for the acute and chronic illnesses varied between illnesses and were based on well-defined clusters of symptoms, resource use, and/or mortality risk.

The impacts on the consumer for each level of severity for each illness were described in terms of patient symptoms, mortality rates, duration of treatment and recovery, frequently used medical treatment, and functional status during treatment and recovery. Functional status during the illness was defined as either in the hospital, in bed at home, or at home not in bed. Table 2 illustrates such descriptions for botulism. The data for these descriptions came from the clinical literature.

DETERMINE TIME SPENT IN SPECIFIC HEALTH STATES

Before the specific impacts of a foodborne illness can be translated into changes in the consumer's overall health status, an exhaustive set of health states must be defined. In this paper, we describe the use of the Rosser and Kind[6] set of health states. Any set of health states that is general enough to be applied to all foodborne illnesses and for which utility (well-being) weights relative to perfect health have been estimated could be used. Table 3 presents the Rosser and Kind health state definitions. They express health status in terms of two dimensions: disability and distress.

Once a set of health states was chosen, the impacts of each foodborne illness were described in terms of time spent in specific health states as a result of the illness. These descriptions are shown for botulism in Table 4 using the Rosser and Kind health state descriptions. A mild case of botulism was estimated to result in five days with ability to work severely limited and with mild distress. A serious case of botulism, in contrast, was estimated to result in 90 days confined to bed in severe distress, 30 days confined to a chair in moderate distress, and 60 days unable to work in mild distress.

ESTIMATE LOSSES IN QUALITY ADJUSTED LIFE YEARS

In order to estimate the quality adjusted life years lost as a result of the foodborne illness, a series of assumptions was made. These include age at exposure to the violation,

Table 1. Sample of Foodborne Illness Caused by Violations of the FD&C Act

Violation	Acute Effects	Chronic Effects	Cancers
1. D & C Red #10	Contact Dermatitis		Bladder
2. Cat Filth/Damage	Toxoplasmosis	Congenital Toxoplasmosis	
3. C. Botulinum	Botulism		
4. Chloroform		Liver Changes	Liver
5. Salmonella	Salmonellosis		
6. Inadequate Pasteurization, LACF	Salmonellosis, Botulism		
7. Sulfite	Allergic Response		

Table 2. Impact of Botulism on Patient

Illness	Symptoms	Duration	Treatment	Functional Status	Fatality Rate
Botulism					
Mild	malaise, weakness, fatigue	5 days	antitoxin	5 house days	0%
Moderate	nausea, vomiting, diarrhea, abdominal pain, fever, malaise, weakness, headache, dizziness	21 days	antitoxin	7 hospital days 7 bed days 7 house days	0%
Severe	same as moderate plus: respiratory paralysis, muscular paralysis, pulmonary infection	180 days	antitoxin respiratory support	90 hospital days 30 bed days 60 house days	22.5%

Sources: FASEB[1]; Mann *et al.*[2]; Todd[3]; Todd[4]; CDC[5].

Table 3. Rosser and Kind[6] Health States

Disability	Distress
1. None	1. None
2. Slight social disability	2. Mild
3. Severe social disability, slight impairment at work	3. Moderate
4. Work severely limited	4. Severe
5. Unable to work	
6. Confined to chair	
7. Confined to bed	
8. Unconscious	

Table 4. Time in Specific Rosser and Kind[6] Health States with Botulism

Illness	Disability	Distress	Duration
Botulism			
Mild	4	2	5 days
Moderate	7	3	7 days
	6	3	7 days
	4	2	7 days
Severe	7	4	90 days
	6	3	30 days
	4	2	60 days

latency period for the illness after exposure, remaining life expectancy at time of illness and state of health at onset of illness and for remaining lifetime. For this study we assumed age at exposure of 30 years, with a 20 year latency period for cancer but no latency period for acute or chronic effects. Remaining life expectancy at 30 and 50 was assumed to be 46 and 26 years respectively, and in the absence of the disease individuals were assumed to remain in perfect health for their remaining lifetime. Lipscomb *et al.*[7] have shown that this last assumption only results in overestimates of the losses associated with illness of about 5 percent.

Using these assumptions, after the times spent in specific health states were estimated for the foodborne illnesses, the estimated utility (well-being) weights shown in Table 5 for the Rosser and Kind index were used to compute estimates of the losses in quality adjusted life years (QALY's) associated with each illness. These estimates are shown for mild, moderate, and severe cases of botulism in Table 6. The estimated losses in quality adjusted life years are much larger for those who die from the disease, 25.5 QALY's discounted at 3 percent (46 QALY's undiscounted), than for those who have a severe case and survive, .647 QALY's.

Table 5. Rosser and Kind[6] Index Utility Weights

Disability	Distress			
	1	2	3	4
1	1.0	0.995	0.990	0.967
2	0.990	0.986	0.973	0.932
3	0.980	0.972	0.956	0.912
4	0.964	0.956	0.942	0.870
5	0.946	0.935	0.900	0.700
6	0.875	0.845	0.680	0.000
7	0.677	0.564	0.000	−1.486
8	−1.028			

Table 6. Losses in Quality Adjusted Life Years from Botulism

Illness	Fatality Rate	Loss for Survivors QALY's* (QALD's)**	Weighted Average Loss QALY's* (QALD's)**
Botulism			
Mild	0%	0.00055 (0.2)	0.00055 (0.2)
Moderate	0%	0.0263 (9.6)	0.0263 (9.6)
Severe	22.5%	0.647 (236.)	6.24 (2,279.)

*QALY is a quality adjusted life year.

**QALD is a quality adjusted life day.

COMPUTE A RELATIVE SEVERITY INDEX

A relative severity index can be computed by choosing one foodborne illness as the reference state with a relative severity index value of 1. In this paper we chose a severe case of botulism as the reference state. The relative severity of mild and moderate cases of botulism were estimated to be $8.8 \times 10E\text{-}05$ and $4.2 \times 10E\text{-}03$, respectively.

The distribution of mild, moderate, and severe cases of botulism expected to be observed from products contaminated with botulinum toxin will vary according to the concentration of botulinum toxin, as well as according to the typical portion size for the food product and consumer characteristics such as age. Thus, in using these severity indices to estimate the hazards associated with different violations in different food products, the index values for the three levels of severity must be combined using weights derived from estimates of these other factor values.

CONCLUSIONS

In this paper we have described a method that can be used to generate a severity ranking for all foodborne illnesses. We have illustrated the use of our method using one foodborne illness only, botulism, and choosing only one of the alternative health status indices that could have been used in this type of analysis. Although not apparent from this single example, the key factor that determines relative severity of an acute illness is its fatality rate. This is also true for cancers, but not for chronic diseases where the degree of functional impairment is of critical importance.

REFERENCES

1. Federation of American Societies for Experimental Biology (FASEB), Identification of Foodborne Illnesses Associated with FD&C Act Violations, Appendix A in Estimating the Value of Consumers' Loss from Foods Violating the FD&C Act, Research Triangle Institute, Prepared for Center for Food Safety and Nutrition, Food and Drug Administration, Contract No. 223-87-2097, September, 1988.
2. J. M. Mann, G. D. Lathrop, and J. A. Bannerman, Economic Impact of a Botulism Outbreak: Importance of the Legal Component in Foodborne Disease, *Journal of the American Medical Association* **249(10)**:1299-1301 (1983).
3. E. C. D. Todd, Economic Loss from Foodborne Disease and Non-Illness Related Recalls Because of Mishandling by Food Processors, *Journal of Food Protection* **48(7)**:621-633 (1985a).
4. E. C. D. Todd, Economic Loss from Foodborne Disease Outbreaks Associated with Food Service Establishments, *Journal of Food Protection* **48(2)**:169-180 (1985b).
5. Centers for Disease Control (CDC), Botulism in the United States, 1979, *The Journal of Infectious Diseases* **142(2)**:302-305 (1980).
6. R. Rosser and P. Kind, A Scale of Valuations of States of Illness: Is There a Social Consensus? *International Journal of Epidemiology* **7(4)**:347-358 (1978).
7. J. Lipscomb, J. T. Kolimaga, P. W. Sperduto, J. K. Minnich, and K. J. Fontenot, Cost-Benefit and Cost-Effectiveness Analyses of Screening for Neural Tube Defects in North Carolina, Draft Report prepared for the State of North Carolina (1983).

A Graphical Display of Risk Information

Stephen L. Brown and Joseph V. Rodricks
ENVIRON Corporation
Washington, DC

ABSTRACT

Cancer risk assessment and management of hazardous air pollutants under the Vinyl Chloride decision requires a two-step process. When regulating a pollutant such as benzene, EPA must first determine whether a proposed level of emissions is "safe" and then in a second step whether it provides an ample margin of safety. Safety is judged in terms of both maximum individual risk and population risk ("cancer incidence"). Both determining safety and setting an ample margin require consideration of uncertainties in risk assessment. This paper proposes a graphical display of maximum individual risk versus population risk, with degree of certainty represented by the size of circles showing various possible estimates of risks. Risk criteria are represented by a criterion band based on risk management precedents. Visual inspection of the diagram can aid in standard setting.

KEYWORDS: Vinyl Chloride, benzene, uncertainty, graphics, cancer risk management

INTRODUCTION

Quantitative cancer risk assessment has become a major tool for federal agencies in their efforts to regulate potentially carcinogenic chemicals in the home, the workplace, and the general environment.[1] Although estimates of risk are only one of several inputs into the process of managing risks, comparisons of various measures of risk to risk criteria or benchmarks are influential in determining the degree of attention that an agency will devote to a situation that poses a potential cancer risk.

One area in which quantitative risk assessment has considerable influence is the development of standards for hazardous air pollutants under Section 112 of the Clean Air Act, administered by the Environmental Protection Agency (EPA). This section[2] is an example of "health-based standards" in which the primary emphasis of the statutory language was on the protection of the public health. Other standards, such as those covering pesticides, are "balancing" standards in the sense that allowable exposures are developed with due attention to the technical feasibility and cost of achieving them, in comparison to the health benefits to be gained by lowering exposures.

Recently the Court of Appeals, in an opinion written by Judge Robert Bork, directed EPA to set standards under Section 112 with a two-step process. In the first step, the Agency must demonstrate that the proposed standard will protect human health, regardless

Risk Analysis, Edited by C. Zervos
Plenum Press, New York, 1991

of the cost of achieving it. Judge Bork made it clear, however, that the Court interpreted the Clean Air Act not to require absolute freedom from risk. Instead, "safety" meant freedom from a level of risks beyond that found acceptable as a part of everyday life. Questions of uncertainty, cost, technical feasibility, and so on must be deferred until a second step, in which the Agency can determine what further reductions in exposure are required, if any, to provide an "ample margin of safety." Because the case involved a complaint over the application of Section 112 to vinyl chloride, it has become known as the Vinyl Chloride decision.[3]

MEASURES OF RISK

Most of the pollutants currently regulated under Section 112 are assumed to be carcinogens, and this paper will focus on the assessment and management of cancer risks. Regulatory decisions under Section 112 have typically considered two kinds of risk: individual risk, often to a highly exposed subset of the population at risk, and population risk or, in EPA terminology, incidence. Individual risk is ordinarily expressed as the lifetime excess probability of developing a cancer from lifetime exposure to the pollutant. Population risk is ordinarily expressed as a hypothetical excess incidence rate of new cancers per year throughout the population at risk. Individual risk may be considered in the decision process so that no group will bear an inequitable share of the risk, while population risk may be considered in order to protect the public health as a whole.

Figure 1 shows a graph of individual risk versus population risk, plotted on scales that are logarithmic in both types of risk. Individual risk, plotted vertically, is labeled "Maximum Individual Risk" to emphasize the idea that such risk is estimated for a highly exposed subset of individuals. In fact, most EPA risk assessments refer to a hypothetical "maximally exposed individual" (MEI) who would spend his whole life at the point of maximum concentration outside the facilities being regulated. No real person would have such exposures, but the MEI exposure does provide a theoretical upper bound on potential exposures. This first figure shows only one point, identified with a star, which represents the combination of maximum individual risk and incidence (population risk) for a hypothetical chemical, as they would be computed under EPA's usual practice. Not only is the exposure to the MEI a conservative estimate for the real exposures for highly exposed individuals, but the computation of risk also entails use of a "plausible upper limit" for the cancer potency factor that relates exposure to lifetime risk.

In a proposed rule for benzene under Section 112,[4] EPA offers four ways of using this point with risk management criteria to identify the need for risk reduction. Two of the proposals (Approaches C and D) use only maximum individual risk as a criterion, at levels of 1 in 10,000 (10^{-4}) or 1 in 1,000,000 (10^{-6}). A third method (Approach B) uses only population risk, at an incidence of 1 cancer per year in the exposed population. The fourth method (Approach A) is less mechanical and may consider uncertainties as well as population and individual risk; it suggests that 10^{-4} individual risk can be used as a potential starting point. Figure 1 shows how the first three criteria can be represented on the risk diagram. For this hypothetical chemical, the risk would be acceptable under the population risk criterion but not under either of the individual risk criteria. It might or might not be acceptable under a case-by-case approach.

Consideration of uncertainty would have to be purely qualitative in any of the four methods proposed by EPA. In fact, only Approach A clearly allows consideration of uncertainty in the first stage decision (determining safety). It would seem that more use can be made of the available information about risk, and that such use will enhance the ability of EPA risk managers to make their decisions and of the public to understand them.

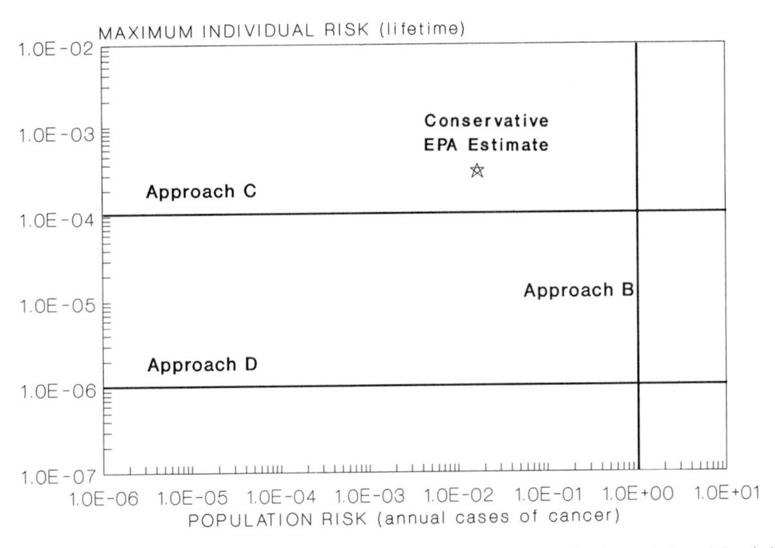

Fig. 1. Display of maximum individual risk versus population risk with risk criteria proposed by the Environmental Protection Agency for the regulation of benzene.

REPRESENTING UNCERTAINTIES

Recent risk assessments by the Office of Air Quality Planning and Standards have acknowledged that differing estimates of risk variables are possible within the bounds of the available data. Special attention is given to different models for estimating cancer potency factors, but alternative estimates of exposure to highly exposed people and to the population as a whole are also possible.

Suppose just three estimates were generated for each important variable (cancer potency factor, exposure of highly exposed people, average exposure for typical people, number of typical people exposed). One estimate would be a most plausible or best estimate of the value of the variable. The others would be a plausible upper bound ("high") and a plausible lower bound ("low"), each representing the tail of the distribution of possible values. In each case, "plausible" means a value generated by deliberation among experts in the various branches of risk assessment, as could be obtained by a panel of EPA's Science Advisory Board, for example. At present, no rigorous statistical approach can produce these values, although the techniques of meta-analysis[5] hold some promise in this regard.

There are 81 ways of combining these values. Calculations for some fictitious but reasonable values for the hypothetical chemical are presented in Table 1. If these values were to be plotted on the risk diagram, a better appreciation of the uncertainties involved in risk assessment for carcinogens is obtained.

Such a display, however, would be misleading in the sense that one could be led to believe that all the points are equally likely to be true. In fact, the points developed with best estimates of the variables are very much more likely to be true than those that use extreme values, either high or low. To deal with this situation, the relative confidence in each of the estimates may be represented by circles whose areas are proportional to the probabilities that the estimates are most nearly true. Table 2 shows the probabilities and circle sizes for various combinations of the estimates. For example, if the best estimate for cancer potency factor were combined with the upper limit for MEI exposure and the lower

Table 1. Sample Calculations for Multiple Estimates of Risk for a Hypothetical Chemical

Variable	High	Best	Low
Cancer Potency Factor (CPF) $(mg/kg/day)^{-1}$	0.15	0.02	0.0004
MEI Exposure (MEI) mg/kg/day	0.0022	0.0016	0.0004
Average Exposure (AE) mg/kg/day	0.00084	0.00056	0.000084
Population Size (PS) No. of people	27000	14000	8000

Sample Calculations:

All high values for variables:
Maximum individual risk = CPF×MEI = 0.15×0.0022 $= 3.30\times10^{-4}$
Population risk = CPF×AE×PS = 0.15×0.00084×27000/70 $= 4.86\times10^{-2}$

All best values for variables:
Maximum individual risk = CPF×MEI = 0.02×0.0016 $= 3.20\times10^{-5}$
Population risk = CPF×AE×PS = 0.02×0.00056×14000/70 $= 2.24\times10^{-3}$

All low values for variables:
Maximum individual risk = CPF×MEI = 0.0004×0.0004 $= 1.60\times10^{-7}$
Population risk = CPF×AE×PS = 0.0004×0.000084×8000/70 $= 3.84\times10^{-6}$

Best CPF, high MEI, low AE, low PS:
Maximum individual risk = CPF×MEI = 0.02×0.0022 $= 4.40\times10^{-4}$
Population risk = CPF×AE×PS = 0.02×0.000084×8000/70 $= 1.92\times10^{-4}$

Table 2. Probabilities of Risk Estimates and Corresponding Circle Sizes

Number of Best Estimates	Number of Extreme Estimates	Probability of Being Most Nearly Correct	Relative Circle Area	Relative Circle Diameter
0	4	0.0016	1.0	1.0
1	3	0.0048	3.0	1.7
2	2	0.0144	9.0	3.0
3	1	0.0432	27.0	5.2
4	0	0.1296	81.0	9.0

Note: Neither the probabilities shown nor the circle sizes associated with them are intended to be precise. They are intended to provide the viewer with a visual sense of the relative plausibility of various estimates of risk.

limits for average population exposure and population at risk, there would be one best estimate and three extreme estimates, for a probability of 0.0048 (about 1/2 percent). These circles are displayed in Fig. 2, in which over half of the points (those with very low probabilities of being true) are omitted. The bulk of the estimates fall considerably lower in risk than the conservative EPA estimate represented by the star. It must be emphasized that this display is for a hypothetical chemical and is not based on real data. In most real EPA decisions, however, estimates of this sort can be generated with little additional effort from the mass of data that must be collected in the course of developing a standard.

UTILITY IN RISK MANAGEMENT

This representation of risks shows uncertainty explicitly and has the potential to be used in risk management under the constraints imposed by the Vinyl Chloride decision. To do so, one must also be able to represent risk criteria on the diagram. As indicated earlier, three of the four decision alternatives presented in the benzene proposal can be so plotted, but it is not clear that any of them captures either historical precedent for risk management or fundamental principles about how individuals and society make risk decisions.

Travis *et al.*[6] analyzed 132 regulatory decisions by various federal government agencies under several statutory authorities and found considerable historical support for individual risk criteria in the range between 10^{-6} and 10^{-3}, although some decisions have declined to regulate higher risks, based in part on the level of the associated population risk. Travis *et al.* show a region of risk acceptability included between two boundaries. Above the higher boundary, risks are virtually never accepted without some sort of regulatory action, whereas below the lower boundary they are considered *de minimis* and are virtually always accepted. Between the boundaries, a risk management decision depends on other factors, such as cost and feasibility of exposure reductions. Figure 3 presents a variation of their display to fit the scales used here. The two regions labeled "impossible" are for populations greater than 250 million (lower right) or smaller than 1 (upper left). Few data points are available for the left side of the figure.

A region of risk acceptability is clearly appropriate in risk management under balancing-type statutes, in which consideration of cost and feasibility can be used to determine where in the region the standard should be set. For decisions about hazardous air pollutants under the Vinyl Chloride interpretation of Section 112, however, a sharper criterion of safety is being considered by EPA for the first-stage decision. This criterion, if adopted, likely would fall somewhere in the region shown by Travis *et al.*[6]

Because some emphasis in risk management has been placed on "natural" criteria such as one in a million, the boundaries shown by Travis *et al.*[6] show sharp breaks in slope. Although it can be argued that these breaks represent some valid choices, the available data do not support them strongly. What does seem clear is that higher individual risks can be accepted when the population risk is small and vice versa. (Stated differently, higher individual risks can be accepted, within limits, if the number of people exposed is small.) The simplest representation of this tradeoff is a linear risk criterion band. A band is proposed rather than a sharp line only to indicate that the location of the criterion is not well known and may vary depending on the type of risk being managed.

The placement, shape, slope, and width of this criterion band are choices ultimately to be made by duly appointed risk managers responsible for the protection of the public health. Nevertheless, we propose a band consistent with historical precedent and with arguments based on fundamental principles.

If the risk criterion band is presented along with the array of risk estimates proposed earlier, a better risk management decision will be possible, as shown in the next three

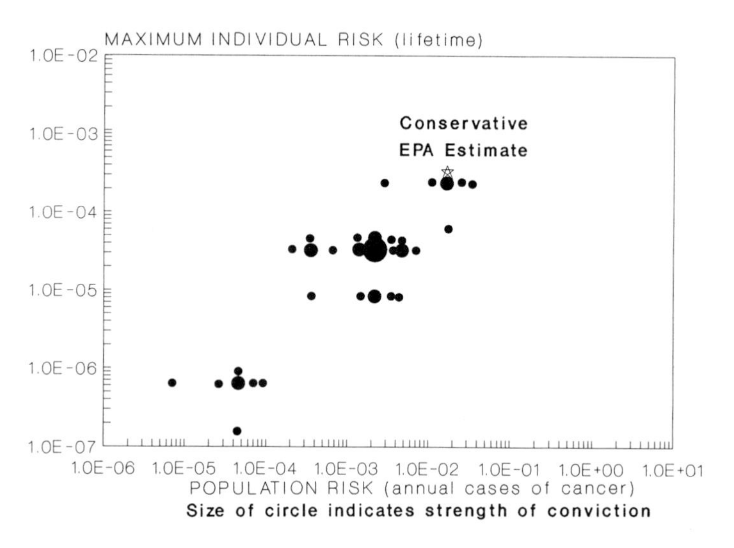

Fig. 2. Display of various estimates of risk for a hypothetical chemical. Circles represent different combinations of cancer potency factor, MEI exposure, average exposure for the population, and size of the population at risk. Size of circle indicates probability that the estimate is most nearly correct.

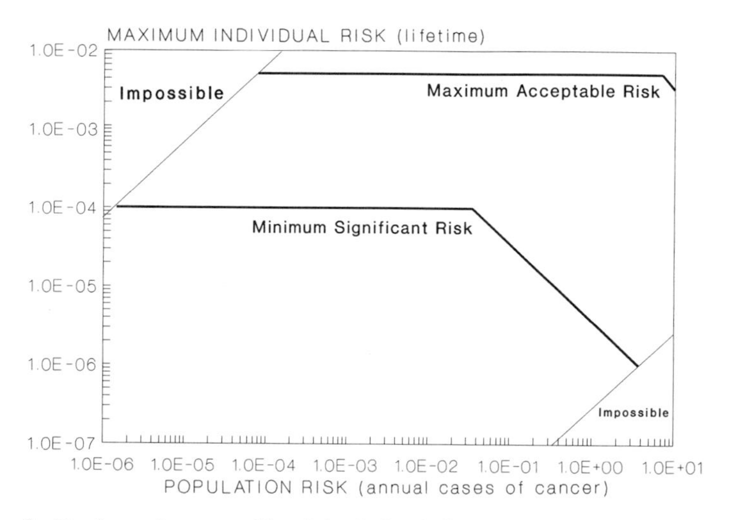

Fig. 3. Region of acceptable risk derived from precedents in federal regulatory decisions. Adapted from Travis *et al.*[6]

figures. Figure 4 shows a situation in which not only the conservative EPA estimate of risks but also the bulk of all risk estimates is above the risk criterion band. In the case of this hypothetical chemical, the risk profile suggests the need for reductions in risk through controls on emissions. In Vinyl Chloride terms, the situation would likely be judged unsafe in the first-stage decision.

Figure 5 shows another hypothetical situation, in which the bulk of risk estimates falls well below the criterion band. Even the conservative EPA estimate does not exceed the criterion, and a reasonably confident decision can be made not to regulate the risks further.

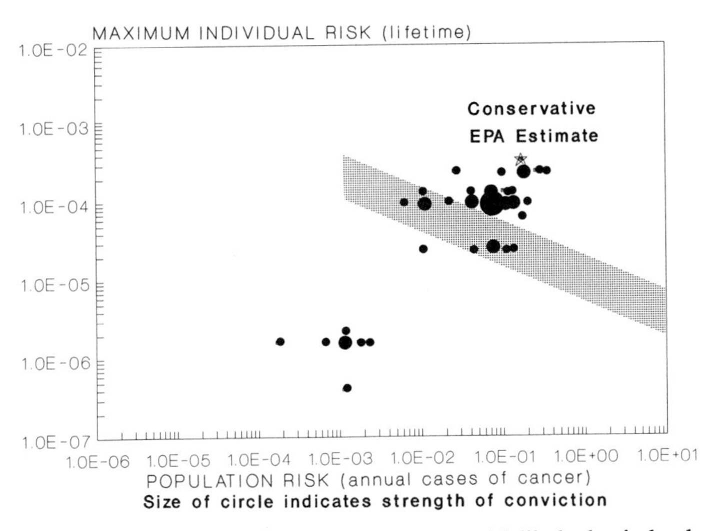

Fig. 4. Hypothetical situation in which risks would likely be judged unsafe under first-stage Vinyl Chloride decision process. Emissions likely should be reduced.

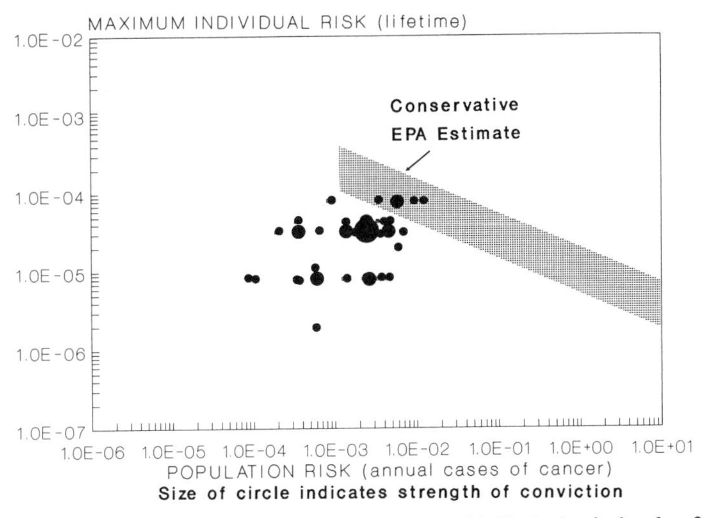

Fig. 5. Hypothetical situation in which risks would likely be judged safe under first-stage Vinyl Chloride decision process. Emissions would likely not need to be reduced.

Figure 6 shows the most interesting hypothesis—one that uses the data points from Fig. 2. Here the bulk of the risk estimates remain below the criterion band, but a few estimates, including the conservative EPA estimate, fall above the criterion. This situation can be interpreted in the following fashion under the two-phase Vinyl Chloride structure. First, the most likely risk estimate, shown by the largest circle, and its close neighbors would be used to define "safety" or "acceptable risk." In the situation shown, current exposures might be considered safe in the Vinyl Chloride sense. In the second stage, the EPA risk manager could examine the distribution of risk estimates above the criterion band and decide whether or not current exposures provide an adequate margin of safety, given the distribution of uncertainties and other factors, such as the cost, feasibility, and risk-reduction benefits of emission controls. For the fictitious data shown, current exposures

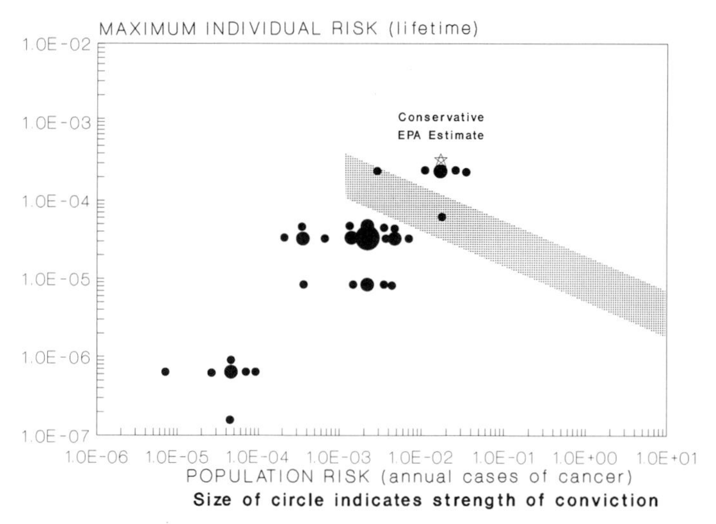

Fig. 6. Hypothetical situation in which risks would likely be judged safe under first-stage Vinyl Chloride decision process, but margin of safety might not be judged adequate under second-stage. Emissions may or may not need to be reduced.

might or might not be considered to provide an adequate margin of safety, depending on the degree of risk aversion the manager felt appropriate.

CONCLUSIONS

The graphical display of risk assessment and risk management information described in this paper is as yet incompletely defined, but it has considerable promise to utilize the available information about cancer risks more fully than is currently the case. Although developed with hazardous air pollutants in mind, it clearly could be used for standard setting not only under other health-based statutes but also for balancing statutes. The further definition of the risk criterion band is the responsibility of the risk managers. Furthermore, the details of producing the display of risk estimates deserve further development. The process described here, by using more of the available data in a comprehensible graphic format, would lead to a more considered control decision that would be easier to justify to all interested parties.

ACKNOWLEDGMENTS

The research leading to this paper was supported in part by the American Petroleum Institute but the conclusions do not necessarily represent API's views. Useful comments on earlier drafts were provided by Terry Yosie, Martha Beauchamp, Robert Strieter, Cosmo DiPerna, Arthur Sampson, and others connected with API's Benzene Issues Group. Mary Landers and Mark Corrales of ENVIRON Corporation conducted much of the research on which the paper was based.

REFERENCES

1. National Research Council, *Risk Assessment in the Federal Government: Managing the Process*, National Academy Press, Washington, DC (1983).
2. National Emissions Standards for Hazardous Air Pollutants, 42 USC 7412.

3. Natural Resources Defense Council vs. Environmental Protection Agency, 824 F. 2d 1146 (1987).
4. U.S. Environmental Protection Agency, National Emissions Standards for Hazardous Air Pollutants; Benzene Emissions from Maleic Anhydride Plants, Ethylbenzene/Styrene Plants, Benzene Storage Vessels, Benzene Equipment Leaks, and Coke By-Product Recovery Plants, Proposed Rule, 53 F.R. 28496-28592, July 28, 1988.
5. R. M. Putzrath and M. E. Ginevan, Effect of Meta-Analysis on the Risk Assessment of Trichloroethylene, Presentation at the 9th Annual Meeting of the American College of Toxicology, Baltimore, MD, October 31-November 2, 1988.
6. C. C. Travis, S. A. Richter, E. A. C. Crouch, R. Wilson, and E. D. Klema, Cancer Risk Management: A Review of 132 Federal Regulatory Decisions, *Environ. Sci. Technol.* **21**:415-420 (1987).

Comparing Human and Animal Cancer Risk Models Using Multistage Theory: Exponential vs. Relative vs. Additive Risk

Robert N. Brown, Carol Brignoli Gable, Linda K. Tollefson, Janet A. Springer, and Ronald J. Lorentzen
Food and Drug Administration
Washington, DC

ABSTRACT

Comparing human and animal cancer risk assessments often results in inconsistencies due to different extrapolation methodologies. Descriptive relative risk models using cumulative dose are typically used in human epidemiological studies, whereas multistage additive risk models using dose rate are typically used in high dose animal studies to extrapolate to human exposures. Biologically motivated nonclonal and clonal multistage risk models are reviewed for their unifying role in consistently comparing human and animal risks and for suggesting alternate cumulative dose epidemiological risk models.

KEYWORDS: Cancer risk, comparative risk, descriptive epidemiology, multistage theory, polynomial exponential

INTRODUCTION

Although animal studies are routinely used for setting upper bounds on human cancer risk, the most appropriate data comes directly from epidemiological cohort studies. However, problems inherent in these cohort studies, such as (1) confounding variables, (2) lack of statistical detection power, (3) difficulty in choosing proper control groups, and (4) uncertainties in the exposure histories, may limit their usefulness in risk assessments. To compensate for many of these problems and the scarcity of human data, continuous exposure lifetime animal experiments are conducted under controlled conditions at high dose to maximize the odds of observing tumors in small animal cohorts.

Several different mathematical models are potentially available to estimate excess risk from both animal and human data (IARC, 1987). With animal studies, linear-at-low-dose models such as the classical nonclonal multistage model are frequently fitted to observed tumor responses while the best estimate of excess risk or upper bound on excess risk is typically conservatively (linearly) extrapolated to lower dose levels corresponding to human exposure (Crump, 1981). Descriptive two-step linear-at-low-dose approaches similar to those of Gaylor and Kodell (1980) yield results comparable to the linearized multistage models, the primary potential differences being whether or how one chooses an upper confidence limit on observed incidence and at what dose one switches to a linear model for the extrapolation to lower doses.

Epidemiological practice in fitting intermittent or short term human exposure data and extrapolating excess risk to other low dose exposure scenarios is less well defined. Within the context of linear-at-low-dose extrapolation models, there are a variety of descriptive epidemiological models which yield different excess risks. For example, cumulative dose additive and multiplicative risk models may yield 2-4 fold variability in excess lifetime risks; in a theoretical analysis of generic exponential, relative, and additive risk models, Hoel (1985) implied even greater variability.

The purpose of this review is to relate the more common descriptive epidemiological models typically used with human studies to the more mechanistically-based multistage models typically used with animal studies and to suggest approaches leading to a more consistent comparison of human and animal risks.

Typical exposure patterns in human studies are quite different from animal studies. Failure to adjust risk models for such differences as age at initial exposure, duration of exposure, and followup time since last exposure will result in well-known biases when extrapolating risks to exposure scenarios different from those used to estimate model parameters (Chen, Kodell, Gaylor, 1988; Kodell, Gaylor, Chen, 1987; Hoel, 1985). These biases will not be considered here. However, to avoid such biases and to clarify the interrelationships between descriptive and mechanistic risk models, models will be compared under the assumption of constant continuous exposure.

MULTISTAGE THEORY

Multistage theory has been the basis for development of both the classical k-stage nonclonal (cell transition or mutation) multistage models and the two-stage clonal (cell mutation and cell growth) multistage models (Armitage and Doll, 1957; Whittemore and Keller, 1978, Moolgavkar, Venzon, Knudsen 1979, 1981; Thorslund, 1987). Information on stages of carcinogenesis, age-specific incidence, short-term exposure, competing mortality, and sex and species differences can be handled conveniently within the framework of multistage theory (Day and Brown, 1980; Crump and Howe, 1984; Brown and Chu, 1983a, 1983b; Chen, Kodell, Gaylor, 1988).

The classical nonclonal multistage model attempts to describe the carcinogenic process as a series of simple somatic cell mutations (transitions) leading to a single malignant cell; however, its growth into a lethal tumor is not explicitly modeled. Nevertheless, this model predicts the log-log age-specific incidence apparently observed for many epithelial tumors in man (Hoel, 1985; Peto, 1977) which appear to follow relatively high kth powers of time t (frequently $k > 5$).

Armitage and Doll (1957) proposed a generalized two-stage model of carcinogenesis based on the assumption of stem cell transformation into an exponentially growing premalignant cell clone which may eventually transform into a single tumor cell. This clonal model accounts for exponential proliferation of preneoplastic cells and predicts tumor incidences that rise steeply with age without requiring the extra high powers of time needed to fit the nonclonal model.

More recently Moolgavkar, Venzon and Knudson (1979,1981) have proposed an even more general two-stage model that predicts cancer incidence to be a function of cell birth and death rates rather than just net cell growth rates. With this model, Moolgavkar is able to describe adult or epithelial tumor rates when model parameters are assumed time-independent and also childhood and hormonally influenced cancer rates when parameters are time-dependent (Moolgavkar, 1983).

Multistage models are nonlinear models and can be computationally unstable for curvilinear incidence data. Other significant uncertainties affecting their use in risk assessment include lack of knowledge of the biological mechanism of toxicity and difficulty of measuring biological parameters. Therefore, scientific prudence and consistency in the protection of public health would seem to require extra care in the conservative implementation of the corresponding risk estimates (e.g., by guaranteeing low dose linearity).

In any case, this paper uses classical k-stage nonclonal and 2-stage clonal multistage theory to better organize and express various formulae for age-specific incidence in both cumulative dose and dose rate forms. These multistage based models will be compared with common descriptive epidemiological models, which are reviewed below.

DESCRIPTIVE EPIDEMIOLOGICAL RISK MODELS

Descriptive linear-at-low-dose epidemiological risk models are not based upon mechanistic biological theory. There are four generic types of descriptive risk models in common use. Following Hoel (1985), the age-specific incidence or hazard function $\lambda(t,z)$ for an individual at age t is typically written as a regression equation in terms of one or more explanatory variables. By assumption, the explanatory variables z are restricted to exposure, written either in dose rate form, d_r, or, more typically, in cumulative dose form, d_c. These formulations fall under the general description of additive (absolute) risk models, relative (multiplicative) risk models, exponential (multiplicative) risk models, and general nonlinear risk models. The generic formulation of the first three descriptive models is

$$\begin{aligned} &(a)\ \lambda(t,z) = \lambda_0(t)+\beta z \\ &(b)\ \lambda(t,z) = \lambda_0(t)+(1+\beta z) \\ &(c)\ \lambda(t,z) = \lambda_0(t)e^{\beta z} \end{aligned} \qquad (1)$$

where $\lambda_0(t)$ is the background incidence rate and β is a regression parameter for the exposure covariate z. Examples of these models are described by Breslow and Day (IARC, 1987).

An example of the general non-linear model is the two-stage MVK model with time-dependent model parameters. Such a model cannot be linearized by simple approximations or transformations of variables.

MULTISTAGE RISK MODELS

Of the two basic types of multistage model in common usage, the k-stage nonclonal model includes only a cell transition (mutation) rate from one stage to the next stage. The clonal model, currently restricted to 2 stages, adds a cell growth (proliferation) rate factor to the first stage. Attention will be limited to the case where both mutation and proliferation rates are time independent.

Nonclonal Model

Nonclonal models can be written in either relative or additive risk form, using either the dose rate or cumulative dose metric ($d_c=d_rt$).

Additive Risk Formulation

If at most two mutation or transition rates are dose related to the carcinogen, age-specific tumor incidence $\lambda(t,z)$ can be expressed as

$$\begin{aligned}\lambda &\cong q_0 t^{k-1} + q_1 d_r t^{k-1} + q_2 d_r^2 t^{k-1} \\ &= q_0 t + q_1 d_r t + q_2 d_r^2 t \quad (k=2)\end{aligned}$$

$$\text{[Additive Risk } (d_r)\text{]} \qquad (2a)$$

or as

$$\begin{aligned}\lambda &\cong q_0 t^{k-1} + q_1 d_c t^{k-2} + q_2 d_c^2 t^{k-3} \\ &= q_0 t + q_1 d_c + q_2 \frac{d_c^2}{t} \quad (k=2)\end{aligned}$$

$$\text{[Additive Risk } (d_c)\text{]} \qquad (2b)$$

where $q_0(t)^{k-1}$ is the background age-specific incidence. It is clear that the first two terms of the multistage model can be regrouped into the form of the descriptive additive risk model (1a), $\lambda(t) = \lambda_0(t) + \beta z$, but only when there are precisely two stages and one of those transitional rates is not dose related (q_2=0). In this case, however, the background rate is $q_0 t$ and yields a poor approximation to age-specific background tumor rates that increase faster than the first power of time.

While multistage theory (2a) implies that excess risk follows a functional form parallel to background risk (dose rate metric), both terms of which are proportional to t^{k-1}, no such parallel linkage is commonly assumed by users of the descriptive additive model—an apparent deficiency of most descriptive additive risk models.

Relative Risk Formulation

In relative risk form, multistage incidence can be given as:

$$\begin{aligned}\lambda &= q_0 t^{k-1}\left(1 + \frac{q_1}{q_0} d_r + \frac{q_2}{q_0} d_r^2\right) \\ &= q_0 t\left(1 + \frac{q_1}{q_0} d_r + \frac{q_2}{q_0} d_r^2\right) \quad (k=2)\end{aligned}$$

$$\text{[Relative Risk } (d_r)\text{]} \qquad (2c)$$

or

$$\begin{aligned}&= q_0 t^{k-1}\left(1 + \frac{q_1}{q_0}\frac{d_c}{t} + \frac{q_2}{q_0}\frac{d_c^2}{t^2}\right) \\ &= q_0 t\left(1 + \frac{q_1}{q_0}\frac{d_c}{t} + \frac{q_2}{q_0}\frac{d_c^2}{t^2}\right) \quad (k=2)\end{aligned}$$

$$\text{[Relative Risk } (d_c)\text{]} \qquad (2d)$$

where the leading factor $q_0 t^{k-1}$ is the background tumor rate and the long expression within parentheses is the standard mortality ratio (SMR) divided by 100. Note that multistage excess incidence (2c) parallels background incidence (dose rate metric), whereas the descriptive relative risk excess incidence (1b) follows a higher power of time than does background incidence. If the descriptive relative risk model is generalized to include higher order powers of cumulative dose, then the discrepancy in functional form between excess and background incidence grows worse. The first observation has been partially noted by Hoel (1985). Although the descriptive relative risk model assumes an incidence linkage not necessarily provided by the descriptive additive risk model, still these discrepancies between excess and background incidence are clearly inconsistent with multistage theory and suggests a potential theoretical defect in the descriptive relative risk approach.

In other words, multistage theory (2d) implies that the powers of time in the excess risk component must decrease inversely with increasing powers of cumulative dose — something seldom, if ever, assumed by descriptive relative risk models.

The standard mortality ratio (SMR) of the nonclonal multistage SMR is constant for a given dose (dose rate metric), whereas that for the descriptive relative risk model increases linearly throughout life. While some observable SMRs may increase early in life, they don't appear to increase forever. Such variability in SMRs appears to be handled better by multistage theory than by descriptive relative risk models; similar discrepancies exist for fractional lifetime exposures where multistage SMR's tend to decline after exposure stops but descriptive relative risk SMRs typically plateau (Hoel, 1985).

In contrast to the additive multistage model, there appear to be no conditions under which the k-stage nonclonal cumulative dose multistage model (2d) reduces to the corresponding generic descriptive relative risk model (1b) (see C. Brown *et al.*, 1983a,1983b, for attempts).

Two-Stage Clonal Multistage Model

The two-stage MVK clonal multistage (CMS) model with time-independent parameters can be expressed as:

$$\lambda = C_0 M_0 M_1 (e^{Gt}-1)/G \tag{3a}$$

where C_0 represents the number of zero stage cells susceptible to the cancer transformation process, M_0 and M_1 represent the zero and first stage cellular transformation or mutation rates to the next stage, and G represents the first stage cellular growth or proliferation rate.

The number of susceptible cells, the cell mutation rate and the cell proliferation rate parameters can be modeled as a spontaneous background value plus possible dose rate related linear increases over background. Thus $C_0 = C_{00}+d_rC_{01}$, $M_0 = M_{00}+M_{01}d_r$, $M_1 = M_{10}+M_{11}d_r$ and $G = G_0+G_1d_r$. For simplicity of exposition, we shall assume that C_0=1 and is not dose related. Letting $q_0 = M_{00}M_{10}$, $q_1 = (M_{00}M_{11}+M_{01}M_{10})$, and $q_2 = (M_{01}M_{11})$, $\lambda(t)$ can be reexpressed as

$$\lambda = (q_0+q_1d_r+q_2d_r^2)(e^{Gt}-1)/G, \tag{3b}$$

or, through a Taylor series expansion, as:

$$\lambda = (q+q_1d_r+q_2d_r^2)t(1+Gt/2+G^2t^2/6+...). \tag{3c}$$

Inspection of the infinite series expansion of the altered exponential factor suggests that

$$te^{(G/2)t} < (e^{Gt}-1)/G < te^{Gt}, \tag{3d}$$

and if time t is expressed in fractional units of the median lifespan, then $G >> 1$ typically (Armitage, 1957). Indeed, since the number of cell doublings in a lifetime (G/ln2) is usually considered to be much greater than 1, a value for G>>1 would appear to be highly likely. Unfortunately, these bounds are not very tight. The lower approximation is relatively precise only when $Gt << 1$.

If we attempt to approximate the altered exponential factor more precisely by a simpler exponential factor, such as $te^{G^* t}$, then it can be shown that at median lifespan (t=1), $G^* = G - \ln G$ would appear to yield a crude but potentially useful approximation to the altered exponential. Using this approximation G^* for the cellular proliferation rate G and assuming that $G^* = G_0^* + G_1^* d_r$ can also be dose related as a background rate plus linear increase, $\lambda(t)$ in (3b) can be expressed as

$$\lambda \cong \left(q_0 + q_1 d_r + q_2 d_r^2\right) te^{G^* t} \tag{3e}$$

$$= \left(q_0 te^{G_0^* t}\right)\left(e^{G_1^* d_r t}\right)\left(1 + \frac{q_1}{q_0} d_r + \frac{q_2}{q_0} d_r^2\right)$$

[Approx. CMS Exp. Relative Risk $(d_r, k = 2)$] (3f)

or as

$$\lambda \cong \left(q_0 te^{G_0^* t}\right)\left(e^{G_1^* d_c}\right)\left(1 + \frac{q_1}{q_0}\frac{d_c}{t} + \frac{q_2}{q_0}\frac{d_c^2}{t^2}\right)$$

[Approx. CMS Exp. Relative Risk $(d_c, k = 2)$] (3g)

Theoretically, it seems clear that the 2-stage clonal model or approximations, with an exponential growth factor, has greater flexibility than a given k-stage nonclonal model to fit background or excess age-specific incidences. Background tumor incidences for most tumors do not appear to follow a simple power of time throughout life—as required by nonclonal models. For example, U.S. mortality statistics indicate age-specific leukemia incidence increases from apparent constant or linear rates in youth to cubic or higher rates in old age. Indeed, the 2-stage clonal model may explain Doll's need for high exponents of time (range of 1-10, mean about 5) to fit background human tumor rates—the high exponents probably reflect exponential cell growth rates (Doll, 1971; Whittemore, 1977; Moolgavkar, 1983). Furthermore, this flexibility extends to the description of excess risks and SMRs. For example, clonal SMRs, contrary to nonclonal SMRs, increase in early life (3f,3g), subsuming one of the strengths of descriptive relative risk models, while allowing for eventual decrease if exposure stops—one of the weaknesses of the descriptive relative risk model.

Special Cases of the 2-Stage Clonal Model

Mutation rates not dose related. If background incidence $\lambda_0(t) = q_0 te^{G_0^* t}$, $\beta = G_1^*$, $z = d_c$ and M_0, M_1 are not dose related ($q_1 = q_2 = 0$), incidence (3g) reduces to a form of the descriptive multiplicative exponential risk model (1c), namely

$$\lambda(t) = \lambda_0(t)e^{\beta z} = \left(q_0 te^{G_0^* t}\right)e^{\beta d_c}$$

[Exponential Risk (d_c)]

Cell proliferation rate is zero. If $G^* = 0$, $\lambda_0 = q_0 t$, $\beta = q_1/q_0$, and $z = d_c$, then incidence reduces to the classical 2-stage nonclonal model; and if only one mutational stage is dose related ($q_2 = 0$), incidence reduces to a special case of the descriptive additive risk model (1a).

Both mutation rates, but not growth rate, are dose related. In this case ($G_0^* \neq 0$, $G_1^* = 0$) incidence is given by

$$\lambda = \left(q_0 t e^{G_0^* t}\right)\left(1 + \frac{q_1}{q_0}\frac{d_c}{t} + \frac{q_2}{q_0}\frac{d_c^2}{t^2}\right)$$

$$\text{[CMS Relative Risk } (d_c, k = 2)] \qquad (3h)$$

$$= \left(q_0 t e^{G_0^* t}\right) + q_1 d_c\left(e^{G_0^* t}\right) + \left(q_2 \frac{d_c^2}{t}\right)\left(e^{G_0^* t}\right)$$

$$\text{[CMS Additive Risk } (d_c, k = 2)] \qquad (3i)$$

with $q_2 = 0$ if one mutation rate is dose related (i.e., under the assumption that each transition rate is restricted to a linear dose relation).

Expressions (3h,3i) can be thought of as clonal generalizations of the classical 2-stage nonclonal cumulative dose model with an exponential time factor added to account for more rapid growth in both the background and excess rates. In addition, it would appear that the more general form (3g) of the 2-stage clonal model yields a new cumulative dose epidemiological risk model that combines the descriptive exponential model with the k=2 nonclonal multistage risk model. Of course (3g) can also be rewritten in its equivalent dose rate and/or additive form. Breslow and Day (IARC, 1987; pp. 136,160,173,183) reference somewhat similar generalized descriptive risk models: (1) multiplicative model, $\lambda = (e^{\alpha_j})(e^{x_{jk}\beta})$; (2) additive relative risk model, $\lambda = (e^{\alpha_j})(1+x_{jk}\beta)$; (3) excess risk model, $\lambda = \lambda_j^* + e^{(\alpha + x_k \beta)}$; (4) and generalized multiplicative exponential risk model, $\lambda = x_1(t)\, \beta_1 e^{y_1(t)\gamma_1} + x_2(t)\, \beta_2 e^{y_2(t)\gamma_2} + \ldots$; where indices j and k refer to time and dose subgroups. However, these models lack either the necessary generality or the mathematical economy of the multistage model and their parameters lack clear mechanistic interpretation.

DISCUSSION

Relationships between dose rate forms of multistage risk models frequently used in animal studies and cumulative dose forms of descriptive models frequently used in human studies have been reviewed in the context of constant continuous exposure and common dose measure (dose rate and cumulative dose). Such context helps minimize confusion over the source of theoretical and computational differences or inconsistencies between the two modeling approaches. Multistage theory as well as specific multistage models or approximations explicitly assumes that excess tumor incidence is a functional perturbation of background incidence and offers a reasonable way to explain, reject or improve upon most descriptive cumulative dose epidemiological risk models. To encourage greater use of consistent risk models for interspecies comparison and extrapolation, several cumulative dose formulations of special cases of multistage risk models or their approximations have been presented for consideration.

Although not pursued herein, simplifications of the 2-stage clonal risk model generalizing common descriptive additive and exponential models may be useful in providing more plausible maximum and minimum upper bounds on extrapolated low dose risks—apparently wider bounds than provided solely by the common descriptive additive and relative risk models alone. However, bounding clonal multistage models by submodels and determining which submodel is more conservative than another may be complicated by the suggestion that the relative magnitudes of excess risk for descriptive additive and exponential models appears to reverse as age increases (Hoel, 1985).

It is particularly noteworthy that the generic descriptive relative risk model (1b) does not appear to be derivable as a special case of the 2-stage clonal model or k-stage nonclonal model and thus may be inconsistent with multistage cancer theory altogether.

In summary, there is a correspondence between some descriptive risk models (e.g., generic additive model and generic exponential model) and the simplest submodels of biologically motivated multistage models. Other descriptive models appear to be less consistent with multistage theory and difficult or impossible to approximate by any multistage submodel (e.g., generic relative risk model). The use of multistage theory and models to interpret, reject or generalize common descriptive epidemiological risk models should encourage the application of more consistent yet biologically defensible risk models to interspecies extrapolation and comparison—especially as the experimental data base allowing such comparisons steadily increases. Hopefully, increasing use of more consistent cross-species risk extrapolation models, such as is possible within the unifying context of multistage theory, should encourage risk assessors to focus increasingly on other, potentially larger sources of human/animal risk uncertainty.

REFERENCES

Armitage, P., and Doll, R., 1957, A Two-Stage Theory of Carcinogenesis in Relation to the Age Distribution of Human Cancer, *British Journal of Cancer* **11**:161-169.

Brown, C. C., and Chu, K. C., 1983a, Implications of the Multistage Theory of Carcinogenesis Applied to Occupational Arsenic Exposure, *J. National Cancer Institute* **70**:455-463.

Brown, C. C., and Chu, K. C., 1983b, A New Method for the Analysis of Cohort Studies: Implications of the Multistage Theory of Carcinogenesis Applied to Occupational Arsenic Exposure, *Environmental Health Perspectives* **50**:293-308.

Chen, J. J., Kodell, R. L., and Gaylor, D. W., 1988, Using the Biological Two-Stage Model to Assess Risk from Short-Term Exposures, *Risk Analysis* **8**:223-230.

Crump, K. S., 1981, An Improved Procedure for Low-Dose Carcinogenic Risk Assessment from Animal Data, *J. Environ. Pathol. Toxicol.* **5**:675-684.

Crump, K. S., and Howe, R. B., 1984, The Multistage Model with a Time-Dependent Dose Pattern: Applications to Carcinogenic Risk Assessment, *Risk Analysis* **4**:163-176.

Day, N. E., and Brown, C. C., 1980, Multistage Models and Primary Prevention of Cancer, *Journal of the National Cancer Institute* **64**:977-989.

Doll, R., 1971, The Age Distribution of Cancer: Implications for Models of Carcinogenesis, *J. Royal Statistical Society* **134**:133-166.

Gaylor, D. W., and Kodell, R. L., 1980, Linear Interpolation Algorithm For Low Dose Risk Assessment Of Toxic Substances, *Journal of Environmental Pathology and Toxicology* **4**:305-312.

Hoel, D. G., 1985, The Impact of Occupational Exposure Patterns on Quantitative Risk Estimation, *Risk Quantification and Regulatory Policy, Banbury Report 19.*

IARC, 1987, *Statistical Methods in Cancer Research, Vol. II: The Design and Analysis of Cohort Studies*, International Agency For Research On Cancer, N. E. Breslow and N. E. Day, eds., IARC Scientific Publications No. 82, distributed in the U.S. by Oxford University Press.

Kodell, R. L., Gaylor, D. W., and Chen, J. J., 1987, Consequences of Using Average Lifetime Dose Rate to Predict Risk from Intermittent Exposures to Carcinogens, *Risk Analysis* **7**:339-345.

Moolgavkar, S. H., and Venzon, D. J., 1979, Two-Event Models for Carcinogenesis: Incidence Curves for Childhood and Adult Tumors, *Mathematical Biosciences* **47**:55-77.

Moolgavkar, S. H., and Knudson, A. G., 1981, Mutation and Cancer: A Model for Human Carcinogenesis, *Journal of the National Cancer Institute* **66**:1037-1052.

Moolgavkar, S. H., 1983, Model for Human Carcinogenesis: Action of Environmental Agents, *Environmental Health Perspectives* **50**:285-291.
Peto, R., 1977, Epidemiology, Multistage Models, and Short-Term Mutagenicity Studies, in *Origins of Human Cancer*, H. H. Hiatt, J. D. Watson, and J. A. Winsten, eds., Cold Spring Harbor Laboratory, Cold Spring Harbor, New York.
Thorslund, T. W., Brown, C. C., and Charnley, G., 1987, The Use of Biologically Motivated Mathematical Models to Predict the Actual Cancer Risk Associated with Environmental Exposure to a Carcinogen, *Risk Analysis* **7**:109-119.
Whittemore, A. S., 1977, The Age Distribution of Human Cancer for Carcinogenic Exposures of Varying Intensity, *American J. Epidemiology* **106**.
Whittemore, A. S., and Keller, J. B., 1978, Quantitative Theories of Carcinogenesis, *SIAM Review* **20**:1-30.

Application of Ridge Regression and Principal Component Analysis to Specialty Glass Data for Encapsulation of Nuclear Waste

V. S. Arakali
West Valley Nuclear Services Co., Inc.
West Valley, NY

ABSTRACT

There are many instances where a large body of data is collected with the purpose of developing an empirical model of a multivariate process. Such a data set may not always lend itself to any robust statistical modeling of the process because of the uncertainties arising from synergic effects of multivariate process. The uncertainty of the models based on such a data set can be assessed by the application of ridge regression analysis. The data set transformed into an orthogonalized set by the application of principal component analysis provides a better base for developing a model for multivariate process. This paper presents the application of principal component analysis to orthogonalize a data set consisting of glass composition data and leach resistance data as its integrity index to contain nuclear waste. An empirical model relating integrity index and the variables derived from principal component analysis of glass composition data is shown to be better than that based on a raw nonorthogonalized data set. Ridge regression is used to study the nonorthogonality of the raw data set.

KEYWORDS: Ridge regression, principal component analysis, orthogonalization of data, statistical modeling, rank reduction

INTRODUCTION

Borosilicate glass is the reference waste form in the United States for the disposal of high-level nuclear wastes. The leach rate for radionuclides from the glass under conditions anticipated in a repository is one of the most important specifications for the waste form. The leaching characteristics of the waste form are dependent on several factors, but primarily the glass composition. To arrive at a suitable glass composition, specific to the nuclear wastes at West Valley, a series of glasses were prepared by varying several critical components and analyzing the glasses for their leaching behavior.

An empirical model based on the existing data relating glass composition and its leach resistance (a measure of its ability to retain waste in glass matrix) would be useful in predicting the leach resistance of a matrix of different composition. In the waste vitrification process, chemicals that make up the waste glass are measured. If a reliable

Risk Analysis, Edited by C. Zervos
Plenum Press, New York, 1991

model exists, the leach resistance of the glass can be predicted from its chemical makeup even before the glass is produced.

In recent years several sophisticated tools for the analysis of large data sets have been reported,[1] although multiple linear regression is one of the most widely used and understood techniques for model development in many fields of science and technology. In multiple regression, the estimate of regression coefficients is based on minimization of the residual sum of the squares. This estimation procedure is a good one provided the data vectors are orthogonal, that is, when the correlation matrix does not deviate from a unit matrix. The effects of nonorthogonality on the coefficient estimate, as explained by Hoerl,[2] can be determined by ridge trace method. If the data vectors are found to be nonorthogonal, the regression coefficient estimates are generally made by deleting the interfering vectors, thereby ignoring the correlation bond. A regrouping of the data vectors can be made to get a better estimate of the coefficients. Application of principal component analysis to orthogonalize the data set has the additional advantage that it reduces the dimensionality of the data set while retaining the variability as much as desired.

In this work, ridge trace method has been applied to the West Valley glass data base to determine the interfering variables which make the coefficients sensitive to the data set from which they are derived. Applying the principal component analysis technique, the data set is orthogonalized and a multiple linear regression model is developed. The prediction capability of the model with raw data and with orthogonalized data is compared.

THE MODEL

Systematic glass development work specific for West Valley nuclear waste is being conducted at the Catholic University of America and Battelle Pacific Northwest Laboratories in terms of specifying a compositional range for processability and durability. The data base[3] consisting of 40 glass types tested at the Vitreous State Laboratory of the Catholic University of America for West Valley vitrification process is used in this study. There are 32 variables representing weight percent of 32 oxides in the glass data. Ridge trace and multiple regression coefficients are estimated using 35 of the 40 glass types. Boron and lithium leach rate estimates are predicted for the remaining 5 glass types.

The standard model for multiple linear regression is

$$Y = XB + E \tag{1}$$

where X is an nxp matrix, E is an error matrix associated with the model, and B is an unknown regression coefficient vector determined for

$$B = X'Y/X'X\,. \tag{2}$$

If $X'X$ is not a unit matrix, the least square estimates are sensitive to the data set on which the coefficients are based. The dependence of B on the data set is analyzed, as explained in Ref. 2, by calculating the least square estimate based on the matrix whose diagonal elements are augmented with small positive values, $0 \leq k \leq 1$,

$$[X\,X' + kI] \tag{3}$$

as a function of the parameter k.

The ridge trace variation of the coefficient B as a function of k, identifying the sensitivity of the estimation to the glass data set, is calculated and shown in Figs. 1 through 3. It is observed from the figures that a slight variation in the data set is likely to give a different estimation for the coefficient. A model based on this data set is not likely to result in correct estimates for the leach rates. This is shown more clearly later when the predicted leach rates for the unknown glass types are compared with measured data.

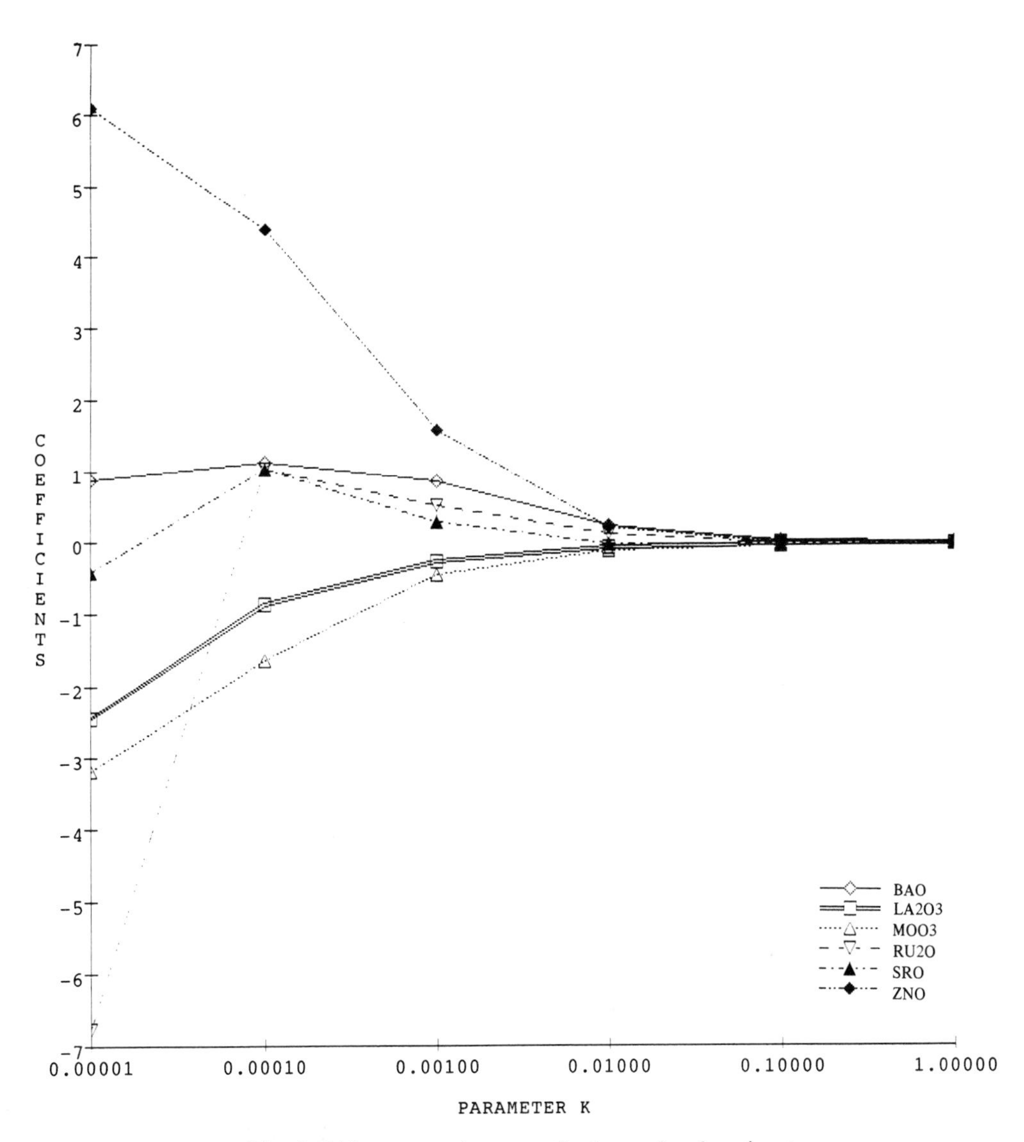

Fig. 1. Ridge regression trace for boron leach estimate.

Grouping the oxides (variables) having approximately positive and negative effects may result in better estimates. The other alternative is to orthogonalize the data set. The method of principal component analysis[4,5] is applied in this study to transform the data set and is shown to generally yield better predictions than the ridge analyses method.

The first step in principal component analysis is to determine a linear combination of oxides (variables) which captures the variability of each oxide in the data set by determining the eigenvectors of the data matrix. The first eigenvector represents a combination that captures the largest fraction of the variability. The second eigenvector captures the largest fraction of the remaining variability and so on. The eigenvector determination is continued until a desired fraction, for example, 95 percent of the total variability, is represented by the eigenvector set. In this study, from the data set consisting of 35 glass types and 32 variables, 7 principal components are extracted retaining more than 95 percent of the variability in the data set. The resulting data set has the advantage of having only 7 dimensions that are mutually orthogonal. The reduction of the dimensionality is very useful

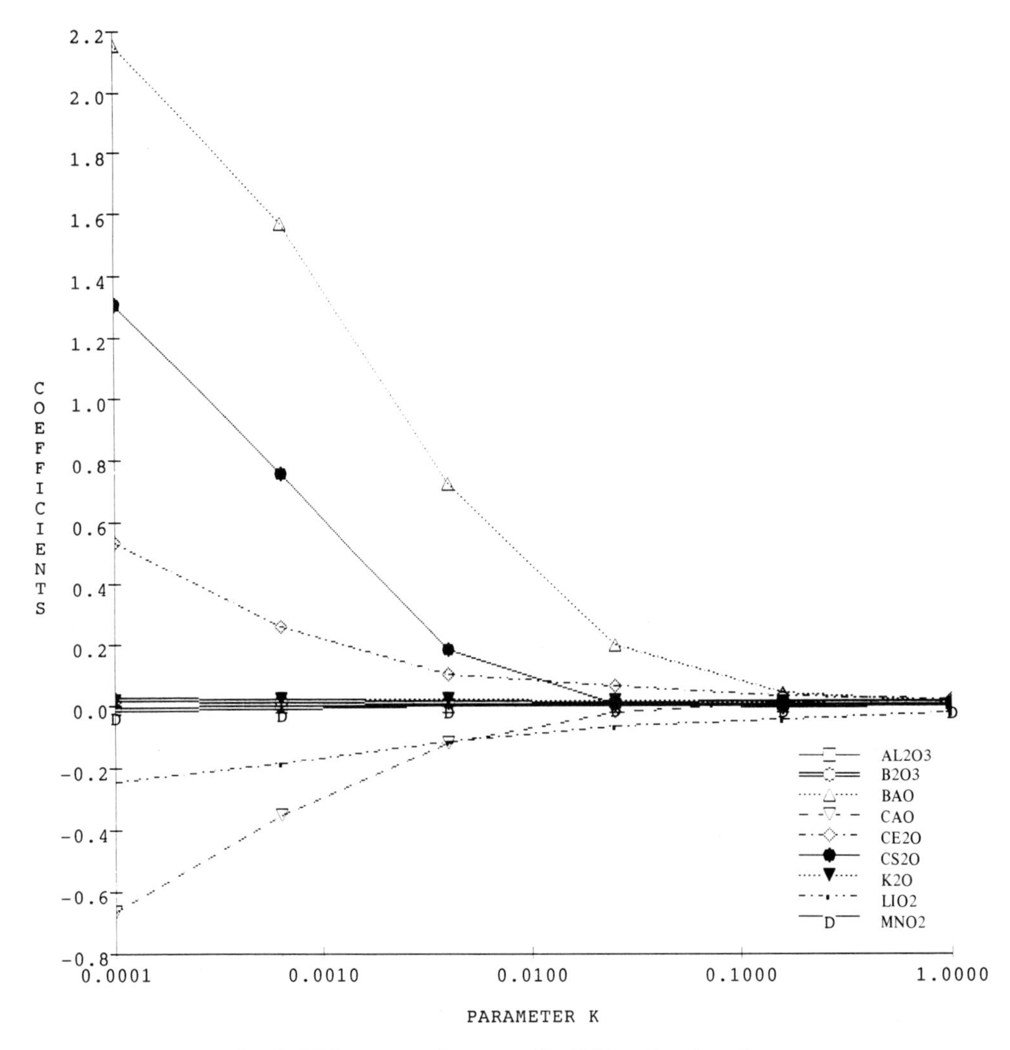

Fig. 2. Ridge regression trace for lithium leach estimate.

when dealing with a data set containing a large number of variables in that it reduces the computation time, especially if a nonlinear regression is needed. For example, a nonlinear regression analysis of the glass data with 32 variables could not be completed even after several hours using a Digital Vax 8200 processor with 12 megabytes of random access memory. But after reducing the variables to 7, it could be completed within a few minutes with the same computer. A new data matrix consisting of 7 variables for 35 glass types is calculated by multiplying the raw data by the eigenvectors. This transformed matrix is the basis for developing separate multiple regression models to estimate boron and lithium leach rates of the 5 glass types not included in determining the model coefficients.

The ridge trace of the transformed data set is, as expected, orthogonal and is shown in Figs. 4 and 5. The stability of the coefficients, with respect to small variations in the data set, is evident from the zero gradient of the ridge trace.

Multivariate regression coefficients to estimate boron and lithium are calculated for both the raw data set and the set obtained by principal component analysis for purpose of comparison and are shown in Tables 1 and 2. Using these regression coefficients, the leach

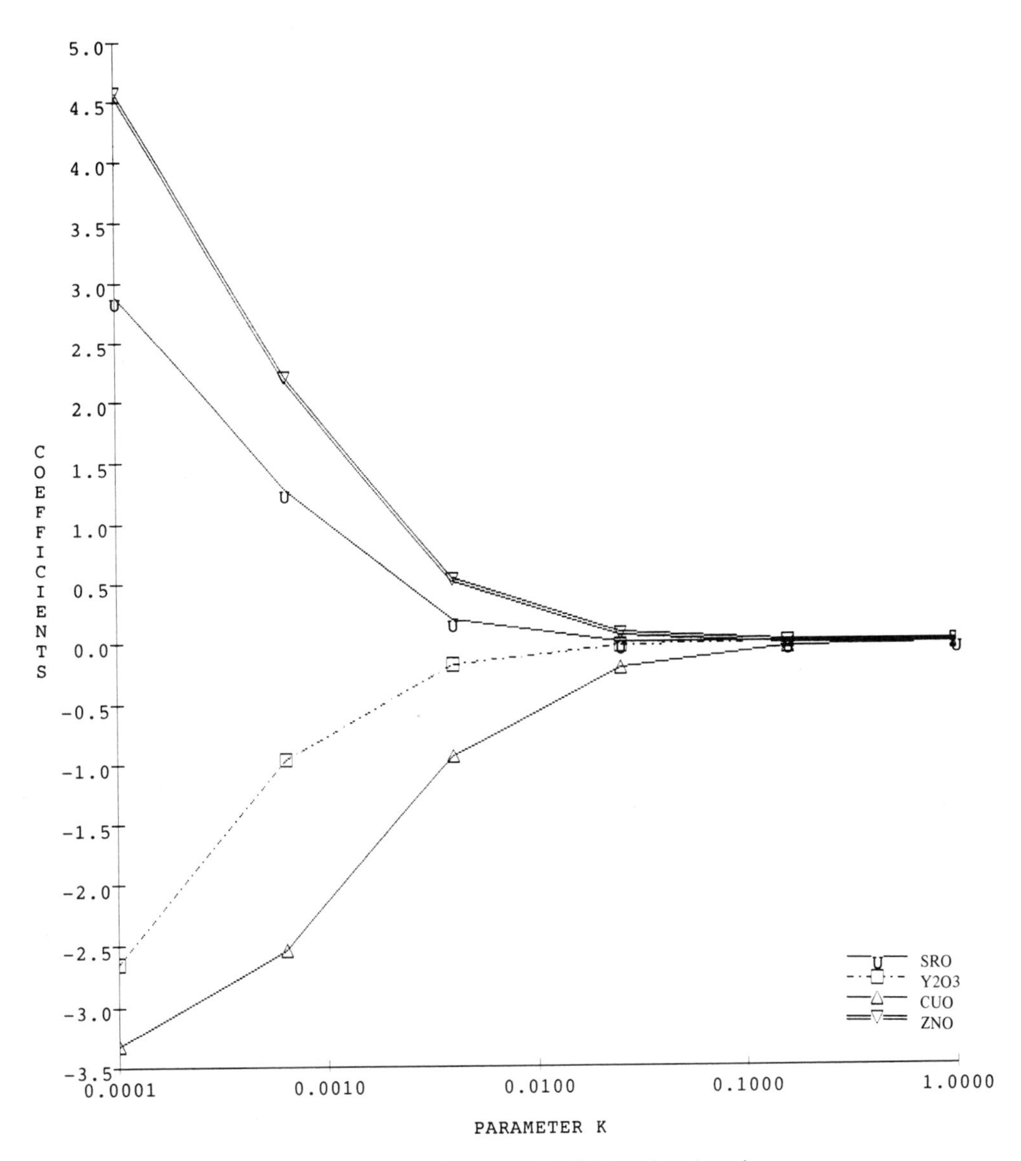

Fig. 3. Ridge regression trace for lithium leach estimate.

rate estimates of boron and lithium for 5 glass types external to the data set employed to determine the coefficients are compared with the model predictions and the measured values in Tables 3 and 4. The predictive capability of PCA transformed orthogonalized data set is clearly better than that based on raw data. Several theoretical and empirical models[6,7] have been developed and more effort is continuing to improve predictability of glass durability estimates. The leach data used in this analysis was developed to find the extremes of durability profile.

CONCLUSION

It is shown in this study that the calculation of ridge trace does provide insight into the interference effects of the variables in the data set. Multiple regression models based on such nonorthogonal data sets do not provide good results.

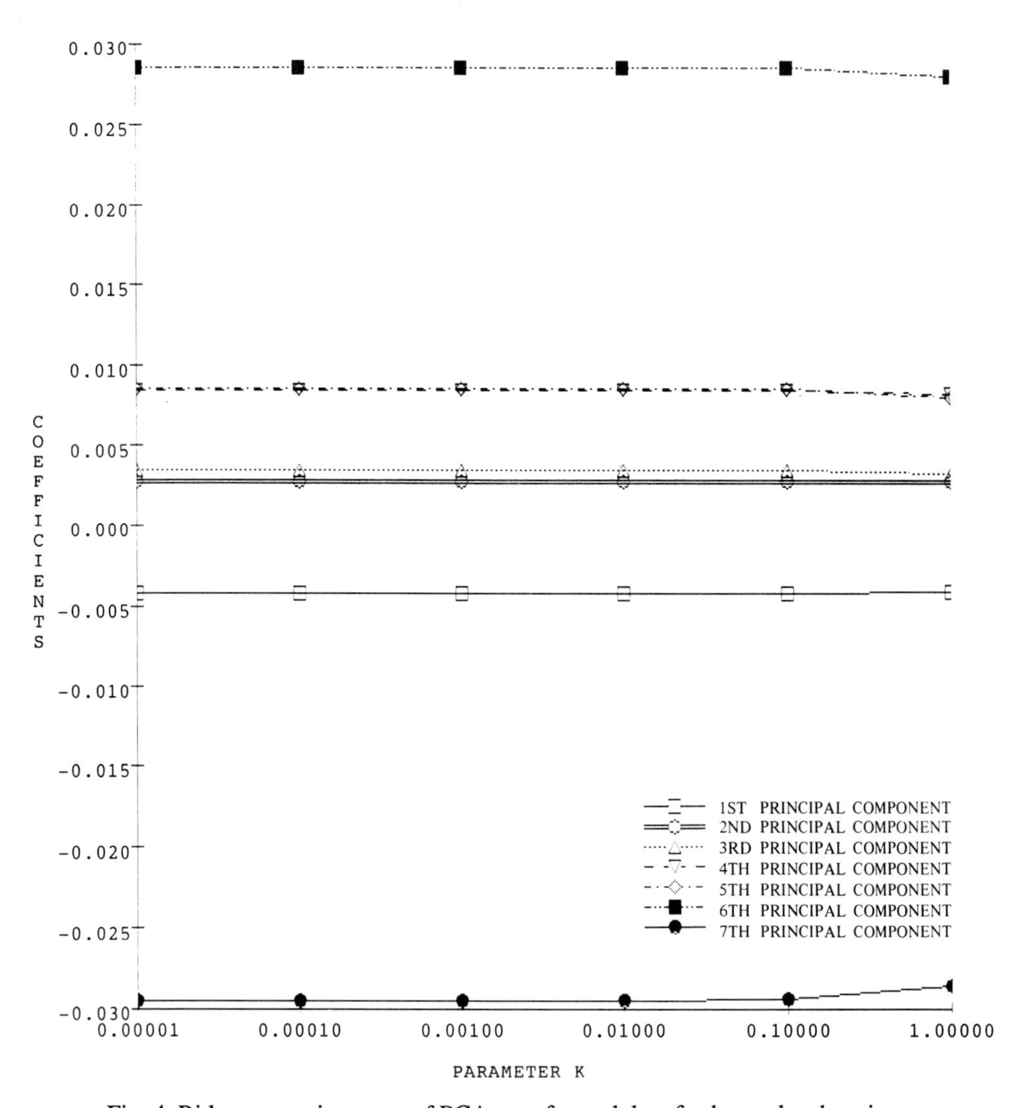

Fig. 4. Ridge regression trace of PCA transformed data for boron leach estimate.

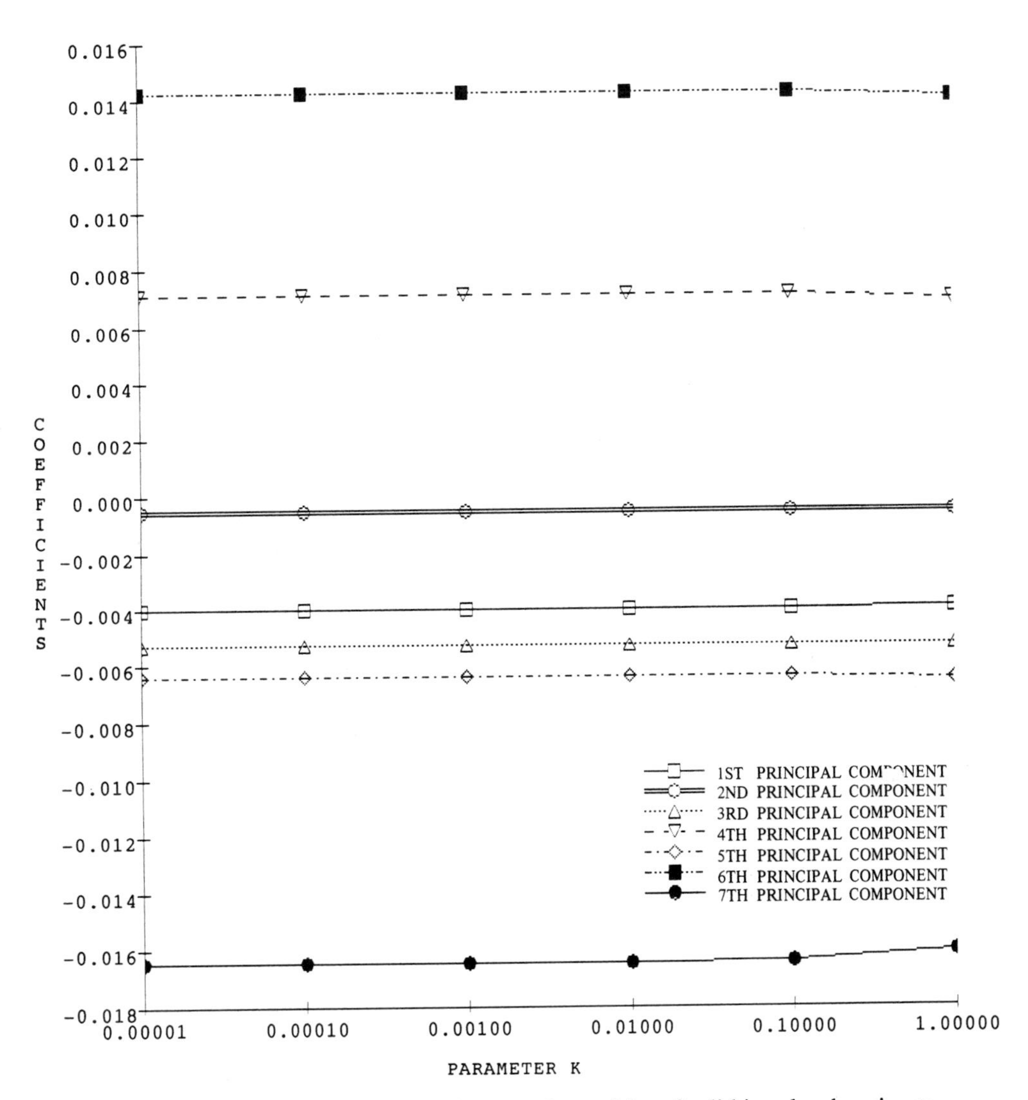

Fig. 5. Ridge regression trace of PCA transformed data for lithium leach estimate.

Table 1. Regression Coefficients for Boron and Lithium Leach Rate Estimate

0	1 Variables	2 Boron Coefficients	3 Lithium Coefficients
1	Al_2O_3	0.014621	–0.004201
2	B_2O_3	–0.034200	–0.026198
3	BaO	–5.435975	–3.026230
4	CaO	1.868396	0.331422
5	Ce_2O	–0.655844	–0.534866
6	Cr_2O_3	4.981633	1.098788
7	Cs_2O	–1.892818	–0.959909
8	Fe_2O_3	0.044729	0.037669
9	K_2O	0.112785	0.096800
10	La_2O_3	–0.002417	2.188380
11	LiO_2	0.526354	0.185589
12	MgO	–0.615132	0.488217
13	MnO_2	0.077356	0.050856
14	MoO_3	–13.286090	8.910022
15	Na_2O	–0.110743	–0.054633
16	Nd_2O_3	6.475422	1.169286
17	NiO	–0.885127	–0.591646
18	P_2O_5	0.066390	0.014295
19	Pd_2O	803.478512	1520.004090
20	Pr_6O_{11}	15.236279	–1.857649
21	RuO_2	–104.449074	–190.553847
22	SiO_2	–0.021216	–0.001706
23	Sm_2O_3	33.017843	67.350806
24	So_3	–6.843444	–5.236436
25	SrO	–19.704778	–8.264869
26	ThO_2	0.020880	–0.029462
27	TiO_2	1.213825	–0.407809
28	UO_2	–0.046665	–0.017693
29	Y_2O_3	–23.799456	–23.201117
30	ZrO_2	–0.537964	0.134303
31	CuO	7.457916	4.764255
32	ZnO	–4.692749	11.776724

Table 2. PCA Based Regression Coefficients for Boron and Lithium Leach Estimate

0	1 Variables	2 Boron Coefficients	3 Lithium Coefficients
1	Component 1	–0.004034	–0.004183
2	Component 2	–0.000525	0.002788
3	Component 3	–0.005298	0.003493
4	Component 4	0.007104	0.008475
5	Component 5	–0.006424	0.008577
6	Component 6	0.014218	0.028544
7	Component 7	–0.016496	–0.029501
8			
9	Maximum VIF	1.000000	1.000000
10	Error SS	0.199281	0.141220

Table 3. Boron Leach Rate Estimation Comparison

0	Glass Type	1 Regression of Raw Data	2 Regression of PCA Transformed Data	3 Measured Data
1	WV28B	–0.07	0.24	0.23
2	WV29	–0.09	0.28	0.21
3	WV29B	0.11	0.28	0.29
4	WV30	0.36	0.26	0.20
5	WV30B	0.59	0.26	0.27

Table 4. Lithium Leach Rate Estimation Comparison

0	Glass Type	1 Regression of Raw Data	2 Regression of PCA Transformed Data	3 Measured Data
1	WV28B	0.44	0.32	0.40
2	WV29	0.02	0.34	0.26
3	WV29B	0.16	0.28	0.35
4	WV30	0.50	0.34	0.28
5	WV30B	–0.14	0.34	0.28

If the interference effects are significant and numerous, application of principal component analysis is a good method for orthogonalization of a correlated data set and for developing the predictive models based on the transformed data set. The ability to reduce the dimensionality and still retain the desired amount of variability in the data set is particularly advantageous in reducing the computational time.

REFERENCES

1. M. A. Sharaf, D. L. Illman, and B. R. Kowalski, *Chemometrics*, Wiley, New York (1986).
2. A. E. Hoerl and R. W. Kennard, Ridge Regression: Biased Estimation for Nonorthogonal Problems, *Technometrics* **12**:1 (1970).
3. J. R. Carrell, Report on West Valley Compositional Variability Glasses, WVST 88-024, Battelle, Pacific Northwest Laboratories, Richland, Washington.
4. S. Wold, M. Sjostorm, R. Carlson, T. Lundsted, S. Hellberg, B. Skagerberg, C. Wikstorm, and J. Ohman, Multivariate Design, *Analytical Chemical Acta* **191**:17-22 (1986).
5. D. Veltkamp, B. Wise, B. Davis, L. Ricker, and B. R. Kowalski, Progress Report on Process Control Model Development for West Valley Vitrification Process for the period from March 17, 1987 to March 17, 1988, Center for Process Analytical Chemistry, University of Washington, Seattle, WA.
6. C. M. Jantzen and M. J. Plodinec, *Journal of Noncrystalline Solids* **67**:207 (1984).
7. X. Feng and Aa. Barkatt, *Waste Management '87* **1**:54 (1987).

The Use of Probabilistic Risk Assessment in Emergency Response Planning for Nuclear Power Plant Accidents

Robert L. Goble
Clark University - CENTED
Worcester, MA 01610

Gordon R. Thompson
Institute for Resource and Security Studies
Cambridge, MA

ABSTRACT

Emergency response plans are in place for all operating US nuclear power plants. These plans are designed to meet criteria which were developed by the federal government in the late 1970s, relying in part upon the results of probabilistic risk assessments (PRAs). However, those criteria do not reflect all of the insights which may be gained from PRAs. We outline some alternative principles and criteria for emergency response planning, drawing upon the strengths, weaknesses and potential for further development of PRA methods.

KEYWORDS: Probabilistic risk assessment, emergency planning, nuclear accidents

INTRODUCTION

The first serious applications of probabilistic risk assessment (PRA) to emergency planning for nuclear power plant accidents were made approximately a decade ago. Like much of the effort in emergency planning, those applications and subsequent refinements of them can be viewed positively — they were a major improvement over the past; or they can be looked at negatively — they have had unclear objectives and are riddled with inconsistencies. This paper summarizes a set of recommendations we have made for substantial improvements in emergency plans and emergency response capabilities. These recommendations are either based on PRA considerations or represent opportunities for the use of PRA methods to improve response capabilities in emergency situations. Our work used existing PRA studies, analyses, and models; we have not attempted new analyses. The work is best viewed within its context — the history of PRA studies of nuclear power plants and the present regulatory requirements for emergency planning for nuclear power accidents.

Support for this work has come in part from the Three Mile Island (TMI) Public Health Fund as a part of a project, coordinated at Clark University, to prepare an emergency plan for the TMI region. The generic recommendations we present here will not necessarily be incorporated in that plan and are only a small portion of the topics dealt with in the project.

SPECIAL CHARACTERISTICS OF NUCLEAR POWER PLANT ACCIDENTS

Much more research and investment in infrastructure have gone into emergency planning for nuclear power plant accidents than for other kinds of technological accidents. In Table 1 we compare properties of severe nuclear plant accidents with typical properties of severe chemical accidents. Nuclear accidents can produce early injuries and fatalities out to distances of several miles or more; they can produce excess exposures, which carry significant risk of cancer, at distances of well over 100 miles. Most chemical accidents generally affect relatively small areas, but the worst accidents can produce early deaths and irreversible injuries at distances approaching those possible for nuclear power plants. Nevertheless there remains a striking difference in the distance scale over which there may be significant contamination. Other differences are important as well: in a nuclear accident, harm can result even when people do not have direct contact with the material released, and perhaps no other major technology generates as much fear in the public.

Is there a disparity between the effort put into nuclear and chemical emergency planning? Perhaps the more pertinent questions are (1) how effective has the nuclear planning effort been? and (2) can the experience with nuclear planning be used effectively in other settings? We believe there are emergency planning lessons for chemical accidents and other hazards to be drawn from the nuclear experience; but the differences in scale, in type of accident, and in the history of nuclear power regulation must be kept in mind.

PROBABILISTIC RISK ASSESSMENTS

Most major probabilistic risk assessments for large industrial accidents have been for nuclear power plants. Assessments are based on assigning probabilities along event trees. Because of the large number of engineering systems in a nuclear power plant and their linkages to each other, these analyses are very complex and demanding. As illustrated in Fig. 1, the analyses are conventionally (and conveniently) separated into three levels. A Level I PRA is an assessment of the probability of occurrence of a sequence of events that will lead to core melt or other major core damage. A Level II PRA is an assessment of the mechanisms and probabilities for passing from core damage to radioactive releases of various sorts. A Level III PRA extends the analysis from radioactivity releases to consequences for human health and welfare.

The first large scale PRAs (Levels I - III) for nuclear power plants were performed 13 years ago in the Reactor Safety Study, often called WASH-1400 or the Rasmussen Report after its principal author.[1] In the years since, WASH-1400 has been the subject of numerous criticisms and reevaluations. Also, more than 20 PRAs of other commercial power plants have been made.[2] Along with the production of these PRAs, the NRC and industry have supported extensive research directed at topics identified by the work on PRAs. The present situation may be summarized as follows:

1. Nuclear power plants in the U.S. differ sufficiently among themselves that the dominant accident sequences and the PRAs are very much specific to individual reactors.

Table 1. Distances of Concern for Nuclear and Chemical Accidents*

	Major Nuclear Accident	Major Chemical Accident
For early deaths	5 miles	3 miles
For irreversible injuries	25 miles	10 miles
Contamination of levels of concern (for cancer and other latent health effects)	200 miles	? (10-20 miles)

Examples

Chernobyl	Evacuation to 18 miles Contamination regulated beyond 500 miles
Bhopal	Deaths and early injuries to 3 miles
Seveso	Detectable contamination to 4 miles

*Typical distances (under moderately adverse meteorology).

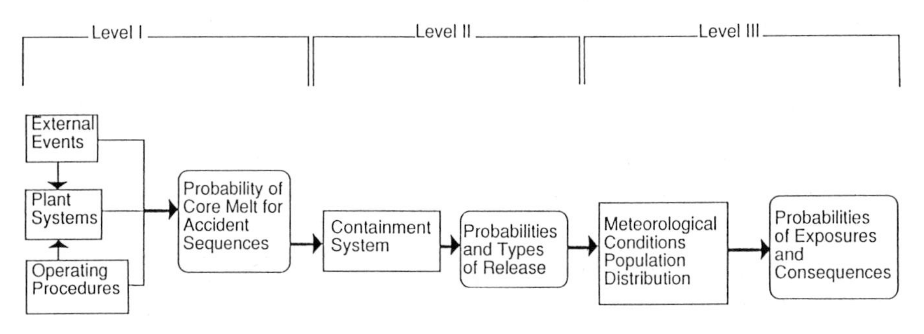

Fig. 1. Levels of probabilistic risk assessment for nuclear power plants.

2. Most estimates of the probability of core melt (or major core damage), i.e., Level I estimates, lie within an order of magnitude of each other; the range is roughly 5×10^{-5} to 5×10^{-4} per reactor year.[2,3]
3. Estimates of the conditional probability of a major release after core melt differ much more; they typically range from 0.003 to 0.3.[1,4]
4. Major criticisms that have been made of WASH-1400 and subsequent PRAs include:[2,5,6]
    a. failure to give a systematic and consistent treatment of uncertainties;
    b. deliberate omission from the calculations of important sources of risk; these include operation of the plant outside normal conditions (this was the initiating problem at Chernobyl), sabotage, and terrorism;

c. inadvertent omission of important sequences; and

d. insufficient attention to the testing of PRA methods and assumptions.

Issues concerning uncertainties and omissions are best considered in the context of how risk assessment is used. The omission of terrorism from PRA calculations is often appropriate, in that the methods are not well suited to deal with this sort of hazard and it can be misleading to make it appear that those risks can easily be compared to, for example, combinations of pump failures. Such comparisons are totally unnecessary if the issue at hand is how to make effective improvements in plant design or operating procedures. If the issue were the absolute risks of a reactor accident, then the omission might well be misleading. Absolute risk estimates, however, have only limited uses.

The three levels of nuclear PRAs differ greatly in the nature of the problem they address, in the methods used, and in the kind and quality of data that support them. Table 2 is a summary characterization of each level.

Level I and Level III are both based on systems (the plant or the meteorological environment) operating for the most part under familiar conditions. The analysis is relatively accessible to testing. For both Level I and Level III, the results depend strongly on local properties, the design of the particular reactor and the local population distribution and meteorology. A Level II analysis is made for systems operating in truly extreme conditions for which there is hardly any actual experience. Because of the complexity of the system, the analysis is based on computer codes which cannot tested easily. Level II analyses are likely to have substantial uncertainties, not only in predicting probabilities of particular classes of events but in predicting the timing of events. Finally, it is important to note that Level III results can be very sensitive to assumptions about emergency response: this is encouraging in that it indicates that emergency planning may do some good.

PRAs can have two important types of application to emergency planning: to assist in the definition of a planning basis and to guide the implementation of particular response measures. We begin by discussing the selection of the planning basis; later we will describe some potential applications of the second type.

ROLE OF PRA IN ESTABLISHING THE PRESENT EMERGENCY PLANNING BASIS

Figure 2 shows the sequence of documents through which WASH-1400 results were applied to emergency planning regulations. The initial activities after publication of WASH-1400 were the work of a joint NRC/EPA Task Force on Emergency Planning, whose report was published as NUREG 0396,[7] and analyses based on WASH-1400 by Aldrich *et al.*[8] which were used by the Task Force. The Task Force recommendations for a planning basis for emergency plans, published late in 1978, became a matter of urgent concern immediately after the accident at TMI, and they were embodied in emergency planning regulations issued in NUREG 0654.[9] There has been considerable controversy and legal maneuvering over the implementation of these regulations and, perhaps for that reason, there have been no changes made in the regulatory planning basis, despite a considerable amount of new information and research.

The Task Force on Emergency Planning considered several possible rationales for establishing a planning basis (see Appendix I in NUREG 0396[7]); these included rationales using "risk, probability, cost effectiveness, and consequence spectrum" as considerations. The Task Force "chose to base the rationale for the planning basis on a spectrum of consequences, tempered by probability considerations." The Task Force rejected risk considerations primarily because it interpreted the use of a risk basis as requiring

Table 2. Features of PRA Levels

Level I	
Typical results:	Probability of core melt 5×10^{-5} to 5×10^{-4} per reactor year
Data base available:	Equipment and system operating experience, other operating experience, all at normal conditions
Calculational basis:	Event tree analysis with probabilities
Major omissions:	Operation outside normal procedures (the initiating event at Chernobyl)
	Malicious acts — sabotage and terrorism
Level II	
Typical results:	Conditional probability of major early release 0.003 to 0.3
Data base available:	TMI — small scale experiments
Calculational basis:	Computer codes simulating complex physical processes at extreme conditions
Level III	
Results depend sensitively on:	Meteorological conditions; population distribution, emergency response measures taken; and nature of release
Data base available:	Extensive meteorological, demographic records
Calculational basis:	Computer dispersion models

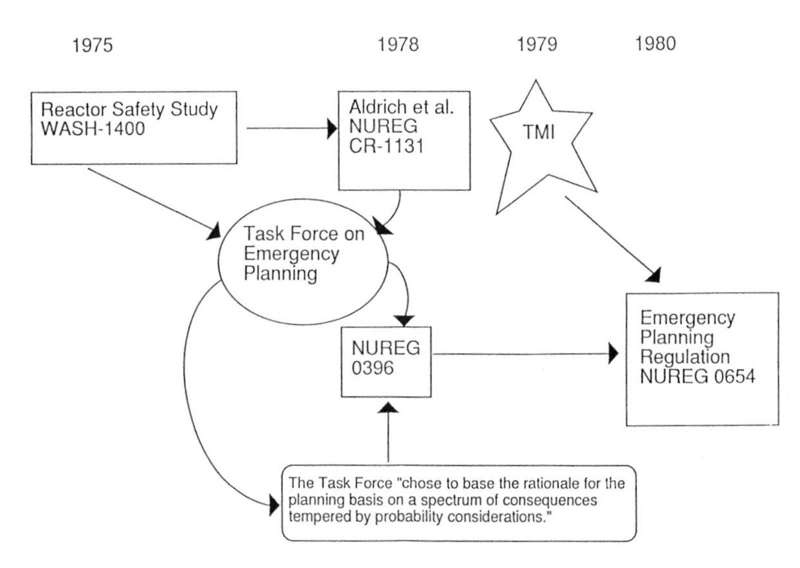

Fig. 2. Critical documents in the incorporation of PRA in emergency planning regulation.

comparisons with non-nuclear emergency planning and it was unwilling to make such comparisons. While the accident consequence spectrum chosen still appears appropriate, the rationale is both limited and in some respects questionable. It does not provide adequate guidance for the formulation of emergency plans. There are two serious deficiencies. One is that emergency planning objectives are not specified well enough to gauge whether a planning effort is adequate. The discussion of Protective Action Guides (PAGs) is representative: "the Task Force concluded that the objective of emergency response plans should be to provide dose savings for a spectrum of accidents that could produce offsite doses in excess of the PAGs." They also observe, "This does not mean that doses above the PAG levels can be prevented or that emergency response plans should have as their objective preventing doses above PAG levels." The second deficiency is closely related to the first: it is that in setting the planning basis no consideration is given to the relative effectiveness of emergency response measures in various accident situations. Risk comparisons between possible accident situations with and without various emergency response capabilities (not comparisons with non-nuclear accidents) provide clearer and more useful guidance for formulating and evaluating plans.

EMERGENCY PLANNING LESSONS FROM A SYSTEMATIC CONSIDERATION OF PRA

Based on the present state of PRAs, risk comparisons indicate that risks of early death and injury and risks for people to exceed the EPA Protective Action Guides (PAGs) are largely concentrated in accidents in which a core melt (or severe core degradation) is accompanied by a large early release. This result appears to hold even for the lower range of estimates of the conditional probability (given core melt) for a large, early release. When combined with the potential opportunities for saving exposures and health effects by evacuation and sheltering, and keeping in mind the Level II uncertainties in predicting the conditional probability, risk comparisons, in our view, imply that:

- If emergency planning is demanded for serious (core melt) accidents, then the most crucial objective is to plan effectively for large, early releases.

This conclusion, in turn, has clear implications for planning criteria:

- The most effective measure is early evacuation. Emergency plans should strive in most circumstances to make it possible to evacuate a region close to the reactor before radioactivity from even a rapidly developing accident arrives.
- In circumstances when it is not feasible to complete an evacuation before a potential arrival of radioactivity, then there is a need to plan to choose appropriate combinations of emergency measures. Planning is needed because sheltering may be a preferable response to an incomplete evacuation and because there are additional risks of moving people into the radioactive pathway.

Based on these considerations it is appropriate to recommend precautionary evacuation of the region at greatest risk around a nuclear plant whenever the risk of a core melt becomes substantial (10% might be a suitable cut off).

A response strategy that uses precautionary evacuation must include the following:

- continuous monitoring of a large number of plant system parameters;
- on line comparison with PRA sequences to identify conditions in which the risk becomes substantial (begins to exceed 10%);
- appropriately designed emergency planning zones;

- an accident classification scheme that focuses on the decision to initiate precautionary evacuation; and
- coherent planning for emergency responses not covered by precautionary evacuation.

Part of using a precautionary strategy is knowing when it might be too late. It is possible that there will not be adequate warning before core melt is already underway. In this situation, the issue is whether it would be better to shelter people for the period until the core penetrates the reactor vessel; there may be a significantly enhanced risk of release at this point, with the likelihood that if a release does not occur soon, it will probably be substantially delayed. Level II PRAs do not, unfortunately, provide very firm guidance on this issue as of now.

The definition of emergency planning zones is based on identifying the geographical areas appropriate for particular measures. We recommend a three zone scheme which is summarized in Table 3. The size of the inner zone is chosen to best implement precautionary evacuation; it is the region in which early deaths and health effects present the most risk, and it is small enough that a rapid evacuation should be feasible in most circumstances.

Emergency classification should be based on plant status and levels of risk rather than on immediate release characteristics. Our proposed rationalization of the existing NRC classification is summarized in Table 4. The most important differences from present practice are a classification level directed specifically to precautionary response and the separation of core melt accidents (with their potential for large effects) from other types of accidental releases of radioactivity.

Table 5 summarizes the differences between our recommendations on precautionary evacuation, on zones and on classification, and existing practice which follows NUREG 0654. It should be kept in mind that many other contemporary workers in emergency planning are taking a similar approach and making related though different packages of recommendations.[10] This evolution has yet to be incorporated in regulations, however.

FURTHER PRA RESEARCH NEEDS

Further research and development of PRAs will be required to implement improvements in emergency response capability similar to these proposals. Much of this research and development work is already in progress but has not been focused on emergency planning needs. We see specific needs in each of the three PRA levels.

Level I — The major need is to develop an analysis of precursors, so that it will be feasible for many accident sequences to identify (on-line) situations in which the probability of core melt exceeds a target value (such as 10%). This is a case in which PRA can contribute directly to the implementation of an emergency response strategy.

Level II — Despite the uncertainties intrinsic to Level II analyses, it would be very useful to better quantify the relative probability of releases over time in the period after the core penetrates the reactor vessel.

Level III — Outside the region of precautionary response, much of the management of protective measures should be based on monitoring and meteorological projection. An important need is to have measures of the risks of misdirecting people because of uncertainties in plume projection. Appropriate measures of uncertainty need to be available on-line and directly tied to the particular conditions at the time of the accident.

Table 3. Recommended Planning Zones for Nuclear Emergency Response

Inner Planning Zone (IPZ) — an area located within five miles of the plant. It is the area of highest risk which requires the most rapid response. The primary emergency preparation is for early evacuation of the entire zone.

Middle Planning Zone (MPZ) — an area located between five and twenty-five miles from the plant. This is an area of lower risk requiring flexible response. The primary emergency preparations are for sheltering and evacuation downwind from the plant.

Outer Planning Zone (OPZ) — an area beyond twenty-five miles from the plant. The primary emergency preparations are for sheltering, followed by evacuation or relocation from hot spots, and protection from radioactivity in food and water.

Table 4. Recommended Classification of Nuclear Accidents

Classification Level	Plant Conditions	Level of Response
Unusual event	An event that might compromise plant safety	Notification of state and federal officials
Alert	Significant increase in probability of core melt Significant possibility of radioactive release without core melt	Activation of emergency response organizations
Projected general emergency	Substantial increase in probability of core melt (probability estimated to be 10% or greater)	Initiation of precautionary emergency response
General emergency	Core melt imminent or ongoing	Appropriate response in all zones
Additional classification for less severe accidents (no core melt)		
Limited area emergency	Release of radioactivity imminent or ongoing, but no core melt	Appropriate emergency response (in inner zone)

Table 5. Comparison Between the Recommended Approach to Emergency Planning and Practice According to NUREG 0654 Regulation

	NUREG 0654	Recommended
Stated objectives:	Dose saving and in some cases life saving	(1) Life saving (2) Exposures reduced below PAGs (3) Dose savings
Initiation of evacuation:	At core melt or when release is expected	When there is substantial (10%) probability of core melt
Planning zones:	2 zones: 0-10 miles, plume protection 10-50 miles, ingestion protection	3 zones: Inner: 0-5 miles Precautionary action Middle: 5-25 miles Flexible response Outer: 25 miles + Plume and ingestion protection
Accident classification:	4 levels based on plant conditions or size of release	4 levels based on likelihood of core melt 1 level for release without core melt

Perhaps now, more than a decade after the development of nuclear PRA methodologies, we are nearing a time when these methods will be used systematically in emergency planning.

REFERENCES

1. U.S. Nuclear Regulatory Commission, Reactor Safety Study, WASH-1400, October 1975.
2. Steven Sholly and Gordon Thompson, The Source Term Debate: A Report by the Union of Concerned Scientists, Union of Concerned Scientists, January 1986.
3. U.S. Nuclear Regulatory Commission, Reactor Risk Reference Document, NUREG-1150 (3 vols.) (Draft), February 1987.
4. B. John Garrick (Study Director) *et al.*, Seabrook Station Probabilistic Safety Assessment, Pickard, Lowe and Garrick Inc., prepared for Public Service Company of New Hampshire and Yankee Atomic Electric Company, 6 volumes, December 1983.
5. H. W. Lewis *et al.*, Risk Assessment Review Group Report to the US Nuclear Regulatory Commission, NUREG/CR-0400, September, 1978.
6. R. Wilson *et al.*, Report to the APS of the Study Group on Radionuclide Release from Severe Accidents at Nuclear Power Plants, *Reviews of Modern Physics* **57(3)**, Part II, July 1985.

7. D. C. Aldrich, P. McGrath, and N. C. Rasmussen, Examination of Offsite Radiological Emergency Protective Measures for Nuclear Reactor Accidents Involving Core Melt, NUREG/CR-1131, 1978.
8. U.S. Nuclear Regulatory Commission and U.S. Environmental Protection Agency, Planning Basis for the Development of State and Local Government Radiological Emergency Response Plans in Support of Light Water Nuclear Power Plants, NUREG-0396, December 1978.
9. U.S. Nuclear Regulatory Commission and Federal Emergency Management Agency, Criteria for Preparation and Evaluation of Radiological Emergency Response Plans and Preparedness in Support of Nuclear Power Plants, NUREG-0654, Rev. 1, November 1980.
10. T. J. McKenna *et al.*, Pilot Program: NRC Severe Reactor Accident Incident Response Training Manual, US Nuclear Regulatory Commission, NUREG-1210, (5 volumes) February 1987.

Risk Tracers: Surrogates for Assessing Health Risks

Sylvia A. Edgerton
PRI Environmental Technologies, Inc.
Honolulu, HI

ABSTRACT

A method is suggested for developing risk tracers for assessing health risks in situations where resources are not available for full scale risk analysis, or where undetectables or complex mixtures confound the analysis. The method consists of using tracer techniques to identify source contributions to ambient concentrations of chemical species. In the case of undetectables, a knowledge of the source contributions and the relative concentrations of chemicals in the source emissions may be used to estimate ambient concentrations of the undetectable and hence exposures. In complex mixtures, the source apportionment determines the relative contribution of each source, and total risks are assessed based on known specific risks associated with exposure to each source type. An example is given for calculating risks from ambient air concentrations of dioxins where the 2,3,7,8-TCDD is reported as undetected, and a source apportionment of the other dibenzo-p-dioxin and dibenzofuran congener groups are used to estimate probable 2,3,7,8-TCDD concentrations. A second example is given to show how the method may be used to calculate risks for exposure to complex polyaromatic hydrocarbon (PAH) mixtures.

KEYWORDS: Risk tracers, 2,3,7,8-TCDD concentrations, polyaromatic hydrocarbon (PAH), dibenzo-p-dioxin, dibenzofuran

INTRODUCTION

Given the tremendous number of chemicals that are released daily into the environment, it is impossible to characterize accurately the risk to human health which each one individually, or a complex mixture of many, might create. A thorough scientific evaluation would be extremely costly and would require more human and laboratory resources than are available today. Even if these resources were available, residual uncertainties would probably still remain quite large. Yet our policy makers must make decisions daily based on limited information and uncertain data analyses; and these decisions are often made in a hostile atmosphere where conflicting interests add only more confusion to the process.

Expanding this situation to the global state of affairs, more and more of the development in the rapidly industrializing countries is going on with very little application of what we in the U.S.A. would consider the basic principles of environmental protection. This may be at least partially due to a backlash from what these countries see as a widening gap between the resources necessary to control chemical releases and the resources they are willing to devote to this area. In the face of ever growing complexity in the risk assessment process, there are many reasons for efforts to be made to simplify the methodology for use in instances where resources are simply not available to conduct detailed analyses. Though a careful and thorough scientific analysis is usually desirable, a simpler, lower-cost analysis, in lieu of no analysis at all, can often illuminate a path for priority risk reduction efforts without frustrating the decision maker with highly technical and costly programs.

Caution, of course, is always necessary in interpreting these mini-analyses, and the limits of their application should always be conveyed to those who would use the results in policy decisions.

Risk indicators could be developed which would combine the probabilities for the occurrence of adverse human health or ecological effects with projected population exposures based on corresponding environmental and biological indicators. The use of risk indicators has been proposed previously for comparing occupational risks[1] and for constructing national risk profiles.[2] Environmental indicators and indices for water and air quality have been used for several decades to reduce the complexity of large quantities of data to a simple form and provide insight into the state of the environment.[3] Biological indicators, found in human blood, tissue, urine, body fat, etc., are commonly used to indicate certain types of exposures which have already occurred. Both generalized environmental and biological indicators are types of risk indicators in that they can provide some qualitative or semi-quantitative measure of the degree of risk. However, due to such factors as the variabilities in human metabolism and population sensitivities, it is often difficult to relate these indicators directly to individual or population exposures.

Environmental risk tracers are defined as chemicals that may or may not be toxic themselves but occur in the environment in predictable proportion to the hazardous substance of interest. A risk tracer is a specific type of risk indicator, one which can be quantitatively related to chemical species or source specific type of risk, and hence can provide a quantitative estimate of the exposure and, given the dose/response relationship, a quantitative estimate of a specific risk itself.

Environmental indicators might provide only a semi-quantitative measure, such as a scale from 1-10, indicating good-bad, or indicating when an "acceptable risk standard" has been exceeded. For example, respirable particle concentrations are an indicator of air quality and could be used as an indicator of health risk; yet this measure alone provides no quantitative information on the chemical nature of the air particles, which vary widely in their toxicological properties, and hence cannot provide any real quantitative estimates of health risk. As another example, benzo(a)pyrene (BaP) is often used by EPA[4] and others as an indicator of products of incomplete combustion (PIC) which are thought to pose an important air quality health risk. However, these products and their mutagenic potential may vary widely depending on the type of combustion, and for a mixture of sources this relationship cannot be simply predicted from (BaP) concentrations.

For an environmental indicator to be a tracer, there must be a well defined empirical relationship between the tracer and the source of risk, and the source emissions profile of hazardous substances must be well characterized. Likewise, for a biological indicator to be a risk tracer, the relationship between the biological quantity measured and the degree of risk must be quantitatively known.

METHODOLOGY FOR DEVELOPMENT OF ENVIRONMENTAL RISK TRACERS

Environmental risk tracers may be characterized as simple or complex depending on the relationship between the tracers, the hazardous substances of interest, and their sources in the environment. The risk tracer model reduces to a simple ratio where the hazardous substance and its tracer have only one source. This condition is rarely met; however, some efforts have been made to use individual tracers as surrogates for health risk.

The U.S. EPA National Emission Standards for Hazardous Air Pollutants (NESHAPS) study used "best fit" compounds, those emitted from similar sources with proportional emission rates or production levels, as surrogates to estimate exposure to 15 substances under evaluation for potential regulation under NESHAPS.[5] No consideration was given, however, to evaluation of multiple source emissions of these "best fit" substances.

A complex mixture of sources, with each source characterized by a profile of multiple chemical species in the emissions, may be resolved by solving a set of linear equations representing the sum of all source contributions to each of the tracer species. The mass concentration of each species, C_i, measured at a receptor will be the sum over all sources of the mass fraction of i in source j, a_{ij}, times the source contribution to that species from source j, S_j. That is

$$C_i = \sum_{j=1}^{p} a_{ij} S_j \tag{1}$$

The set of linear equations C are solved using least squares techniques for the source contributions, S. This type of model is referred to as the Chemical Mass Balance (CMB) model.[6,7] Other types of receptor oriented techniques have been described[8,9] and successfully applied to apportion the sources of air particulates, polyaromatic hydrocarbons and volatile organics.

By using tracer techniques to identify the sources contributions to chemical species in the environment, along with source profiles which contain the relative emissions of these chemicals and hazardous substances of interest, estimates can be made of hazardous substance exposure and risk in instances where their actual measure is impossible or too costly. Several examples of the use of these techniques in risk assessment will be given. In the first example, it is of interest to estimate the risk of exposure to polychlorinated dibenzo-p-dioxins (PCDD) and polychlorinated dibenzofurans (PCDF) in the atmosphere.

The concentrations of many of the congeners are known; however, the ambient concentration of the 2,3,7,8-TCDD isomer, which contributes to most the health risk, is usually below the analytical detection limits for this substance. An analysis of potential sources of PCDD and PCDF is used to estimate (infer) the concentration of 2,3,7,8-TCDD and hence to estimate the health risk. In example 2, a method is presented for estimating health risks from organic air pollutants by assessing the sources contributing to those pollutants.

Example 1. Estimates of Health Risks from Airborne Dioxins and Furans

A recent study was conducted by Battelle Columbus Division[10] to determine the health risk associated with ambient concentrations of PCDD and PCDF in ambient air in Ohio. Several ambient air samples were collected in urban areas downwind of suspected sources, such as municipal and sewage sludge incinerators, and analyzed for total concentrations of the tetra- through octa-PCDD and PCDF congener groups and for 16 specific 2,3,7,8-TCDD isomers. With detection limits as low as 12 fg/m^3 (1 fg is 10^{-15} gm), no 2,3,7,8-TCDD was detected in any of the samples.

In a mixture of PCDD and PCDF, 2,3,7,8-TCDD is generally considered to be the major contributor to the mixture's toxicity. Potential health risks from exposure to these substances are generally calculated using the toxic equivalency method of Bellian and Barnes.[11] In the method, the concentrations of each homologue and/or congener group present in the mixture is multiplied by a toxicity equivalence factor (TEF) associated with that group. For example, relative to 2,3,7,8-TCDD, which has a TEF of one, other TCDDs have a TEF of 0.01 and OCDDs have a TEF of zero. The ambient concentrations of 2,3,7,8-TCDD are generally so low that they are below most achievable detection limits. In the most conservative assumption, the concentration of 2,3,7,8-TCDD could be considered equal to its detection limit. However, this would likely overestimate the risk, whereas an assumption that the concentration is zero would underestimate the risk.

A preferred method would be the estimation of probable concentrations of 2,3,7,8-TCDD based on the concentrations of the other congener/or homologue groups compared with those expected from the distribution in the emission profiles of the contributing sources. The concentrations of 2,3,7,8-TCDD are high enough in the source emissions to be well above detection. A source apportionment study was conducted on the Ohio air samples,[12] and the expected concentrations of 2,3,7,8-TCDD in the ambient samples was inferred.

Figure 1 shows the estimated 2,3,7,8-TCDD concentrations for a sample which consists primarily of municipal incinerator emissions. The concentration in toxic equivalents at two sites is shown in Table 1 assuming the concentration of the undetected 2,3,7,8-TCDD is (A) zero, (B) equal to the detection limits, (C) as estimated by calculation from the distribution predicted from the source apportionment.

The expected 2,3,7,8-TCDD equivalents (shown under assumption C) are 1.5 to 27 times greater than those calculated assuming the lack of detection implies zero concentration (shown under assumption A). If the concentrations are assumed equal to the detection limits (B above) both samples appear to be about equal in toxicity, whereas in fact the sample from Site 1 is probably at least 10 times more toxic than that from Site 2. Using EPA's 1987 risk factor 2,3,7,8-TCDD, Site 1 appears to present a risk of about 10^{-5}, which might be considered "unacceptable," but under assumption C, the risk is about 10^{-6}, which would probably be considered acceptable. The use of source profiles to predict ambient profiles provides a far more logical solution to the problem of assessing risk from undetectable, but possibly non-negligible, hazards.

Example 2. Estimates of Health Risks from Airborne Organics

The concentrations of organic compounds in ambient air are of particular interest due to the fact that many are suspected human carcinogens. These compounds exist both in the particulate and gaseous phase in ambient air, and include such classes as aliphatic hydrocarbons, polycyclic aromatic hydrocarbons (PAHs), carboxylic acids, aza-arenes, and nitro-PAH. The PAH and their nitrogen analogs are probably the best studied of the particulate and semivolatile organic fractions due to the preponderance of experimental data documenting their existence in ambient air and their potentially carcinogenic effects. Because the sampling and analysis for these compounds is very costly, it is of interest to know to what extent compound specific information is necessary for assessing the health risk of exposure to suspended organic particulate material in the ambient air.

PAHs are formed during most types of combustion processes and are thus present in almost every environment populated by humans. Some worldwide contribution to atmospheric PAH may be produced naturally by vegetation; however, it is not likely that

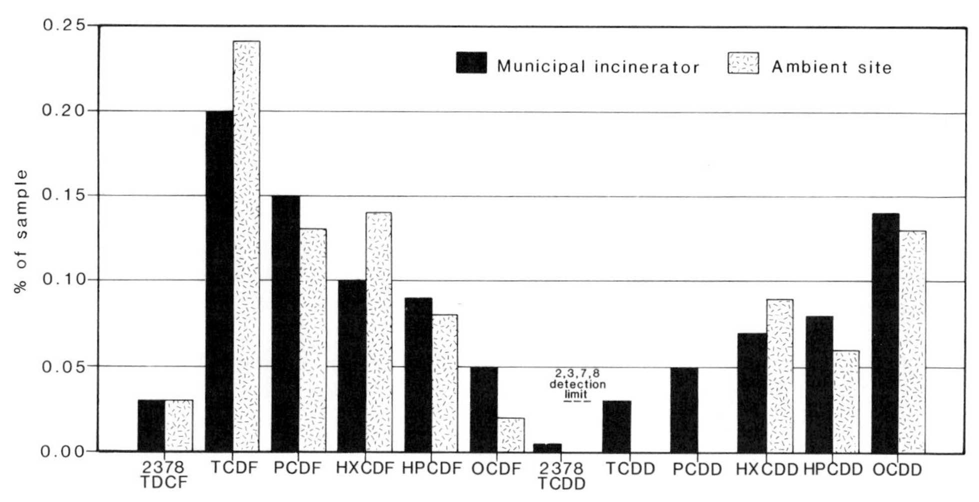

Fig. 1. A comparison of the municipal incinerator profile with that of an ambient sample. The amount of 2,3,7,8-TCDD is below the detection limit but can be estimated from the source profile.

Table 1. 2,3,7,8-TCDD Equivalent Exposure Levels (fg/m^3) for Two Sites in Ohio

	Concentration Assumption for Undetectables		
	Zero	Detection Limit	Source Apportionment
Site 1	81.4	314.9	133.1
Site 2	0.4	255.4	10.9

this source contributes significantly to the high concentrations of PAH found in urban air and in indoor air during home heating and cooking. While ambient air PAH measurements in the U.S. may range from 0.1 to 100 ng/m^3, current studies being conducted by the U.S. EPA have shown that PAH concentrations inside homes in China, in an area with a high lung cancer rate, may reach as high as 10 µg/m^3 (10,000 ng/m^3) and can account for up to 23% of the mutagenicity of the vapor and particulate phase organics sampled.[13] Usually the specific compounds which contribute to the majority of the mutagenicity of a atmospheric sample are not identified.

The biological activities of the individual compounds are often dependent on the concentrations of other related and sometimes non-related compounds present. Therefore, a quantitative assessment of cancer risk from PAH, or from organic compounds in ambient air, must take into account the concentrations of tens or maybe hundreds of compounds present in the complex mixture. Added to this difficulty is the task of extrapolating short-term in vitro animal experiments to the biomedical risk of humans. This is not only a laborious process but also stretches the current potential of analytical chemical methods and of the available toxicological and pharmacological techniques. The mutagenic activities of the fractionated compound classes, such as acids, bases, and neutrals (aliphatics, aromatics and polar neutrals), have been determined for many combustion products[14] and vary greatly by source category. This type of research points to a more source-oriented, rather than substance-oriented approach to risk assessment.

An alternative method to the direct analysis of ambient air samples for specific toxic contaminants is the analysis of source influence in ambient air samples and the application of prior knowledge relating to contaminants or health hazards present in specific source emissions. If the contribution of the sources to the concentrations of total organic material can be quantitatively determined, using receptor modeling techniques,[15] their contribution to the total cancer potency can also be estimated using comparative potencies methods[14,16,17] and combined with specific source-exposure models.[18]

The comparative potency method assumes that the ratio of the unit risk from source i, r_i, to the unit risk of a reference source, r_o, which is known from epidemiological studies, is approximately equal to the ratio of the potencies, p, of each as measured in short-term bioassay studies. That is:

$$r_i = r_o \frac{p_i}{p_o} \tag{2}$$

Assuming that the total risk can be approximated by a linear sum of the risks from the individual sources (in reality one must correct for synergistic and/or antagonistic response to the mixture), the total risk, R_T, summed over j sources is

$$\begin{aligned} R_T &= R_o + \sum_j R_j \\ &= r_o \left\{ D_o + \sum_j \frac{p_j}{p_o} D_j \right\} \end{aligned} \tag{3}$$

where R_o is the known risk from the reference source and the risk from the jth source, R_j is calculated as the unit risk of source j, r_j, times the dosage received from source j, D_j. The D's are determined by the receptor-exposure analysis which apportions the specific source contributions to the exposure and the dose-exposure relationship. Therefore, if the mixture of source contributions and the relative potency of each source is known, it may be possible to estimate the total risk without a complex chemical analysis for all possible hazardous organic compounds. Assessing the synergisms and antagonisms of source mixtures may actually be simpler than assessing those associated with various combinations of individual hazardous chemical substances.

If only one source type is present, a single tracer may be used to represent exposure to a predictable mixture of hazardous substances. Recent research has shown pyrene, fluoranthene, and phenanthrene to be good tracers for total PAH and PAH derivatives in indoor air.[19]

In another study where air pollutant concentrations were dominated by one type of source, residential wood burning, extractable organics and fine particulate concentrations correlated highly with the mutagenicity of air samples.[20] Using tracer techniques, estimates of risk can often be made with measures far simpler and less costly than those involving the complex characterization of each individual component in the mixture. Risk estimates for complex mixtures of sources, or for sources which cannot be easily characterized, however, may require analytical methods of much greater specificity and higher costs. Methods for analyzing for airborne organics range from thermo-optical methods for quantifying total organic particulate material on filter samples (about $40/sample) to solvent extraction, fractionation, and GC/MS analysis for specific compounds (about $1000/sample).

Although the specific value of employing more sophisticated analytical methodologies for detecting organics in air and in reducing the uncertainties in risk

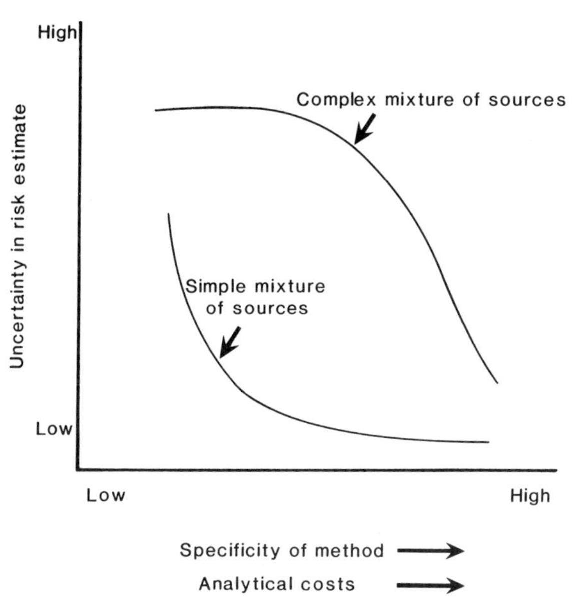

Fig. 2. High cost analyses may be necessary to reduce the risk uncertainty in a complex mixture of chemical sources, as more specific risk tracers are needed to resolve source contributions. For a simple mixture, a single tracer may be enough to provide a good risk estimate.

estimates is actually a function of the chemical mixture itself, a general relationship is expected to be as shown in Fig. 2.

CONCLUSIONS

Given the ever increasing complexity and costs associated with assessing the public health risks from environmental contaminants, there is tremendous incentive to develop methods that can provide risk estimates based on less intensive and less costly analyses. The use of risk tracers as surrogates for more complex measurements of hazard is suggested. Risk tracers are developed primarily to characterize the sources of hazardous materials, and, given the hazardous substance emission profile from each source, it is possible to estimate quantitatively the risks from multiple hazards based on the tracer measurement(s) alone. Risk tracers should be especially useful in the absence of sufficient financial or analytical resources for more complex analyses.

REFERENCES

1. Kenneth Solomon and Stanley C. Abraham, The Index of Harm: A Useful measure for Comparing Occupational Risk Across Industries, *Health Physics* **38**:375-391 (1980).
2. Jeanne X. Kasperson and Roger E. Kasperson, Priorities in Profile: Managing Risks in Developing Countries, *Risk Abstracts* **4(3)**, (July, 1987)
3. Wayne R. Ott, *Environmental Indices: Theory and Practice*, Ann Arbor Science Publishers, Ann Arbor, MI (1978).

4. Elaine Haemisegger, Alan Jones, Bern Steigerwald, and Vivian Thomson, The Air Toxics Problem in the United States: An Analysis of Cancer Risks for Selected Pollutants, EPA-450/l-85-001 (1985).
5. Robert M. Schell, Estimation of the Public Health Risks Associated With Exposure to Ambient Concentrations of 87 Substances, Office of Air Quality Planning and Standards, U.S. EPA, Research Triangle Park, NC (July, 1984).
6. John G. Watson, Chemical Element Balance Receptor Model Methodology for Assessing the Sources of Fine and Total Suspended Particulate Matter in Portland, Oregon, Ph.D. Dissertation, Oregon Graduate Center, Beaverton, Oregon (1979).
7. John G. Watson, John A. Cooper, and James J. Huntzicker, The Effective Variance Weighting for Least Squares Calculations Applied to the Mass Balance Receptor Model, *Atmos. Environ.* **18**:1347-1355 (1984).
8. Ronald C. Henry, Charles W. Lewis, Philip K. Hopke, and Hugh J. Williamson, Review of Receptor Model Fundamentals, *Atmos. Environ.* **18**:1507-1515 (1984).
9. Philip K. Hopke, *Receptor Modeling in Environmental Chemistry*, John Wiley and Sons, New York (1985).
10. S. A. Edgerton, J. M. Czuczwa, J. D. Rench, D. A. Egan, R. F. Hodanbosi, and P. J. Koval, Determination of Polychlorinated Dibenzo-p-Dioxins and Dibenzofurans and Associated Health Risks in Ambient Air in Ohio, presented at the APCA Annual Meeting in Dallas, TX, Paper 88-77.1 (June, 1988)
11. Judith S. Bellian and Donald G. Barnes, Interim Procedures for Estimating Risks Associated with Exposures to Mixtures of Chlorinated Dibenzo-p-Dioxins and Dibenzofurans, EPA/625/3-87/012 (March, 1987).
12. Sylvia A. Edgerton and Jean M. Czuczwa, Source Apportionment of Dioxins and Dibenzofurans in Ambient Air in Ohio, in *Receptor Models in Air Resource Management*, John Watson, ed., Air Pollution Control Association Press, Pittsburgh, PA (1988).
13. Jane Chuang, Battelle Columbus Division, Columbus, OH, Personal communication, September, 1988a.
14. Joellen Lewtas, Marcia G. Nishioka, and Bruce A. Petersen, Identification and Comparative Risk Assessment of Airborne Carcinogens From Combustion Sources, EPA/600/D-86/013 (January, 1986).
15. J. M. Daisey, P. J. Lioy, and T. J. Kneip, Receptor Models for Airborne Organic Species, EPA/600/3-85/014, PB85-172583 (1985).
16. J. E. Harris, Diesel Emissions and Lung Cancer, *Risk Analysis* **3**:88-100 (1983).
17. Roy E. Albert, Joellen Lewtas, Stephen Newnow, Todd W. Thorslund, and Elizabeth Anderson, Comparative Potency Method for Cancer Risk Assessment: Application to Diesel Particulate Emissions, *Risk Analysis* **3**:101-117 (1983).
18. Sylvia Edgerton, Estimating Specific Source Exposures to Toxic Air Pollutants from Measurement of Toxic Air Pollutants, proceedings of the EPA/APCA Symposium, Raleigh, NC (March, 1986).
19. J. C. Chuang, G. A. Mack, J. W. Stockrahm, S. W. Hannan, C. Bridges, and M. R. Kuhlman, Field Evaluation of Sampling and Analysis for Organic Air Pollutants in Indoor Air, EPA/600/4-88/028 (1988b).
20. R. R. Watts, R. J. Drago, R. G. Merrill, R. W. Williams, E. Perry, and J. Lewtas, Wood Smoke Impacted Air: Mutagenicity and Chemical Analysis of Ambient Air in a Residential Area of Juneau, Alaska, *J. Air Pollut. Control Assoc.* **38**:652-660 (1988).

Science Advisory Board's Judgments in the Assessment of the Risk of Environmental Contaminants[a]

C. Richard Cothern
U.S. Environmental Protection Agency
Washington, DC

ABSTRACT

The assessment of risk due to environmental contaminants depends, in part, on scientific data. When such data are incomplete, as is usually the case, assumptions based on scientific judgments are made to analyze the consequences. Specifically, when health related data needed to assess the risk posed by environmental contaminants are missing or incomplete, it becomes necessary to make assumptions using scientific judgment to estimate the risk. The present discussion presents a few of the consensus judgments of the Science Advisory Board of the U. S. Environmental Protection Agency concerning the health effects and risk for some environmental contaminants. Because of the uncertainties in current scientific knowledge for many environmental contaminants, judgments differ and there is no right or wrong opinion.

KEYWORDS: Dose delivery, environmental contaminants, exposure route, pharmacokinetics, risk assessment, scientific judgments

INTRODUCTION

In the process of developing regulations to protect human health and the environment, the U. S. Environmental Protection Agency (EPA) considers a wide variety and range of information and scientific data that sometimes appear to be conflicting. One endeavor where scientific data are important is in the assessment of the risk to human health from environmental contaminants. For no contaminant are data complete, and there are usually significant gaps and uncertainties in the available data. To assess any risk on the basis of incomplete data, scientific judgment is needed. However, scientists can and sometimes do disagree on specifics of individual judgments that are a part of the assessment process. Such disagreements can lead to controversy. Controversy is expected and is a desirable part of the intellectual process in the development of new ideas and should not be confused with controversies in non-science areas. Examples of science controversies include discussions regarding the modification of risk assessments in cases where the environmental contaminant is a cancer promoter, induces a non-fatal rather than a fatal

---

a. The thoughts and ideas expressed here are those of the Science Advisory Board and do not necessarily reflect policies of the U.S. Environmental Protection Agency.

cancer, or acts by a carcinogenesis mechanism that occurs in test animal but not in humans. See Refs. 1-5 for recent publications that discuss these and other controversies in more detail.

One major role of the EPA Science Advisory Board (SAB) is to give informed opinion based on independent review of background documents for regulatory decisions and on issues that arise in the analysis of scientific data relating to environmental health risk assessments.

Examples of the documents reviewed recently by the Environmental Health Committee of EPA's SAB include health criteria documents for acrylamide, arsenic, barium, copper, 1,2-dichloroethylene, ethylbenzene, paradichlorobenzene, PCBs, perchloroethylene, phosgene, selenium, styrene, trichloroethylene and xylene. In addition, reviews have been conducted of such topics as thyroid follicular cell carcinoma, guidelines for male and female reproductivity and rules being developed to regulate the filtration of and coliform level in drinking water. The Committee has also reviewed research in the area of neurotoxicology methods, water distribution systems and disinfection of drinking water. The SAB reviews such documents and issues, especially in cases of conflicting claims, and advises the EPA Administrator regarding its perspective on the adequacy and reliability of the technical basis for rules and regulations. In the present discussion, a few issues on which the SAB has given advice recently will be discussed using the context of such risk assessment components as carcinogenicity, exposure, mixtures (relative toxicity of components) and pharmacokinetics.

IS IT A HUMAN CARCINOGEN?

One of the more difficult tasks in the development of health risk assessments for environmental contaminants is answering the question, "Is it a human carcinogen?" In most cases, only animal bioassay data are available, and the mechanism leading to tumors is not known. If a contaminant causes cancer in animals, it is not known if it will also cause cancer in humans. Any assumption that animal test results predict specific human health effects involves scientific judgment. Examples where such assumptions are not well supported by human studies include lead (cancer in rats and mice but not in humans, except at very high levels), arsenic (cancer in humans but not in animals) and thalidomide and aspirin (birth defects in humans but not in many common laboratory animals). See also a recent comparison of animal and human cancer risks.[6] However, these instances are regarded as anomalies, and the general assumption is that if a contaminant causes cancer in animals, it may also do so in humans (although the organ or system involved may be different).

In deciding the likelihood that a contaminant may cause cancer to humans, EPA has developed guidelines that involve categorizing scientific judgment in a weight-of-evidence scheme. This scheme involves the categories: (A) human carcinogen; (B) probable human carcinogen; (C) possible human carcinogen; (D) not classifiable as to human carcinogenicity; and (E) evidence of non-carcinogenicity to humans.[7]

Perhaps one of the best known areas of disagreement among scientists is in the interpretation or connotation of the descriptors "possible" and "probable" used in the weight-of-evidence scheme. Examples of environmental contaminants whose weight of evidence classifications using the EPA categorization seem to be problematic or difficult and whose health criteria documents have been reviewed recently by the SAB include dichloroethylene, trichloroethylene, perchloroethylene and paradichlorobenzene.

The Environmental Health Committee (EHC) of the SAB and its subcommittees view the weight-of-evidence categories as a continuum that ranges from clear evidence that a contaminant is a human carcinogen (e.g., ionizing radiation, arsenic, benzene, hexavalent chromium compounds, coke oven emissions, nickel subsulfide from smelting operations and vinyl chloride, among others) to the absence of evidence that a contaminant is a human carcinogen (e.g., Endrin). The categories B (probable) and C (possible) are portions of the continuum lying between the two extremes and themselves represent a continuum. Thus these categories are not viewed as discrete and disconnected boxes but as part of a continuous range.

Trichloroethylene is an example of an environmental contaminant with a low tumorigenic potency in animals as demonstrated by tumor responses in bioassays. There are no human data for the carcinogenicity of trichloroethylene. In the judgment of SAB scientists trichloroethylene has the potential to cause cancer in humans. The SAB concluded, however, that "the overall weight of evidence lies on the continuum between B2 and C ...," adding the judgmental comment that the potency appears low.

Besides concern about relatively low carcinogenic potency, the lack of understanding about the mechanism involved may make scientists uneasy about their judgments. In some cases mechanisms have been suggested and theories of action proposed. In August 1987, the EHC/SAB and its Halogenated Organics Subcommittee (HOS) held a workshop to examine some of the mechanisms which could be involved in the generation of mouse liver and rat kidney tumors. Subject areas discussed in the workshop included alpha-2u-globulin production, peroxisome proliferation and oncogene activation. It is not the objective of this paper to review that workshop or the general subject of cancer mechanisms. However, some idea of progress in this area can be found in Refs. 8-26, which were available at the workshop.

The mechanism by which peroxisome proliferators, such as hypolipidemic drugs, could cause cancer is not proven. It is hypothesized that the carcinogenicity is mediated through increased oxidase stress. There is an increase in the production of free radicals that could possibly result in DNA damage. The free radicals might activate oncogenes, and amplification of genes of the peroximal fatty acid oxidation system near an oncogene is also possible. Also, the peroxisome proliferation receptor itself might activate an oncogene. If carcinogenesis is directly related to the ability of these compounds to induce peroxisome proliferation, then carcinogenic risk could be predicted with some assurance by assaying the peroxisome proliferation. The workshop participants emphasized that risks are more likely related to hepatic hyperplasia than to peroxisome proliferation.

It has been strongly suggested that an important mechanism in production of a specific tumor type in male rat kidneys involves alpha-2u-globulin. The following sequence is the suggested mechanistic pathway. First, alpha-2u-globulin is synthesized by the liver and secreted into the blood stream. Then a xenobiotic may be metabolized in the liver and the alpha-2u-globulin binds with a metabolite. This conjugate is filtered in the glomerulus, the proximal tubular epithelium reabsorbs it, and it accumulates there. It is hypothesized that the conjugate is more difficult to metabolize than the alpha-2u-globulin alone. This conjugate then accumulates and is injurious to the cell. Most of these cells are in the P2 segment of the kidney. The alpha-2u-globulin overload results in increased apoptosis (programmed cell death), followed by increased replication to replace the lost cells. The new cells are functional and thus develop the protein overload. The xenobiotic presumably mediates the alpha-2u-globulin overload, but is not otherwise a prerequisite to toxicity and tumorogenic response. Alpha-2u-globulin infused into normal female rats induces replicative rate increases comparable to those seen in males. The biochemical peculiarities of the male rat are also reflected microscopically as hyaline droplets in the cytoplasm.

Alpha-2u-globulin overloads these droplets not found in female rats or in humans so far as we know now. Thus male rat kidney tumors may not be indicative of the potential for human carcinogenicity. Activated oncogenes have been studied in chemically induced and spontaneously occurring mouse liver tumors and provide information at the molecular level to aid in risk assessment.[27]

Prior to the workshop, the HOS of the EHC/SAB had reviewed the health criteria document for ortho-, meta- and paradichlorobenzene. The EPA staff had earlier classified paradichlorobenzene as a B2 carcinogen. The alpha-2u-globulin mediated mechanism was reported for the rat kidney tumors, and there was an absence of positive genotoxicity studies for paradichlorobenzene. For these reasons most of the HOS members, using their scientific judgment, recommended reclassifing para-dichlorobenzene as a category C carcinogen. The original B2 classification had in the meantime been the conclusion, based on the evidence, of scientists and management in EPA's Office of Drinking Water, which was preparing to propose a standard for para-dichlorobenzene. These differences of opinion represent the reality of current scientific knowledge, and the opinions cannot be considered right or wrong.

Another environmental contaminant that has been difficult to classify using the weight-of-evidence scheme is perchloroethylene. In this case, among other endpoints, tumors were found in the male rat kidneys. However the experiment was not conducted in such a way as to determine if alpha-2u-globulin or hyaline droplets were present. Thus, the evidence is suggestive but not conclusive. To provide focus for the workshop in August, the EPA Administrator formally asked the SAB three questions.

The two first questions and the responses to them are presented below. While these responses have general applicability, they specifically express the SAB's judgment[28] regarding perchloroethylene. The third question concerned research recommendations in light of the uncertainties.

> *Question 1:* **Assuming that not all animal tumors are of equal significance to evaluating human hazard, what is the SAB's current consensus position, based on scientific evidence or professional judgment, of the relative significance of male rat kidney or mouse hepatocellular tumors for human risk assessment?**
>
> *Concerning the alpha-2u-globulin mediated mechanism the SAB response was: "From available scientific evidence, this mechanism appears to be unique to male rats." Concerning peroxisome proliferators they concluded that "a causal relationship for this mechanism is plausible but unproven. The Board's consensus on the significance of mouse liver tumors is that mechanistic explanations are not sufficiently well developed and validated at this time to change EPA's present approach expressed in its risk assessment guidelines for carcinogenicity. It concludes that the generation of mouse liver tumors by chemicals is an important predictor of potential risks to humans (emphasis added). Of the several mechanistic models under consideration (including regenerative hyperplasia, oncogene activation, and trihalomethyl radical formation), the one most promising for immediate application to risk assessment is characterized by proliferation of peroxisomes, an intracellular organelle, in the liver." However, further research is required to be more definitive about this mechanism.*
>
> *Question 2:* **What is the Board's view of the approach taken by EPA in using its guidelines to infer human carcinogenic potential from the total body of scientific evidence on perchloroethylene?**
>
> *The SAB response was, in part: "The issues regarding the application of the risk assessment guidelines appear not to represent disagreement among scientists about scientific evidence but, rather, the consequence of attempting*

to fit the weights of evidence into necessarily arbitrary categories of risk. Since the weights of evidence, and uncertainties associated with such evidence, for perchloroethylene and other compounds fall within a range of scientifically defensible choices, it may not be possible, in some instances, to fit them neatly into only one risk category. Moreover, the more incomplete the data, the less precision one can expect in classifying a compound within EPA's cancer guidelines. In addition, the type of evidence that places a compound in a particular category may vary considerably from substance to substance within that category. For perchloroethylene, as with trichloroethylene, the Science Advisory Board concludes that the overall weight of evidence lies on the continuum between the categories B2 and C of EPA's risk assessment guidelines for cancer."

In many cases there are few or no bioassay data for an environmental contaminant. One such case, 1,2-dichloroethylene, came to the EHC for review. The EPA proposed to use a surrogate, 1,1-dichloroethylene, to infer risk. The Committee concluded that it was scientifically unsound to use a surrogate, but political realities may dictate that course when there is a need to make a regulatory decision on a chemical for which direct data do not exist in sufficient quantity or quality.

EXPOSURE ROUTE

Although EPA may be concerned about a chemical contaminant in a specific medium, it is important to recognize that exposure to the chemical may not be limited to that medium. For example, a volatile substance such as xylene is released from drinking water to indoor air from the washing of clothes and dishes, taking baths and showers, and flushing toilets. Another exposure route is ingestion of tap water. In its review of the criteria document for xylene, the SAB noted that EPA had not included the potential for exposure via inhalation in its estimates. Because of the importance of this exposure route the Risk Assessment Forum at EPA is currently examining this problem for a wide range of volatile substances. Setting the standard for xylene is also interesting because standards suggested by conventional analysis of the bioassay data indicate a value above the odor threshold. Most people would not drink the water if it had such an odor, and thus it may be wiser to set the standard at or below the odor threshold. Thus, xylene is a case where a standard based on aesthetics is more stringent than one based on toxicity.

MIXTURES

Development of a regulatory standard for a mixture, such as polychlorinated biphenyls (PCBs), presents difficulties such as those of measurement (separation, standards cost) and prediction of health effects for a potentially wide range of toxicities. The SAB concluded that the scientific data for the health effects of PCBs, although by no means complete, was adequate for developing a scale of toxicity similar to the toxicity equivalence factors (TEFs) developed by the Risk Assessment Forum for chlorinated dibenzo-p-dioxins and dibenzofurans.[29] The risk of cancer for a particular mixture of PCBs can be more realistically estimated using this procedure that gives the toxicity for separate isomers relative to the most toxic. It must be remembered, however, that this will not necessarily bear any relation to other types of toxicity, e.g., adverse effects on *in utero* development.

PHARMACOKINETICS

In the last few years it has become increasingly recognized that it is desirable to base quantitative risk estimates on the delivered dose, or more specifically the concentration of contaminant at the tissue site of the toxic action, rather than on the applied dose or ambient concentration.[30,31] Uncertainty in quantitative risk assessments may be reduced by knowing more about the effects of different conditions of exposure on the amount and pattern of delivered dose. For example, examination of delivered doses may be more useful in comparing the toxic results of exposures by different routes of administration than simple exposure levels. In some cases including pharamacokinetic data can produce more accurate risk assessments.[31]

The projection of human risks by extrapolation from experimental animal studies conducted at high doses by artificial exposure regimes to low dose human exposures is rendered potentially more reliable and biologically meaningful. Of course, the examination of delivered doses does not answer all questions about extrapolation in risk assessment. For example, the equivalency of doses across species is determined not only by relative dose delivery but also by any species differences in reactivity or susceptibility to a given delivered dose and by metabolic differences. Similarly, the extrapolation of effects from high to low doses or from acute to chronic exposures depends not only on the delivered dose differences resulting from the various circumstances but also on the relative toxicological effects of different degrees and durations of tissue exposure to the contaminant and from differences in metabolism from species to species. Given the usefulness of delivered dose information, how is it to be obtained? Direct experimentation usually is not possible in the case of human exposures, and it is not acceptable from an ethical viewpoint. In any case, experimental results apply only to the particular experimental conditions of the individual experiment, and delivered dose estimates are needed for a variety of situations, many of which cannot easily be studied in the laboratory. Use of delivered doses in quantitative risk assessment has become a practical possibility only since the advent of physiologically based pharmacokinetic models and the computer resources on which to run them.

Pharmacokinetics describes the disposition of a contaminant and its metabolites in the body over time, including the processes of absorption, distribution, biotransformation, and excretion. Physiologically based pharmacokinetic models are mathematical descriptions of these processes, expressed in terms of physiologically meaningful and experimentally measurable rates (such as blood flows, breathing rates and metabolic rates) and capacities (such as blood and tissue volumes). Given the proper data, mathematical models can be developed which quantitatively describe the fraction of a compound that is absorbed, that moves through the body, that is metabolically activated or detoxified and eliminated. Such models are both descriptive and predictive; when properly formulated and tested, they may be used to predict delivered doses under conditions of exposure different from those initially tested, such as different routes of administration, different exposure concentrations, and different time patterns of exposure. Finally, models developed for one species may be used in predicting delivered doses in another, untested species, by employing data and knowledge of comparative physiology to scale the various physiological parameters. Systematically varying parameters that are known to vary among individuals, with age or with sex (e.g., enzyme activities) provide a means to predict the impact of inter-individual or species variability.

There are limitations on this approach due to the lack of data on metabolic and age mediated differences that prevent extended effective use of this model.

The application of a physiologically based pharmacokinetic (PBPK) model in a recent EPA publication[32] was observed by the HOS/EHC to be generally well conceptualized and organized. The Committee has for some time advised EPA to use such an approach and was pleased to see this first step in that direction. The Subcommittee further observed that "This application — of pharmacokinetics — represents a novel approach that can sharpen EPA's ability to refine risk estimates in the future. The Subcommittee commends EPA for incorporation of such information into the weight of evidence determination of the carcinogenic potential of dichloromethane. Adoption of the Reitz-Andersen model, with certain modifications, is a positive step forward for the Agency's risk assessment process. The critical analyses of the constraints of the model are thoroughly discussed and scientifically balanced. EPA, for example, is justified in adjusting the estimates of Reitz-Anderson for breathing rates traditionally used in EPA models. The rationale for using surface area factor adjustment, and contrary arguments, are clearly described." More data will be required to validate these models more completely.

DISCUSSION

Many of the judgments described in this paper are examples of the characteristics listed in a recent address to the Society for Risk Analysis (Houston, Texas, November 1987) by the former Director of the SAB, Terry Yosie (now the Vice President for Environmental Affairs of the American Petroleum Institute) in his description of the post-conservative risk assessment era. Some of these characteristics include the increasingly fragile nature of the decision making process, the increasing view that risk assessment and risk management are a continuum rather than separate entities, an increasing reliance by EPA on the scientific community, a longer time for decisions, and the substitution of scientific data for conservative assumptions.

With the emergence of new scientific data and information, new controversies are likely to emerge, increasing the fragility of the risk assessment process. The area of cancer mechanisms promises to be an active area of research and possible controversy. To the extent the alpha-2u-globulin mechanism applies, a clear case may be demonstrated where the presence of animal tumors does not predict the likelihood that a chemical will cause cancer in humans and require massive redirection of regulatory energies. However, seldom do tumors appear only in male rat kidneys and this will not likely reduce the fragility of the weight-of-evidence decisions. New scientific evidence often brings new differences of opinion, and these controversies will continue to provide for a fragile decision making situation. Not only do risk assessment and risk management fall on a continuum, but so also do other aspects of quantitative risk assessment. The SAB has concluded that the weight-of-evidence scheme is also a continuum. In some cases, these decisions may even transcend the scientific evidence on a continuum into the policy area. This situation was described by Weinberg as transcientific.[33] Decisions concerning conversion of animal bioassay data to predictions of human cancer may always be based on some scientific evidence along with assumptions based on scientific judgments, and those described here also have this character.

Future decisions in risk assessment will be more completely based on scientific evidence, as has been shown here in the areas of pharmacokinetics and in the analysis of the carcinogenic potential of mixtures such as PCBs. However the emergence of more information regarding complex mixtures or categories, such as in the case of PCBs, will require more analysis, lengthening the time needed for analysis, and will result in even longer times being required for regulatory decisions.

The SAB will continue to be part of the post-conservative risk assessment movement, encouraging better and more complete scientific analysis and continuing re-assessment as new data become available. The increasing reliance on scientific data and the broader use of scientific judgment recommended by the SAB will become more a part of the decision making process. If Yosie is correct, then among other things it will become increasingly difficult to bring closure to scientific controversies.

Some topics likely to be reviewed by the SAB in the future include methods of modifying risk assessment to allow for differences between tumor initiators and promoters, the importance of practical thresholds for carcinogens (where the dose-response curve suddenly drops to a lower value — not zero as would be the case in a real threshold), and possible adjustments in risk factors to compensate for a non-fatal cancer or to compare different endpoints (such as neurological, immunological, reproductive, developmental and cancer), and weigh their relative risks.

ACKNOWLEDGEMENTS

Thanks to Dr. Jerry Blancato of EPA's Office of Research and Development for contributing the background discussion of pharmacokinetics in this paper and to Eleanor Merrick for her editorial comments and suggestions.

REFERENCES

1. *New York Times*, EPA Reassesses the Cancer Risk of Many Chemicals (January 4, 1988); Differing Roles of Cancer Agents Are Studied (January 5, 1988); and Assessing the Risky Job of Risk Assessment (January 24, 1988).
2. F. Perera, EPA Cancer Risk Assessments, *Science*, p. 1227 (1988).
3. P. Abelson, Cancer Phobia, *Science* **237**:473 (1987).
4. W. North and T. F. Yosie, Risk Assessment: What It Is, How It Works, *EPA Journal* **13**:13-15 (1987).
5. T. F. Yosie, EPA's Risk Assessment Culture, *Environ. Sci. Technol.* **21**:526-531 (1987).
6. B. C. Allen, A. M. Shipp, K. S. Crump, B. Kilian, M. Hogg, J. Tudor, and B. Keller, Investigation of Cancer Risk Assessment Methods, Clement Associates, Inc., Ruston, LA (1987).
7. Federal Register, 51 FR 33992, September 24, 1986.
8. C. L. Alden, A Review of Unique Male Rat Hydrocarbon Nephropathy, *Toxicologic Pathology* **14**:109-111 (1986)
9. M. Charbonneau, B. G. Short, E. A. Lock, and J. A. Swenberg, Mechanism of Petroleum-Induced Sex-Specific Protein Droplet Nephropathy and Renal Cell Proliferation in Fischer-344 Rats: Relevance to Humans, Chemical Industry Institute of Technology, RTP, NC (unpublished manuscript).
10. R. L. Kanerva and C. L. Alden, Review of Kidney Sections from a Subchronic d-limonene Oral Dosing Study Conducted by the National Cancer Institute, *Fd. Chem. Toxic* **25**:355-358 (1987a).
11. R. L. Kanerva, G. M. Ridder, L. C. Stone, and C. L. Alden, Characterization of Spontaneous and Decalin-Induced Hyaline Droplets in Kidneys of Adult Male Rats, *Fd. Chem. Toxic.* **25**:63-82 (1987b).
12. R. L. Kanerva, G. M. Ridder, F. R. Lefever, and C. L. Alden, Comparison of Short-Term Renal Effects Due to Oral Administration of Decalin or d-limonene in Young Adult Male Fischer-344 Rats, *Fd. Chem. Toxic.* **25**:345-353 (1987c).
13. R. L. Kanerva, M. S. K. McCracken, L. C. Stone, and C. L. Alden, Morphagenesis of Decalin-Induced Renal Alterations in the Male Rat, The Proctor and Gamble Company, Miami Valley Laboratories, Cincinnati, OH (unpublished report).
14. R. R. Maronpot, J. K. Haseman, G. A. Boorman, S. E. Eustis, G. N. Rao, and J. E. Huff, Liver Lesions in B6C3F1 Mice: the National Toxicology Program, Experience and Position, *Arch. Toxicol. Suppl.* **10**:10-26 (1987).
15. M. A. Mehlman, C. P. Hemstreet, III, J. J. Thorpe, and N. K. Weaver, eds., *Renal Effects of Petroleum Hydrocarbons*, Princeton Scientific Publishers, Inc., Princeton, NJ (1984).
16. R. Montesano, H. Bartsch, H. Vainio, J. Wilbourn, and H. Yamasaki, eds., Long-Term and Short-Term Assays for Carcinogens: A Critical Appraisal, International Agency for Research on Cancer (WHO), IARC Publication No. 83 (1986).

17. Nutrition Foundation, The Relevance of Mouse Liver Hepatoma to Human Carcinogenic Risk, A Report of the International Expert Advisory Committee to the Nutrition Foundation, Washington, DC, September, 1983.
18. J. A. Popp, ed., *Mouse Liver Neoplasia*, Hemosphere Publishing Corp., New York (1984).
19. D. P. Rall, Carcinogenicity of p-dichlorobenzene, *Science* **236**:897 (1987).
20. M. S. Rao and J. K. Reddy, Peroxisome Proliferation and Hepatocarcinogenesis, *Carcinogenesis* **8**:631-636 (1987).
21. L. C. Stone, R. L. Kanerva, J. L. Burns, and C. L. Alden, Decalin-Induced Nephrotoxicity: Light and Electron Microscopic Examination of the Effects of Oral Dosing on the Development of Kidney Lesions in the Rat, *Fd. Chem. Toxic.* **25**:43-52 (1987).
22. L. C. Stone, M. S. McCracken, R. L. Kanerva, and C. L. Alden, Development of a Short-Term Model of Decalin Inhalation Nephrotoxicity in the Male Rat, The Proctor and Gamble Company, Miami Valley Laboratories, Cincinnati, OH (unpublished manuscript).
23. U.S. Consumer Product Safety Commission, Chronic Hazard Advisory Panel on Di(2-Ethylhexl)Phthlate(DEHP), September, 1985.
24. U.S. Environmental Protection Agency, Proliferative Hepatocellular Lesions of the Rat, Risk Assessment Forum, EPA/625/3-86/011, February, 1986.
25. J. M. Ward, R. A. Griesemer, and E. K. Weisburger, The Mouse Liver Tumor as an Endpoint in Carcinogenesis Tests, *Toxicology and Applied Pharmacology* **51**:389-397 (1979).
26. J. M. Ward, B. A. Diwan, M. Ohshima, H. Hu, H. M. Schuller, and J. M. Rick, Tumor-Initiating and Promoting Activities of Di(2-ethylhexyl)Phthalate *in vivo* and *in vitro*, *Environmental Health Prospectives* **65**:279-291 (1986).
27. S. H. Reynolds, S. J. Towers, R. M. Patterson, R. R. Maronpon, S. A. Aaronson, and M. A. Anderson, Activated Oncogenes in B6C3F1 Mouse Liver Tumors: Implications for Risk Assessment, *Science* **237**:1309-1316 (1987).
28. Science Advisory Board, SAB-EHC-88-011, U. S. Environmental Protection Agency, (A-101F), Washington, DC (1988).
29. Risk Assessment Forum, Interim Procedures for Estimating Risks Associated with Exposures to Mixtures of Chlorinated dibenzo-p-dioxins and -dibenzofurans (CDDs and CDFs), U.S. Environmental Protection Agency, EPA/625/3-87/012 (1987).
30. National Academy of Sciences (NAS), *Pharmacokinetics in Risk Assessments, Drinking Water and Health*, Vol. 8, National Academy Press, Washington, DC (1987).
31. A. S. Whittemore, S. C. Grosser, and A. Silvers, Pharmacokinetics in Low Dose Extrapolation Using Animal Cancer Data, *Fund. Appl. Tox.* **7**:183-190 (1986).
32. U.S. Environmental Protection Agency, Update to the Health Assessment Document and Addendum for Dichloromethane (Methylene Chloride): Pharmacokinetics, Mechanisms of Action and Epidemiology, EPA/600/8-87/030A, Washington, DC (1987).
33. A. Weinberg, Science and Transcience, *Minerva* **10**:209-212 (1972).

The Impact of Risk Management Legislation on Small Counties

Raymond F. Boykin
California State University, Chico
Chico, CA

ABSTRACT

With the growing concern for hazardous materials and the way they are processed, stored, transported, and disposed of, numerous states have passed legislation dealing with these materials. In California, this legislation is known as the Risk Management and Prevention Program (RMPP). This paper deals with the impact that this new legislation has on small counties and their ability to deal with the level of responsibility required. A survey was performed to assess the level of RMPP implementation in all counties in California.

KEYWORDS: Risk management, risk legislation, hazardous materials

INTRODUCTION

With the growing amount of environmental legislation dealing with toxic chemicals in the last several years, small counties are experiencing a crisis in managing the situation. In California, several laws have been passed recently dealing with acutely hazardous materials. These laws now make up Article II of Chapter 6.95, State of California Health and Safety Code (hereafter known as the RMPP — Risk Management and Prevention Program.) This code requires county and/or municipal agencies (local fire departments or county health and environmental departments) to administer a risk management and prevention program. There are two specific requirements.

1. All facilities than handle at one time amounts of any extremely hazardous materials equal to or in excess of 500 pounds, 55 gallons, or 200 cubic feet of gas must submit an Acutely Hazardous Materials (AHM) Registration form to the local Administrative Agency (AA). An extremely hazardous substance is any chemical found on the U.S. EPA list of extremely hazardous substances [40 CFR (Code of Federal Regulations) part 355, Sections 302 and 304]. Local government may develop more stringent threshold standards and U.S. EPA, pursuant to Title III, may have lower threshold planning quantities.

2. The local AA may request the submission of an RMPP from facility operators as required. In most cases this will only include facilities which handle quantities of AHMs above the threshold quantities. However, the local AA has the authority to require an RMPP even if the amount of the AHM is less than the state threshold

Risk Analysis, Edited by C. Zervos
Plenum Press, New York, 1991

minimum, when the amount of material is perceived as presenting a significant risk to the public.

RISK MANAGEMENT AND PREVENTION PROGRAM

A guidance document for the preparation of an RMPP is being developed by a technical advisory committee, chaired by Dr. Fred Lercari (Office of Emergency Services, State of California). This document details the necessary elements of the RMPP as required by the state's health and safety code. Currently, the RMPP includes the following.

1. A list and a description of all AHM accidents in the last three years and corrective measures taken.
2. A list and a description of all AHM equipment.
3. Current design, operating, and maintenance procedures that deal with AHM accident risk.
4. Detection, monitoring, and control systems in the AHM facility.
5. The ongoing AHM risk management program.

The RMPP is to be supported by a hazard analysis which will include a hazard identification study, an external events impact analysis, a hazard likelihood assessment, and an offsite consequence analysis. The language in this part of the health and safety code is vague and confusing to individuals with little exposure to risk assessment methodologies. The guidance document that is being developed at this time will attempt to define this part of the RMPP. The AA also has the authority to request any additional technical information it deems to be important for the evaluation of the RMPP.

REGULATORY IMPACT

As can be seen from the cursory review of the health and safety code dealing with acutely hazardous material risk management, the impacts on the local AAs and the facility operators could be immense. For the local AA, the technical expertise for reviewing the RMPPs is very limited. Only a few of the larger counties in California have a staff with the technical ability to assess the RMPP. To substantiate this situation a survey of AAs was conducted. In the survey, all identified AAs were asked if they had an existing AHM registration program (the first requirement in the health and safety code). The survey questionnaire also asked if they were implementing the RMPP.

Survey Results

The survey included all AAs in California with responsibility for implementation of the RMPP. The responsible county level agencies were divided into two groups by total county population. All counties with less than 200,000 residents were labeled small counties (34); counties with more than 200,000 residents were labeled large counties (24). The results of the survey were sorted and tabulated by county size. Tables 1 through 3 present the results of the survey.

Of the counties responding, 55% have an active RMPP program. However, several of the counties with no current program stated that they were in the planning phases of developing a program.

Through subsequent communications with large county health officials, it was discovered that the single no response county does have an active program but failed to

Table 1. RMPP Survey Results — State Totals

	Number	Percentage (%)
No Response	7	12
No Current Program	23	40
Active Program	28	48

Table 2. RMPP Survey Results — Large Countries

	Number	Percentage (%)
No Response	1	4
No Current Program	4	17
Active Program	19	79

Table 3. RMPP Survey Results — Small Countries

	Number	Percentage (%)
No Response	6	18
No Current Program	19	56
Active Program	9	26

respond to the survey. If it was included in the active program category, then over 83% of the large counties would have active programs.

As can be seen from the survey data, large counties are much more likely to have a RMPP program in place than small counties. The survey indicated that of those counties responding, 83% of the large counties have an active program compared to only 32% of the small counties. An interesting fact that also surfaced during the survey was that 3 of the small counties have not even designated a responsible agency.

A majority of the small counties having no current program indicated in the survey that they had not yet begun to collect the AHM data required under Chapter 6.95 of the California Health and Safety Code. This data collection requirement in the code stipulated a January 1, 1988 compliance date. The survey was conducted in the later part of April 1988.

After the survey, several small counties were contacted informally to discuss the RMPP implementation issue. None of the counties contacted had any individual on their staff that understood the full technical requirements of the RMPP. Also, two of the large counties have indicated in discussions following the survey that they have no person on their staff with the experience they feel is necessary to review the RMPP document adequately.

FINANCIAL IMPACT

As with many new regulations in California, the local government is responsible for implementation and funding. No state financial support has been provided to assist the local AAs to implement and manage this program. It is evident from a recent discussion with several different county officials that this could create a situation where a company in a large county will be required to submit more rigorous RMPP and technical support documents than a company in a small county.

The smaller counties will not be able to afford the thorough review that an RMPP may receive in a larger county. A recently planned review of one RMPP in a large California county is expected to cost over $100,000. This amount could represent the entire annual health and safety budget for numerous small counties in California.

SUMMARY AND CONCLUSIONS

The total impact of the new risk management legislation in California has not been felt. Most counties, large and small, are still in the process of trying to determine the best course of action. However, the initial survey results are disheartening. At this time, the technical and financial capability to implement the RMPP does not exist in a majority of the counties in California.

It is not clear what the financial implications will be for industry. This legislation originally targeted chemical and allied industries. However, this sweeping legislation, with the large number of AHMs that it is attempting to regulate, is also impacting everyone from the local pest controller and dry cleaner to the large semiconductor manufacturer.

Community-Level Use of Risk Analysis: A Case Study

D. Amaral, R. Hetes, F. Lynn, and D. Austin
University of North Carolina
Chapel Hill, NC

ABSTRACT

The first few months of implementation of the risk analysis component of SARA Title III by Durham County, North Carolina, are described. Members of a subcommittee of the Local Emergency Planning Committee (LEPC) investigated the sources of potential release of extremely hazardous substances in the county, projected zones of vulnerability using specialized software, and identified segments of the community having the highest priority for emergency planning. Without the expert technical assistance that was volunteered or donated, the members of the Subcommittee could not have fulfilled their mission of using risk analysis to support the planning requirements of the law. The process of analysis itself may be credited with reduction of potential risk in the community.

KEYWORDS: Risk analysis, Local Emergency Planning Committee (LEPC), SARA Title III, community groups, emergency planning

INTRODUCTION

In 1986, in the wake of the Bhopal, India tragedy, in which more than 4,000 residents were killed because of exposure to methylisocyanate spewed from a Union Carbide pesticide plant, the U.S. Congress passed the Emergency Planning and Community Right-to-Know Law (Title III of the Superfund Amendments and Reauthorization Act). The purpose of Title III, as it is often called, was to provide citizens and emergency planners and responders information about hazardous substances that were being stored and used in their localities. If they knew what lay in their midst, they would be better prepared to handle an accident when it occurred and to give affected neighbors appropriate instructions on how to proceed. They would be able to work with facilities in an effort to prevent emergencies.

The law called for the creation of Local Emergency Planning Committees (LEPCs) and State Emergency Response Commissions (SERCs), which were to be broadly representative of the community and which were to receive data from companies on the amounts and locations of hazardous substances. In addition, the law required companies to submit annually to the State Emergency Response Commission and the U.S. EPA a list of the names and amounts of toxic chemicals they released into the air and water as part of regular plant operations. Title III allowed states to decide the geographic jurisdiction of a

LEPC. In North Carolina, the county unit was selected. Other states chose smaller units, while yet others declared their entire state one LEPC.

In North Carolina, the Division of Emergency Management was the lead agency for administering Title III. It prepared extensive guidelines[1] for local committees, with, *inter alia*, instructions to establish subcommittees, including one on hazard, vulnerability, and risk analysis. This paper analyzes the efforts of Durham County's Hazard, Vulnerability, and Risk Analysis Subcommittee to use the data provided by Title III to conduct a hazard or risk assessment. The assessment was conducted in order to identify places in the community particularly vulnerable to leaks or explosions.

Durham county (pop. 166,510) includes within its borders old and dying industries, e.g., tobacco and textiles, as well as high-tech companies, e.g., IBM and the experimental laboratories in Research Triangle Park. Even before the passage of the federal legislation, the city of Durham (pop. 150,000), had enacted the first Community Right-to-Know Law in the South, responding to a 1983 explosion requiring evacuation at a hazardous waste facility called Armageddon. With state and local funding, a citizen advisory board had, in addition, supervised a quantitative assessment of the hazards that the Armageddon plant posed.

Representation to be accorded groups, agencies and businesses on the Durham LEPC became one of very few issues briefly contested during the organizational process. In the initial formation of the LEPC, Durham Emergency Management staff appointed only one "community" representative—a staff attorney with the local legal services office—as suggested in State Emergency Response Commission (SERC) guidelines. However, that representative apprised several other community groups of their potential interest in the LEPC's deliberations and lobbied successfully for their representation on the LEPC. This explains why both the Durham LEPC and the Hazard, Vulnerability, and Risk Analysis Subcommittee (Subcommittee) composition was weighted more heavily on the side of community group representatives than were other LEPCs across the state.

Within the LEPC itself, eight community groups were represented—the overall LEPC composition is given in Table 1. Of the 42 members of the LEPC, eight were community group representatives, 16 were representatives of regulated facilities, and 14 represented providers of emergency services. Additionally, with funding from the Bauman Family Foundation, staff from the UNC-Chapel Hill Institute for Environmental Studies provided technical assistance to the LEPC and the Subcommittee.

Within the Subcommittee, the four community group representatives composed 25% of the total committee and 33% of the effective working Subcommittee.

Of the four community group representatives on the Subcommittee, three had relatively high levels of expertise in the risk assessment area and access to resources useful to the subcommittee. A representative of the local Sierra Club chapter was an environmental engineer working with the Research Triangle Institute on EPA waste disposal regulations. A representative of the League of Women Voters had extensive experience with environmental issues and access to computer expertise. A representative of a local political issues group was a Ph.D. student in environmental engineering. Only two representatives of regulated facilities regularly attended Subcommittee meetings. Each had technical hazard analysis backgrounds and positions in their firms; one was appointed chair of the committee.

In summary, the composition of the Subcommittee was relatively homogeneous in the area of technical expertise, while still representative of several important groups in the community. It is worth noting, however, that of the 11 firms which were eventually identified through the risk-screening process as users of "extremely hazardous substances"

Table 1. Composition of the LEPC and Subcommittee in Durham County
Number of Representatives, by Group

Committee or Subcommittee	Regulated Facility	Emergency Services Provider	Citizen Group	Media	I.E.S. Staff	Total
LEPC	16	14	8	2	3	43
Subcommittee	6	3	4	0	3	16
Subcommittee Effective Working Group*	2	2	3	0	3	10

*Includes only persons attending more than one meeting of the Subcommittee.

at levels which warranted further attention, only one was represented on the Subcommittee. (Five were represented on the LEPC as a whole, although there was a representative of Research Triangle Park, where several others were located.) The lack of representation of regulated facilities on the Subcommittee negated some of the potential benefits of participation in the hazard analysis process.

FORMATION OF HAZARD, VULNERABILITY, AND RISK ANALYSIS SUBCOMMITTEE

On April 6, 1988, the Subcommittee of the Durham County LEPC was officially formed. This Subcommittee has the responsibility to carry out analyses comprised of three major elements: hazard identification, vulnerability analysis, and risk analysis. These analyses provide the foundations for the work and activities of other subcommittees and the LEPC as a whole.

Hazard identification consists of the assessment of any situation that has the potential for causing injury to life, or damage to property and the environment. Hazard identification provides information on the identity, properties, location and quantity of chemicals within a region.

Vulnerability analysis describes the geographic area that might be affected if an incident were to occur. Major elements of vulnerability analysis are the identification of a vulnerable zone (the area most likely to receive the impact of a release), the human population within that zone, and critical facilities (e.g., hospitals, schools, nursing homes) or environmental features within that zone.

Risk analysis builds upon the previous two analyses and estimates the likelihood of an incident occurring and the severity of the consequences from such an incident.

THE SUBCOMMITTEE WISH LIST

The Subcommittee began meeting approximately six months before the deadline for the LEPC plan. The SERC guidelines were distributed but did not provide sufficient detail with which to begin analysis. Subcommittee members had some experience—enough to begin designing the analysis they wanted to see done. In several brainstorming sessions, Subcommittee members outlined the kind of information they wanted to obtain and delegated tasks to obtain data, maps and documents that might be needed. They also outlined the calculations they wanted to perform and began making plans to generate quantitative results that would inform the LEPC about the risks in the county.

An early problem was too much enthusiasm and not enough direction. Plans were made to obtain vast quantities of data without much regard for its usefulness. Of even greater concern was the lack of a concept among the members of what the whole LEPC could or would do with the information aggregated by the Subcommittee. A few meetings were spent recognizing these issues and addressing them. Some of the documents available from the state and the county suggested that the direct action for which planning would take place would be evacuation.[2,3] Indirectly, LEPC activities might lead facilities to take actions to reduce risks. No clear authority for the LEPC to require risk reduction could be identified by members of the Subcommittee.

The Subcommittee also recognized early on that there would be no resources for computing, staff work, materials or support available through SARA Title III. Several of the members arranged for their employers to provide resources such as photocopying, meeting space, and access to personal computers with spreadsheet software. These, and much of the members' time, were all donated voluntarily to permit the Subcommittee to function.

In designing its approach to analysis, the Subcommittee listed categories of harm that were of potential concern. These included long- and short-term harm to people, property, wildlife and the ecosystem. Members were concerned about the potential of emergency releases to contaminate the water supply and sensitive environmental areas, as much as the vulnerability of schools, hospitals, nursing homes, day care facilities and residential communities. They wanted to be able to calculate the total impact to each of these categories, in both acute and chronic terms, from the information obtained through the reporting requirements of the law. Information on facilities, substances, amounts and types of hazards would be filed with the LEPC in a few months, and they wanted to be able to take that information, make some calculations, and recommend priorities to the Planning Subcommittee.

The Subcommittee members described their desired calculations for each facility in a graph of likelihood of release vs. potential harm. Of highest priority would be facilities graphed furthest from the origin. The committee envisioned being able to plot each facility and place zones of low, medium and high overall risk within the graph. Members were concerned that much judgment would be required to determine what constituted a low or a high risk and were not at all certain how to go about determining this. In addition, it was not clear how to estimate the frequency or likelihood of a release from any given facility. A sketch of the graph drawn in one of the committee meetings is shown in Fig. 1.

Committee members wanted to be able to quantify risks for each category of potential harm and rate the categories relative to one another. In other words, they needed a way to trade off risks to one category, such as wildlife, with risks to another category, such as people in nursing homes. They discussed the possibility of developing weighting schemes that would allow them to represent the overall risk across all categories. Very quickly, the members realized that they would never be able to obtain the information needed to quantify such things as the response in wildlife to contamination from accidental releases, and that starting with risks to humans would be an appropriate approach, given their task and the potential actions likely to be considered in the plan. For a brief period, however, the members were speaking as if what they really wanted to be able to do was a full multi-attribute risk assessment to rank the facilities in the county.

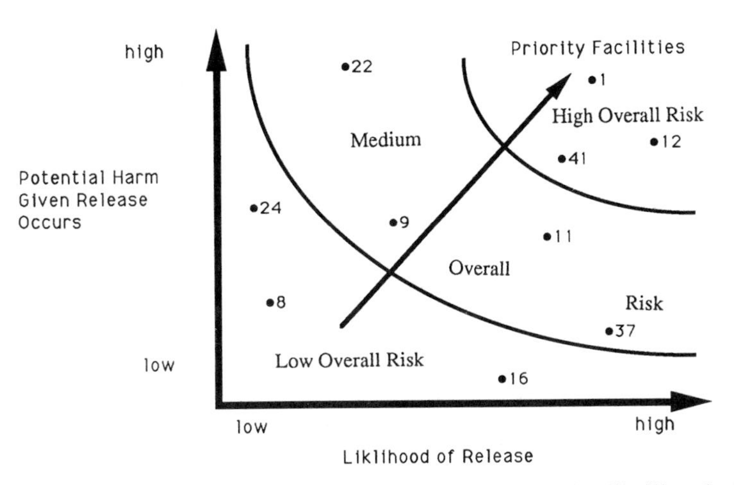

Fig. 1. Priority should be given to facilities for which both the likelihood of a release is high and the potential for harm given the occurrence of a release is also high. Points on graph are hypothetical facility numbers.

The authors provided some technical assistance at this stage, redirecting the efforts of the members, and helped focus them on tasks that would be tractable, given the purpose of the committee, the time constraints, and the information likely to be available. The authors had access to draft guidance documents being developed by the EPA and distributed copies of the sections concerning how to do a screening analysis. With this initial guidance in hand, the committee redefined its immediate tasks and got to work collecting data and putting facilities onto overlay maps.

The EPA guidelines[3] directed Subcommittee members to calculate the radius of vulnerability around a facility from data about the potential release. Tables are provided that give radii for discrete combinations of assumptions about the hazardous concentration in air, wind speed and type of terrain, and the amount of substance released. Appendices lead the reader to calculate the concentration level and release rate to use in reading the tables. The method used to generate the tables is not accurate below 0.1 miles or above 10 miles, and this is quickly observed when using the tables. It is not clear what one should do with a handful of facilities for which the radii are all greater than 10 miles. How does one discriminate?

Finding the information needed to do these calculations and actually doing them are tedious and error-prone tasks. Although the directions are straightforward, the task requires some technical background and some judgment about how to make assumptions and approximations appropriate to the physical situation. The only chemicals for which data are given to calculate radii are the substances on the EPA's Extremely Hazardous Substances list. Just locating the chemicals reported by the facilities in this list was a challenge to most of the members of the Subcommittee.

At about the same time that the committee began struggling with this screening analysis by hand, the authors learned of the availability of the CAMEO (Computer Aided Management of Emergency Operations) software and arranged to have it demonstrated during one of the Subcommittee meetings.[4] The authors assisted in implementing the Macintosh version to do the screening analysis. The screening analysis support provided in

CAMEO is identical to the approach in the EPA guidelines, using a radius of vulnerability calculated from the hazardous concentration and the same assumptions about the release conditions.

The CAMEO software facilitated the data gathering process. Most useful was the ability to identify the EHS list of chemicals automatically and look up the hazardous concentration to use in calculating the vulnerability zones. The software outputs have the same characteristic limitations as the hand calculations. For example, the technique is still limited to calculating radii between 0.1 and 10 miles.

HAZARD IDENTIFICATION

As part of the hazard identification process, the Subcommittee reviewed the Tier I and Tier II forms submitted under the requirements of SARA, Sections 311 and 312. A total of 59 reports were submitted from industries within the county. Twenty-one facilities reported information on the hazard group only (Tier I), 18 reported the presence of fuel storage only, and 20 reported information on specific chemicals (of these, three reported more than 50 chemicals; the others had less than 12 chemicals per facility).

Preliminary studies did not include the 3 facilities having greater than 50 chemicals. Review of the other facilities indicated that 43 different chemicals had been reported. Of these, 15 are on the Extremely Hazardous Substances list. Eight facilities reported chemicals listed as Extremely Hazardous Substances. The most frequently reported chemicals, excluding fuels, within the county (by number of facilities, not quantity) are shown in Table 2.

To identify the facilities which had not filed either Tier I or II forms but which still may have stored hazardous materials, a review of county records was undertaken by Standard Industrial Classification (SIC) codes and is presently being interpreted. Additionally, a review of existing records identified 465 gas stations in Durham County.

Other categories of fixed facilities which have been identified as potential handlers and storers of hazardous materials include hazardous waste generators regulated under The Resource Conservation and Recovery Act (RCRA) and farms or agricultural enterprises storing large quantities of fuels and pesticides. The Subcommittee has contacted both the Solid and Hazardous Waste Branch, North Carolina Department of Human Resources, and the Durham County Agriculture Extension for further information.

A review of reports[5] of past incidents has shown that transportation incidents involving gasoline and other petroleum products represent a significant portion of the risk from hazardous materials. The Subcommittee has targeted this as an issue of concern and has initiated efforts to obtain information on the type, quantity and route of transit of hazardous substances within the county. As this information is not presently available, the Subcommittee has made a request to the SERC to develop and implement a strategy to collect it. Until it becomes available, the vulnerability and risk analyses for transportation hazards cannot be done with confidence. When information is available on major hazardous materials transportation routes (both road and rail), transportation hazard identification will be carried out.

Initially the routes of concern are the major transportation routes, Interstates 40 and 85, and the railroad system. The interstates are known to be common transit routes for hazardous materials through Durham County, and Norfolk Southern and CSX are known to use the railway system through Durham County to transport hazardous materials. Hazardous material incidents have occurred on these routes in the past. Other local routes will be identified as more information becomes available.

Table 2. Most Frequently Reported Chemicals in Durham County

Sodium Hydroxide	Hydrogen Chloride*
Sulfuric Acid*	Hydrogen Fluoride*
Nitrogen	Carbon Dioxide
Argon	Hydrogen
Oxygen	Carbofuran*
Chlorine*	

*Chemicals listed in the EHS list.

VULNERABILITY ANALYSIS

The Subcommittee identified what were considered to be sensitive human sub-populations for hazardous materials incidents. These included schools, hospitals, nursing homes and day care centers. Once identified, they were also located on an overlay to a base map of the county. Environmental receptors of concern include surface waters and natural and cultural resources (e.g., sensitive habitat based on the county's natural resources inventory). The locations of these potential receptors were also plotted on an overlay to the county map.

The CAMEO software calculates zones of vulnerability based on the properties of chemicals present and quantity expected to be released in an incident. Areas are calculated based on dispersion predictions (under worst-case meteorological conditions), health information [e.g., levels Immediately Dangerous to Life and Health (IDLH)], occupational Threshold Limit Values (TLV), and any other relevant data, and the maximum quantity of chemicals stored at a particular site.

The CAMEO screening database and software package is limited to those substances designated as Extremely Hazardous. A preliminary calculation was made for the eight facilities (excluding the three with greater than 50 chemicals), and vulnerability zones of greater than 10 miles for each were calculated based on available information and conservative screening assumptions.

For this initial screening, the information input was limited to what was available at that time, which may lead to greatly exaggerated results. The quantity of chemicals was the upper value of the range of the code designated on the Tier II form. Actual total quantity stored may be significantly less, and the quantity in any one vessel (the maximum expected to be released) may be smaller still. For example, one facility reduced its actual inventory of chemicals by several orders of magnitude from the time of reporting. As a result, its vulnerability zone was reduced to less than 0.1 miles. Because of this, the Subcommittee has identified as a priority task obtaining more detailed information on actual quantities stored (both total amount and maximum single vessel or container). A letter requesting more detailed reporting is being developed for distribution to improve this database and thus obtain more realistic vulnerability zone predictions.

Additionally, the default meteorological conditions used for this screening may not be realistic. A revision of meteorological stability conditions in the calculation greatly changed the predicted vulnerability zone. While CAMEO can only directly calculate vulnerability zones for extremely hazardous substances, it does have an air model to calculate the same for other chemicals. This process, while much more tedious, will be carried out for facilities and chemicals indicated to be of sufficient concern to warrant such attention.

RISK ANALYSIS

The evaluation to date has shown that some facilities pose greater hazards than others within Durham County and require greater attention. However, due to lack of data, it is difficult to draw firm conclusions at this time. The initial screening has indicated what is required for further refinements: more detailed information on quantities of chemicals present and a better-defined most likely worst-case scenario for use in the severity and likelihood determinations. The three facilities having greater than 50 chemicals are assumed to be critical facilities unless an initial screening currently in progress indicates otherwise.

The only conclusion which can be reached from this initial hazard screening exercise is that none of the remaining seven facilities can be removed from consideration as critical. It is not known how many facilities should have reported but did not.

When realistic vulnerability zones are obtained, a designation of the level of risk (level of concern) can be made, depending on the area of vulnerability. The areas of vulnerability for fixed facilities will be plotted on an overlay of a map of the county. By comparing the overlays for the facilities and sensitive receptors, one can determine what population and receptors are within the predicted vulnerability zone. In this way, facilities will be designated as critical facilities in regard to the potential for harm (contained within the vulnerability zone). Sensitive receptors at risk will also be identified and targeted for planning efforts to reduce risk and to develop evacuation and response plans. The Subcommittee has passed a motion to select a community in an area of concern to become a model for others in the development of evacuation plans and overall planning. A community or neighborhood within East Durham will be selected to begin this process.

One feature of CAMEO not yet implemented by the Subcommittee is the large database of hazardous substances not on the EPA's EHS list. When combined with the more sophisticated atmospheric dispersion model also provided in CAMEO, this database will allow members to examine other substances reported by the facilities in the county and obtain more detailed information about the vulnerability zones. For example, at the screening level, the calculations produce a simple radius. The air model produces a teardrop-shaped prediction of the zone that is probably more realistic. This capability comes at the cost of a requirement for more sophisticated input data, which the Subcommittee may or may not be able to obtain.

Neither the EPA guidelines nor the CAMEO software provide help on the prediction of the likelihood of releases from facilities. This task is almost beyond the capabilities of the Subcommittee members. Past emergency and transportation accident records are hardly useful in predicting the next Bhopal-like event to occur in Durham. For this knowledge, the members realize that they will need to obtain support from the technical staff of the facilities, who can explain potential weaknesses in the processes, storage practices, etc. Obtaining candid cooperation in this endeavor will be very challenging and will require additional screening to make sure the effort is directed to the most appropriate facilities.

EXPECTATIONS ABOUT TITLE III

From the experience of the Durham County LEPC, it appears that the expectations raised by the scope of Title III may be unrealistic. Even though Subcommittee members brought talent, training, motivation and personal resources to their tasks, the requirements for doing a complete risk analysis may have exceeded their capabilities. The biggest limitations have been lack of time and access to useful information. Adequate amounts of each of these may never be available, so in reflecting on whether doing risk analysis is worthwhile, it helps to consider the benefits that have come from the experience of the Subcommittee.

If the conduct and the results of the risk analysis are to be more realistic and informative, several additional needs must be met. Better guidance and training is needed, and much sooner. Participants might not have been able to accomplish nearly this much without the assistance of the authors. We can say this with confidence, since the EPA documents and workshops were not made generally available until late summer, leaving almost no time in which to actually conduct the analysis. The access to educational opportunities has also been severely limited. Finally, better information is needed from the facilities, such as actual quantities and maximum container size, before meaningful risk calculations can be produced.

The Durham experience is not typical for North Carolina and probably not for the country, but it is instructive and suggests ways to make the hazard assessment phase of Title III more workable. Durham's tradition of citizen activism and cooperation between government, citizens, and industry is important in understanding the success of the Risk Assessment and Hazard Evaluation Subcommittee. The temptation in Title III is to turn the process of implementation over to paid staff. This did not happen in Durham. While the Durham assistant emergency manager was an active member of the Subcommittee, the bulk of the work was conducted by citizen volunteers and industry representatives. They spent many volunteered hours plotting maps and crunching numbers through a computer. While the U.S. EPA and NOAA provided manuals and software, without the technical assistance and time volunteered by faculty, staff and students from neighboring UNC-CH, the vulnerability and risk scenarios would not have been conducted with the degree of precision that they were.

The Durham experience shows the importance of involving the entire community. Enlarging the LEPC to include more citizen group representatives is important to the group's vitality. The subcommittee was regularly attended by 8-10 members, and attendance at the LEPC's regular meetings ranged from 30 to 50.

Of these benefits, perhaps the most significant is that the risk analysis activity itself performed as a communication and consensus generating tool. The participants in the screening analysis brought together the pieces of information about their county for the first time, and as a group could begin to see where the most vulnerable communities might be located. As they worked together to create the lists of hospitals, schools, gas stations, and industrial facilities, and the screening zones around the facilities, and as they began to put this information to use, the members were building a structure for future risk analyses. They were sharing information, identifying needs, and observing the implications of the initial analysis together. Given the make-up of the representation on the Subcommittee, this experience alone is remarkable and demonstrates how Title III is working to build community cooperation that may eventually lead to a significant reduction in risk.

It may be unrealistic, however, to expect most LEPCs to have the hardware and software, and more importantly the skills to conduct the type of hazard assessment EPA would like to have. Title III did not provide funds for the committee. The North Carolina legislature allocated money for staff to serve LEPCs. Durham's regional planner, however, was not involved in the hazard assessment exercise as he was hired late in the process. In Durham, the Emergency Management Assistance Agency (EMAA) committed staff time. Industry has recently contributed a computer to the EMAA office.

Hazard evaluation can be conducted at the local level. Ideally, industries should conduct the assessments themselves and provide the information to the community.

Evidently some large companies have provided such assessments in other U.S. communities. If this is not possible, however, LEPCs will need to obtain funds through fees on industry to buy software and hardware and, if necessary, get technical assistance to understand and run the software programs.

While the conduct of the hazards assessment is important, it could prove to be a sterile exercise unless it is successfully incorporated into the emergency plan and used to work with industry to improve the storage and handling of hazardous materials. This is the next step in Durham's efforts to prevent the accidents and leaks that have occurred in the past and could happen in Durham in the future.

REFERENCES

1. North Carolina Division of Emergency Management, *Guidebook for Local Emergency Planning Committees.*
2. National Response Team, *Hazardous Materials Emergency Planning Guide*, March 1987.
3. U.S. EPA, FEMA, and U.S. DOT, *Technical Guidance for Hazards Analysis: Emergency Planning for Extremely Hazardous Substances*, December 1987.
4. National Oceanic and Atmospheric Administration and U.S. EPA, *The CAMEO™ II Manual: Advance Copy*, May 1988.
5. Durham County Office of Emergency Management, *Incident Reports*, 1985-1988.

Diffusion of Emergency Warning: Comparing Empirical and Simulation Results

George O. Rogers and John H. Sorensen
Oak Ridge National Laboratory
Oak Ridge, TN

ABSTRACT

As officials consider emergency warning systems to alert the public to potential danger in areas surrounding hazardous facilities, the issue of warning system effectiveness is of critical importance. The purpose of this paper is to present the results of an analysis on the timing of warning system information dissemination including the alert of the public and delivery of a warning message. A general model of the diffusion of emergency warning is specified as a logistic function. Alternative warning systems are characterized in terms of the parameters of the model, which generally constrain the diffusion process to account for judged maximum penetration of each system for various locations and likelihood of the public's being in those places by time of day. The results indicate that either telephone ring-down warning systems or tone-alert radio systems combined with sirens provide the most effective warning system under conditions of either very rapid onset, close proximity or both. These results indicate that single technology system provide adequate warning effectiveness when available warning time (after detection and the decision to warn) extends to as much as an hour. Moreover, telephone ring-down systems provide similar coverage at approximately 30 minutes of available public warning time.

KEYWORDS: Emergency warning, warning diffusion, chemical spills, warning systems, warning contagion

INTRODUCTION

Under the Emergency Planning and Community Right to Know Act [also known as Title III of the Superfund Amendments and Reauthorization Act (SARA)], communities are required to develop emergency response plans for fixed-site facilities that store hazardous chemicals. A critical part of that planning is the means to warn the public in the event of a release. Emergency warning systems for potentially hazardous facilities must be effective, and effectiveness depends on a number of factors. How many people will be alerted to hazards presented by potential emergencies? How will they know what to do in response to such signals? When will they receive the warning? This paper analyzes the dissemination of warning information; it deals with alerting the public and delivering a warning message.

A general logistic model for the diffusion of emergency warning is specified. Each alternative warning system is characterized in terms of the influence of the model parameters on the maximum penetration of each system. The parameters include locations

Risk Analysis, Edited by C. Zervos
Plenum Press, New York, 1991

and the likelihood of the public's being in those places by time of day. There are four independent warning systems that are considered separately:

1. a system consisting of sirens and alarms, prompting people to obtain additional warning information from the media;
2. a system comprised of tone-alert radios which are centrally activated and subsequently broadcast a warning message;
3. a system using automatic-dialing telephone systems, which hang up all telephones in the system, block out incoming calls, and then ring the phones and play a warning message; and
4. a dual media and route alerting system in which the Emergency Broadcast System (EBS) is activated and officials go through areas at risk to disseminate the warning.

Alternatives are then combined to achieve maximum warning system effectiveness. These two combined systems are as follows:

1. a combination siren- and tone-alert-radio system and
2. a telephone ring-down and siren system.

The probability that people located at various distances from a hazardous facility will receive a warning before exposure to airborne releases of toxic materials is compared for each warning system under three scenarios of hazard-onset speed. This analysis integrates a complex set of information to assist emergency managers in selecting effective emergency warning systems for use in conjunction with potentially hazardous facilities.

THE WARNING PROCESS

Warning people of impending danger encompasses two conceptually distinct aspects—alerting and notification. Alerting deals with the ability of emergency officials to make people aware of an imminent hazard. Alerting frequently involves the technical ability to break routine acoustic environments to cue people to seek additional information. In contrast, notification focuses on how people interpret the warning message. People's interpretation of the warning message is critically important in their selection of appropriate behavior in response to emergency warnings.

Emergency warning messages are received through a series of pathways that color their meaning. Some of this coloring is the result of cognitive processes; some is the result of the social structure. People interact with others, forming social networks, even though the forms of these networks vary. The routine and established nature of social networks has led to widely accepted generalizations concerning their function in society.[1,2,3,4] Social networks also function in emergency situations and shape the response to emergency warnings. Two general propositions are strongly supported by the disaster literature.[5]

1. People respond to emergency warnings in the context of prior experience and the existing social and physical environs that interact with the warning message; and
2. The extent to which the warning message is received depends on the nature of the warning message and the prior behaviors of all social actors.

Emergency warning messages are processed in the context of the social network. This means that people have pre-existing estimates of the threats presented by their environments. Furthermore, these estimates, together with personal experience, provide the basis for selecting behavior (i.e., whether to accept, ignore, disseminate, challenge, or confirm the warning message).[6]

One of the results of an emergency warning is the recognition of threat, which creates psychological discomfort. Many people alleviate this discomfort by reducing the uncertainty associated with the message.[7] The warning process (Fig. 1) involves factors that affect both the message and the characteristics of the receiver[8] or the sender and receiver.[9] Once the warning is received, its content is evaluated in terms of the certainty and ambiguity associated with the event—its estimated severity, timing and location of impact. This evaluation considers the likelihood of personal impact (will it affect me?), timing of impact (when will it occur?), and its anticipated effects (is the threat significant?).[10,11] The evaluation of the warning message leads to the determination of its relevance, which in turn leads to the perception of personal risk. If the message content is deemed irrelevant (I am not at risk), no emergency response is likely to ensue. However, should the warning message be considered relevant (I may be at risk), the message is processed in the context of prior disaster experience, relative proximity to the source of disaster, confidence in the source of warning, interpretation of the warning, and discussion with members of the social network. The warning message is processed in the context of the existing social structure, which leads to the initial perception of threat. The cumulative process provides the foundation for the selection and evaluation of emergency response behavior.

However, the warning response process is not a linear stimulus-response process.[12] The first issuance of warning sets in motion an information-seeking process by which people attempt to confirm and reconfirm the contents of the warning,[13] and to discover what friends, neighbors, or relatives are doing in response to the warning.[9] As a result, members of the public become part of the informal warning system by disseminating the message further.[8]

Public response to emergency warnings is heavily influenced by warning content. Janis[14] describes effective warning messages as requiring a balance between fear-arousing and fear-reducing statements. Fear-arousing statements provide sufficient description of the impending danger to evoke vivid mental images of the potential crises which reduce the chance of surprise as the event evolves. Fear-reducing statements present the realistic mitigating factors of the situation, while providing information concerning realistic responses by both authorities and individuals. The fear-arousing content of the warning message alerts the public to the potential for harm, whereas the fear-reducing content provides notification of appropriate avoidance, protective, and mitigative emergency actions. Empirical research provides ample evidence of the message factors that shape response.[9] These factors include credibility of the warning source; clarity, consistency, accuracy, and detail of the information; and frequency of the message issuance.

DIFFUSION OF EMERGENCY WARNINGS

The diffusion of emergency warnings resembles diffusion of other types of information or communication, except that it occurs over a shorter time period. The basic mathematical function is a logistic function. The cumulative proportion of people receiving the warning forms an S-curve which is determined by the exponential form of the initial alerting process and the logistic form of the subsequent contagion of the warning and message through the population.[8]

The alerting, characterized as a "broadcast process" that disseminates the emergency warning, is centralized in the sense that many are alerted simultaneously. Contagion, on the other hand, is characterized as a "birth process" whereby people first hear of the event and then sequentially tell others.[15] The general mathematical specification of the diffusion curve is

$$dn/dt = k[a_1(N - n)] + (1 - k)\,[a_2 n(N - n)]\,.$$

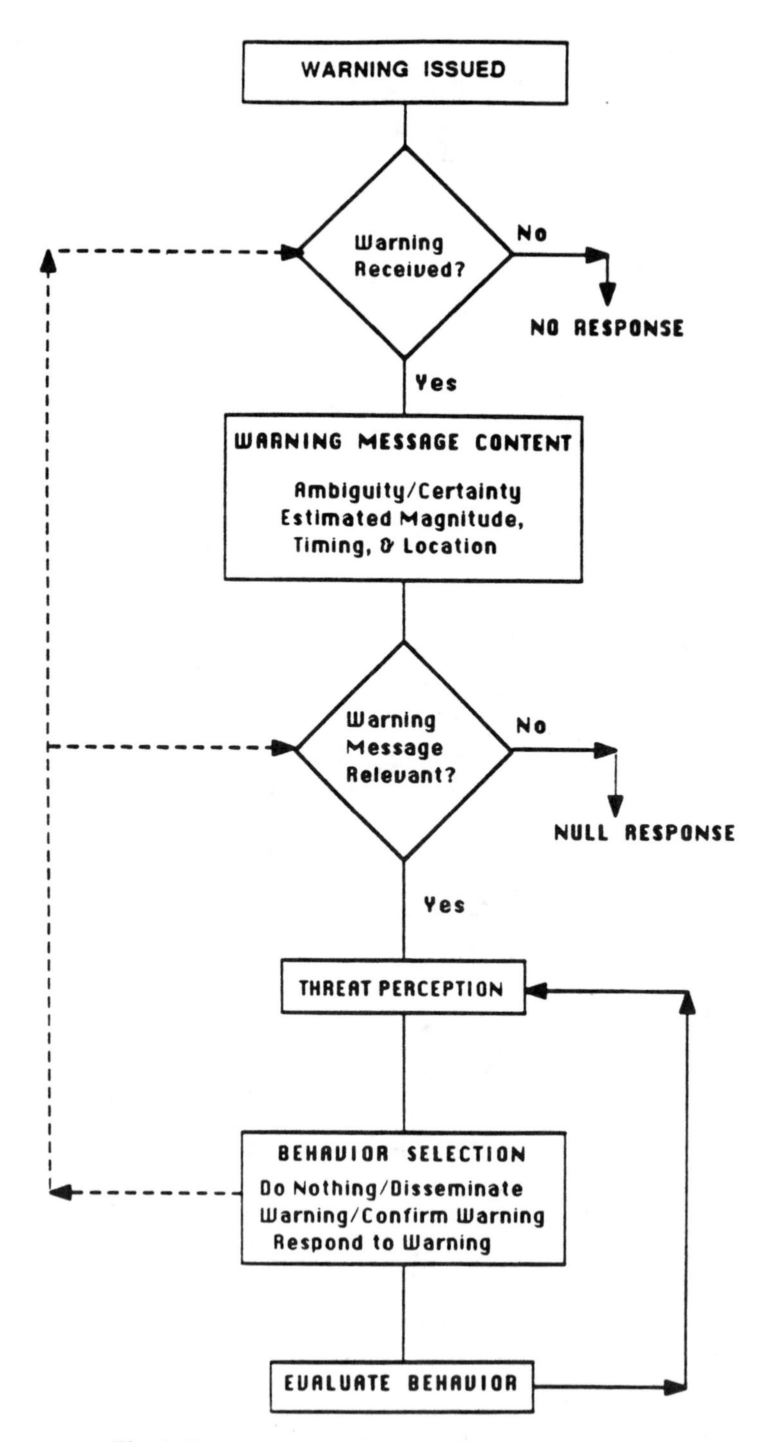

Fig. 1. Emergency warning and response process.

where k is the portion of the population alerted via the broadcast process, that is, the proportion of people who are alerted to the potential for harm who immediately recognize the meaning of the alert signal. The quantity $(1 - k)$ represents the proportion of people left to be warned. The broadcast parameter, a_1, summarizes the efficiency of the alerting process, and the birth parameter, a_2, summarizes the effectiveness of the contagion process. N is the proportion of the population to be warned, and n is the proportion warned at the beginning of each period $(t_0,t_1,...,t_i,...)$. Because each warning system provides differing degrees of information concerning the appropriate action to protect oneself from harm, or to mitigate the potential for harm, the broadcast and birth parameters represent the dependence of each system on alerting and contagion, respectively. For example, the contagion parameter for a siren system will be relatively high because it depends on recipients taking an active role in their own warning (i.e., they must do something). Usually this entails seeking further information via another (secondary) source.

DATA AND METHODS

Ideally, the process of estimating diffusion curves would first gather data concerning the timing of individual receipt of warnings in historical warning events that used different warning systems and then fit a logistic curve to the data and empirically derive the parameters. Unfortunately, due to methodological problems, reliable data of this kind do not exist. The most serious problem is obtaining data that are relatively free of recall problems. One such problem is the "suspended" time often reported by disaster victims. Typical interpretations of duration are seldom valid in emergencies.[16,17,18] Another form of this problem occurs as a function of time and the dissipation of accuracy in time estimates. Another problem is simply that the heterogeneity of accidents and disasters makes cross-hazard comparison, or even comparison within a single hazard (when other significant differences exist), difficult at best.

The method used here first specifies the parameters of the model based on the character of these warning systems, which are based on a limited set of data from warning events. The diffusion curve is then mathematically generated. And finally, they are fit to some limited data from several different disasters. This method provides a greater validity than would be obtained through simulation alone. The parameters are assigned to reflect the qualitative differences in warning systems. The results of this procedure are summarized in Table 1.

These warning diffusion curves are then compared with four warning cases where reasonably continuous data concerning receipt of first warning were collected: First, warning in two communities 20 miles (i.e., Toutle/Silverlake) and another that is approximately 35 miles (i.e., Woodland) from the cone of Mt. St. Helens as reported by Lindell and Perry.[19] Toutle and Silverlake are less than a mile apart and lie in flood plains of rivers that drain the Mt. St. Helens area; these were combined into a single sample. Woodland is on the Lewis River on the southwest side of the mountain. The second case involves two train derailments in western Pennsylvania, one in Pittsburgh and the other in Confluence.

Approximately 10 percent of the residents of Toutle, Silverlake and Woodland were sampled. The interviews were conducted in August and September 1980, approximately 10 to 18 weeks after the May 18, 1980 eruption. The completion rate for interviews conducted in Toutle/Silverlake was 89%, while the completion rate in Woodland was 90%. The data collection method is described in greater detail by Perry, Greene and Lindell.[20]

Two surveys of residents in the Bloomfield section of Pittsburgh were conducted by the University Center for Social and Urban Research at the University of Pittsburgh (UCSUR). The self-administered mail-back survey was distributed to 750 households in the

Table 1. Model Parameters Used to Estimate Diffusion of Warnings

System	k	Alerting Parameter		Contagion Parameter		30-minute limit	Release rate (%)
		Dependency	a_1	Dependency	a_2		
Sirens	0.2	Low	0.2	High	0.3	0.75	0.3
Tone-alert radios	0.4	High	0.3	Low	0.2	0.90	0.1
Media	0.3	Moderate	0.2	Moderate	0.25	0.50	0.5
Telephones	0.4	Very high	0.35	Low	0.2	0.93	0.1
Siren and tone-alert	0.4	High	0.3	High	0.3	0.95	0.1
Siren and telephone	0.4	Very high	0.35	High	0.3	0.95	0.1

emergency area in mid-June 1987, approximately 9 weeks after the April 11, 1987 accident. These households proportionally represent the 1980 population residing in each Census tract in the affected area of the city. Households were selected from each street in each Census tract in the affected area to assure even coverage. No follow-up letter or contact was initiated by UCSUR, although the cover letter gave contact information for respondent-initiated follow-up. A total of 220 questionnaires were returned by mid-August, yielding a response rate of 29.3%. In addition, 129 telephone interviews of area residents were made between July 14 and 22, 1987. A non-systematic, non-random procedure was used by UCSUR to represent each street in the impacted area. A total of 214 working residential telephones were selected, representing households in the affected area and not selected for study via the mail-back survey. A three call-back procedure is employed by UCSUR, which means three attempts to complete the interview are made at various times-of-the-day and days-of-the-week for each selected number. This procedure yielded an effective response rate of 60.3%. When combined, the two surveys represent 7000 households in the Bloomfield area; 349 completed instruments constitute a combined response rate of 36.2%.

Approximately 12% of the listed and unlisted residential telephone numbers in Confluence were sampled. The interviews were conducted from October 20 to 28, 1987, approximately 22 weeks after the May 6, 1987 accident and precautionary evacuation. Interviews with 106 residents of Confluence resulted in an 89.8% response rate. The method is discussed in greater detail by Snyder and Schlarb.[21]

SPECIFYING THE DIFFUSION MODEL

As with any simulation process, the selection of the parameters of the model is critical and tends to become the central focus of discussion of the simulation results. Alternative parameters for such simulations can be examined, adjusted, and analyzed as more empirical evidence becomes available.

The proportion of people receiving the alert signal and immediately recognizing its meaning, k, depends on the capability of the warning system to produce a signal that will be heard and understood immediately. The choice of k reflects the partition between people fully warned via the warning system (broadcast), including both alerting and notification, and those warned through contagion, requiring a secondary step of notification (birth). Warning systems which alert people to the potential for harm and which clearly and immediately notify them of appropriate protective action depend on the broadcast process. Telephone and tone-alert radio systems and systems combining telephones and tone-alert radios with sirens are the systems that are most dependent on the broadcast process. At the other end of the spectrum, siren systems depend on a second step in the warning process that requires the recipient to acquire information concerning appropriate action from another (secondary) source. Media-based systems are moderately dependent on the broadcast process.

Warning systems that include systems based on telephone and radio-alert are least dependent on the contagion process. Siren-based systems, however, are highly dependent on contagion in that people are not likely to know what to do. Media-based systems are moderately dependent on contagion. Because some members of society cannot be expected to understand the meaning of warning signals regardless of their effectiveness, all emergency warning systems depend on the contagion process to some extent. For example, no one expects all children to comprehend the warning message and be able to carry out protective action. Dependency on contagion also occurs because of the complexity of the warning process. Emergency warning is not a simple stimulus-response situation. The simplified warning process depicted in Figure 1 represents a complex of social and psychological processes which suggest that people will seek additional information to reduce uncertainty.[8,9,11,]

The alerting parameter, a_1, depends on the efficiency of the broadcast process. It reflects the ability of the warning system to reduce uncertainty through the broadcast process. The alerting parameter, a_1, represents the proportion of previously unwarned people who are warned (including both alerting and notification) during the period t_i to t_{i+1} via the broadcast process. The selection of the exponential growth curve thus represents the efficiency of the broadcast process in providing complete warning.

The most efficient warning system is a telephone system because most people hear and answer phones when they ring. Furthermore, nearly all will listen to the message, particularly if the message makes it clear that "this is an emergency." The telephone system also offers the recipient two-way communication via information numbers, further reducing uncertainty by providing additional information. Tone-alert radios are slightly less efficient than the telephones because some people will not hear the radio activate, some will have trouble understanding the message, and radios are one-way communication channels. Although these differences are subtle, they are likely to reduce efficiency. The media has a low alerting parameter because at any given time, including peak use hours, the vast majority of people are not engaged with the electronic media. Media-based systems work only if the recipient happens to be listening at the time of warning. This means that people must act by coincidence prior to the warning.

Siren systems are less efficient than other systems for a variety of reasons. The most important reason is the dependence of siren-based systems on an active participation in the warning process. People must do something immediately to find out what the siren means, which protective actions are required, and how to take them. A number of factors contribute to one's not hearing the siren(s), not recognizing its meaning or not recognizing that a warning situation exists when the siren is heard.

The contagion parameter, a_2, is based on the efficiency of the birth process. It reflects the ability of the warning system to reduce uncertainty through the contagion of warning. The contagion parameter, a_2, represents the proportion of previously unwarned people who are warned (including both alerting and notification) during the period t_i to t_{i+1} via the birth process. The selection of the logistic growth curve represents the efficiency of the birth process in providing complete warning.

Siren systems are evaluated as highly dependent on people's search for additional information to determine the meaning of the siren signal. However, once such information is sought, which is represented as $1 - k$, the notification is assumed to be quite effective (i.e., a_2 is relatively high). This occurs because people actively seeking information are more receptive of the information provided (i.e., they are listening).

Media-based warning systems are characterized by a process in which people hear a warning and tell others to listen. Hence, these systems are moderately dependent on the birth process for initial alerting, even though they are relatively effective in notifying people who are tuned in about what to do. Both media- and siren-based systems depend on contagion $(1 - k)$. However, the former requires contagion for initial alerting that an emergency exists, and the latter requires it for notification of appropriate protective actions to be taken. Because siren-based systems represent official warning, they are expected to be slightly more efficient than media-based systems that require social network alerting. Systems based on tone-alert radios and autodial telephones are least dependent on contagion $(1 - k)$; in addition, they can provide information only to limited numbers of people at one time. They are therefore judged to have the least efficient contagion process, represented by low contagion parameters.

Limits on the diffusion rates were imposed based on judgments of the level of warning that could theoretically occur in the next 30 minutes (t_i to t_{i+30}) under good warning conditions. These limits were derived from empirical observations and their extrapolation.[22] Because warning is a cumulative process, all systems are expected to warn almost 100% of the population at some point. The initial limits imposed on each system are presented in Table 1. To represent the cumulative nature of the process, the initial limits are gradually released throughout the warning period. This is equivalent to recognizing that the capability to warn people in the next 30 minutes depends in part on the number warned in previous periods. For example, warning in the next 30 minutes has only 30 minutes initially, but 10 minutes into the warning period, the cumulative warning window time is 40 minutes. The release rate values in Table 1 allow the limits imposed on each system to increase, approaching 100% of the population warned in the long run. Conceptually, the release rate characterizes the constraints associated with different warning systems.

Because of the synergistic effect associated with combined systems, the parameter specification for them selects the least restrictive release rate associated with the two combined systems. This reflects the complementary nature of the combined systems, providing the primary reason for using the two systems. All emergency warning systems depend on the contagion process.

ADJUSTING FOR LOCATION AND TIME OF DAY

Warning systems are generally characterized by their ability to alert people and transfer information. The penetration of the emergency warning systems varies for people in different locations and engaged in different activities. Each warning system has a different penetration capability in five fundamental locations/activities: (1) home asleep, (2) indoors at home or in the neighborhood, (3) outdoors in neighborhood, (4) in transit, and (5) working or shopping. In addition, two activities are allowed to "override" the other locations/activities, that is, watching television and listening to the radio. Such electronic-media-"exposed" activities are relevant for warning because some of the systems depend on these forms of media. Figure 2 summarizes the average percentage of the population in these location/activity categories over a 24-hour period starting with 12 midnight.[23] Table 2 provides estimates of the percentage of the population reached by each warning system

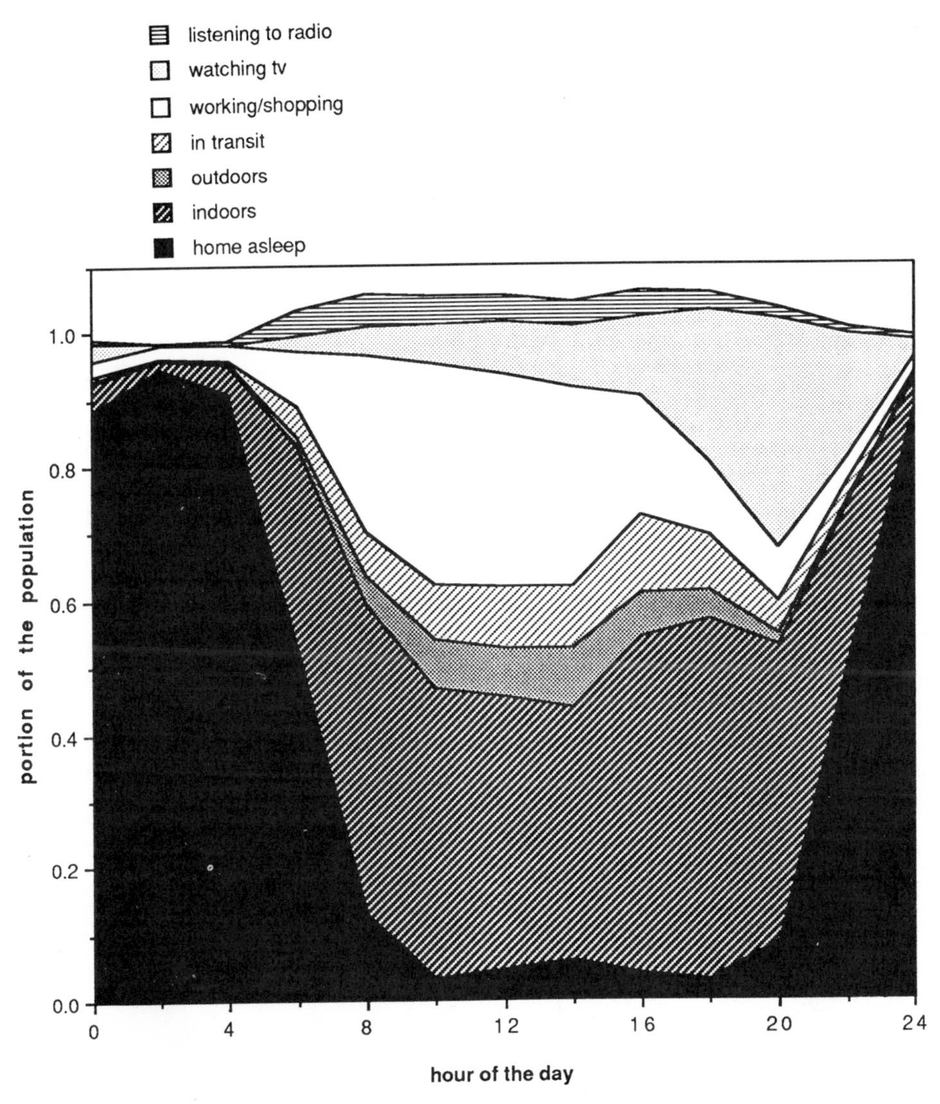

Fig. 2. Average time budget.

while engaged in the different activities. The effect of these locations is presented in greater detail in Ref. 24. The logical process is illustrated through the discussion of the effects of being at home asleep.

One of the most vulnerable positions, at least in terms of perception, occurs when people are at home asleep. In a regional survey, Nehnevajsa[25] asked people what kinds of things awaken them at night, for example, between 2 a.m. and 4 a.m. The results indicated that 69.1% of the residents in southwestern Pennsylvania are aroused from sleep by sirens in their area, and 93.3% reported that telephone calls wake them up. These empirical data are used as estimates of the penetration rate for the siren and alarm and the telephone ring-down systems, respectively. Because tone-alert radios are similar to telephones but may or may not be physically located in the bedroom, as are many phones, the penetration rate for tone-alert radios is estimated at 85%. Furthermore, because media and the emergency broadcast system are dependent on having either a radio or a TV on at the time of warning

Table 2. Warning Systems Effectiveness by Location and Activity

Location/Activities Alarms	Alternative Warning Systems				Siren and Alarm Systems Combined With	
	Sirens and Radios	Tone-Alert Phones	Auto-Dial Media	EBS/ Radios	Tone-Alert Phones	Auto-Dial
Assumed Penetration by Location/Activity						
Home asleep*	0.691	0.85	0.933	0.0	0.90	0.933
Indoors at home or in neighborhood	0.80	0.90	0.95	0.40	0.90	0.95
Outdoors in neighborhood	0.90	0.0	0.0	0.20	0.90	0.90
In transit	0.90	0.0	0.0	0.20	0.90	0.90
Working or shopping	0.60	0.70	0.80	0.10	0.70	0.80
Television	N/A	N/A	N/A	1.0	N/A	N/A
Radio	N/A	N/A	N/A	1.0	N/A	N/A
Time-Adjusted Warning System Effectiveness						
Annual average	0.665	0.685	0.745	0.287	0.784	0.826

*Reported arousal by sirens and telephones is derived from a survey in 1985 by the University of Pittsburgh, Center for Social and Urban Research. (See Ref. 25.)

and because most people do not sleep with them on, the penetration rate is assumed to be zero for media/EBS warning systems.

Existing data are used to estimate directly the parameters of some systems and logically extended to reflect the known characteristics of the other warning systems. People who are watching television or listening to the radio are assumed to be engaged with the media, so that they would be warned even if they are doing other things while they are watching TV or listening to the radio. For example, people that are working around the house while listening to the radio would be likely to receive emergency warning broadcast on that medium.

ADJUSTING FOR HOW PEOPLE SPEND THEIR TIME

The probability that people would be located in a specific location was estimated on the basis of data collected by the Survey Research Center at the University of Michigan for a national probability sample of U.S. households in 1975 and again in 1981.[23,26] This analysis employs a daily schedule data structure.[27] Figure 2 summarizes the average annual daily time budget.

Each type of warning system is evaluated in terms of the likelihood that people in the different locations will be warned; moreover, the locational capabilities of each system are mapped onto the probability that people will be in these locations at various times of the day. This mapping of locational system effectiveness on the likelihood of the presence of people in these locations provides a relative effectiveness in terms of the likelihood that people will be engaged in various activities in various locations (Table 2).

The warning dissemination process is adjusted to account for time-dependent activities by multiplying the location activity adjustment factor in Table 2 by the average portion of the population engaged in each activity in a 24-hour period. This value represents the portion of the population in each activity assumed to receive the warning. This is then summed for each warning system to achieve the time-adjusted warning system effectiveness score. The resulting score is then used to weight the original alerting parameter (a_1) in the diffusion model. This weighting reduces the influence that the initial alert has on diffusion according to the average distribution of people in various activities who would not receive an initial alert. The time adjusted model was run with these parameters to derive the adjusted curves of Fig. 3. This procedure can also be altered slightly to produce time-specific curves to reflect the locations/activities of the population for any 2-hour period.

EMPIRICAL FIT WITH EXISTING DATA

The warning diffusion curves, which are now adjusted for location-specific penetration on the basis of the likelihood that people will be in a specific location, are presented, with six empirical cases of emergency warnings. The first case represents an emergency warning summary of the Big Thompson Flood of 1977.[28] The study found that approximately 30% of the population a received warning in a manner other than by seeing the water coming. It is difficult to estimate how much time was spent warning people. The incident suggests that downstream residents received a 45-minute warning time, whereas residents further upstream had only a 15-minute warning. The average of 30 minutes is employed here. The second observation is the Fillmore Flood, in which 72% of the population at risk were warned in about 60 minutes.[10] There are two observations at the 2-hour mark: one reports a complete warning of nearly 100% during the Mississauga chemical accident;[29] in the other incident, the Sumner flood, 84% of the population were warned in about a 2-hour period.[10] Two additional cases are reported with an approximately 2.5-hour warning time: a 96% warning is reported by Perry and Mushkatel[30] in response to a nitric acid spill in Denver, Colorado; in the Mt. Vernon, Washington, chemical accident, 82% were notified as the result of emergency response effort.[30] Figure 4 qualitatively compares siren- and media/EBS-based warning systems with these empirically observed emergency warnings.

The data from the two train derailments and Mt. St. Helens concerning the receipt of warning are compared with the siren- and media-based systems in Fig. 5 in terms of the cumulative proportion warned by time into the event. The measurement difficulties are clearly evidenced by the proportion of respondents that reported receiving warning prior to the occurrence of the train derailments. This seems to occur at least partially because of the way people think about and recall time. For example, the noontime Pittsburgh event actually occurred at 12:25 p.m., but many of those reporting warning receipt prior to that time said they were warned at noon. It is not hard to construct that many people would recall the time in terms of what they were doing at the time (e.g., eating lunch) and report it as noon (i.e., 12:00 p.m.). The proportion warned initially (i.e., at the time of the eruption) is assumed to be zero in the communities impacted by the eruption of Mt. St. Helens.

The communities of Toutle and Silverlake were assessed at greater risk prior to the eruption than Woodland. As a consequence the sheriff's office made special efforts to make

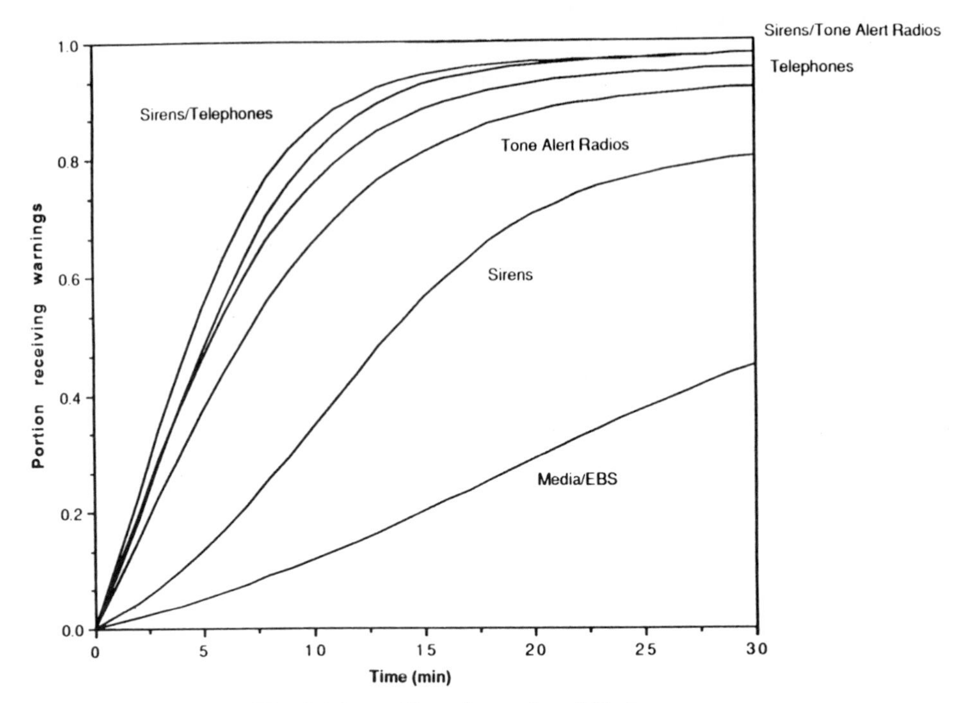

Fig. 3. Time adjusted warning diffusion.

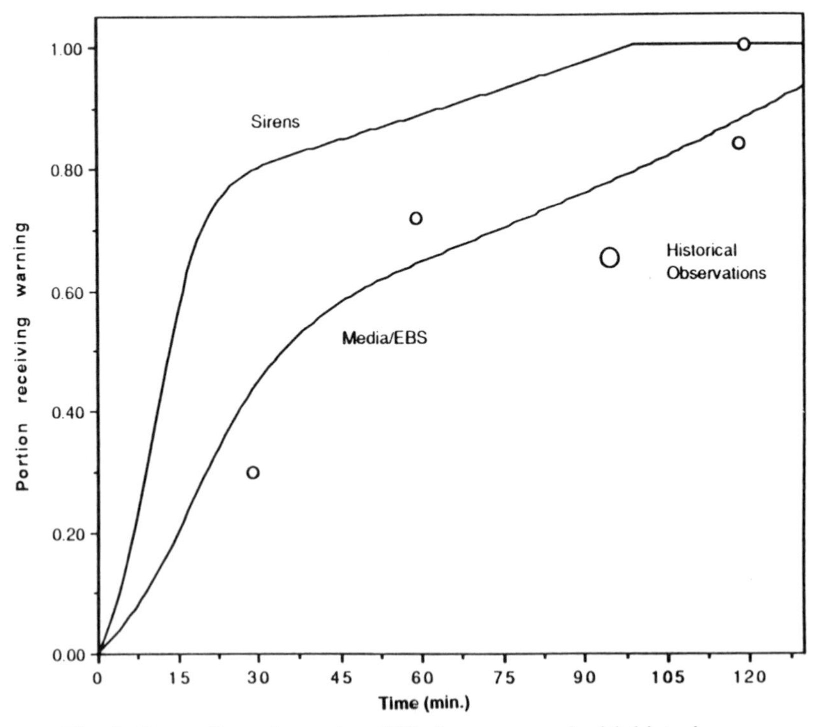

Fig. 4. Time adjusted warning diffusion compared with historic cases.

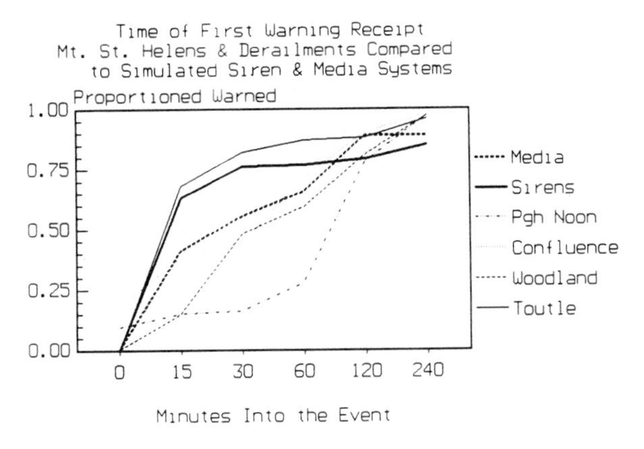

Fig. 5. Time of first warning receipt.

residents of these areas aware of the hazard. Hence, it was anticipated that residents of the Toutle/Silverlake area would receive warning more quickly than Woodland area residents, because of the effort to setup a warning system and because of the social networks known to emerge in disasters. Toutle/Silverlake residents were expected to rely more on officials and neighbors than Woodland, where media sources were deemed more important. The data indicate that social networks were the most frequently cited source of first awareness in both cases, with recognition of environmental clues being the second most cited source in Toutle/Silverlake and media being the second most cited source of warning in Woodland.[19] The result is that social network warning sources stimulated on the basis of direct environmental evidence (i.e., in Toutle and Silverlake) generated 82% coverage in 30 minutes, while the media driven social network warning system (i.e., in Woodland) reached 81% in two hours.

Both train derailment warning situations consisted primarily of route-alerting and door-to-door warning systems. Each is characterized by an S-shaped curve, with the Confluence warning reportedly approaching 90% warned in about two hours and the Pittsburgh event reportedly approaching 80% warned in about three hours. However, because of methodological uncertainties it is possible to identify only people that positively report having received some kind of warning. It is not possible to identify those not receiving warning. While the warning situations in Confluence and Pittsburgh are characterized by rapid dissemination in the first hour and half of the event, only 12.5% report being warned in the first 15 minutes in Pittsburgh while 36.8% reported being warned in the same period in Confluence. This may be a function of a number of factors, including the type of event, the size of the area to be warned, distance from the source, the time of day, or a bias associated with attributable experience gained vicariously in Confluence when the Pittsburgh event occurred about a month earlier. In Confluence, almost 70% report receiving warning in the first hour, while only 23% report having received a warning in the same period in Pittsburgh. Neither event is characterized by complete (100%) warning, and both indicate that very rapid onset emergencies can result in people being engulfed in danger prior to receiving warning.

WARNING SYSTEM EFFECTIVENESS

From an emergency management standpoint, the most appropriate measure of effectiveness is the ability of a warning system to provide populations at risk with adequate time to respond appropriately to the situation. Hence it is not necessarily the time it takes to warn people but the timing with respect to the onset of hazard that provides a measurement of warning system effectiveness. For example, a warning system that takes only 10 minutes to warn a population that will be exposed to hazard in 8 minutes is certainly less effective than a system that provides warning in 1 hour when exposure occurs in 1-1/2 hours.

Three hypothetical situations are posited to compare the onset of hazard emanating from a source at a rate of 1, 3, and 6 meters per second. These could occur as a flash flood brought on by a cloudburst or a dam failure upstream, such as those at Buffalo Creek or the Teton Dam failure; as a toxic-vapor cloud emanating from a noxious facility; or as a transportation accident, such as the accidents in Mississauga, Ontario; Bhopal, India; or Institute, West Virginia. In the case of airborne toxins, the variable rates are attributable to differing meteorological conditions and, in particular, wind speed. The variable rates of downstream exposure in river basins are the consequence of various hydrological characteristics, such as vertical drop per kilometer.

Because the warning systems examined here are concerned with public warning, they do not treat time needed for hazard detection or communication and decision making by authorities as a variable factor. It is assumed that the process of deciding to warn takes an average of 10 minutes and that the warning procedure begins at that point in time. If the decision time is longer or shorter, the numbers reported would change, but the overall relative performance would remain unchanged. Such organizational decision-making time is variable, given the events in question. At Bhopal, approximately 20 minutes elapsed prior to any alarm, and the public alarm was apparently shut down completely for nearly 30 minutes after that.[31] In the Cheyenne flash flood, public warnings began to be issued 5 minutes after detection.[32] This analysis considers a critical area of 35 km from the hazard source. Beyond 35 km, no specialized warning effort would be needed, because sufficient time would exist to disseminate a warning using an ad hoc procedure.

The probability of warning people prior to exposure at various distances is estimated by combining the estimates based on the models for each warning system alternative with hypothetical "downwind/downstream" times (Table 3). The most important insight provided by these results is that the amount of time it takes an organization to decide to warn, which includes hazard detection, is critical to warning system effectiveness. The results in Table 3 demonstrate the critical nature of organizational decision-making under conditions wherein warning time is most limited. People cannot fully protect themselves from hazard when they do not receive warning before exposure to emerging emergency conditions.

A second significant implication of the analysis concerns the feasibility of alternative forms of population protection. Many fatalities from floods result when people attempt to evacuate or cross a flooded stream in an automobile.[32] In chemical emergencies, eight out of every 100 evacuees are injured by inhalation of toxic vapors.[33] Alternatives to formal evacuation in fast-onset events include escape and sheltering. Escape is the movement on foot out of the flooding area or the toxic plume.[34] Sheltering involves moving to a secure place in a structure and taking steps to keep the hazard agent from entering the structure. In chemical incidents, sheltering may be an extremely effective way of self-protection.[35] Our analysis supports both actions as practical alternatives to formal evacuations because of the relatively short time to implement these actions.

The combination of either telephone ring-down or tone-alert radio warning systems with sirens provides the most effective warning system under conditions of very rapid onset (e.g., 6 meters/second), close proximity, or both. These results indicate that alternative individual systems provide adequate warning effectiveness when available warning time (after detection and the decision to warn) extends to as much as an hour and that tone-alert radios and telephone ring-down systems provide similar coverage at approximately 30 minutes of available public warning time.

Table 3. Available Time and Distance for Warning System Alternative

Warning System	Distance in kilometers				
	1-2	2-5	5-10	10-20	20-35
Onset speed of 1 m/sec: minutes (+0.5) =	15.5	48.8	115.5	240.5	448.8
A. Sirens and alarms	0.563	0.855	1.000	1.000	1.000
B. Tone-alert radios	0.811	0.939	0.999	0.999	0.999
C. Auto-dial telephones	0.882	0.971	1.000	1.000	1.000
Media/EBS	0.199	0.595	0.843	0.927	1.000
A and B	0.925	0.993	1.000	1.000	1.000
A and C	0.941	0.993	1.000	1.000	1.000
Onset speed of 3 m/sec: minutes (+0.5) =	-1.2	10.0	32.2	73.9	143.3
A. Sirens and alarms	0.0	0.296	0.809	0.922	1.000
B. Tone-alert radios	0.0	0.610	0.922	0.963	0.999
C. Auto-dial telephones	0.0	0.713	0.955	0.996	1.000
Media/EBS	0.0	0.102	0.473	0.693	0.893
A and B	0.0	0.759	0.977	1.000	1.000
A and C	0.0	0.816	0.977	1.000	1.000
Onset speed of 6 m/sec: minutes (+0.5) =	-5.3	0.3	11.4	32.2	66.9
A. Sirens and alarms	0.0	0.0	0.390	0.809	0.903
B. Tone-alert radios	0.0	0.0	0.697	0.922	0.957
C. Auto-dial telephones	0.0	0.0	0.792	0.955	0.989
Media/EBS	0.0	0.0	0.132	0.473	0.668
A and B	0.0	0.0	0.842	0.977	1.000
A and C	0.0	0.0	0.882	0.977	1.000

The results indicate that a combination warning system is the most effective system in the 10-km radius. Given an instantaneous release (e.g., of water from a dam failure or toxic chemical from an accident) at low-onset speeds, most people in the 10-km zone will receive a warning. At the onset speed of 3 meters per second, the combination systems do not lead to adequate warnings within 2 km but perform well within the 5- to 10-km range. Under very-rapid-onset, it will be difficult to adequately warn people within 5 km.

Within 35 km, some multiple-method warning systems may also be desirable, although 100% overlap is not necessary. A combination of sirens, tone alerts and media/EBS warning could be used to warn populations within 10 to 20 km. The exact mix needs to be determined on the bases of local geography, potential hazard and population distribution. Beyond 20 km, it seems appropriate to rely principally on the media/EBS systems, except for institutional populations, which require prompt notification in the entire emergency planning zone.

This analysis provides a preliminary basis for planning warning systems for fast-moving events, such as dam failures or chemical spills or explosions, and for assessing the effectiveness of warning systems currently being used. Although this analysis has focused on the timing of warning, it is recognized that the organizational structure for issuing the warning and the style and content of the warning and the possible availability of protective actions are also critical factors in the overall effectiveness of the systems. As society creates more and more potential hazards, such as industrial facilities, chemical weapons, biotech facilities, nuclear power plants, and other unforeseen technologies, the need for careful planning for emergency warnings increases in importance.

REFERENCES

1. T. Parsons, T., *The Social System*, The Free Press, NY (1951).
2. M. Granovetter, The Strength of Weak Ties, *American Journal of Sociology* **78**:1360-1380 (1973).
3. P. Blau, *Inequality and Heterogeneity: A Primitive Theory of Social Structure*, The Free Press, NY (1977).
4. R. Burt, Social Contagion and Innovation: Cohesion versus Structural Equivalence, *American Journal of Sociology* **92**:1287-1335 (1987).
5. H. Williams, Human Factors in Warning and Response Systems, in *The Threat of Impending Disaster*, G. Groesser *et al.*, eds., pp. 79-104, MIT Press, Cambridge, MA (1964).
6. E. Baker, Predicting Response to Hurricane Warnings: A Reanalysis of Data from Four Studies, *Mass Emergencies* **4**:9-24 (1979).
7. I. Janis and L. Mann, Emergency Decision Making: A Theoretical Analysis of Responses to Disaster Warnings, *Journal of Human Stress* **3**:35-48 (June 1977).
8. G. Rogers and J. Nehnevajsa, Warning Human Populations of Technological Hazard, in *Proceedings of the ANS Topical Meeting on Radiological Accidents*, CONF-860932, pp. 357-362, Oak Ridge National Laboratory, Oak Ridge, TN (1987).
9. D. Mileti and J. Sorensen, Why People Take Precautions Against Natural Disasters, in *Taking Care: Why People Take Precautions*, pp. 189-207, N. Weinstein, ed., Cambridge University Press, Cambridge (1987).
10. R. Perry, M. Lindell, and M. Greene, *Evacuation Planning in Emergency Management*, Lexington Books, Lexington, MA (1981).
11. R. Perry and A. Mushkatel, *Disaster Management: Warning Response and Community Relocation*, Quorum Books, Westport, CT (1984).
12. D. Mileti, *Natural Hazard Warning Systems in the United States*, Institute of Behavioral Science, University of Colorado, Boulder, CO (1975).
13. R. Leik T. Carter, and J. Clark, *Community Response to Natural Hazard Warnings: Final Report*, University of Minnesota, Minneapolis, MN (1981).
14. I. Janis, *Psychological Stress*, John Wiley and Sons, NY (1958).
15. C. Lave and J. March, *An Introduction to Models in the Social Sciences*, Harper & Row, New York (1975).
16. John P. Keating, Elizabeth F. Loftus, and Michele Manber, Emergency evacuations during fires: Psychological considerations, in *Advances in Applied Social Psychology*, Vol. 2, pp. 83-100, R. F. Kidd and M. J. Saks, eds., Lawrence Erlbaum Associates, Hillsdale, NJ (1983).
17. G. O. Rogers, Role Conflict in Crises of Limited Forewarning, *Journal of Applied Sociology* **3(1)**:33-50 (1986).
18. G. Rogers and J. Nehnevajsa, *Behavior and Attitudes Under Crisis Conditions: Selected Issues and Findings*, U.S. Government Printing Office, Washington, DC (1984).
19. M. Lindell and R. Perry, Warning Mechanisms in Emergency Response Systems, *International Journal of Mass Emergencies and Disasters* **5(2)**:137-153 (1987).

20. R. Perry, M. Greene, and M. Lindell, *Human Response to Volcanic Eruption*, Battelle Human Affairs Research Centers, Seattle (1980).
21. P. Snyder and J. Schlarb, A Case Study of a Voluntary Preventative Evacuation: The May 1987 Train Derailment in Confluence, Pennsylvania, Annual Meeting of the North Central Sociological Association (April 1988).
22. J. S. Sorensen and D. Mileti, Warning and Evacuation: Answering Some Basic Questions, draft manuscript under review (1988).
23. F. Juster *et al.*, 1975 - 1981 Time Use Longitudinal Panel Study, The University of Michigan, Institute for Social Research, Survey Research Center, Ann Arbor (1983).
24. G. Rogers and J. Sorensen, Diffusion of Emergency Warnings, *Environmental Professional* **10**;281-294 (1988).
25. J. Nehnevajsa, Western Pennsylvania: Some Issues in Warning the Population Under Emergency Conditions, University of Pittsburgh, Center for Social and Urban Research (1985).
26. J. Robinson, *How Americans Use Time*, Praeger, New York (1977).
27. Norman P. Hummon, Linda Mauro, and George O. Rogers, Time Budget Analysis and Risk Management: Estimating the Probabilities of Event Schedules of American Adults, in *Enhancing Risk Management and Decision Making*, Lester B. Lave, ed., Plenum Press, New York (1987).
28. E. Gruntfest, *What People Did During the Big Thompson Flood*, Working Paper 32, Institute of Behavioral Science, University of Colorado, Boulder, CO (1977).
29. Ian Burton, Mel Kliman, David Powell, Larry Schmidt, Peter Timmerman, Peter Victor, Anne Whyte, and Joanne Wojick, The Mississauga Evacuation, Final Report, Institute for Environmental Studies, University of Toronto, Toronto (1981).
30. R. Perry and A. Mushkatel, *Minority Citizens in Disaster*, University of Georgia Press, Athens (1986).
31. W. Morehouse and M. Subramanian, The Bhopal Tragedy, Council on International and Public Affairs, New York (1986).
32. J. Sorensen, Warning Systems in the 1985 Cheyenne Flash Flood, in *What We Have Learned Since the Big Thompson Flood*, E. Gruntfest, ed., Institute of Behavioral Science, University of Colorado, Boulder (1987a).
33. Sorensen, J., Evacuations Due to Off-Site Releases from Chemical Accidents: Experience from 1980 to 1984, *Journal of Hazardous Materials* **14**:247-257 (1987b).
34. R. Prugh, Mitigation of Vapor Cloud Hazards, *Plant/Operations Progress* **4**:95-104 (1985).
35. G. Purdy, and P. Davies, Toxic Gas Incidents—Some Important Considerations in Emergency Planning, *I.CEM.E Symposium Series* **94**:257-268 (1985).

APPENDIX A: DESCRIPTION OF TRAIN DERAILMENT ACCIDENTS AT PITTSBURGH AND CONFLUENCE, PENNSYLVANIA

Pittsburgh Phosphorous Oxychloride Release

On Saturday, April 11, 1987 at 12:29 p.m., a westbound Conrail freight train derailed in Pittsburgh, Pennsylvania. In the process of derailing the westbound train sideswiped an eastbound train causing it to derail. Four tank cars containing hazardous materials on the eastbound train were derailed. Sparks resulting from the accident ignited a fire, however, "...contrary to reports circulated at the time of the accident, none of the hazardous materials ignited" (Railroad Accident Investigation Report, No. A-63-87, Consolidated Rail Corporation, Pittsburgh, Pennsylvania, April 11, 1987). Because of the involvement of hazardous materials, Pittsburgh emergency personnel initiated an evacuation upon arrival at the scene; about 20 minutes after the accident. Some local residents in immediately adjacent areas had already begun to evacuate. Up to 22,000 people were evacuated as the initial evacuation area was expanded to accommodate changing weather conditions. The fire was extinguished by 3:30 p.m., however, the primary concern centered around a derailed tank car containing phosphorus oxychloride. This tank car developed a crack in the dome permitting between 30 and 100 gallons of lading to escape. Emergency response teams inserted a tennis ball in the vent pipe to prevent further release and neutralized the chemicals that had escaped with hot ash and sand. By 5:50 p.m., the affected areas had been declared safe and the initial evacuation order was rescinded. Emergency officials planned a second precautionary evacuation for 1:00 p.m. the following day to upright the leaking tank car; however, a close inspection of the damaged tank car shortly after midnight detected continued degradation of the tank car. At 1:30 a.m., an evacuation order affecting between 14,000 and 16,000 residents within a half mile of the scene was issued. This second evacuation order was not rescinded until 4:30 p.m. on Sunday, April 12, 1987. Approximately 25 people were treated for eye and throat irritation at area hospitals, and three people were hospitalized during the course of the accident.

Confluence Precautionary Evacuation

On Wednesday, May 6, 1987 at 4:00 a.m., 21 of 27 "empty" tank cars carrying product residues, including propane, chlorine, caustic soda, carbon disulfide, methyl chloride, chloroform and isobutane derailed in Confluence, Pennsylvania. Because tank cars carrying residue can haul up to 3% of the load, emergency officials had no way to determine the exact amount of products remained in cars. Upon examination of the train's manifest, emergency management officials initiated a precautionary evacuation of the 986 residents. A three-minute non-stop siren blast was sounded, which primarily alerted the volunteer firemen as residents could not be expected to know what the siren blast meant. At approximately 4:30 a.m., a door-to-door and portable loudspeaker alert and notification of the emergency began using volunteer firemen and untrained volunteers. Public shelters were set up in the area's high school, local school buses and ambulances provided transportation for those needing it, and within 45 minutes the evacuation was complete. Assistance from area-wide emergency personnel sealed two leaking propane tankers by 9:48 a.m., but the chance of explosion and/or fire during wreckage cleanup prevented return until 6:10 p.m.

A Comparison of Successful and Unsuccessful Public Involvement: A Practitioner's Viewpoint

James L. Creighton
Creighton & Creighton, Inc.
Palo Alto, CA

ABSTRACT

This paper—based on a practitioner's experience rather than empirical research—describes those attributes which make public involvement programs successful or unsuccessful. Among the attributes discussed are the character of the issue, the existing political climate in the affected community, the planning and timing of the public involvement activities, the credibility of the sponsoring entity, the certainty with which the consequences of the proposed actions can be predicted and the effects of the decision on various interests in the community. These points are illustrated with examples from both successful and unsuccessful public involvement programs. Examples are given of ways to overcome existing conditions not conducive to successful public involvement.

KEYWORDS: Public involvement, public, decision-making, effectiveness, comparisons

DEFINING SUCCESS

The obvious starting point in talking about successful versus unsuccessful public involvement is the question: what is successful public involvement? The question is obvious, but the answer is not.

Here are four possible outcomes of public involvement. Which of these outcomes is a success?

- The public accepts the program which the agency wants to carry out.
- The public clearly prefers one of a list of options, any of which would be acceptable to the agency.
- The public is in agreement that it doesn't want the program proposed by the agency.
- Everybody has a chance to be heard, but it is clear that the public is divided as to which decision is appropriate.

If we want to be "pure" in our approach to public involvement—which is to say that the job of public involvement is to ascertain clearly how the public feels and incorporate the public's perceptions into the decision making—then the first three of these outcomes are successful. Even in the fourth outcome we get a good reading of public opinion, but it is

Risk Analysis, Edited by C. Zervos
Plenum Press, New York, 1991

very hard to incorporate the public's views in a decision if all we know is that the public is bitterly divided. My experience suggests, though, that agencies prefer the first outcome—their proposal is accepted. Public involvement specialists would tend to support the second outcome as a more legitimate form of public involvement. Some of the more enlightened agencies have also come to live with the second outcome. But most agencies consider either the third or fourth outcome—the public is clearly opposed or clearly divided—as signs of unsuccessful public involvement.

The participants have yet a different perspective. For some participants, merely to be listened to makes the public involvement successful. For others, the measure of success is the degree to which they can influence the decision. Using this definition of success, they will look at the substantive decision and measure their success accordingly. No matter how effective the process in listening to and responding to public concerns, if the decision doesn't go far enough in their desired direction, they will judge the public involvement unsuccessful and the agency unresponsive.

The point is simply that success is in the eye of the beholder. Most systems for evaluating public involvement assume that there is a single objective measure of the success of the program. The hard, messy reality is that everybody who participates has a different set of criteria for the success of the public involvement program. The only evaluation systems I have seen which seem credible are systems which specify the criteria of several stakeholders, and then assess how well the program met those specified goals. My bias is that no system of measurement begins to reflect reality accurately until it evaluates from the perspective of multiple stakeholders.

MY OWN CRITERIA

If success is in the eye of the beholder, then before I start talking about some of the factors determining whether programs are successful, I'd better share what success means to this beholder. My own criteria of success are as follows:

A program is successful to the extent that it

1. gives an accurate reading of public sentiment,
2. results in programs which reflect this sentiment, and
3. contributes to a consensus.

The first criterion must be met for a program to be successful. The minimum a public involvement program should accomplish is to provide an accurate expression of public opinion. I have to qualify this somewhat. Pragmatically, I would have to rephrase that to say that, at a minimum, it must give an accurate reading of those people who care about the issue. Unless an issue is extremely significant in a community, the average citizen will defer to those people who care about the issue. At a community level, the difference between a very small issue and a highly controversial issue is the difference between 50 active people caring about the issue and 5,000. If this is an issue in which 5,000 people are interested, then the public involvement program must reflect the opinions of those 5,000. But if it is an issue that 500 people care about, then I'm more worried about whether I did a good job of hearing the 500 than I am worrying about the missing 4500. But a clear implication is that a good public involvement program tells you whether the interested public is 50 people or 5000 people.

The second criterion—the degree to which the public's opinions are reflected in decision making—makes the difference between a passable program and a truly good program. Having said this, I can quickly begin to make all kinds of qualifying statements.

There are issues where there is a clear community consensus which is at odds with the national consensus or even federal law. There are issues which by their nature are all or nothing decisions, so there is little way the public can influence the decision, unless the decision is to drop the proposed action entirely. But despite these and many other qualifiers I can give you, I can't think of any public involvement programs that I consider fully satisfactory where the participation of the public did not have a material bearing on the outcome.

The third criterion—the program's contribution to consensus on the issue—is something I hold out as more of a desirable end than an essential requirement. One of the valuable functions of public participation and numerous dispute resolution techniques such as mediation is that they contribute to community consensus. Although I believe a program can be considered fully successful if it meets the first two standards, I want, in addition, for the public involvement to help pull people together rather than drive them apart. As a minimum it should meet the standard used by doctors. It should "do no harm" to the cohesiveness of the community.

FACTORS WHICH INFLUENCE SUCCESS

Now I want to turn to a discussion of those factors which contribute to the success or failure of a public involvement program. One thing which will be immediately apparent in this discussion is that many of these factors are largely outside the control of the people conducting the public involvement, or even the agency itself. I think this reflects reality. There are times when we've done a thorough and totally conscientious public involvement program only to have it blow up in our faces, due to factors outside our control. Other times I've been involved in programs which were fully adequate but a trifle mundane, in which we came out looking as if we walked on water. One reason for identifying those external factors which contribute to success or failure is that some of them, at least, are within the control of the agencies but well outside the purview of what is normally thought of as public involvement. Agencies need a very broad perspective on the factors which make the difference in the success or failure of a program. Another reason is, while I don't want to let anyone off the hook who's done a lousy job of public involvement, there are people out there who think they are a failure when what went wrong had little to do with how conscientious or capable they were in implementing their public involvement program.

For convenience I've grouped the factors into four categories: (1) the character of the issue, (2) the culture and history of the sponsoring agency, (3) the existing political climate in the community, and (4) the planning and timing of the public involvement activities. My observations are presented as propositions, although, as suggested in my title, they rest on nothing but my experience as a practitioner.

The Character of the Issue

Public involvement is more likely to be successful if:

1. *There are multiple options, not just a single option.* If there is only one way the problem can be solved, it is very hard for the agency to escape slipping into either a "selling" posture or a defensive posture. Either posture sets up a "we/they" relationship with the public, increases the public's fears of being manipulated, and focuses the discussion on the proposed solution without first getting emotional commitment that there is a problem. Sometimes the fault lies in the way the agency has defined its options. Often there are options, but the agency would prefer not to address them. But there are times when it is just the nature of the issue that only one solution is possible.

2. *The outcomes of the action are well-understood and can be accurately assessed.* When I look back on the issues on which I conducted public involvement in the 1970s—whether to build a freeway, dam or airport, or how to manage a forest—they look downright sane in comparison to today's issues. Today's issues always seem to be questions involving risk, probability, and uncertainty—which can be little surprise to this audience. Things start to get crazy when there are no fixed points. Uncertainty about risk increases fears, undermines the credibility of the agency, and leaves no firm ground for resolving issues. As you all know too well, it also lends itself to demagoguery.

3. *The technology involved is familiar.* In many ways this is a corollary of the factor above. If the technology involved is new or exotic, people are less likely to accept your assessment of the outcomes and more likely to fear unanticipated consequences.

4. *The issue is confined to the local community and is not a part of a larger national debate.* You cannot be involved today in any issue involving nuclear power or nuclear waste without it becoming messy. There's just no way it can remain a local issue. There are too many interests involved, with too high stakes, for resolution of the issue at a local level. Anytime the broader outside world sits in judgment on the decision, it becomes very difficult to run public involvement in the local community, because they aren't the only public which counts.

5. *The duration of the decision-making process is limited.* Most people in the public cannot relate to decision-making processes that last three to five years or more. The longer the process, the harder it is to maintain interest, the more risk there is that people will become suspicious that work done in technical phases of the study unfairly foreclosed options, and the more danger there is that new actors will get involved who want to reopen every decision which was made previously.

The Culture and History of the Agency

Public involvement is more likely to be successful if:

1. *The agency is a credible source of information.* The simple question is: when the agency provides information to the public, will the public trust the information? Credibility in this instance has two components: *competence* and *objectivity*. There are many agencies which have technically competent staff but are so associated with advocacy for certain kinds of solutions or projects that the public doesn't trust their data. Once an agency is seen as an advocate for a particular outcome, then the public suspects that technical work is being done to support the outcome the agency wants. As an example, do you really trust the local airport to accurately report noise from airplanes? Do you trust a chemical company to assess the risk from its products?

2. *The perceived values of the agency are consistent with the solutions being considered.* Agencies have histories, and the public remembers those histories. As agencies change missions or take on new missions, they often find themselves asking the public to trust them to carry out a program which seems inconsistent with the agency's history. Some of the public's suspicion may be unfair, may be five or ten years out of date, or may be well-founded, based on a pragmatic understanding that it takes five or ten years before the reality of an agency catches up with the new rhetoric of its management. But in evaluating credibility, the public looks hard at the question of whether it is believable that this agency would be willing or even able to

implement some of the solutions being proposed. Some of the nation's water development agencies, for example, are now presenting themselves as willing and able to implement non-structural or regulatory programs. Will the public believe them?

3. *The perceived values of the agency are consistent with an open, participative process.* The process of public involvement is not value-neutral. There is a clear preference in public involvement for openness, candor, equality, democracy, participation, and so on. The preeminent value of many agencies is control, and given that value, they have a history of being reluctant to share information, of emphasizing centralized, directive decision making, and of preferring to deal with the power establishment rather than the general public. This is as much a part of the history of the agency as the kinds of projects it has carried out. Just as an agency which has been associated solely with structural solutions is somewhat suspect when it claims willingness to consider non-structural approaches, agencies which have a history of closed, directive decision making are suspect when they claim willingness to engage in open dialogue with the public. The first case is a lack of credibility regarding the *content* of the decision, the second a lack of credibility about the agency's willingness to engage in an open *process*.

The Political Climate Within the Community

Public involvement is more likely to be successful if:

1. *The community itself is cohesive.* Obviously it's going to be easier to achieve agreement on a plan or direction if the community itself is not so divided that it is incapable of agreement not just on this issue but virtually any issue. Communities go through periods where there is a generalized sense of direction that is largely accepted by everyone, followed by periods where there is bitter division. If you reach the community at a time when the battle is already raging, your program is very likely to get caught up in the controversy and battle for power which already exists. If your program deals with issues identical to those already being debated in the community, you can count on problems. In the parlance of sociologists, you're "reinforcing the existing cleavages" in the community.

2. *The existing social and political leadership of the community are trusted to represent the community.* This point is closely related to the one above. During times when there is a general agreement on direction and the social and political leadership is perceived as competent, the general public will accept decisions made by community leaders. But during times when communities are debating about future direction, significant portions of the public will not accept decisions made by the social and political leadership. It's clearly easier to achieve a consensus when you're working with a small number of people than when you must work with numerous competing groups. If you rely on the leadership of a community during times of major change in a community, you may find that the people you consulted with have been swept from office and the community no longer considers itself bound by what occurred previously.

3. *The issue is not being used to gain political advantage in local politics.* If the subject of a public involvement program happens to coincide with a major debate in a community, then there is a considerable possibility that people will use the issue to try to gain political power. If, for example, a project could pose some risk to the community, an ambitious candidate may well exaggerate the risk in an effort to convince the community that he or she is better able to represent them when dealing with evildoers from outside.

The Planning and Timing of the Public Involvement Activities

At last we reach the realm where agencies have considerable control over the factors which determine the success of failure of the programs.

Public involvement is more likely to be successful if:

1. *The public involvement activities are an integral part of the decision-making process.* Public involvement activities which are just an "add-on," just tacked on to the side of an existing decision-making process, are far less likely to be successful. They might—with luck—give you a reasonable reading of public opinion. They will fail miserably, however, in meeting the other goals I identified earlier for successful public involvement programs—demonstrating a clear connection between public comment and the outcome of the decision-making process, and contributing to a consensus. In effective public involvement, the public involvement activities are an integral part of the decision-making process. You know why you are going to the public at a particular point in time, what particular segment of the public you have to reach, and what information you have to get from them. In the same way that you could not pass key decision points without certain economic or engineering studies completed, you should not be able to pass those points without your public involvement activities also being completed.

2. *The active interested public is included early in the decision-making process.* Every manual or guide on public involvement—including my own—stresses the need to involve the public early in the decision-making process. This is an admonishment based on the early days of public involvement when agencies tried to involve the public late in the game, after most of the alternatives had already been discarded, and the agency was deeply committed to a single answer. This was and remains a prescription for failure. On the other hand, I've seen agencies "burn out" the interest of the public by trying to involve the general public intensively during Year One of a five-year study. So you'll find the admonishment above qualified to specify the "active interested" public.

3. *The techniques chosen are appropriate to the portions of the public you're trying to reach and to the information you're trying to obtain from the public.* You could write a whole book on this topic—in fact I have—but the key point is that when you select your techniques you need to have thought through where you are in the decision-making process, what information you need to get to the public, what information you need to get from the public, and who is the public for this particular phase of your decision-making process. This provides the context which allows you to discriminate which technique is appropriate.

4. *As much care and attention goes into anticipating the questions the public will have as into reacting to the questions once they're been raised.* Typically a public involvement consultant is called upon to advise on public involvement techniques, but increasingly I find myself spending at least as much time talking about what the issues will be and what work, such as additional studies, have to be done if the agency is going to be credible in addressing the issue. For example, if you are a utility company siting a transmission line, you are not going to be credible if—in a day where people are talking about possible links between electromagnetic fields and cancer—you cannot answer questions such as: What are the magnetic fields which will be generated by this line? What is the scientific evidence regarding the link between electromagnetic fields and cancer? Would burying these lines reduce the fields? How much would it cost to bury the lines? What impact would burying have on rates? You should have the answers going in. Otherwise the issue will grow, you will not be credible, and "the other side" will always be on the offensive.

GAINING CONTROL OVER EXTERNAL FACTORS

As noted previously, many of the factors I've discussed remain outside the control of the agency and certainly outside the control of the public involvement specialist. I am identifying these factors, however, in the hope that if you recognize the role they play in determining your success, you'll do what you can about them.

1. Carefully evaluate your decision-making process to see if you can increase the number of options, increase certainty regarding outcomes, increase confidence in the technology, and either confine the issues locally or get the involvement of national groups from the beginning.

2. If you know you have credibility problems, allow for this by using credibility-building procedures like peer review boards, advisory groups, National Academy of Science reviews and so on. Also, lean over backwards throughout the program to provide total visibility and complete access to information.

3. Find out as much as you can about the community before you start your program, so you don't set off the land mines from lack of awareness.

4. If the community is divided, be sure you establish communication links to both or all sides, not just the power establishment.

Successful public involvement isn't determined just by what techniques you use. Fundamentally, success depends on your method of making decisions and the sensitivity you show to the political context in which those decisions are being made.

Elicitation of Natural Language Representations of Uncertainty Using Computer Technology

Bruce Tonn and Richard Goeltz
Oak Ridge National Laboratory
Oak Ridge, TN

Cheryl Travis
University of Tennessee
Knoxville, TN

ABSTRACT

Knowledge elicitation is an important aspect of risk analysis. Knowledge about risks must be accurately elicited from experts for use in risk assessments. Knowledge and perceptions of risks must also be accurately elicited from the public in order to perform policy analysis and develop and implement programs intelligently. Oak Ridge National Laboratory is developing computer technology to elicit knowledge from experts and the public effectively and efficiently. This paper discusses software developed to elicit natural language representations of uncertainty. The software is written in Common Lisp and resides on VAX Computer Systems and Symbolics Lisp machines. The software has three goals: to determine (1) preferences for using natural language terms for representing uncertainty, (2) likelihood rankings of the terms, and (3) the way likelihood estimates are combined to form new terms. The first two goals relate to providing useful results for those interested in risk communication. The third relates to providing cognitive data to further our understanding of people's decision making under uncertainty. The software is used to elicit natural language terms used to express the likelihood that various agents will cause cancer in humans and that cancer will result in various maladies, and the likelihood of everyday events.

KEYWORDS: Uncertainty, knowledge elicitation, computer technology, risk perception

INTRODUCTION

Risk analysis is a complex, challenging field. To be successful, it must embrace a multitude of disciplines, from the physical to the social. It has been shown historically that new tools and measurement devices designed for the physical sciences have almost always generated important advances in our understanding of nature. We believe that new technologies and methodologies being developed for the social sciences will, by analogy, generate important advances in the practice of risk analysis. This paper explores the potential benefits of using computer technology for knowledge elicitation.

Knowledge elicitation is a term used to represent a process whereby cognitive structures held by experts or individuals about a particular subject are inferred from data collected through a question and answer method. Knowledge elicitation or acquisition is the key process in the development of expert systems, which are computer systems designed to make decisions like human experts (e.g., physicians, loan officers, computer technicians). Through many hours of questions and answers, knowledge is elicited from human experts in such a manner that the data have rigorous structure, are manipulable by computer software, and are faithful to the terminology and concepts used by the expert.

Expert systems have many potential applications in risk analysis as do more general applications of knowledge elicitation methods. This paper in particular is concerned with eliciting knowledge from the public about risk beliefs and especially about natural language terminology used to represent uncertainty. Thus we are concerned with eliciting terminology and cognitive structures from individuals under the assumption that such data are comparable in structure and in use to expert knowledge.

Given these definitions, we can now discuss three differences between knowledge elicitation and traditional social science surveys, interviews, and pencil and paper instruments. First, knowledge elicitation yields more complex types of data. The data are not yes-no, Likert Scale (e.g., 1-7), or multiple choice. For the most part, the data are not opinions or approval ratings, although the notion of salience may play an important role in representing risk beliefs. Instead, the data may be procedural in describing how the world works, (e.g., smoking causes cancer), semantic in describing how the world is put together (e.g., the EPA is a kind of large public organization), factual in describing the state of the world (e.g., the probability of surviving AIDS for more than five years is 20%), or cognitive in describing how the mind works (e.g., how an individual may combine probabilities).

As a second difference, knowledge elicitation is more structured than open-ended and anthropological interviews. During interviews, the interviewer can lead the interviewee in any number of manners which may not be particularly predictable at the beginning. However, the notes and protocols may be sketchy, wordy, and complex. It may be extremely difficult and time consuming to translate free-flowing natural language data into forms amenable to computer representation, analysis, and manipulation. Computerized knowledge elicitation may not yield the same wealth of information in the same time as an interview or be as free flowing as an interview, but the data will be more structured.

Computerized knowledge elicitation offers flexibility and power not available in surveys and interviews. For example, people need not be given extreme limitations in response modes. Computers can be programmed with tens if not hundreds of acceptable responses and only interfere with an elicitation if an unacceptable response is given. This is the approach followed in the experiments described below. Well designed computerized elicitations can tailor-make questions for each person depending on past answers. Powerful systems can analyze data in real-time to identify inconsistencies or anomalies in the data and give the person the opportunity to provide more consistent answers. In contrast, it would be very tedious to tailor-make pencil and paper surveys and human interviewers may not be able to be so thorough during an interview.

Oak Ridge National Laboratory has developed several automated knowledge elicitation systems that could benefit risk analysis. One, known as ARK for Acquiring and Reasoning about Knowledge, elicits procedural and semantic knowledge about how the world works.[1] ARK has been used to collect information about people's beliefs about the consequences of two risk agents, AIDS and toxic waste.[2]

Another set of programs is known as LES, for Likelihood Elicitation System. LES elicits from people uncertainty assessments and data on how people manipulate their assessments. One application of the technology involved elicitation of probability estimates about everyday events and conjunctions of these events.[3] This paper next describes the computer method used to elicit natural language representations of uncertainty about everyday events and about causes and effects related to cancer. Then some results useful to risk communication researchers are presented.

TECHNOLOGY

LES is written in Common Lisp. This language is supported by very powerful workstation development environments which allow efficient code development. Common Lisp is also suited for advanced artificial intelligence methods, such as machine learning, which may be incorporated into future versions of LES. Finally, Common Lisp is well suited to handling symbolic information, such as natural language representations of uncertainty.

LES is actually a software shell that can be easily primed to explore any number of uncertainty contexts and heuristics. There are two major elements to LES, Session 1 and Session 2. The former concentrates on eliciting likelihood estimates of simple propositions (e.g., the likelihood of smoking causing cancer) whereas the latter elicits likelihood estimates of complex propositions (e.g., the likelihood of being wakened at night by outside noises and going to the grocery store that day). Currently, complex propositions can be conjunctions or disjunctions of two simple propositions. The software can be easily modified to handle other kinds of complex propositions.

Questions can be posed about any topic. This work involves two topic areas, cancer and daily events. In the first session of the cancer experiment, individuals answer 25 questions about the likelihood of a risk agent, such as mercury, causing cancer in a human being and 25 questions about the likelihood of cancer resulting in a change in one's physical well-being, such as depression. In the daily event experiment, 31 questions are asked about the likelihood of everyday events, such as going to the grocery store or flossing one's teeth. In the second session of the cancer experiment, the complex questions elicit the likelihood of a risk agent causing cancer AND cancer resulting in a change in physical well-being. In the daily event experiment, the complex questions pose conjunctions of events.

Likelihood estimates can be elicited in numerous modalities. This research utilized natural language modalities as opposed to eliciting numbers representing probabilities, chances, percentage of time, certainty or possibility. Figure 1 presents an example of a session 2 question for the daily event experiment using natural language terms. The subject is given a screen containing valid terms. The top terms are modifiers and must be used with one of the six basic terms: certain, uncertain, likely, unlikely, possible, and impossible. The modifiers were drawn from risk analysis work by Schmucker.[4] Any modifiers can be used on any basic term. "Not" can also be used with or without a modifier. As a result, the subject has the opportunity to specify any of 324 possible terms and the computer will ensure that a valid term is entered.

Computer technology also benefits the reliability of the data in two other ways. First, in each first session, the subject is given the chance to edit answers. Special screens come up with answers to the simple questions and highlight to the subject the desirability of reviewing one's answers. Data are automatically collected on edits made. Second, in each second session, LES analyzes the consistency of the complex, in this case conjunctive, questions with respect to one another. If an answer is inconsistent, the subject is asked if he or she agrees with the answer. If not, the answer to the conjunctive question is deleted and the related session 1 answers are reviewed. An inconsistent answer is one in which the subject's estimate of the conjunctive probability of two terms that have lower or equal single probabilities compared to another pair of two terms is higher than the subject's estimate of the conjunctive probability of the latter pair.

What is the likelihood of BOTH events happening:

that you will have a good day at school or work

AND

that you or someone you live with will vacuum your home

The TX hedge can be one of the following:

very	fairly	virtually	rather	almost
somewhat	kind of	sort of	mostly	basically
extremely	really	more or less	essentially	technically
strictly	roughly	relatively	practically	especially
for the most part		largely	barely	reasonably
typically	highly			

The TX term can be one of the following:

likely	unlikely
certain	uncertain
possible	impossible

<tx, ?> possible

Fig. 1. Example of a session 2 question; daily event experiment.

The previous paragraph begs the question of how probabilities can be assigned to natural language terms. At the end of each first session, LES asks each subject to rank order all the terms that individual used. A screen is presented and the subject ranks the terms from most unlikely to most likely. Operationally, the subject picks a term number and moves it to a new ranking number. For example, the term "certain" could be 12th in the list of 15 terms. LES would allow the subject to rank this term number 1 or 2 or anywhere from 1 to 15. If a new term is used in session 2, LES immediately asks the subject to rank the term. Data are collected on each ranking operation of each subject. Thus LES is able to elicit directly data on likelihoods and indirectly on sorting heuristics. This would not be possible with pencil and paper studies.

Also not possible with pencil and paper studies is the ability of LES to tailor-make each second session. Each complex question is based on that individual's answers during session 1 where high, medium, and low assessments of likelihood are paired with other high, medium, and low assessments. This is done to determine whether the magnitude of assessments influences the heuristics used to combine them. A maximum of 36 second session questions are tailor-made for each individual along these lines.

RESULTS

Natural language representations of uncertainty were elicited from two groups of subjects: 42 subjects from Oak Ridge National Laboratory participated in the cancer experiment; and 15 subjects from the University of Tennessee-Knoxville participated in the daily event experiment. Each subject completed session 1 and session 2 during the same sitting, which lasted approximately 45 minutes. The experimenter offered only a brief introduction to the software and the goals of the study. The experimenter only intervened to ensure that the subjects rank-ordered their terms in session 1.

Results presented below describe individuals' use of terms, interpolations of the probability associated with each term, semantical usage of the terms, individuals' uncertainty discernment, and the way people form conjunctions of natural language representations of uncertainty not in accordance with normative theory.

Table 1 presents a listing of the most frequently used natural language terms. Most used are the terms ‘possible’ and ‘unlikely’. The majority of the most frequently used terms are not modified and are less specific rather than more specific. For example ‘possible’ is less specific that ‘highly possible’. These observations are consistent across the two experiments. One interpretation is that less specific answers are more easily elicited than very specific answers. This could be because people do not possess more specific assessments or because the experimental situation prevented construction of more specific answers.

One difference between the two experiments relates to concept utilization. In the cancer experiment, possibility/impossibility was the prevalent concept whereas in the daily event experiment, likely/unlikely was the prevalent concept. This can be expected because people’s knowledge of cancer is not likely to be as first-hand as with respect to daily events. Thus cause and effects are ‘possible’ whereas events are ‘likely’. In the cancer experiment, only 49% of the elicitations had modifiers. The rate is 67% for the daily event experiment. These results further support the observation that the subjects may feel they know more about the likelihoods of daily events. In both experiments, the most frequently used modifier was ‘very’, at 24% and 26% of the modifiers used in the cancer and daily event experiments, respectively. Four other frequently used modifiers were ‘somewhat’ (12%, 17%), ‘highly’ (16%, 12%), ‘extremely’ (7%, 10%), and ‘fairly’ (9%, 10%). The modifier ‘not’ was used less than 1% of the time in both experiments. Thus the elicited knowledge is in some sense positive rather than negative.

Probability estimates for the natural language terms were derived from the rankings. For each person’s terms, the most likely term was assigned a probability of 1.0 and the lowest term a 0.0. If the person had used n terms, then the remaining $n-2$ terms were given the boundaries of $n-1$ interpolated equal intervals. For example, if the person had used only three terms, certain, possible, and impossible, then this method would yield probabilities for these terms of 1.0, 0.5 and 0.0. The probabilities for each term for each individual were then averaged together. Table 2 contains the results.

The results are informative in several respects. First, one can see that terms containing ‘possibility’ are found in the middle. This use of possibility is consistent with the theory of insufficient reasoning: if one possesses no knowledge about an event or truth of a proposition, then it is acceptable to assign a probability of 0.5. Second, the interpolations are generally consistent with past research where subjects were simply asked to associate probabilities with words.[5,6]

Third, one can begin to estimate the effect of modifiers. For example, the effect of modifying ‘likely’ by ‘very’ is relatively large but the marginal change from ‘very likely’ to ‘highly likely’ is small. Indeed, the relationships between modifiers and basic terms can become quite complex. Table 3 illustrates mirror relationships between terms. ‘Certain’ and ‘uncertain’ are not mirror images of each other, even when modified. ‘Possible’ and ‘impossible’ likewise are not mirror images. If anything, ‘certain’ matches better with ‘impossible’ and ‘uncertain’ matches better with ‘possible’. Only ‘likely’ and ‘unlikely’ possess mirroring characteristics. These results indicate that natural language is at once both extremely expressive and idiosyncratic.

The subjects varied considerably on their use of the language. As Fig. 2 indicates, it appears that in the daily event experiment, where people have more definite knowledge, more terms were used by each individual than in the cancer experiment. In the cancer experiment almost as many subjects used only 1-5 terms as used 16-20 terms and 26+ terms. It is unclear whether this observation is due to a difference in knowledge levels between subjects or due to differences in preferences for language use. In any case, a more expressive risk communication language could be useful for some people but wasted on others. Of course, a more expressive language could offer more risk of using terms about which people have different definitions.

Table 1. Most Frequently Used Natural Language Terms by Experiment (Percent of Answers)

Term	Cancer Experiment (N=3229)		Cancer Experiment (N=1005)	
	% of Ans.	Freq. Rank	% of Ans.	Freq. Rank
Possible	18.0	1	10.3	2
Unlikely	10.9	2	11.0	1
Impossible	7.5	3	1.5	20
Likely	6.4	4	6.8	4
Uncertain	5.9	5	0.5	32
Highly Unlikely	4.1	6	5.9	5
Very Likely	4.1	7	7.4	3
Very Possible	3.4	8	3.4	8
Very Unlikely	3.3	9	4.6	6
Somewhat Likely	2.6	10	3.4	8
Highly Likely	2.1	11	0.8	24
Somewhat Possible	2.1	11	4.1	7
Certain	2.0	13	2.4	12
Virtually Impossible	2.0	13	0.4	36
Rather Unlikely	1.6	15	1.2	21
Fairly Likely	1.4	16	2.0	15
Extremely Unlikely	1.4	17	2.1	13
Highly Possible	1.3	18	1.2	21
Fairly Possible	1.2	19	1.7	17
Almost Impossible	1.1	20	0.7	26
Somewhat Unlikely	1.0	21	3.4	8
Fairly Unlikely	0.8	25	2.7	11
Extremely Likely	0.8	26	1.6	18
Very Certain	0.7	28	1.9	16
Almost Certain	0.5	30	1.6	18
Extremely Certain	0.3	45	2.1	13

Table 2. Probability Interpolations of Selected Terms

	Cancer Exper.	Daily Exper.	Lichtenstein and Newman (1967)	Beyth-Maron (1982)
Certain	0.98	0.95		0.99
Highly Likely	0.90	0.85		
Very Likely	0.88	0.80	0.87	
Rather Likely	0.79	0.68	0.69	
Likely	0.77	0.68	0.72	0.61
Fairly Likely	0.73	0.71	0.66	
Somewhat Likely	0.69	0.56	0.59	
Very Possible	0.68	0.59		
Possible	0.60	0.55	0.37	0.54
Somewhat Possible	0.56	0.47		
Uncertain	0.36	0.54	0.40	
Rather Unlikely	0.34	0.19	0.24	
Fairly Unlikely	0.32	0.33	0.25	
Somewhat Unlikely	0.28	0.38	0.31	
Unlikely	0.27	0.29	0.18	
Very Unlikely	0.22	0.18	0.09	
Highly Unlikely	0.19	0.27		
Virtually Unlikely	0.06	0.07		
Impossible	0.02	0.04		

Table 3. Mirror Image Term Probabilities by Experiment

Terms	Cancer Experiment	Daily Event Experiment
Certain	0.98	0.95
Uncertain	0.36	0.54
Very Certain	0.94	0.92
Very Uncertain	0.36	---
Likely	0.77	0.68
Unlikely	0.28	0.29
Very Likely	0.88	0.80
Very Unlikely	0.22	0.18
Possible	0.60	0.55
Impossible	0.02	0.04
Very Possible	0.68	0.59
Very Impossible	0.07	0.03

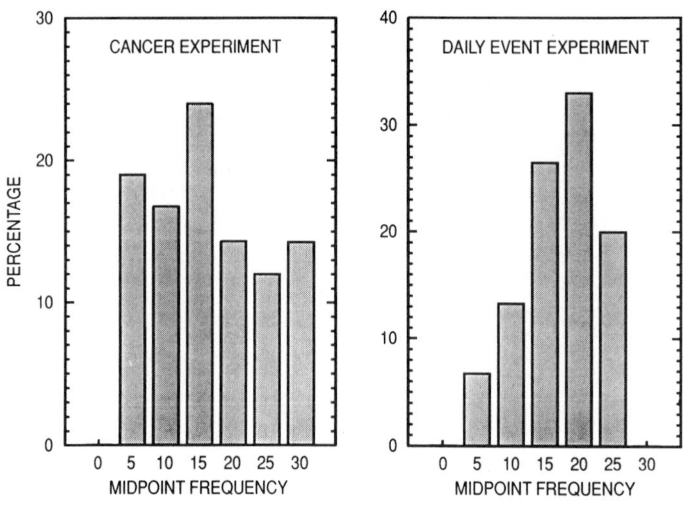

Fig. 2. Number of terms used by subjects by experiment.

The last results pertain to rules of conjunction *not* used by subjects. The data in Table 4 could only have been collected via our automated knowledge acquisition method. The observations row refers to the average answers subjects gave for second session questions. The rules refer to answers the subjects would have been expected to give if they had used those rules to answer the second session questions. For example, if a second session question had been "What is the likelihood of smoking causing cancer and cancer causing depression" and the subject's answers to those simple questions had been 0.90 and 0.90 (interpolated), then using the product rule the answer would have been 0.81. The subject could have given any answer, interpolated, between 0.0 and 1.0.

On average, people do not use the product, average, minimum and maximum rules. Of course, the product rule is the normatively correct rule. Only in the high/high conjunctive questions is the product rule close to the actual average. Usually, the observed average changes relative to the rule predictions as the magnitudes of the simple likelihoods change. For the cancer experiment, the minimum rule closely describes conjunctions when a low likelihood is involved whereas in the daily event experiment the average rule seems to be closest. The goal here is not to say exactly how people process uncertainties but to highlight, in a time honored tradition, how people do not process uncertainties and state that the elicitation capabilities of LES provide new kinds of data to study this question.

DISCUSSION

This study highlights advantages of knowledge elicitation techniques for risk analysis. First, the knowledge elicited from the subjects pertains to likelihoods concerning cause and effect relationships and event occurrence instead of opinions and perceptions. Second, the resulting data sets are complex; they contain each subject's rank orderings of natural language representations of uncertainty, edits made to answers, sorting instructions, and information on the consistency of their answers. Such data require non-standard analysis techniques and approaches. Third, the flexibility of the computer in collecting data is quite evident. LES is able to tailor-make question and answer sessions and perform data analysis in real time, thus enabling the collection of unique and more reliable data. Fourth, the knowledge elicitation approach fostered the collection of rigorously defined data. All information collected from the subjects fits into prearranged data fields immediately available for analysis.

Table 4. Comparison of Uncertainty Combinations to Rules by Experiment

	Magnitude of Terms Combined*					
	High/High		High/Low		High/Medium	
Observation/Rule	C	DE	C	DE	C	DE
Observations	0.74	0.67	0.29	0.29	0.62	0.52
Product Rule	0.71	0.74	0.09	0.10	0.42	0.40
Average Rule	0.84	0.86	0.48	0.47	0.67	0.66
Minimum Rule	0.78	0.81	0.11	0.12	0.49	0.47
Maximum Rule	0.90	0.90	0.85	0.82	0.84	0.85
	Low/High		Low/Low		Low/Medium	
	C	DE	C	DE	C	DE
Observation	0.28	0.33	0.16	0.12	0.27	0.27
Product Rule	0.11	0.10	0.01	0.02	0.07	0.07
Average Rule	0.49	0.48	0.12	0.12	0.31	0.31
Minimum Rule	0.13	0.12	0.06	0.08	0.14	0.15
Maximum Rule	0.84	0.85	0.18	0.16	0.48	0.47
	Med./High		Med./Low		Medium/Medium	
	C	DE	C	DE	C	DE
Observation	0.53	0.56	0.26	0.29	0.50	0.46
Product Rule	0.40	0.40	0.06	0.06	0.24	0.25
Average Rule	0.66	0.65	0.30	0.30	0.49	0.49
Minimum Rule	0.48	0.48	0.11	0.14	0.44	0.44
Maximum Rule	0.84	0.83	0.49	0.46	0.54	0.55

*Low = 0.0 to 0.33; Medium = 0.34 to 0.66; High = 0.67 to 1.0.

This study provides useful information for risk analysis and especially for risk communication. For example, subjects frequently use the concept of 'possibility' when representing uncertainty. Risk information communicated in terms of probability to people who think in terms of possibility may not be communicated properly. Subjects prefer to use simple, ordinary modifiers such as 'very' and 'highly' in their language, although the impacts of modifiers depend very much on the concept being modified. In general, first level modifiers, such as modifying 'likely' with 'very', carry more weight than second level modifiers, such as modifying 'likely' with 'highly' instead of 'very'.

Uncertainty language is exceedingly complex. Concepts do not, in general, possess mirror images. For example, 'possible' is not a mirror image of 'impossible'. People utilize a tremendous range of concepts and discernment. It is just as likely that a person will use 6 to 10 natural language terms to represent uncertainty as that he will use over 25 terms. Future research could attempt to determine whether this range is due to a lack of knowledge to discern or a preference for simplicity.

Lastly, the data make possible an analysis into heuristics used to combine estimates of uncertainty. The results indicate that people do not utilize normatively acceptable rules. Future research should strive to extend this work to determine whether people process uncertainties at least in minimally acceptable ways. Such research would need to define what is minimally acceptable and be able to classify people based on their heuristics.

REFERENCES

1. B. Tonn and L. Arrowood, ARK-Acquiring and Reasoning About Knowledge, Proceedings of the Third Annual Expert Systems in Government Conference, Washington, DC, October 21-23, 1987.
2. B. Tonn, C. Travis, L. Arrowood, R. Goeltz, and C. Mann, Analysis of Individual Risk Belief Structures, in *Advances in Risk Analysis: Risk Assessment in Setting National Priorities*, Proceedings of the 1987 Annual Meeting of the Society for Risk Analysis, Houston, TX, James J. Bonin and Donald E. Stevenson, eds., pp. 431-441 (1989).
3. B. Tonn and R. Goeltz, An Experiment in Combining Estimates of Uncertainty, in *Advances in Risk Analysis: New Risks, Issues and Management*, Proceedings of the 1986 Annual Meeting of the Society for Risk Analysis, Boston, MA, Louis A. Cox, Jr., and Paolo F. Ricci, eds., pp. 403-412 (1990).
4. K. Schmucker, *Fuzzy Sets, Natural Language Computations, and Risk Analysis*, Computer Science Press, Rockville, MD.
5. R. Beyth-Marom, How Probable is Probable? A Numerical Translation of Verbal Probability Expressions, *Journal of Forecasting* **1**:257-269 (1982).
6. S. Lichtenstein and J. R. Newman, Empirical Scaling of Common Verbal Phrases Associated with Numerical Probabilities, *Psychon. Sci.* **9**:563-564 (1967).

Social Conflict Assessment in the Design of Risk Management Systems

Michael L. Poirier Elliott
Georgia Institute of Technology
Atlanta, GA

ABSTRACT

Risk management strategies frequently generate conflict. This conflict results not only from differences in interests associated with expected outcomes, but just as fundamentally from divergent assessments, perceptions and values associated with risk management. These differences impair communication and creativity in decision making and inhibit decisive action. To effectively design, implement and administer policy, the risk manager must therefore generate cooperation amongst the individuals and organizations that can block action. An effective risk management system is consequently also a conflict management and consensus building system. Hence, methods for more effectively coping with conflict in risk management systems are needed. This paper examines the root sources of risk-based conflict, develops methods for assessing potential conflict as part of a risk management process, and presents an alternative approach to designing risk management systems built upon concepts of both risk assessment and social conflict assessment. The approach focuses analysis on a wider range of concerns than is typically envisioned by risk analysts, and is imbedded in models of policy making and dispute resolution. Based upon simulations involving risk managers and policymakers in waste management systems, the approach shows promise of facilitating workable risk management policy.

KEYWORDS: Risk management, dispute resolution, hazardous waste, risk perception, simulations

INTRODUCTION

In recent years, conflict over risk and its management has increased dramatically. In fields as disparate as genetic research, toxic substance control and technology management, disagreements have erupted over the risks involved, the margins for safety that the government ought to ensure, the approaches necessary to ensure these safety margins, and the appropriate government response in light of uncertainty.[1,2] As a consequence, policy making for many aspects of risk management no longer functions effectively.[3]

Substantial improvements in our risk management capacity therefore depend on our ability either to abate or resolve conflict. To move forward, we must build a workable social consensus. To do so will require a deeper understanding of the sources and consequences of this conflict, as well as the development of improved processes of conflict resolution.[4]

An understanding of conflict associated with risk management is, however, difficult to achieve. The techniques we have employed, while expanding our knowledge considerably, do not allow us to examine social conflict as a dynamic process. Problems differ by discipline and technique. Experiments in social psychology allow for in-depth assessments but are generally restricted to small numbers of subjects. These techniques therefore cannot be used to analyze the interactions between and among competing interest groups that are an essential feature of public policy risk management disputes. Survey studies elicit an individual's perceptions but do not impose a shared context through which an individual can evaluate those perceptions and judge their likely response. Case study analysis and anthropological assessments provide a broader view but do not allow for interventions or experimentations that might test assumptions about the dynamics of conflict.

This paper proposes an alternative approach to risk management research, one that is designed to probe the dynamics of conflict directly. Based on principles of action research and social learning theory, the proposed strategy couples: (1) systematic conflict assessment to (2) multi-party experimental simulations and (3) interventions into actual disputes. The conflict assessment and interventions allow the analyst/intervenor to explore more fully conflict under field conditions. In turn, gaming experimentation allows alternative strategies to be tested in order to clarify the patterns of risk perception, their impact on behavior in conflicts, the sensitivity of those patterns to various public policy options, and the possibility of developing consensus when perceptions of risk vary widely. Gaming simulations provide a structure for exploring risk management disputes in both their wholeness and in detail. Because simulations are holistic, they provide a laboratory for studying linkages otherwise left uncovered, linkages which appear only when interactions actually take place. Because simulations are controllable, specific alternatives can be introduced, tested and probed.

To help illustrate the potential for this approach, the paper also describes an application of these techniques to the hazardous waste facility siting issue.[5,6] In hazardous waste management, substantial disagreement exists over the significance of risks associated with new treatment facilities and the appropriateness of control strategies.[7,8,9] While the lay public generally supports the necessity of siting new treatment facilities, residents of potential host communities remain fearful that these facilities may prove dangerous.[10] At the same time, many professional risk managers believe that lay fears are unwarranted. To these managers, state of the art hazardous waste treatment facilities pose few risks to a host community.[11,12,13] The analysis, however, has not proved compelling to those who hold a different view. As such, hazardous waste facility siting debates share many of the classic elements associated with risk management disputes, and thus can well illustrate the applicability of conflict assessment techniques to risk management research.

THE APPLICATION OF CONFLICT ASSESSMENT TO RISK MANAGEMENT DISPUTES

In political and economic decision making, conflict emerges out of differences between groups. Like all public policy conflicts, risk management decisions create controversy because they aggravate disagreements over the social contract within which public decisions are made. By the social contract, I mean the basic elements and processes of social exchange which allocates resources and power in society. In the public policy arena, this contract has four basic elements:[14]

1. social structures, which regulate the basic allocation of resources in society;

2. decision-making procedures, which establish ongoing rules for policy making and alter control over political and private decision making;

3. substantive issues, which focus on the outcome of individual decisions; and

4. uncertainty, which alters expectations of future outcomes.

Structural conflicts focus on basic power relationships and on the fundamentals of political decision making — on issues of equity, justice, majority rule and minority rights. In the management of hazardous waste, some community groups are now making claims that the solution to hazardous waste lies not in improved treatment of wastes but rather in reduction in waste generation. These groups further argue that to achieve waste minimization, the state should intervene directly into the industrial production process by banning the production of whole classes of hazardous substances and processes which generate hazardous wastes. This form of environmental and community populism therefore argues that no treatment facilities should be built, because treatment facilities create a market demand for waste and hence compete with waste minimization efforts. As such, this contention is structural because it calls into question the fundamental relationship between a private corporation and the community in which the corporation is located.

Procedural conflicts focus on the ways by which political decisions are made within a particular social order. Procedures act as gates to decision making power, controlling the flow of information, establishing rules of evidence, and altering the ability of individuals to influence policymakers. Disputes over community participation in facility siting decisions are procedural because they claim that a technical process, in and of itself, cannot be trusted to reach a decision that will protect the public interest. In addition, other procedural characteristics also make these disputes intrinsically difficult to resolve. Because benefits are diffuse, support for facilities is minimal in both the electorate and the industrial users of these facilities. Active proponents of these facilities, then, tend to be restricted to state government and the developer. Both are compromised as advocates, the first because the state must also regulate the facility once constructed and the second because the developer must seek to maximize profit in order to operate successfully in an open, competitive market. At the same time, opponents tend to be disorganized and fractionated. While they typically are residents of the same local community, most opponents involved in a hazardous waste dispute organize themselves as the dispute unfolds. Such groups are frequently reactive, with disorganized leadership selected on an ad hoc basis. Thus, the legitimacy of both proponents and opponents is questioned by others in the dispute. Neither side trusts the other.

Substantive conflicts focus on the consequences of decisions. Disputants, recognizing that political decisions essentially involve trading off the interests of one group with those of another, seek to use decision making procedures to maximize their own interests. The impasse over siting emerges in part from a displacement between the interests of proponents and the interests of opponents. Benefits of a hazardous waste facility are spread widely across a region, with no single beneficiary (excluding the developer of the facility) feeling especially well rewarded. At the same time, the risks and costs are concentrated in a very small area of the host community.[16] In the political arena, diffuse regional support is counteracted by concentrated local opposition. Since decisions about whether to require the creation of a waste minimization program within specific industries, to impose new regulations on waste management or to permit construction of a waste treatment facility directly affect the interests of numerous individuals, differences between the interests of various groups causes substantive conflict to emerge. Further, while proponents typically seek to focus the dispute on matters of substance, opponents focus on values, perceptions and principles as much as on substance. The dialogue is distorted because neither side accepts the definition of the issues as proposed by the other. As a result, even setting an agenda for discussion and agreeing on a process for resolving differences is difficult.

Uncertainty-based conflicts focus on the likelihood of future consequences. Even when parties can agree on structural, procedural and substantive grounds, they may be unable to reach an agreement because they interpret risks and uncertainties differently and do not agree what future consequences will be. Disagreements over the likely impacts of waste treatment facilities are clearly uncertainty-based.

In risk management literature, discussions of conflict almost invariably focus on the uncertainty-based sources of conflict. While it is undoubtedly true that uncertainty and risk perception play a dominant role in these conflicts, we should not underestimate the importance of structural, procedural and substantive aspects of risk management disputes.

Conflict assessment examines the patterns of conflict across each of these potential sources. Local opposition to hazardous waste facilities, for example, neither begins nor ends with issues of risk. Community opposition is based on structural, procedural and substantive elements as well. Structurally, opponents argue that private enterprise does not have the right to place communities involuntarily at risk, particularly since many of the risks associated with wastes could be reduced at the source. Procedurally, opponents argue that once sited, a facility and its treatment activities become a permanent neighbor. Because local residents do not necessarily accept decisions made at the state level that exclude local participation, opponents argue that the siting decision is the only significant control a community has over a waste treatment facility, and therefore encourage the local community to exercise this power by excluding the facility. Substantively, while support for better treatment processes and improved hazardous waste management facilities is almost universal, local opposition to specific sites is equally widespread.[15] This dichotomy emerges because hazardous waste facilities, like prisons and power plants, are regionally beneficial but locally noxious. Siting decisions are therefore redistributive: the location of the benefits is isolated from the location of the risks and involves the transfer of costs from one jurisdiction to another.[16]

This then is the context for understanding the impact of uncertainty and risk on facility siting disputes: even in the absence of issues of risk, the dispute would be difficult to resolve. The dispute is characterized by

- little agreement on the issues that could make up an agenda for resolving differences,
- widely divergent interests and competitive goals,
- amorphous and fractionated parties, selected on an ad hoc basis, and
- a relationship between the parties that is short lived and antagonistic.

The uncertainty associated with siting hazardous waste facilities complicates the resolution of these disputes even further.[17,18] This uncertainty causes risk to emerge as a discrete issue in the debate, decreases the ability of participants to evaluate the viability of management techniques, gives rise to important differences in perceptions of impact, and raises issues of the appropriate public policy response in light of uncertainty and risk.

This general assessment of risk management conflicts suggests the range of issues that must be dealt with if we are to resolve risk-based disputes. The issues are not solely ones related to uncertainty, but are based on important elements of structure, decision making and substance as well. This assessment, however, can only sensitize us as to the types of issues we are likely to expect in any risk management dispute. If we are to understand more fully the interrelationships between risk perception, risk management preferences and conflict behavior, we must focus on specific behaviors within the context of risk-based conflict and its management. More specifically, we must assess how different groups function within the phenomena of risk policymaking and conflict. An innovative approach to assessing these relations lies in the design and deployment of experimental simulations. These simulations are described in the next section. We then return to a discussion of the findings of these simulations in the following section.

EXPERIMENTAL SIMULATIONS AS A RESEARCH TOOL IN CONFLICT ASSESSMENT

Simulations were designed to learn more about resolving conflicts that grow out of differing perceptions of risk. How are these perceptions fine tuned? Do conflicts in risk perception stem mostly from disagreements about the ability (or willingness) of government and industry to accurately predict impacts, to detect harmful impacts before they reach crisis proportions, to prevent adverse impacts, or to mitigate harmful impacts if they do occur? Are we more concerned with proposed technological improvements that limit the likelihood of hazard or with organizational arrangements for coping with the risks inherent in all technological systems? What is the efficacy of alternative strategies for managing risk?

To facilitate this analysis, the simulations were designed to accomplish four purposes: to communicate information to the participants, to simulate a realistic risk management controversy within the circumstances of a hazardous waste siting process, to promote dialogue and interaction amongst the participants, and to extract information and opinions from the participants.

Simulations were restricted to communities in which a hazardous waste dispute had not occurred. In public policy disputes, the details of an individual's perceptions can be quickly submerged in the rhetoric of a dispute. In struggles, people become strategic. The language they use for communicating their concerns is hard to separate from their position in the dispute. The simulations were designed to examine perceptions in light of disputes, but to do so before the language for describing those perceptions had become stylized by the debate.

The communities were selected on the basis of a few minimal criteria applicable to the siting of hazardous waste treatment facilities. Each community must be readily accessible to an interstate highway and contain large tracts of undeveloped land. Densely populated cities and highly sensitive ecologies were excluded. Selection generally adhered to state criteria for acceptability of sites.

Participants from these two communities were identified from four interest groups: public officials, businessmen, environmentalists, and landowners. On average, eighteen participants took part in each simulation. All participants were from the community in which the simulation was run and shared a commitment to and experience with the political life of the town.

Each simulation had three phases: presenting the siting proposals, discussing and selecting a negotiating partner, and making tradeoffs. The researcher presented participants with a proposal for a rotary kiln incinerator to be sited in their community. Using diagrams and pictures, the characteristics of the facility were described in detail. Three hazardous waste management firms were then presented as competing for permission to build this facility. Incorporated into each package was one of the three major approaches to risk management. Finally, participants were presented with a range of possible compensation proposals, divided into groups of approximately six individuals, and given the freedom to make tradeoffs among the safety and compensation features as they wished.

Close observation and documentation of the simulations provided an important component of the research data. This study therefore incorporated three research tools specifically designed to explore perceptions that motivated observed behavior. Each individual was given a pre-simulation test of general perceptions about and preferences for risk and hazardous waste treatment, two questionnaires probing changes in their perceptions (to be answered as the simulation proceeded), and a post-simulation interview.

Before commencement of the simulations, the attitudes and perceptions of each participant were evaluated using a simple questionnaire. The questionnaire was aimed at determining attitudes towards hazardous waste, industrial development, environmental protection, the state and federal governments, and public regulation of industry. Beliefs about risk management options and knowledge about hazardous waste were also explored. The questionnaire was designed to facilitate evaluation of group behavior in light of individual preconceptions.

During the simulation, each individual was provided with two voting questionnaires. The form was designed as a simple recording device to assist the individual in reflecting on his or her ongoing perceptions of the siting process. The record was confidential and was used as a basis for exploring perceptions that public statements did not reveal.

After the simulations were completed, each individual was interviewed privately. The sixty to ninety minute interviews were used to integrate the results of the questionnaires and observed behavior. The interviews were designed to provide a time for "picking the minds" of the participants. The simulations had greatly enhanced the understanding of these city officials, business people, environmentalists and land owners about hazardous waste facility siting. Interviews probed the trade-offs that participants made during the simulation and examined the relative importance of the various factors that shaped their risk perceptions. Participants were questioned about perceptions, decision making, discrepancies between perceptions and behavior, the relative value of different approaches to risk management, the suggestions they had for improving the siting process, and their reaction to other, untested proposals.

The realism of the simulation and its ability to elicit meaningful comments are difficult to evaluate. It can only be truly experienced from within — as it was by the researchers and the participants — for it is essentially a sophisticated form of communication and interaction among these individuals. But fully a third of the participants in each city made spontaneous comments about the simulation. The flavor of these comments can be summarized with the statements of three individuals.

> I take this exercise seriously. I've tried to give you input, to tell you what you need to hear because it is what I as an official feel really reflects what is best for the town without shirking responsibility for the problem. But it's really hard to grapple with a problem that's so damned important.
>
> A Selectman

> The game was marvelous. It really put us in places where we had to push and think about these problems. The things that individuals felt were most important were really brought out into the foreground and discussed.
>
> A Conservation Commissioner

> Is anyone really considering putting a hazardous waste treatment plant in Essexton? We talked about this in our group. Yes, we have the land. Yes, we have the wind currents that would carry any air pollution away from populated areas. There's 400 acres of open land available in close proximity to a railroad, with a super highway coming right in. A plant like this could conceivably be sited here. The proposal was very realistic.
>
> An Industrial Process Engineer

PERCEPTION AND MANAGEMENT IN THE EVOLUTION OF CONFLICT

Because of the seeming intractability of perceptions held by both the lay public and technical experts, the dynamics of risk perception have attracted considerable research interest.[19,20,21] Most of this literature focuses on differences between lay perceptions and predictions made using technical models of analysis.[22,23,24,25] Implicitly, two aspects of risk management are emphasized:

- Prediction: Do we know enough to forecast the likely effects of a hazardous waste treatment facility? Is this knowledge being impartially examined and presented?
- Prevention: Can we design systems for effectively reducing the potential risk? Will these systems be reliably managed?

As revealed by the simulations and interviews described above, however, many individuals are concerned with a richer array of risk management options. In particular, two additional aspects of risk are emphasized:

- Detection: If hazardous conditions develop, do we have the means to detect these changes? If so, will that data be collected and scrutinized so as to detect changes quickly?
- Mitigation: If serious hazards are detected, do we know how to reverse the dangers and the negative impacts? Will these mitigation measures be applied with sufficient speed and skill to be effective?

This research suggests that, as a vehicle for managing the hazards associated with waste treatment facilities, laypeople generally prefer strategies of risk detection and mitigation to strategies of risk prediction and prevention. Likewise, most laypeople prefer strategies that strengthen social control mechanisms to those that strengthen technological control mechanisms. How might we explain these differences between expert and lay perceptions and preferences for risk management strategies?

The Technical Conception of Risk

Measurement and analysis are the tools of engineers and scientists. Without them, knowledge about hazards cannot be given meaningful (and testable) structure. With them, hazards are potentially predictable and controllable. To be useful to technical experts, however, indicators of risk must be measurable. Implicit in technical measures of riskiness are presumptions that different risks can be equated inasmuch as their expected outcome is the same and that risks can be ordered by measures of expected outcome. Within technical definitions of significant outcomes (i.e., expected deaths) and models of cause and effect are imbedded a preferred method of coping. If risks are caused by predictable physical reactions, then they are best prevented with predictable physical systems. The coping mechanism is one of engineered controls, of estimating the requisite probabilities, and designing for appropriate safety.

Within this model of risk management, much room for disagreement exists. It is not just that laypeople perceive differently than experts; experts argue among themselves. This is not surprising: the scientific method is based on premises that theories are held tentatively, contingent on the development of contrary evidence and new interpretation. These debates are part of the evolution of science. In an attempt to weed out error and inappropriate behavior, the scientific community regulates which perceived facts and theories are to be considered legitimate and which are not. The quality of these debates is controlled by means of independent experiments and peer review. For many of society's most fearsome risks, however, agreed upon facts and criteria of competence are lacking. Quality control is therefore difficult to ensure because quality is at times impossible to define. As in the Love Canal debate, the result is polarization and suppression of tentative viewpoints, even within the scientific community.

This is not to say that rigorous analysis has no place in resolving ambiguities in risk problems. Rather, it suggests that under conditions of public policy conflict, technical analysis can make no claim to a precision it cannot offer, for a problem it can only partially define. The power of technical analysts to design risk management systems, and to convince a skeptical public of their reliability, is limited by their potential fallibility and by the existence of highly informed public who are capable of challenging the assumptions, techniques and limitations of the analysis. Moreover, the scientific process for resolving differences of opinion among scientists, which is difficult to apply even among those who espouse its value, cannot provide the sole support for a risk management system, the legitimacy of which must be based on an entirely different process of decision making.

Despite these limitations, technical experts can do much to inform the risk management debate. Their methods of analysis yield the most precise predictions of unwanted consequences and provide the overview needed to design systems for preventing hazards. These skills are essential to operators of facilities. In addition, opposition to facility siting does not spring from claims that these skills are unnecessary but rather that they are insufficient as currently conceived.

Lay Conceptions of Risk: A Variety of Perspectives

We know much about how lay publics generally perceive and react to risk but very little about variation amongst individuals in a conflict situation. Amongst the lay public, neither perception nor evaluation of risk is as monolithic as first appears. Distinctions within the public are extremely important to conflict management because any attempt to resolve conflict must act upon the variety of perspectives. The simulations identify three distinct patterns. This variety exists because lay conceptions of risk are not bound to risks that are measurable and hence are neither as precise nor as restricted as those of engineers and scientists. Laypersons are concerned less with expected outcomes, which tend to average out rare events, than they are with variability, the possibility of extreme outcomes, and uncertainty. The extent to which individuals focus on extreme outcomes rather than expected outcomes is in fact a good indicator of their acceptance of proposed facilities.

The three types of lay publics identified include what I call sponsors, guardians and preservationists. Sponsors focus most strongly on expected outcomes, preservationists most strongly on potentially catastrophic events, and guardians moderately on both. These differences come about not because sponsors are more rational than preservationists or even that they think more like scientists and engineers. Rather, they come about because sponsors trust the current systems for managing risks and believe in their spokespersons. They accept the logic of experts because management of these risks is part of the standard operating procedure for which experts are trained. The risks are simply not exceptional and hence do not require special attention.

To guardians and preservationists, on the other hand, the risks associated with hazardous waste treatment facilities are exceptional and do require special attention. These hazards are viewed as more threatening than most. To introduce them into a community is to invite loss of control. Guardians focus on health and safety consequences. To place their town in jeopardy by accepting an unwarranted hazard, even one in which the probability is small, is to shirk responsibility to their community. At the same time that guardians perceive the risks to be significant, however, they also perceive them to be potentially controllable. They wish to protect the quality of life in the community without foreclosing change and believe that technical expertise is necessary but hardly sufficient for effectively controlling risks. They strongly promote systems for detecting and mitigating hazards, coupled to systems for holding management accountable and responsive to community concerns.

In addition to these health and safety concerns of guardians, preservationists also focus on aesthetic and cultural consequences. Much more pervasively, an uncertain future provokes anxiety in preservationists. Preservationists believe the risks to be unpredictable, generally oppose any development that changes the character of the town, and are frustrated by the ambiguity inherent in the use of technical analysis and prevention technology. While skeptical about the value of systems for monitoring or for holding management accountable, they are even more skeptical of the effectiveness of existing safety technologies in the absence of improved managerial systems. They feel powerless to control the future should they allow a treatment facility to be sited. In the face of this uncertainty, they prefer to exercise control over the present by denying permission to site the facility.

Because of this basic concern for extreme outcomes and loss of control, guardians and preservationists do not find technical analysis very compelling. These analyses, generally based on the premise that expected outcome is the most appropriate indicator of risk and physical systems the most important causes of hazards, focus on neither the consequences nor the causes of greatest concern to guardians and preservationists. Rather, guardians and preservationists focus on systems for foreclosing worst case scenarios and for retaining community control over the processes that lead to these extreme outcomes. For the most part, they believe that in well designed treatment facilities, risks are most reliably controlled by means of systems for detecting and mitigating hazards and for managing the treatment facility. These future-oriented, management-based solutions form the basis for coping with rare but extreme outcomes as well as more common consequences.

These three groups each included approximately a third of the participants. While this rough equivalency cannot be said to exist throughout the community, it does suggest that each of these groups will be a significant force in the local politics of facility siting. At this point, we can speculate that unless sponsors are motivated to promote the proposal actively, the concerns of guardians for risk and safety are ameliorated, and the opposition of preservationists is minimized, a proposed facility will face stiff opposition from local residents. In a strategy for siting a facility which seeks to engage each of these groups, the nuances in their perceptions of risk must be carefully considered.

We are left, therefore, with the dichotomy discussed above. While technical experts define risk management as a problem of prediction and prevention, many of the lay residents who currently oppose the siting of a hazardous waste facility (especially the guardians) define risk management as a problem of detection and mitigation. The differences have important implications both for risk management and for resolving siting disputes. While prediction/prevention systems seek present control over future events and focus on engineering solutions, detection/mitigation systems seek to foreshorten uncertainty through flexible systems capable of adjusting to changes over time and hence focus on resilient and error correcting management systems.

We are also left with a far more fundamental dichotomy. In the context of public policy dispute, the perceptions associated with different actors in the process vary considerably. Yet, *a priori*, many of these differing perceptions cannot be disproved by widely accepted scientific rationality. Furthermore, the perceptions are closely linked to risk evaluations and to preferences associated with risk management options. The interrelationship between these various elements makes interventions based on "education" of the lay public highly ineffective. Furthermore, given the pervasiveness and variety of these perceptions and preferences at the local levels of governance, attempts to compel acceptance of hazardous waste treatment facilities or other risk management options seems unworkable.

Both from the simulations and from actual interventions into risk management conflict, it appears that these conflicts cannot be resolved in the absence of an open dialogue, one in which all significant participants in the process are involved.[26,27] Only in such a process can we deal with the complex interrelationships between perceptions and risk management preferences, between interests and empowerment issues. These conflict management principles, as they emerged both from participants in the simulations and from lay residents and public officials associated with risk management conflict in their local decision making, are summarized in the next section.

HOW CAN WE MOVE FORWARD?

In this final section, we discuss a process of dispute resolution that seeks to adapt multi-party dispute resolution techniques to the specific characteristics associated with hazardous waste facility siting disputes. The process envisioned has nine distinct tasks.

Identify parties with a stake. Before any process of dispute resolution can begin, a system of identifying parties with a stake must be in place. While we cannot necessarily predict who will actively advocate or oppose a particular siting proposal, we can accurately identify those parties with a stake in the decision. Inclusion of all major stakeholders will help both to legitimize the consensus building process and foreclose unexpected controversy over final agreements.

Ensure appropriate representation of the parties. Siting disputes are multipartied and complex. Direct involvement of all affected individuals in the dispute resolution process would be extremely cumbersome. As a consequence, individuals must be grouped by common interests and representatives selected for participation. Three conditions are most important: representatives must be perceived as legitimate spokespersons, they must be open to scrutiny by those people they represent, and the process itself must offer some opportunities for wider participation.

Select a mediator. In facility siting disputes, a mediator is indispensable. Especially in complex disputes, communication amongst the many stakeholders is extremely cumbersome at best. If issues are to be addressed in an efficient manner, a neutral facilitator will be needed to organize the process, run meetings, facilitate dialogue, and provide other supports to effective communication and consensus building.

While the services of a mediator may well be needed before representatives of the stakeholders are assembled, final selection must wait until this assembly. Ultimately, a mediator's effectiveness depends on his or her relationship to the various stakeholders. For this reason, the decision to employ a mediator must meet with the approval of these stakeholders.

Build the capacity of the represented parties to engage in meaningful negotiation. The ability of stakeholders to engage in negotiation differs considerably amongst the various parties. Most community groups will have little or no experience in negotiations. Further, the representatives of these groups may have constituencies that are disorganized and fractionated. At the same time, while developers and state agencies are more likely to be experienced negotiators, the circumstances of this negotiation will differ considerably from past experience.

The mediator will therefore need to build the capacity of these parties to engage in meaningful negotiation. Three types of assistance are likely to be necessary: development of rudimentary skills in multiparty bargaining, provision of technical assistance for understanding issues, and support for vertical team bargaining. In particular, vertical team bargaining is an important component, for it allows representatives of various interests to build consensus amongst the people they represent and to involve them in decision making. This link is essential if the formation of splinter groups is to be avoided.

In addition, the mediator will need to design a consensus building process that provides ongoing support to groups as needed.

Define the issues. Before discussion can begin on the substance of the dispute, a clear sense of the issues, as defined by each of the stakeholders, must be developed. Clearly, the differences in interests, values and perceptions discussed in this paper require careful exploration if solutions are to be designed which take these differences into consideration. Differences in assumptions will need to be confronted directly, so that a deeper understanding of the issues can be developed.

Generate alternatives for further consideration. Options for siting facilities can be generated through structured brain storming, task forces and other techniques. Options to be considered must be appropriate to the policy decisions under consideration (e.g., source reduction cannot be the sole solution to a facility siting issue if the represented stakeholders do not include waste generators and similar groups), but care must be taken in precluding alternatives prematurely (e.g., a source reduction planning process can be a partial solution to a facility siting issue). The discussion must be open to a wide range of alternative risk management techniques, as well as other aspects of facility siting of interest to various stakeholders.

Jointly assess impacts of the alternatives. Once alternatives are outlined, information will be needed to decide between them. Participants in the consensus building process will need to formulate the questions of greatest importance and decide on an approach for resolving remaining uncertainties. Clearly, assessments of impacts will not yield definitive answers, but the problems associated with traditional technical assessments can alleviated. Approaches such as joint fact finding (the joint design of new studies by participants, including determination of scope, assumptions and boundaries of analysis and selection of consultants) and data mediation of existing analyses can improve communication around issues created by technical analysis.

Expand options. Alternatives, once assessed, are subject to refinement and redesign. The most difficult task of dispute resolution, that of converting a general agreement over goals and objectives into a consensus around the design of particular options to be pursued, must now be conducted. Options must be pieced together to handle the many complex components of the issues.

Options are not limited to the design of risk management systems and mitigation measures, but also include compensation measures. Compensation is frequently an efficient approach for dealing with the redistributive effects of residual impacts. Compensation is not, however, a substitute for fully exploring options for mitigating impacts. Compensation, raised too early in the dispute resolution process, can damage trust and credibility by raising the spector of selling health for privilege.

Design agreements. In addition to specifying the substance of the agreement in detail, the consensus building process needs to specify an implementation plan that is responsive to the high degree of uncertainty inherent in the siting of hazardous waste facilities. Evaluation criteria should be developed against which consistency with the substantive intent of the agreement can be monitored. Likewise, a monitoring system will need to be designed. Finally, contingency agreements are useful for dealing with the remaining uncertainty concerning both impacts and the implementation of the agreement.

CONCLUSIONS

The actual effectiveness of the consensus building process cannot be known in the absence of an attempt to employ it. Innovative modifications to the systems for managing risks have not been an item of negotiation in past siting disputes. Based on the reflections of local residents, however, this process cuts to the very core of the current deadlock in public risk management by working with differences in perceptions, rather than assuming inevitable conflict between them. Further, the process of dispute resolution is designed to cope with characteristics intrinsically associated with risk management systems and to do so in ways that are acceptable to both local and facility operators. In so doing, the process holds open the promise of more effective risk management by both altering the sources of risk and promoting the acceptance of treatment facilities.

ACKNOWLEDGMENTS

This study would not have been possible without the support of the Joint Center for Urban Studies of M.I.T. and Harvard University, the William and Flora Hewlett Foundation (through the Harvard Program on Negotiation) and the Andrew W. Mellon Foundation (through the M.I.T. Center for International Studies). Many individuals gave generously of their creativity and talents to this research, especially Lawrence Susskind, Lawrence Bacow, Gary Hack, and Joseph Ferreira of M.I.T., and Michael O'Hare and Howard Raiffa of Harvard University. Special thanks to Gail Bingham, Tim Mealy and other members of the Conservation Foundation for their support.

REFERENCES

1. M. Douglas and A. Wildavsky, *Risk and Culture*, University of California Press, Berkeley, CA (1982).
2. T. Page, A Generic View of Toxic Chemicals and Similar Risks, *Ecology Law Quarterly* **7(2)**:207-244 (1978).
3. W. Clark, Witches, Floods, and Wonder Drugs: Historical Perspectives on Risk Management, in *Societal Risk Assessment: How Safe Is Safe Enough?* R. Schwing and W. Andrew, Jr., Plenum Press, NY (1980).
4. L. Susskind and A. Weinstein, Towards a Theory of Environmental Dispute Resolution, *Boston College Environmental Affairs Law Review* **9(2)**:311-357 (1980).
5. M. Elliott, Coping with Conflicting Perceptions of Risk in Hazardous Waste Facility Siting Disputes, unpublished doctoral dissertation, M.I.T. Department of Urban and Regional Planning, Cambridge, MA (1984a).
6. M. Elliott, Improving Community Acceptance of Hazardous Waste Facilities Through Alternative Systems for Mitigating and Managing Risk, *Hazardous Waste* **1(3)**:397-410 (1984b).
7. R. Anderson and M. Greenberg, Hazardous Waste Facility Siting, *Journal of the American Planning Association* **48**:204-218 (1982).
8. L. Bacow and J. Milkey, Overcoming Local Opposition to Hazardous Waste Facilities: The Massachusetts Approach, *The Harvard Environmental Law Review* **6(2)**:265-305 (1982).
9. J. Lester and A. O'M. Bowman, *The Politics of Hazardous Waste Management*, Duke University Press, Durham, NC (1983).
10. D. Morell and C. Pollak, *Siting Hazardous Waste Facilities: Local Opposition and the Myth of Preemption*, Ballinger, Cambridge, MA (1982).
11. Massachusetts Department of Environmental Management, *Hazardous Waste Management in Massachusetts*, Commonwealth of Massachusetts, Boston (1981).

12. Massachusetts Department of Environmental Management, *Kommunekemi: The Danish National Hazardous Waste Treatment System*, Commonwealth of Massachusetts, Boston (1982a).
13. Massachusetts Department of Environmental Management, *Analysis of Operation and Emissions from Typical Hazardous Waste Treatment Processes*, Commonwealth of Massachusetts, Boston (1982b).
14. M. Elliott, Conflict Resolution, in *Urban Planning*, A. Catanese and J. Snyder, eds., McGraw-Hill, NY (1988).
15. U.S. Environmental Protection Agency, *Siting of Hazardous Waste Management Facilities and Public Opposition*, Government Printing Office, SW-809, Washington, DC (1979).
16. M. O'Hare, L. Bacow, and D. Sanderson, *Facility Siting*, Van Nostrand, NY (1983).
17. T. O'Riordan, Risk Perception Studies and Policy Priorities, *Risk Analysis* **2(2)**:95-100 (1982).
18. H. Otway and K. Thomas, Reflections on Risk Perception and Policy, *Risk Analysis* **2(2)**:69-82 (1982).
19. B. Fischhoff, S. Lichtenstein, P. Slovic, S. Derby, and R. Keeney, *Acceptable Risk*, Cambridge University Press, NY (1981).
20. D. Kahneman, P. Slovic and A. Tversky, eds., *Judgments Under Uncertainty: Heuristics and Biases*, Cambridge University Press, Cambridge (1982).
21. C. Hohenemser, R. Kates and P. Slovic, The Nature of Technological Hazard, *Science* **220**:378-384 (1983).
22. W. Lowrance, *Of Acceptable Risk*, William Kaufmann, Los Altos, CA (1976).
23. R. Nisbett and L. Ross, *Human Inference: Strategies and Shortcomings of Social Judgment*, Prentice-Hall, Englewood Cliffs (1980).
24. W. Rowe, *An Anatomy of Risk*, John Wiley, NY (1977).
25. R. Schwing and W. Albers, Jr., eds., *Societal Risk Assessment: How Safe Is Safe Enough?* Plenum Press, NY (1980).
26. D. Nelkin and M. Pollack, Problems and Procedures in the Regulation of Technological Risk, in *Societal Risk Assessment*, R. Schwing and W. Albers, Jr., eds., Plenum Press, NY (1980).
27. B. Wynne, Technology, Risk and Participation: On the Social Treatment of Uncertainty, in *Society, Technology and Risk Assessment*, J. Conrad, ed., Academic Press, NY (1980).

A New Limit-Line Approach to Compare Large Scale Societal Accidents

Hector A. Munera
Cisatec Ltd. and Instituto Ser de Investigacion
Bogota, Columbia

George Yadigaroglu
Nuclear Engineering Laboratory
Zurich, Switzerland

ABSTRACT

Frequency-consequence curves (f-c curves) are often used for the comparison of societal risks. Under this approach, nuclear power is a completely acceptable technology. Public reaction to such conclusion is ascribed to "irrationality" or to empirical limitations. Assumptions implicit in f-c curves are briefly discussed.

To avoid the limitations of f-c curves, the paper proposes a disaggregation of large scale accidents into two components: the frequency of accidents and the probability distribution of consequences conditional upon the occurrence of an accident. From historical data, it was found that natural and familiar technological accidents cluster in two areas separated by an empty gap. Surprisingly, nuclear power and natural gas lie in the gap.

For regulatory purposes, the problem of aggregating accident rates and the consequences given an accident can be circumvented by establishing two separate criteria, one for each component. Historical data may be used as a guide for the numerical targets; in particular, it is suggested that the envelope of common technological accidents may provide a guide towards defining a regulatorily tolerable limit-line for the magnitude of less-common technological accidents.

KEYWORDS: Societal risk, limit-lines, f-c curves, risk comparisons, safety goals, high-consequence accidents

INTRODUCTION

The increasingly rapid adoption of new technologies has resulted in numerous improvements in the so-called quality of life and has reduced certain everyday risks, e.g., the risks from infectious diseases, travel, and food poisoning. But new technologies have also introduced new categories of risks that are sometimes subtle and difficult to quantify, e.g., the various risks associated with the use of pharmaceutical products and pesticides.

Risk Analysis, Edited by C. Zervos
Plenum Press, New York, 1991

Certain technologies involving the handling of vast amounts of energy are displacing other well established ones; for example, burning of coal or oil for electricity production has yielded ground to nuclear power; transportation of liquefied natural gas (LNG) has become an alternative to the transportation of coal or oil by conventional means. Although these trends tend to diminish traditional risks such as those associated with mining, conventional transportation, and air pollution, they introduce new, unfamiliar risks[a] such as those related to radioactive contamination from severe nuclear accidents and catastrophic explosions of LNG carrying vessels.

We are fully aware that societal risk is a multifaceted problem with quantifiable and unquantifiable components. However, for clarity, in the following we concentrate on only one aspect: large scale accidents leading to early fatalities. We define as large scale accident any event causing at least ten fatalities.[b]

To handle multidimensional consequences two possible approaches are: (a) to carry out for each dimension a separate analysis similar to the one suggested here for early deaths; or (b) to aggregate all relevant accident attributes in a single index, i.e., a multi-dimensional value function as discussed in chapter 3 of Keeney and Raiffa (1976),[1] to obtain therefrom the appropriate (multidimensional) probability distribution. The two approaches are discussed by Munera.[2]

In this paper we stress the difference between natural and man-made accidents. The public seems to be particularly sensitive to the consequences of large-scale technological accidents. One of the reasons for this may be that there is no historical perspective for such man-made catastrophes; until recently the technologies that could produce large-scale accidents were simply nonexistent. On the contrary the public is accustomed to the catastrophic consequences of large-scale natural disasters such as earthquakes or floods. These seem to be accepted, tolerated or endured. California is the example of a state where living conditions are considered as very desirable in spite of its well-known high seismicity risk.

Another important aspect is an empirical fact: the public perception of numerous small accidents in comparison to infrequent large-scale accidents. In the mind of most persons (and in everyday public decision making) an accident that could kill 10,000 persons with a frequency of occurrence once every 10,000 years is not equivalent to the death of a person every year. What seems to have an important weight is the potential for unlikely but very high consequence events. We see nothing "irrational" in this belief. Simply, it is a manifestation of a mathematical truth: to describe a probability distribution the mean does not suffice in general.

With the plausible purpose of taking into account the whole probability distribution of large scale societal accidents, frequency-consequence curves (f-c curves) were proposed in the Reactor Safety Study (RSS).[3] According to f-c curves like those reproduced in Fig. 1, nuclear power should be a widely acceptable technology. Public outcry following this RSS's suggestion is typically interpreted as caused by uncertainty in data and lack-of-completeness in counting accident sequences,[4,5] the theoretical foundations of f-c curves receiving only occasional attention.[6]

---

a. In this paper *risk* is used as a generic term without any technical meaning. The (Webster) dictionary definition is "dangerous chance; chance of injury, damage or loss." In addition, risk also implies the potential for future unknown unfavorable conditions and/or situations and/or outcomes.

b. This is a rather arbitrary definition dictated to us by the statistical data immediately available. Other definitions of "large scale accident" are, of course, possible, e.g., events causing at least one early fatality, or some arbitrary monetary or environmental damage, and so on.

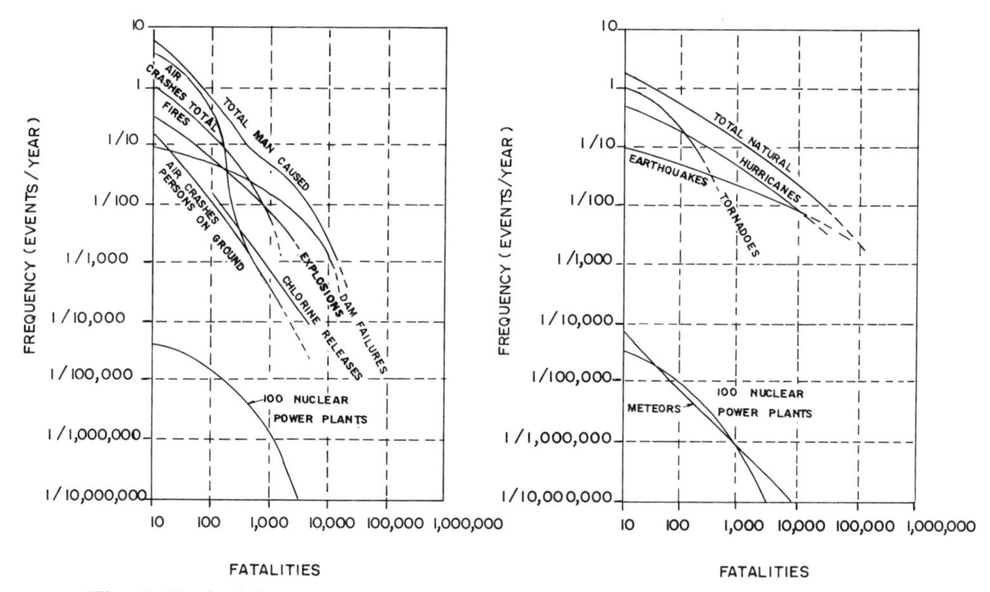

Fig. 1. Typical f-c curves currently used for risk comparisons (taken from Figs. 1-1 and 1-2 of Ref. 3, page 2 of the Executive Summary). Note that if plotted on the same graph, natural and technological risks are intermingled.

In the following discussion, we first propose a disaggregation of large scale accidents into two components: the frequency of undesirable events and the probability distribution of consequences conditional upon the occurrence of such an event. We then interpret f-c curves in the context of the previous model and discuss some assumptions implicit in its intended use. Next from historical data, we show that natural and common technological accidents cluster in two different areas separated by a gap. Surprisingly, in this gap lie some of the most controversial modern technologies, namely nuclear power and natural gas. Thence, we suggest that the envelope of common technological accidents may provide a guide towards defining a limit-line eventually useful for regulatory purposes.

CHARACTERIZATION OF LARGE SCALE SOCIETAL ACCIDENTS

A technological system (TS) is defined as a class of similar devices, used with the same purpose, in some geographical or political region, e.g., aircraft, nuclear power, hydro power in a given country. Further specification may be required as small aircraft/large aircraft, or light water reactors/heavy water reactors, or earth dams/concrete dams, and so forth.

In this paper societal risk (see footnote a, page 168) associated with a TS is characterized by the random duplet (N,X), where:

- N is the total number of accidents, A, during an observation period t; and
- X is the conditional probability distribution of consequences, given that accident A has occurred.

Typically, the empirical probability distribution of A is unknown; in some cases, however, it may be reasonable to assume a Poisson law. For the case of one-parameter probability laws, the probability density function (pdf) is characterized by the mathematical equation plus one numerical value, say the expected value or mean. We assume that the mean is described by the accident rate λ, whose empirical estimate is s/t, where s is the sum of all events that occurred during t.[c] The accident rate in a given geographical area reflects, among other things, the probability of accident per unit time or time surrogate (year, kilometer, passenger-km, etc.) multiplied by the number of units.

X is an empirical pdf derived from historical data by listing the number of events n causing x or more immediate fatalities during an observation period t. This period t should be long enough to have a significant number of events, but short enough to reflect current technological and safety practices. For example, Coppola and Hall[7] used $t = 20$ years for technological accidents, and $t = 40$ years for natural disasters. The distribution of X may be obtained, for instance, by plotting $F^* = n/s$ vs x, where F^* is an empirical complementary cumulative probability distribution function, CCPDF (see Figs. 2-4).

FREQUENCY-CONSEQUENCE CURVES

The current practice is to describe natural and technological risks capable of producing large scale accidents by listing the number of events (n) observed during a specified time-period t (say, 20 years) resulting in x or more victims. Following the RSS[3] most analyses of large scale accidents have adopted a graphical representation whereby n/t is plotted against x. These graphs are the so-called frequency-consequence curves. As seen in Fig. 1, no particular pattern appears in the f-c curves that could hint at what a societally tolerable risk level could be.

In the context of the model described in previously, it is obvious that f-c curves are but plots of λF^* vs x, i.e., they represent empirical accident rates above a given level of consequence x. This means that f-c curves implicitly aggregate the two random variables N and X in a multiplicative fashion, using two different levels of detail: N is reduced to the deterministic parameter λ thus losing the shape of the corresponding pdf, whereas the shape of X's pdf is maintained. The above remark partially coincides with the Royal Society's view[6] that f-c curves are also a form of average comparison.

The well-established theory of first-degree stochastic dominance, FDSD,[8-10] and the weaker form of zero-degree stochastic dominance[11,12] ordinally compare dimensionless probability distribution functions. For the case of unfavorable consequences of interest in risk analysis, represented by CCPDFs as in Figs. 2 and 3, lower curves are preferable. This argument, however, cannot be directly invoked for the comparison of the f-c curves in Fig. 1 because they are not CCPDFs. If proponents and users of f-c curves want the theoretical backing of FDSD, some additional assumptions are required as discussed elsewhere by Munera.[2]

Many of the proposed and/or adopted quantitative safety criteria for nuclear power plants (NPPs) are based on limit-lines, somehow related to f-c curves as reviewed elsewhere.[13,14] We turn now to an alternative interpretation of the same actuarial data-base used by the RSS[3] and updated by Coppola and Hall.[7]

---

c. When referring to random quantities, the name of the quantity is a capital letter, whereas particular values are represented by lower-case letters.

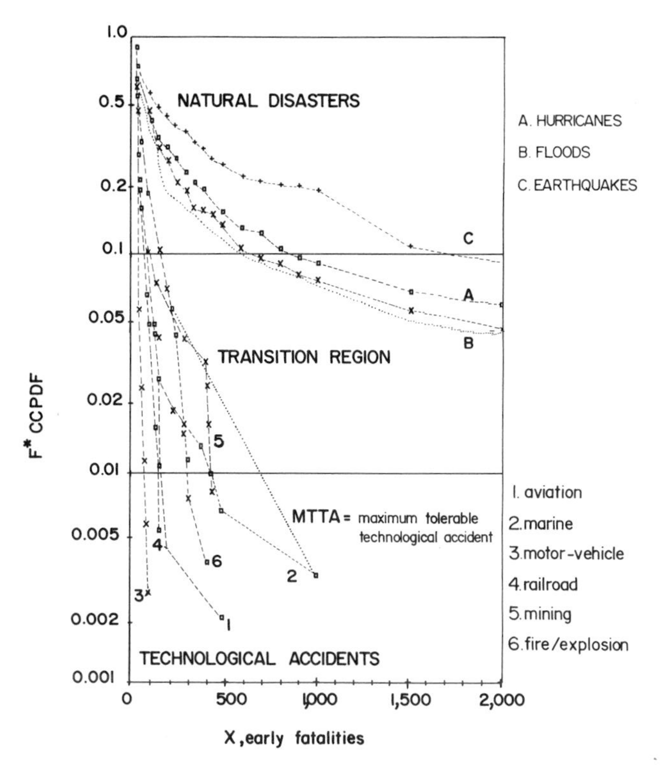

Fig. 2. Natural and technological disasters. CCPDFs obtained from historical data for the whole world in period 1938-1977.[7]

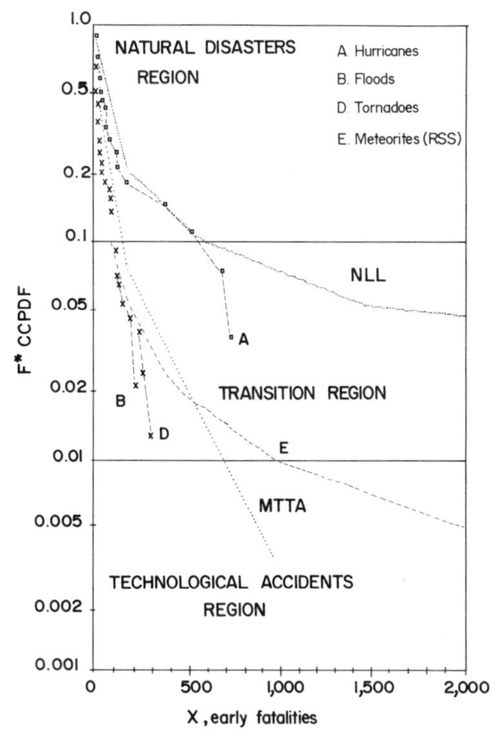

Fig. 3. Natural disasters in the USA. CCPDFs obtained from historical data for the period 1938-1977.[7]

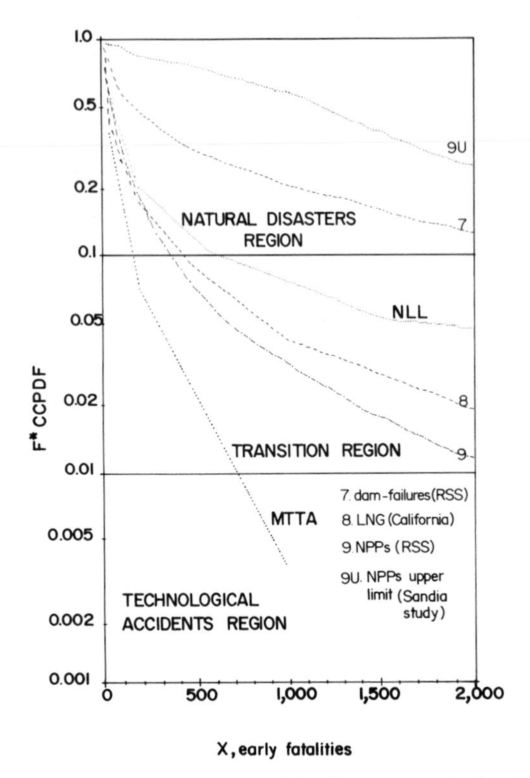

Fig. 4. Technological accidents in the USA. Curves are derived from calculated data collated in Ref. 7.

NATURAL VS TECHNOLOGICAL ACCIDENTS

Frequent Accidents

We reanalyzed[15,16] the empirical data collated by Coppola and Hall[7] for natural disasters (hurricanes, floods, earthquakes, tornadoes) and technological accidents (transport, mining, fire and explosion) with the following results:

a. There is no particular pattern for λ, which spans a rather short interval: 4 to 24 events/year for the total world, and 0.1 to 5 events/year for the USA, as seen in Table 1. Differences between the USA and the total world may be explained by the different number of units and — possibly in some instances — by a lower probability of accident per unit.

b. There is a striking pattern for the total world plots of F^* vs X. Three regions are clearly identified: natural disasters (above), technological accidents (below), and an intermediate empty zone (see Fig. 2). The transition zone is limited above by the lower envelope for natural disasters (Natural Lower-Limit, NLL) and below by the upper envelope for technological accidents, discussed next. Since the technological accidents shown in Fig. 2 are due to familiar technologies,[d] it is suggested that the envelope of F^* may constitute a societally maximum tolerable

d. The typical societal reaction to a familiar accident is to ask for more safety, but not to stop or forbid the technology.

Table 1. Accident Rates for Natural and Technological Disasters[a]

	Historical Accident Rate, Events/Year		
	Total World	(World - USA)	USA
Natural Disasters, Period 1938-77 (t = 40 years)			
A. Hurricanes	5.20	4.50	0.70
B. Floods	8.15	7.03	1.12
C. Earthquakes	4.22	4.12	0.10
D. Tornadoes	-----	-----	1.98
E. Meteorites	-----	-----	0.0001[b]
Technological Accidents, Period 1959-78 (t = 20 years)			
1. Aircraft	23.30	18.25	5.05
2. Marine	15.05	13.10	1.95
3. Motor-vehicle	18.00	16.80	1.20
4. Rail-road	9.35	9.00	0.35
5. Mining	6.05	5.30	0.75
6. Fire and explosion	13.05	9.45	3.60
7. Dam failure	-----	-----	0.20
	-----	-----	0.078[b]
	0.59	0.45	0.14[c]
8. LNG transport New York Harbor	-----	-----	0.017[d]
California sites	-----	-----	0.0015[d]
9. Nuclear power	-----	-----	0.00003[b]

[a]All figures from the actuarial data compiled by Coppola and Hall,[7] except as noted.

[b]Calculated from the RSS.[3]

[c]Worldwide: 13 disasters with more than 10 fatalities in the period 1959-80. Disasters in the USA: 3 (see Table II.2 in Ref. 17).

[d]Calculated from Coppola and Hall.[7]

technological accident (MTTA). This suggestion does not imply that accidents should be accepted or just endured by society. Indeed, efforts should be made to decrease the severity of the consequences of both natural and technological disasters (the viability of this suggestion is exemplified by the USA, as discussed in the following).

c. The CCPDFs for technological accidents in the USA (Fig. 3) are slightly lower than those for the total world shown in Fig. 2, but not enough to justify a separate analysis. The same observation is implicit in Coppola and Hall[7]; they noted that f-c curves in the USA are more or less "parallel" (hence, similar) to the rest of the world (the parallel shift is due to different accident rates λ). Contrarywise, the CCPDFs for natural disasters are significantly lower in the USA than in the rest of the world, as seen in Fig. 3. It is conjectured that the shorter high-consequence tail is a result of preventive measures (flood control, for instance) and sophisticated warning and rescue systems (not always available elsewhere).

It is noteworthy that the curves for tornadoes and floods lie below the MTTA and are qualitatively similar to technological CCPDFs. Given that tornado and flood-prone areas are inhabited and have undergone recent urban development in the U.S.A., it is reasonable to argue that such risks are also tolerable to the U.S. society. These remarks lend further support to the concept of MTTA.

Less-Frequent Technological Accidents

Risk studies of technologies without a sufficient historical data-base for accidents typically report f-c curves. According to our definition of accident, $F^* = 1$ at $X = 10$. Then, the frequency at $X = 10$ equals λ. Dividing the different frequencies by λ the CCPDF immediately obtains as shown in Fig. 4 for the USA.[3,7,18]

The CCPDF for dam failures (see Fig. 4) obtained from the RSS[3] is almost identical to the total world curve for earthquakes (see Fig. 2), excepting the very-high-consequence tail. At least in some countries,[17,19] societal concern for dam-failures is not particularly strong. If this localized observation is more or less general, then it may be conjectured that such disasters are perceived as closer to nature than to technology.

The CCPDF for LNG transport lies above the MTTA, but below NLL (Fig. 4), and is very similar to the average curve for NPPs also shown in Fig. 4. Considerable public controversy has surrounded the development of and/or site-selection for both LNG and NPPs. Again, this fact lends support to the concept of "tolerable" accident, represented here by the MTTA. We note in passing that the upper part of the uncertainty band for NPPs obtained in the Sandia Siting Study[18] lies well inside the region for natural accidents, whereas the lower limit is below the MTTA.

POTENTIAL REGULATORY APPLICATIONS

The aggregation of the two random components of societal risk is often done in an implicit and informal manner. For example, the "technical definition of risk" in the RSS[3] implicitly assumes that the appropriate index to evaluate each separate component is the mean of the distribution, and further assumes that the appropriate aggregation is multiplicative. For a discussion of some hidden assumptions in several indices used for societal and technical risk comparisons see Munera.[2]

Limit-line approaches make an explicit effort at avoiding some of the assumptions mentioned in the previous paragraph, but the results are not much better. For instance, one current limit-line approach uses f-c curves and selects an arbitrary shape of λF^* vs x, that purportedly takes into account the so-called "societal risk-aversion." All steps of such procedure are potentially controversial: the selection of λ as a proxy for N, the multiplicative aggregation of λ and F^*, the linearity of these two components, the shape of the limit-line and its relative position. For further discussion see Munera and Yadigaroglu.[13]

Given the current state-of-the-art in non-deterministic decision making, it seems fairly difficult to find universally acceptable aggregation procedures for N and X. Hence, we suggest that a sufficient and technically feasible approach to get around the aggregation problem is to establish two separate and independent criteria:

1. *Probability-consequence limit-line* (which limits the consequences given an accident). Its theoretical justification is the concept of first-degree stochastic dominance,[2,8-12,14] whereas the empirical justification is the MTTA. Depending upon her particular circumstances every society would opt for regulatorily tolerable technological accident (RTTA) (see Fig. 5 for an example). Note that we are not

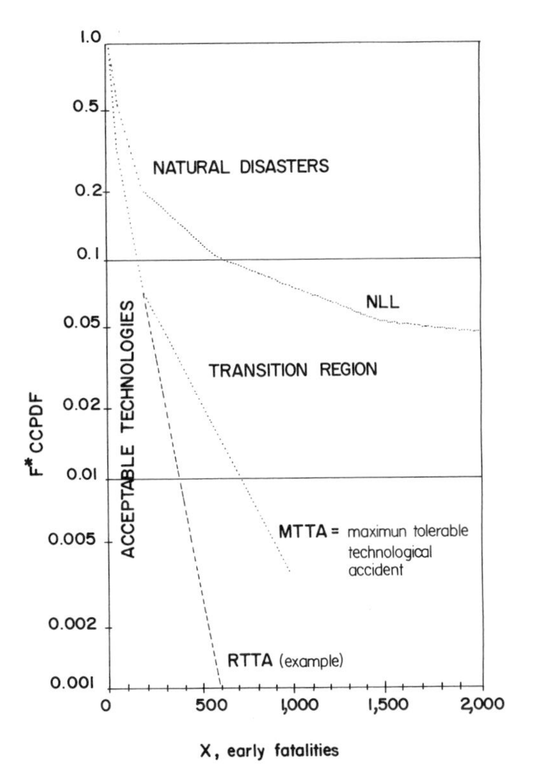

Fig. 5. RTTA limit-lines. Examples of (imaginary) regulatorily tolerable technological accidents. The RTTA divides the space in two regions: acceptable technologies below, and unacceptable above the RTTA.

saying that an accident should be acceptable to society, we are just suggesting a limit that might be tolerable to or endurable by society, thus establishing a guide for regulatory purposes.

2. *Probability of large scale accidents*. As mentioned earlier, this is related to λ. A detailed analysis of empirical data may suggest the order of magnitude of a societally tolerable probability of an accident, e.g., that the probability of a large scale accident (as defined here) be less than 1 in 10,000 per year (or per plant lifetime, etc). One example of such approach is the core-melt limit adopted in the U.S. as a design objective.[20]

The limit-line we are suggesting is a proper probability distribution function, founded on well established theoretical criteria.[8,9,10] It is an ordinal method of measurement being, therefore, much weaker in the required assumptions than any cardinal approach—like the expected value, or the theory of utility in the sense of von Neumann and Morgenstern[21] or the linearized moments model.[11,22,23]

Adoption of such set of dual criteria for regulatory purposes avoids the problem of aggregation, which is two-fold: (a) trade-off between N and X (or in simple words, frequency vs severity of accidents), and (b) individual and public perception/acceptance of N and X.

The proposed approach is "objective" in the sense that there is historical experience and data for a spectrum of different societal risks that may suggest limits for both criteria. On the other hand, it may be unnecessarily restrictive by leaving out the possibility of trading out accident rates against the severity of consequences. In common with all stochastic dominance approaches, the RTTA induces a partial ordering, i.e., not all probability distributions may be compared (that is, if the CCPDF of a project crosses the RTTA, the two probability distributions are non-comparable. Of course, for regulatory purposes a conservative approach is to reject the project, but that is a pragmatic decision, not a theoretically based outcome).

As a final remark, the proposal advanced herein has the merit of defining a criterion limiting the consequences, which from the point of view of public perception of risks seems to be the most salient component. Indeed, when there is an accident the immediate reaction is to ask what was the total number of victims. Concern for the accident rate usually comes up as an afterthought.

CONCLUSION

The empirical data underlying widely used frequency-consequence curves was reinterpreted as an accident rate and a conditional probability of consequences, given an accident. Three regions were identified in the graph of the complementary cumulative probability distribution function of X (CCPDF): natural disasters, technological accidents, and a transition empty region.

For regulatory purposes, the problem of aggregating accident rates and the consequences given an accident (i.e., the CCPDF) can be circumvented by establishing two separate criteria, one for each component. Depending upon each society, the two criteria may be required to hold independently, or may be linked in a lexicographical ordering. Historical data may be used as a guide for the numerical targets; in particular, it is suggested that the envelope of common technological accidents may provide a guide towards defining a regulatorily tolerable limit-line for the magnitude of less common technological accidents.

Our analysis was based on the periods 1938-77 for natural disasters and 1959-78 for technological accidents. Use of more recent data may add detail to the high-consequence low-probability region (several important events have occurred in the last decade, e.g., aircraft accidents, large oil fires, chemical accidents (Bhopal, the contamination of the Rhine), and nuclear accidents (Chernobyl). Such analysis may lead to establishing an upper cut-off point for the magnitude of an accident. Two possible approaches are to (1) set a limit on the probability, and (2) set a cut-off point on the maximum consequence based on physical considerations regarding the technological system, the population distribution, the accident sequences, etc. Munera[2] has argued that events occurring 1 time in 10^9 years are for all practical purposes impossible. For regulatory purposes every society might select a limiting probability in the range of 1 in 10^6 years to 1 in 10^9 years.

REFERENCES

1. R. L. Keeney and H. Raiffa, *Decisions with Multiple Objectives: Preferences and Value Tradeoffs*, John Wiley and Sons, New York (1976).
2. H. A. Munera, A Theory for Technological Risk Comparisons, in *Risikountersuchungen als Entscheidungsintrument—Risk Analysis as a Decision Tool*, G. Yadigaroglu and S. Chakraborthy, eds., Verlag TUeV Rheinland, Cologne (1985).

3. US NRC, Reactor Safety Study, WASH-1400 (NUREG 75/014), US Nuclear Regulatory Commission, Washington, DC (October 1975).
4. Union of Concerned Scientists, The Risks of Nuclear Power Reactors: A Review of the NRC Reactor Safety Study WASH-1400 (NUREG-75/014), H. W. Kendall, Study Director, Union of Concerned Scientists, Cambridge, MA (August 1977).
5. US NRC, Risk Assessment Review Group Report to the U.S. Nuclear Regulatory Commission, H. W. Lewis, Chairman, NUREG/CR-0400, US Nuclear Regulatory Commission, Washington, DC (September 1978).
6. The Royal Society, Risk Assessment, A Report of a Royal Society's Study Group, London (January 1983).
7. A. Coppola and R. E. Hall, A Risk Comparison, NUREG/CR-1916, US Nuclear Regulatory Commission, Washington, DC (February 1981).
8. J. Hader and W. R. Russell, Stochastic Dominance and Diversification, *J. Econ. Th.* **3**:288-305 (1971).
9. M. Rothschild and J. E. Stiglitz, Increasing Risk I: A Definition, *J. Econ. Th.* **2**:225-243 (1970). Addendum to previous paper, *J. Econ. Th.* **5**:306 (1972). Increasing Risk II: Its Economic Consequences, *J. Econ. Th.* **3**:66-84 (1971).
10. K. Borch, Utility and Stochastic Dominance, in *Expected Utility Hypotheses and the Allais Paradox*, M. Allais and O. Hagen, eds., D. Reidel Publishing Co., Dordrecht (1979).
11. H. A. Munera and G. Yadigaroglu, A New Methodology to Quantify Risk Perception, *Nucl. Sci. Eng.* **75**:211-224 (1980).
12. H. A. Munera, On Absolute Preference and Stochastic Dominance, *Theory and Decision* **21**:85-88 (1986).
13. H. A. Munera and G. Yadigaroglu, Quantitative Safety Goals for Nuclear Power Plants: Critical Review and Reformulation within a Unified Theory, in *Implications of Probabilistic Risk Assessment*, M. C. Cullingford, S. M. Shah and J. H. Gittus, eds., Elsevier Applied Science, London and New York (1987). Also in *Res Mechanica* **24**:233-263 (1988).
14. H. A. Munera and G. Yadigaroglu, On Farmer's Line, Probability Density Functions, and Overall Risk, *Nucl. Tech.* **74**:229-232 (August 1986).
15. H. A. Munera, A Quantitative Comparison of Natural and Technological Societal Risks, in *Probabilistic Safety Assessment and Risk Management PSA' 87*, Vol. III, European Nuclear Society and Swiss Nuclear Society, eds., Verlag TUeV Rheinland, Cologne (1987).
16. G. Yadigaroglu and H. A. Munera, Large Scale Accidents and Public Acceptance of Risks, presented at ENVRISK-88, Como, Italy (May 11-13, 1988).
17. H. A. Munera, On the Perception by the General Public in Colombia of the Risks Associated with Electrical Power Generation, Instituto Ser de Investigacion, Bogota (December 1982).
18. T. S. Margulies and R. M. Blond, Variability of Site-Reactor Risk, *Risk Analysis* **4**:89-95 (June 1984).
19. H. A. Munera, Actual and Perceived Low-Probability Hazards from Hydro and Nuclear Electric Power Generation, in *Risks and Benefits of Energy Systems*, International Atomic Energy Agency, Vienna (1984).
20. US NRC, Safety Goals for Nuclear Power Plant Operation, NUREG-0880, Rev. 1, U.S. Nuclear Regulatory Commission, Washington DC (May 1983).
21. J. von Neumann and O. Morgenstern, *Theory of Games and Economic Behavior*, Princeton University Press, 3rd. Ed. Science Editions, John Wiley and Sons, New York (1964).
22. H. A. Munera, Modeling of Individual Risk Attitudes in Decision Making under Uncertainty: An Application to Nuclear Power, Ph.D. dissertation, Department of Engineering, University of California, Berkeley, CA (September 1978).
23. H. A. Munera, The Generalized Means Model (GMM) for Non-Deterministic Decision Making: Its Normative and Descriptive Power, Including Sketch of the Representation Theorem, *Theory and Decision* **18**:173-202 (1985).

Beyond Risk Analysis: Aspects of the Theory of Individual Choice Under Risk

Michael D. Weiss
U.S. Department of Agriculture
Washington, DC

ABSTRACT

Risk analysts are concerned primarily with *determining* risks—with establishing the probability of undesirable events. Yet, once risks are known, decision makers are still faced with the task of choosing among competing risky courses of action. How can they make these choices in a rational manner? This question has been much studied by economists and psychologists, particularly under the rubric of "expected utility theory." In this paper, some of the basic concepts of this subject are investigated from a mathematical perspective. The paper focuses on two main topics: (1) how risk and certainty are represented in expected utility theory, and why; and (2) the independence of behavior under certainty from behavior under "continuous" risk.

KEYWORDS: Choice under risk, expected utility axioms, lotteries

INTRODUCTION

Risk analysts have traditionally been concerned primarily with determining risks—with establishing the probabilities of undesirable events. Yet the determination of such probabilities is not so much an end as a beginning. Once risks are known, even if imprecisely, decision makers—whether affected citizens or government policy makers—are still faced with the task of choosing among competing courses of action.

Consider the situation of a farmer who must decide what type of pesticide to employ in his operation. For each level of application of available pesticides, technical studies may have led to an accurate determination of the probabilities of various adverse health effects on the user. Yet this information does not solve the farmer's "risk problem." For suppose that he can choose between two pesticides known to have differing probability distributions of health effects (as measured, say, along some severity axis such as lifetime medical costs). If his choice were merely between a higher and a lower probability of harm, his decision would be automatic. However, in choosing between two entire *distributions* of probability, he may have to make such judgments as whether he prefers a higher average level of harm mitigated by a zero probability of death as against a lower average level of harm associated with a small but positive probability of death.

Such judgments lie beyond the purview of traditional risk analysis. Yet it is often in just such judgments that the knowledge generated by risk analysts is put to use. Thus the manner in which such judgments are made should be a matter of keen concern to risk analysts.

Now, an individual's preferences among probability distributions might at first appear to be an entirely subjective matter. However, economists long ago discerned order within this seeming disorder. In a pathbreaking work, von Neumann and Morgenstern[1] showed that, if one takes as given a preference ranking of probability distributions satisfying several plausible axioms of rational behavior, one can always construct a numerical-valued function U of probability distributions such that (1) $U(D_1) > U(D_2)$ if and only if D_1 is strictly preferred to D_2 and (2) $U[pD_1 + (1-p)D_2] = pU(D_1) + (1-p)U(D_2)$ whenever $0 \leq p \leq 1$ and D_1, D_2 lie within the domain of the ranking. Condition (1) stipulates that the function U is a numerical representation of the individual's risk preferences, containing the same information as his formal ranking but in a different form. Functions satisfying (1) are called "utility functions." Condition (2) is a linearity property reminiscent of taking expected values. Accordingly, the entire subject has come to be called the theory of "expected utility."

While the empirical applicability of expected utility theory has come under increasing criticism and various alternative approaches have appeared (see Fishburn[2] for a review), the theory has remained the most widely used paradigm for analyzing individual choice under risk. Yet, despite the prominence of the subject, the pertinent literature—particularly the more applied literature—has not always been conducive to understanding. Some commonly claimed results have depended on incomplete arguments or hidden assumptions. Concepts have sometimes been identified inappropriately with special cases. Overall, a clear sense of the mathematical interrelationships of the basic ideas has not been adequately communicated.

The aim of this paper is to clarify several basic aspects of expected utility theory. The paper will focus on two topics: (1) the form in which risk is represented in expected utility theory, and (2) the independence between an individual's choices under certainty and his choices under some forms of risk. Many of the points discussed, while well-known to a relatively small number of economic theorists (for example, see Fishburn[3]), are not well understood by most applied economists, even those using risk concepts in their empirical work. Other observations presented here arise from apparently new perspectives.[4,5] It is hoped that the clarifications provided will ease the path of risk analysts who may wish to familiarize themselves with the economic theory of choice under risk.

COMPOUND LOTTERIES, CONVEXITY, AND THE REPRESENTATION OF RISK

The theory of preferences under risk concerns choices that individuals make when confronted with alternative risky prospects. In economics, these risky objects of choice are customarily called "lotteries." A lottery may intuitively be conceived of as a game of chance in which various prizes occur with preassigned probabilities. These prizes may be a scalar (such as money) or even other lotteries (that is, the opportunity to play other lotteries and receive *their* prizes). In the latter case, one speaks of a "compound" lottery.

Consider the example of a farmer who applies an experimental herbicide having a probability p of success and a probability $1 - p$ of failure. If the first case occurs, he faces a spectrum of possible profits depending, for example, on weather and other unpredictable factors. In the second case, there is another (lower) spectrum of possible profits. In effect, with probability p, the farmer receives one profit lottery as a prize, and with probability $1 - p$, another. This situation has the form of a compound lottery.

The concept of lottery used in expected utility theory is governed by an important convention: two lotteries are considered "equivalent" if they have the same sets of ultimate prizes occurring under the same probability laws, regardless of the processes by which these prizes are achieved. In short, the internal compound structure of a lottery is ignored. The risky objects of choice are not individual lotteries as one intuitively conceives them in everyday life but, rather, are *equivalence classes* of individual lotteries.

It might at first appear that one could define a lottery (or, more precisely, the corresponding equivalence class) mathematically as simply a random variable whose possible values were the various ultimate prizes, those occurring according to the desired probability law. However, the calculation of an overall random variable to represent an empirical compound lottery in terms of its constituent lotteries would be quite complicated. Thus, random variables are not very convenient as mathematical representations of lotteries. Rather, it turns out that *cumulative probability distribution functions (c.d.f.'s)* are more tractable representations.

Recall that, if X is a random variable on a probability space with probability measure P, then the c.d.f. of X is the function F_X defined by $F_X(r) = P(X \leq r)$ for all (real) numbers r. In words: $F_X(r)$ is the probability that the random variable X takes a value less than or equal to r. F_X contains all the probabilistic information inherent in X, but in a more convenient format. It can be shown (1) to be nondecreasing, (2) to be continuous on the right at each point r, and (3) to satisfy $\lim_{r \to -\infty} F_X(r) = 0$ and $\lim_{r \to \infty} F_X(r) = 1$. Conversely, if F is any numerical function satisfying conditions (1) - (3), then there exists a random variable of which F is the c.d.f. Thus, the set of all c.d.f.'s is merely the set of all functions satisfying conditions (1) - (3). We define a *lottery* as a c.d.f., that is, a numerical function F satisfying conditions (1) - (3).

Bearing in mind the distinction between the empirical, everyday concept of lottery and our mathematical representation of it, consider an empirical compound lottery $\mathcal{L}$ that offers empirical lotteries $\mathcal{L}_1$ and $\mathcal{L}_2$ as prizes with probabilities p and $1 - p$, respectively. Then, if the c.d.f.'s L_1 and L_2 are taken to represent $\mathcal{L}_1$ and $\mathcal{L}_2$, respectively, the c.d.f. $pL_1 + (1-p)L_2$ will represent $\mathcal{L}$. (Note that we are using the algebra of functions here; $pL_1 + (1-p)L_2$ is a function whose value at any number r is $pL_1(r) + (1-p)L_2(r)$. Note also that $pL_1 + (1-p)L_2$ is indeed a c.d.f.; this fact is readily proved by reference to the defining properties (1) - (3).) *This simple relationship—the representation of compound empirical lotteries by convex combinations of c.d.f.'s—is central to the usefulness of c.d.f.'s as mathematical representations of empirical lotteries.*

The importance of this relationship between the empirical notion of a compound lottery and the formal concept of a convex combination of lotteries (c.d.f.'s) is exhibited in another aspect of expected utility theory. For another basic assumption of this subject is that the individual's choice set—the set of risks over which his preferences extend—is closed under the formation of compound lotteries. Expressed mathematically, and in view of the previous discussion, this requirement is simply: whenever $0 \leq p \leq 1$ and the choice set contains the lotteries L_1 and L_2, then it must contain $pL_1 + (1-p)L_2$. Observe, however, that the set of all numerical functions, endowed with the usual operations of addition and subtraction of functions and multiplication of functions by numbers, is a *vector space*[6] containing all lotteries as elements. Moreover, within this vector space, the convex combination $pL_1 + (1-p)L_2$ is a point on the line segment joining L_1 and L_2; indeed, $pL_1 + (1-p)L_2$ traces out this line segment as p runs from 0 to 1. Thus the requirement that the choice set be closed under the formation of compound lotteries amounts to the requirement that, whenever the choice set contains two points, it must also contain the line segment joining them. But this is precisely the requirement that the choice set be *convex.*[7]

Now, as noted earlier, when a preference ranking of lotteries satisfies the von Neumann-Morgenstern axioms of behavior under risk, there exists a utility function U satisfying what is essentially the central equation of expected utility theory—the linearity property (in our current notation)

$$U\left[pL_1 + (1-p)L_2\right] = pU(L_1) + (1-p)U(L_2) \ .$$

The foregoing discussion provides an intuitive interpretation for this property. For, if L_1 and L_2 are in the choice set (in which case $U(L_1)$ and $U(L_2)$ are both defined), the convexity of the choice set ensures that $U[pL_1 + (1-p)L_2]$ is also defined. Moreover, if $pL_1 + (1-p)L_2$ is interpreted as a compound lottery offering lottery prizes L_1 and L_2 with probabilities p and $1 - p$, respectively, then the linearity property simply asserts that the utility of a compound lottery is p times the utility of its first component lottery plus $1 - p$ times the utility of its second.

More General Representations of Risk

The definition of lotteries as c.d.f.'s contains the implicit assumption that a lottery's ultimate prizes can be represented by numbers. Indeed, if F is a lottery and t is a real number, we are interpreting $F(t)$ as the probability that the lottery will provide an ultimate prize in the interval $(-\infty,t]$. Thus, in the approach detailed here, the number line represents the set of possible prizes.

In many practical applications, however, a more general definition of a lottery is required. If, for example, in the case previously discussed of a farmer choosing between pesticides, each pesticide was associated with not only a probability distribution of health effects but also a probability distribution indicating its effectiveness in raising crop yield, the farmer would need to consult his preferences among not *one*-dimensional but *two*-dimensional (joint) probability distributions.

Fortunately, it is possible to define lotteries so that quite general types of objects are permissible as ultimate prizes. One such definition characterizes a lottery as a probability measure defined on a set of prizes. To understand how this approach relates to our own, observe that there is a natural one-to-one correspondence between the set of all c.d.f.'s F and the set of all Borel probability measures m on the number line, defined by

$$m\left[(-\infty, t]\right] = F(t)$$

(see Chung[8]). For any c.d.f. F, this formula determines a unique Borel probability measure m on the number line (that is, in effect, on our set of prizes) that contains the same probabilistic information as F, but in a different format. Essentially, while F associates a (cumulative) probability with each *number* t, the probability measure m assigns probabilities directly to *sets* of numbers. In this sense, m plays somewhat the same role as integrating a probability density function over various sets. However, probability measures are more general; for example, they can assign positive probability to a single point (such as when characterizing a "certainty") whereas a probability density function cannot. The adjective "Borel" simply indicates which sets are assigned probabilities by m.

Clearly, the above correspondence associates convex combinations of c.d.f.'s with convex combinations of the corresponding measures; thus, Borel probability measures on the number line share the ability of c.d.f.'s to represent empirical compound lotteries conveniently in terms of their component lotteries. Although the use of point functions such as c.d.f.'s does offer computational advantages, there would have been no *conceptual* barrier to our originally defining lotteries to be Borel probability measures on the number line. Similarly, given a set consisting of *any* objects considered prizes, one could define a lottery to be a probability measure on that set.[9] Much of the advanced economics literature on risk theory uses this approach.

An even more general definition of lottery is implicit in Herstein and Milnor.[10] There a "mixture set" is defined as any set of objects that are capable of being combined with one another, and with weights in [0,1], to form analogs of convex combinations. Convex sets of c.d.f.'s, convex sets of n-dimensional (joint) c.d.f.'s, and convex sets of probability measures are subsumed as special cases.

Representing Certainty

Certainty is merely a special case of risk. When risks are represented by c.d.f.'s, a certainty is represented by a lottery having a single, guaranteed prize, say r. Formally, then, a certainty is represented in expected utility theory by a *degenerate* lottery F_r given by

$$F_r(t) = \begin{cases} 0 & \text{if } t < r \\ 1 & \text{if } t \geq r. \end{cases}$$

It is natural to inquire whether the number r could itself be used to represent the notion of "r with certainty" by "identifying" r with the function F_r. After all, simplifications of this sort are used throughout mathematics, as when the real number b is identified with the complex number $(b,0)$. However, the identification of r with F_r cannot succeed within expected utility theory. For, suppose U were a linear utility function representing an individual's risk preferences over his choice set, and suppose that (as is frequently the case) certainties were among his choices. Then, for any numbers r, s and any p satisfying $0 \leq p \leq 1$, one would have

$$U\Big[pF_r + (1-p)F_s\Big] = pU(F_r) + (1-p)U(F_s) \ .$$

If, now, the identification between numbers and degenerate lotteries were allowed, this equation would reduce to

$$U\Big[pr + (1-p)s\Big] = pU(r) + (1-p)U(s) \ ,$$

from which would follow the special case

$$\begin{aligned} U(p) &= U\Big[p \cdot 1 + (1-p) \cdot 0\Big] \\ &= pU(1) + (1-p)U(0) \\ &= p[U(1) - U(0)] + U(0) \ . \end{aligned}$$

Consequently, U would be linear on the interval [0,1], and one would be forced to conclude that, in cases in which the individual has continuous risk preferences,[9,11] U must, at least over [0,1], be risk neutral (i.e., the individual would always be indifferent between a risk and a certainty equal to the mean payoff value of the risk[11]). Such a conclusion would be logically insupportable. Thus, the proposed identification cannot be allowed.

BEHAVIOR UNDER CERTAINTY VERSUS BEHAVIOR UNDER RISK

Though a few economic theorists know better, there remains a widespread impression in the less theoretical risk literature that, under the von Neumann-Morgenstern axioms of expected utility theory (or under the more succinct axiom system of Herstein and Milnor[10]), the values of a linear utility function under certainty determine its values (and thus the individual's preferences) under risk. Specifically, suppose U is a linear utility function defined over a choice set. Suppose further that the choice set contains all degenerate lotteries (representing certainties). Then, a numerical function u, called the "induced utility function," can be defined from U by the rule

$$u(r) = U(F_r)$$

for each r. It is often claimed, in effect, that U can be recovered from u and that, in fact, U has an "expected utility integral" form given by

$$U(L) = \int_{-\infty}^{\infty} u(t)dL(t) \qquad (L \text{ in the choice set}) .$$

(Note that this integral is of Stieltjes type.[12])

In this section, it is shown that these characterizations are not accurate. Rather, unless the axioms are augmented by additional assumptions, an individual's utility function over certainty is, in a broad range of cases, actually *independent* of his preferences among continuous lotteries (lotteries that are continuous functions in the ordinary sense, such as normal c.d.f.'s).

The demonstration of this assertion begins with a definition. A lottery D is called *discrete* if it can be expressed as a convex combination

$$D = \sum_{i=1}^{\infty} p_i F_{r_i} \quad \left(0 \leq p_i \leq 1; \sum_{i=1}^{\infty} p_i = 1\right)$$

of a sequence of degenerate lotteries F_{r_i}.

Now, it is a fact well-known in probability theory that any lottery L can be expressed as a convex combination

$$L = p_L L_d + (1 - p_L) L_c \quad (0 \leq p_L \leq 1)$$

of a *discrete* lottery L_d and a *continuous* lottery L_c. It follows that, for any linear utility function U defined at L, L_d, and L_c, we have

$$U(L) = p_L U(L_d) + (1 - p_L) U(L_c) \ .$$

However, the decomposition of L into $p_L L_d + (1-p_L)L_c$ is also known to be *unique* in the sense that p_L is unique, L_d is unique if $p_L \neq 0$, and L_c is unique if $p_L \neq 1$. Consequently, the function U_2 defined on the original choice set by

$$\begin{aligned} U_2(L) &= p_L U(L_d) + (1 - p_L)[U + 1](L_c) \\ &= p_L U(L_d) + (1 - p_L) U(L_c) + 1 - p_L \end{aligned}$$

is well-defined. U_2 is easily seen to be linear, and it is a utility function representing the preference ranking defined by: "L is strictly preferred to L^* if and only if $U_2(L) > U_2(L^*)$." Moreover, U_2 agrees with U at degenerate lotteries (i.e., U_2 and U have the same induced utility function u). (To establish this point, note that, since every degenerate lottery F_r is discrete, the number p_{F_r} and the lottery $[F_r]_d$ appearing in the canonical convex decomposition of F_r must satisfy $p_{F_r} = 1$ and $[F_r]_d = F_r$. Thus, $U_2(F_r) = U(F_r) = u(r)$.) Yet, U_2 and U are distinct functions whenever the choice set contains at least one continuous lottery L, for then $p_L = 0$, $L = L_c$, and $U_2(L) = U(L_c) + 1 \neq U(L)$. Hence, it has been demonstrated that, whenever the choice set contains continuous lotteries, distinct linear utility functions defined over this set can take the same values at degenerate lotteries. It follows that it is not generally possible to determine a linear utility function from its values over certainty.

REFERENCES

1. John von Neumann and Oskar Morgenstern, *Theory of Games and Economic Behavior* (second edition), Princeton University Press, Princeton (1947).
2. Peter C. Fishburn, *Nonlinear Preference and Utility Theory*, Johns Hopkins University Press, Baltimore (1988).
3. Peter C. Fishburn, Unbounded Expected Utility, *Annals of Statistics* **3**:884-896 (1975).
4. Michael D. Weiss, *Conceptual Foundations of Risk Theory*, Technical Bulletin No. 1731, Economic Research Service, U.S. Department of Agriculture (1987).
5. Michael D. Weiss, Expected Utility Theory Without Continuous Preferences, in *Risk, Decision and Rationality*, B. Munier, ed., pp. 115-126, D. Reidel Publishing Co., Dordrecht (1988).
6. K. Hoffman and R. Kunze, *Linear Algebra*, Prentice-Hall, Englewood Cliffs (1961).
7. Erwin Kreyszig, *Introductory Functional Analysis with Applications*, Wiley, New York (1978).
8. Kai Lai Chung, *A Course in Probability Theory* (second edition), Academic Press, New York (1974).
9. Jean-Michel Grandmont, Continuity Properties of a von Neumann-Morgenstern Utility, *Journal of Economic Theory* **4**:45-57 (1972).
10. I. N. Herstein and John Milnor, An Axiomatic Approach to Measurable Utility, *Econometrica* **21**:291-297 (1953).
11. Michael D. Weiss, Risk Aversion in Agricultural Policy Analysis: A Closer Look at Meaning, Modeling, and Measurement, in *New Risks: Issues and Management, Advances in Risk Analysis*, Vol. 6, pp. 159-166, L. A. Cox, Jr. and P. F. Ricci, eds., Plenum Press, New York (1990).
12. Walter Rudin, *Principles of Mathematical Analysis* (second edition), McGraw-Hill, New York (1964).

Risk Assessment and Risk Management: Their Separation Should Not Mean Divorce

Richard Wilson and William Clark
Harvard University
Cambridge, MA

ABSTRACT

In 1980 and 1982, two committees of the National Academy of Sciences recommended a separation of risk assessment and risk management. This has, in some cases, been taken too liberally, with the risk manager failing to understand the complexities of the risk assessment. Some undesirable consequences are suggested.

KEYWORDS: Risk assessment, risk management

INTRODUCTION

One hundred and fifty years ago, life was simpler. The same individual:

- performed the science,
- proposed the technology,
- analyzed the risk,
- proposed the standards ,
- recommended legislation, and
- testified before Parliament or Congress.

If he did well, he was knighted or raised to the peerage for his efforts. Such honors went to Sir William Barrett, the sanitary engineer, and Lord Kelvin, the thermodynamicist and shipping expert.

But even then there was opposition to technical progress. Maurice Tubiana records that Louis Pasteur held up the main drainage in Paris because of his objection to peoples' sewage, full of dangerous microbes, being taken under other peoples' houses and streets and possibly spreading disease.

Those were what are often called the "good old days," although the "bad old days" seems a better description.

Risk Analysis, Edited by C. Zervos
Plenum Press, New York, 1991

Nowadays different people do each of the jobs required for technological development and as a consequence we face the problem of encouraging proper flow of information between the participants in the process.

The genesis of this paper was a few discussions between the two authors in 1987 and 1988. We had differences in approach and realized that it might be interesting to discuss our differences before this audience. However, logistic matters prevented Dr. Clark from coming to the meeting and made it impossible for us to discuss the paper in detail in the few days before the meeting when the paper was finally written.

BACKGROUND

In 1979/80 a committee of the National Academy of Sciences under the chairmanship of Professor Howard Raiffa met to discuss risk in society. This committee made several important recommendations. Among them were that scientific data collection should be separated from risk assessment and risk assessment separated from risk management.

Although the full report was never published — only an executive summary was published[1] — it had considerable influence because William Ruckelshaus, a member of the committee, later became head of the EPA.

In 1981/82 a second NAS/NRC Committee, under the chairmanship of Dr. Stallones, issued the report "Risk Assessment in the Federal Government: Managing the Process."[2] The chart in Fig. 1 shows the suggested procedure. It repeats the earlier NAS recommendation of separating the functions of risk assessment and risk management. Although the full report contains most of the caveats and foresees many of the problems noted in this paper, few people got beyond this first figure. The last NAS report, combined with the fact that William Ruckelshaus became administrator of EPA, led to the adoption by EPA of the task separation principle.

Even at the time last NAS/NRC report first came out, we had problems with it. As Fig. 1 shows, information appears to flow only one way, from hazard evaluation to risk assessment to risk management. The separation of hazard evaluation from risk estimation and dose-response evaluation is, we believe, wrong. If the start of the process were hazard postulation, we would have no problem. One of us has emphasized the problem in several forums. What is the hazard of a new, untested chemical? One does not know until one has done a preliminary dose-response and a risk assessment. Yet to suggest that there may be no hazard because one has not yet performed the next steps of risk assessment may obviously allow some risky chemicals to be accepted.

Although the report itself has appropriate cautionary words, these are not often read and the diagram is used as the sole indicator of the recommendations. The rigid adherence to these steps by federal agencies has led to a hiatus in regulation and ignoring of the suggestion by Schneiderman and Mantel[3] that we should provide incentives for good experiments.

In 1985 the EPA produced a modified diagram (Fig. 2) illustrating an overlap between risk assessment and risk management and, more importantly, a feedback line from the management to the assessment phase.

In a book published in early 1982,[4] one of us had a more complex diagram illustrating several steps (Fig. 3). This diagram emphasizes that the risk assessor has to make assumptions (which should be clearly stated) and that the risk should include an uncertainty estimate. The comparison of risk, benefit, and cost is suggested to be part of the assessment.

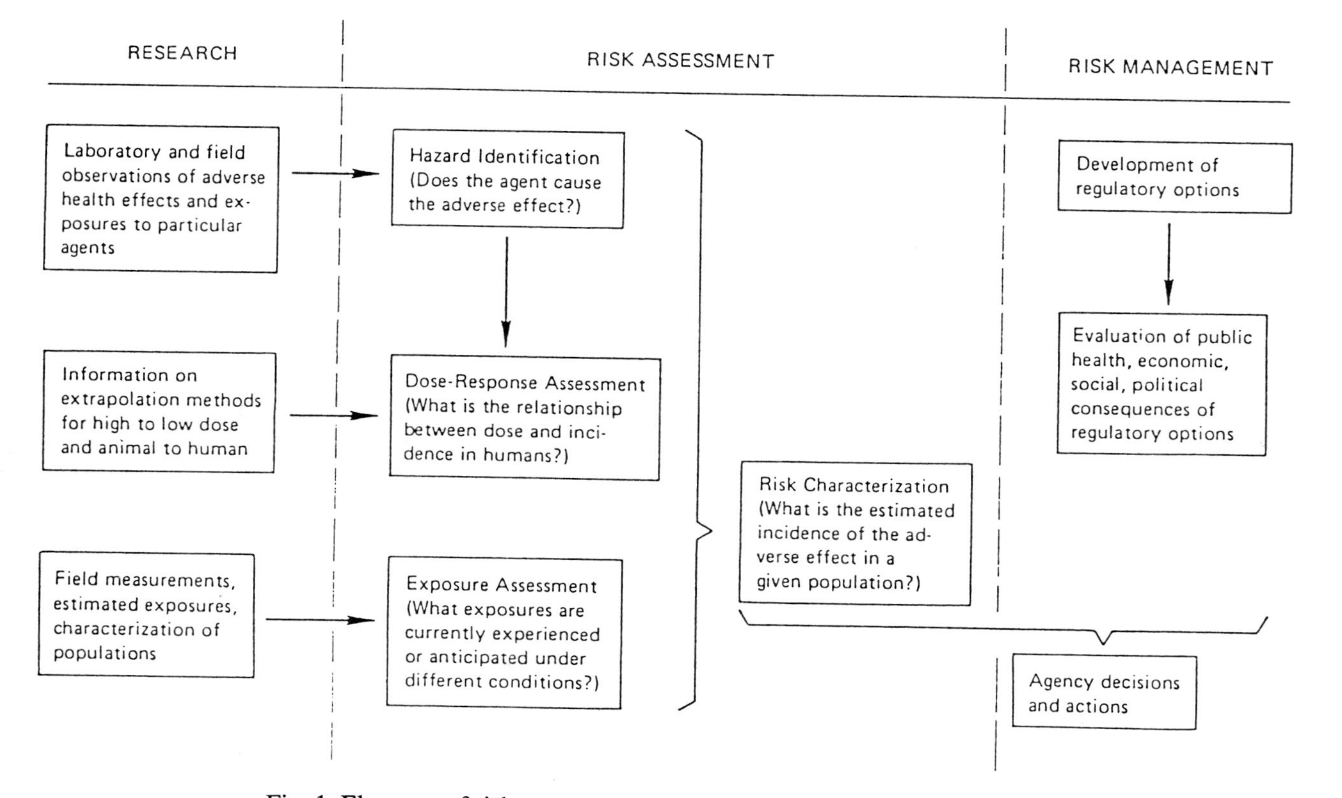

Fig. 1. Elements of risk assessment and risk management. (Source: NAS.[2])

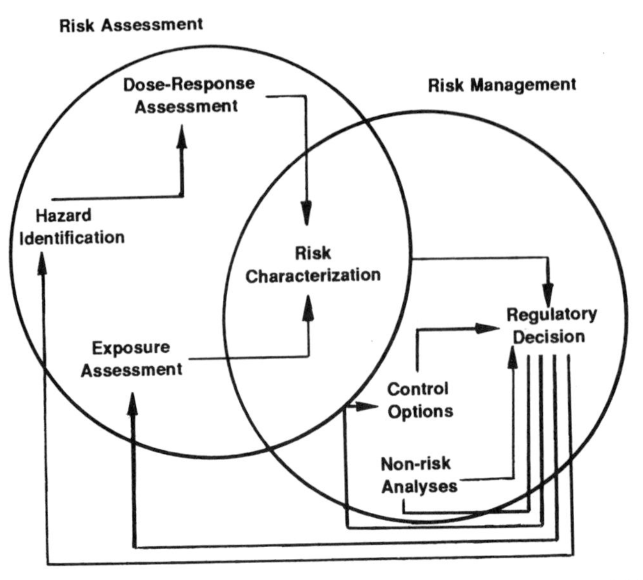

Fig. 2. Risk assessment/risk management distinctions. (Source: EPA, 1987.)

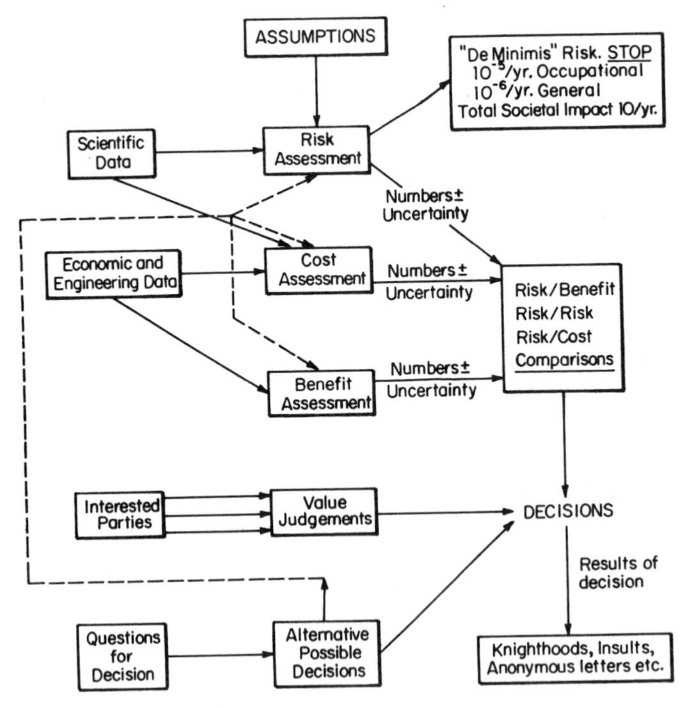

Fig. 3. Idealized scheme for risk analysis. (Source: Crouch and Wilson.[5])

More importantly the feedback line showing how a decision maker may tell the assessor the questions for decision and the lines showing how the values of interested parties are taken into account are explicitly shown.

The separation suggested by the NAS/NRC was always intended to be a functional separation only. It has several advantages:

1. Scientists are left free to do what we all know they do best when left to themselves and to follow interesting developments, no matter where they lead. In response to a question, scientists always have the option to say "I don't know."

2. The risk assessor does not have the option to say "I don't know" in response to a legitimate question. He must state the answer as well as he can, with all the uncertainties, and state clearly his assumptions.

3. The division between the risk assessor and the risk manager discourages interested parties from imposing their values on the assessor and/or influencing him/her unduly. This, perhaps, is the most important reason for the functional separation and one which most influenced William Ruckelshaus. Prior to 1980 some federal agencies were allowing just such undesirable things to happen.

Unfortunately, problems have also developed with the separatist approach.

1. Risk managers have used the separation as an excuse not to understand the science and to insist on a "simple" statement of risk as a single number. All too often, risk managers do not ask for a discussion of possible technological options. They only asks for an assessment of one of them. Moreover they can get cut off from assessment matters they do not want to hear.

2. Risk assessors have used the separation as an excuse to avoid understanding the decision process and the nature of the decision that the assessment is supposed to support.

3. Scientists have used the separation as an excuse to go off into a corner and do irrelevant research.

In our view a good way around these problems is to insist that the information flow be public. The flow of science to the assessor is usually by peer reviewed journals, and this is fairly satisfactory. The flow of assessment to the decision maker is less satisfactory. Although EPA assessments are rapidly improving, they often do not clearly state assumptions, enumerate uncertainties, give a range of values, express dissenting views, and provide perspective by a comparison of risks.

We give an example of the way a risk assessor can usurp the function of a manager if he does not trust the manager. The example may be historical, it may be apocryphal but it is instructive nonetheless. The puritan, Oliver Cromwell, who was Lord Protector at the time of the Commonwealth of England, passed a draconian law making it illegal to kiss in public. The penalty was death. Enforcement questions were decided by a judge and jury. The separation of function was that the jury (the assessors) decided on the fact, the judge (the manager) decided what law applied. In one case the facts were obvious. The jury had seen the defendants commit the crime. But knowing, and disliking, the penalty, they usurped the judge's function and found the defendant not guilty.

Most twentieth century people would feel that the jury (risk assessor) were right to usurp the function of the risk manager.

Twentieth century examples are easy to find. Some of our colleagues in the Harvard School of Public Health and Harvard Medical School do not like to talk about a "risk" of air pollution when it is below a level at which adverse effects are observed in man. They fear that such talk puts unreasonable pressure to reduce the numerical value of the air quality standard unnecessarily. Yet they agree with us that industry do what it reasonably can to reduce emissions, even in locations where the standards are easily met.

An alternate set of flow diagram for decision about risk are given in Fig. 4 from a book by Kates *et al.*[5] These authors emphasize the human needs, the places where the method of meeting these needs can be altered and the loops where further scientific information should be gathered or assessments made. This general example is shown in more detail for pesticide use in Fig. 5.

Kates' flow diagrams are not entirely satisfactory either. They would, in our view, be a completely appropriate description of a process where one person carries out all steps, but they fail to address the question of who is to balance the value judgments of the interested parties and what type of person is to perform which steps.

A combination of the two might be to use the Kates *et al.* procedure as a possible enumeration of the number of cycles around the loop of the Fig. 3 of Crouch and Wilson.[4]

EPA has followed the recommended NAS procedure much more than FDA or OSHA, and in fact we have heard major criticisms of the NAS procedure from both FDA and OSHA representatives. Typically they state that "it is impossible to separate risk assessment and risk management." Possible reasons for the EPA/FDA difference are that the EPA:

- is a younger agency;
- is run by a lawyer, not a scientist;
- administers multiple laws under multiple constraints and objectives; and
- believes that one assessment can often be used for a number of different decisions.

We now illustrate these comments by discussing four general decisions.

DRINKING WATER

Drinking water can have several contaminants. We list them below, with approximate yearly death rate in the whole U.S., based on the EPA analysis procedure which is admittedly conservative.

Contaminant	Death Rate All U.S. (Conservative)
Bacteria	$0 - 10^6$
Chloroform (from chlorination)	1,000
Radon	50
All other industrial pollutants	5

We all hope and expect that the first (bacteria) has been cut to zero by chlorination. We include it here to emphasize that chlorination is highly desirable, although it produces

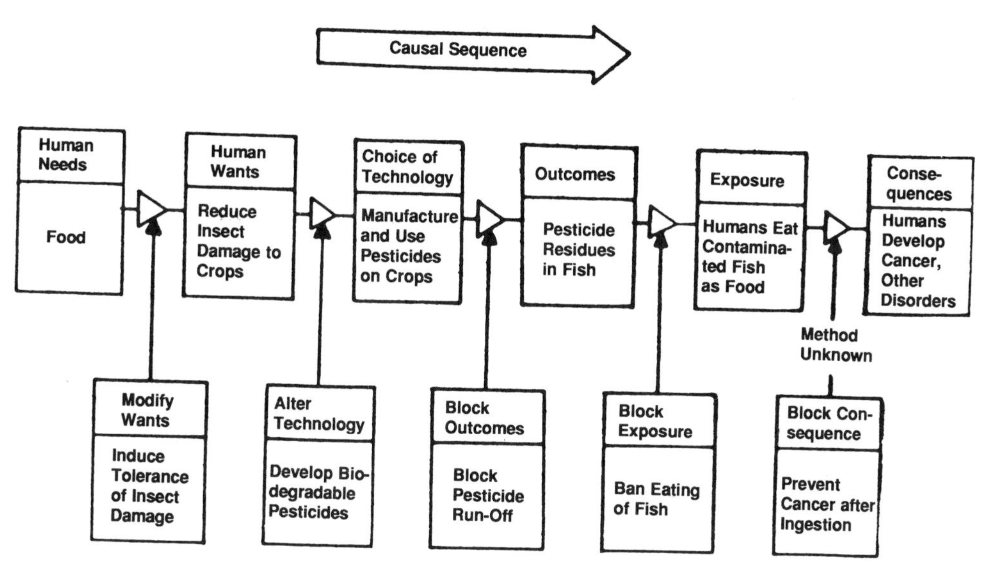

Fig. 4. Hazard structure of pesticide use, illustrating the importance of upstream intervention when downstream intervention is hindered by insufficient knowledge. (Source: Robert Kates *et al.*[4])

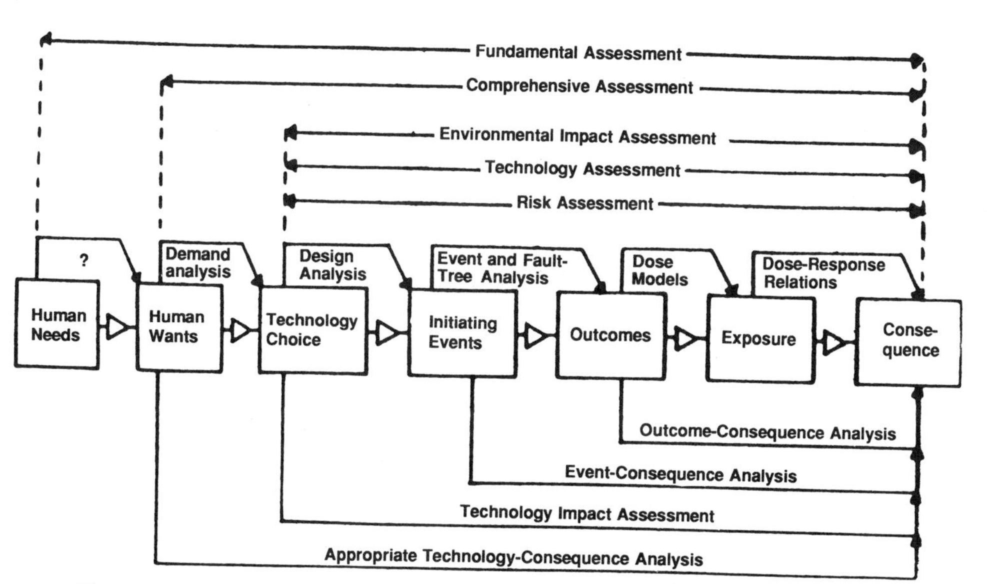

Fig. 5. Modes of analysis is illustrated via the causal structure model of hazards. (Source: R. Kates *et al.*[4])

chloroform at an average level of 50 μg/ℓ. Our major complaint is that until recently the risk assessments for drinking water have not made these matters clear; it has been unclear to the public that the risk manager in setting his standards has known and understood these facts.

ETHYLENE DIBROMIDE

"Position Document No. 4" on ethylene dibromide that was prepared by EPA staff to illuminate the decision on whether or not to ban EDB was one of the worst that we have ever seen. Risks are stated numerically in at least four separate places. Different numbers are used, three of them to four significant figures. Three of them differ by a factor of up to three, one of them (clearly an editing error) is off by a factor of over 100. There is no discussion of the differences and the reason therefore.

There is a large uncertainty in the risk assessment for EDB because almost all of the animals got tumors at the doses that they sustained. This can be overcome by using a time-to-tumor procedure for calculating the potency. The Carcinogen Assessment group of EPA had assumed (pessimistically) that cancers develop as a high power of age (about the 15th power if we understand the assessment correctly). On the other hand, Gold *et al.*[5] in their data bases use a more realistic age dependence and find a carcinogenic potency about 30 times smaller.

There is only a brief discussion of alternate fumigants and no risk assessment for any of the in spite of the legislative requirement of the Federal Insecticide, Fungicide and Rodenticide Act (FIFRA) that benefits and alternatives be considered. One month after the EDB decision and the appalling document on which it based was made public, a bioassay of one alternative appeared in the refereed scientific literature, showing that the risk of this alternative was comparable to the risk of EDB. All of this was made public, but too late for anyone to comment in time to influence the decision.

FOOD ADDITIVES

The FDA, with a scientist at its head, tends to combine risk assessment and risk management. An excellent example is the saccharin decision published in the Federal Register on April 15, 1977. There an excellent risk assessment is given for saccharin, interwoven with reasons for the decision that the Commissioner, Dr. Donald Kennedy, made. There is an important exception. The color additive decision was illuminated by an excellent assessment by a group of scientists under the chairmanship of Dr. Ronald Hart. This was an unusually complete separation of assessment and management because many of the committee members were independent of FDA. Ironically, Commissioner Young's decision to accept the risk of color additives as *de minimis*, based on this assessment, was found to be contrary to the explicit requirements of law as expressed in the Delaney Clause.

One of us[6] has repeatedly needled the FDA because they regulate artificial food additives at a calculated risk level of 10^{-6} per life (calculated conservatively for a gluttenous consumer). Yet they accept natural materials such as aflatoxin B1 at higher levels in peanut butter, even when the peanut butter is used as an additive to food and not as the food itself.

Of course, the FDA has a directive from Congress to be especially careful about food additives; but this should not stop it from explaining to the public the decision process and, more importantly, the risks.

Recently the FDA has, to its credit, been discussing the relative risks of the natural diet and artificial additives[7] and explaining that the diet is at least 1000 times worse.

We note that this is a case where the desired openness is achieved by a management decision in an agency where the managers can and do understand all the details of the assessments. Moreover, they are personally deeply committed to acting in a "goldfish bowl."

CARBON DIOXIDE AND GLOBAL WARMING

The issue of carbon dioxide release and the consequent global warming fits, in our view, the Kates *et al.* flow scheme better than the NAS scheme. However, even that is too simple.

There are (at least) two human needs that contribute to the CO_2 problem: a need for energy and a need for food. Therefore we need two entries on the left-hand side of Fig. 4. The decisions on energy technology often lead to fossil fuel burning, CO_2 production, CO_2 concentration increase in the atmosphere, global warming and perhaps melting of a polar ice cap. Decisions on growing of food can lead to a demand for more agriculture, deforestation and similarly to ecological disasters.

It is harder to describe a place where the risk assessment and the risk management functions can be separated for these decisions.

The issues of global climate change may well be the most important environmental decisions of the century. Accordingly, scientists have been actively involved at all levels of the discussions and have appeared on the same meeting program as heads of state. Therefore one of the purposes of the NAS risk assessment procedures, to act as a medium of communication between the scientist and risk manager, may well be unnecessary.

The EPA did attempt a risk assessment, a draft of which has appeared (in 16 volumes!). Compared to the summaries at many scientific conferences, this draft, in our view, is inferior both in its discussion of both science and risk. Presently, conferences are a superior data resource and recent international agreements suggest that the EPA administrator has acted wisely, although he did not wait for a final assessment.

CONCLUSION

We conclude that it would be an error to endorse as definitive any particular procedure for making decisions about risk. It is even hard to put into one pattern a description of existing procedures.

The important features of any procedure should, in our view, include:

- a clear description of the science;
- a clear description of the risk;
- a place for the public to express its values;
- an opportunity for experts to point out errors and omissions with a reasonable expectation that they will be considered; and
- the basis for the decision by the risk manager who makes the decision on behalf of the public.

REFERENCES

1. NAS, *Risk and Decision Making: Perspectives and Research*, National Academy Press, Washington, DC (1980).
2. NAS, *Risk Assessment in the Federal Government: Managing the Process*, National Academy Press, Washington, DC (1982).
3. M. Schneiderman and N. Mantel, The Delaney Clause and a Scheme for Rewarding Good Experimentation, *Preventative Medicine* **2**:165 (1973).
4. R. Kates *et al.*, *Perilous Progress: Managing the Risks of Technology*, Westview Press, Boulder, CO (1985).
5. E. A. C. Crouch and R. Wilson, *Risk/Benefit Analysis*, Ballinger Publishing Company, Cambridge, MA (1982).
6. L. S. Gold *et al.*, A Carcinogenic Potency Database of the Standardized Results of Animal Bioassays, *Envir. Hlth. Perspect.* **58**:9 (1984).
7. R. Wilson, Talk at Symposium on "Sensitivity of the Method," Alexandria, VA, January 1986.
8. R. Scheuplein, Talk at American Bar Association Meeting, Oct. 21, 1988.

The Assessment of Incineration Risks (AIR) Model

D. B. Chambers
SENES Consultants Limited
Richmond Hill, Ontario, Canada

J. D. Phyper
Steltech
Hamilton, Canada

B. Powers and M. A. Rawlings
SENES Consultants Limited
Richmond Hill, Ontario, Canada

R. F. Willes
CanTox, Inc.
Oakville, Ontario, Canada

ABSTRACT

The Assessment of Incinerator Risks (AIR) model was developed to help assess the risk associated with air emissions from municipal and industrial incinerators. The AIR model evaluates both direct and indirect exposure pathways. The model incorporates Monte Carlo methods for analysis of uncertainty in risk calculation. The results of an example application are presented.

KEYWORDS: Background, exposure, incineration, pathways, risk, uncertainty, Assessment of Incinerator Risks (AIR) model

INTRODUCTION

Incineration has an important role to play in the management of municipal refuse. However, in recent years, public concern over dioxins/furans, polychlorinated bipheny's (PCB's) and elevated metal levels has heightened the controversy surrounding the potential risks associated with municipal waste incineration. Many people living near incinerators are concerned that they will be exposed to levels of hazardous compounds which could potentially result in cancer or other illnesses to either themselves or their children.

The Assessment of Incinerator Risks (AIR) model was developed by SENES Consultants Limited for use in the development of the Metropolitan Toronto Solid Waste Environmental Assessment Plan (SWEAP). CanTox Inc. provided the toxicological analysis. To date, the AIR model has been used to assess five municipal and industrial

Risk Analysis, Edited by C. Zervos
Plenum Press, New York, 1991

incinerators. These include a sewage sludge incinerator, an existing municipal refuse incinerator, a proposed municipal Refuse-Fired Steam Plant, an industrial Energy from Waste (EFW) incinerator, and a generic incineration facility employing Best Available Technology (BAT) based on Swedish emission criteria. This paper focuses on the results obtained for the existing municipal refuse incinerator, which has been recently closed because of a perception of an existing risk to public health.

The AIR model was designed to provide analysis of long-term risks to local residents both from the direct and indirect long-term exposures to incinerator air emissions. It permits Monte-Carlo analyses of the input data used in the exposure pathways analysis but does not address risks associated with worker exposure, the disposal, storage or transportation of the incinerator ash, or runoff from the facility.

The four-stage approach followed in assessing the risk from incineration consisted of the following steps:

- Characterization of emissions in terms of discharge rates and concentrations of substances;
- Determination of the environmental dispersion and fate of each substance emitted, so that concentrations in various environmental compartments (such as air, water, soil, and food) can be predicted;
- Estimation of exposure /doses for each substance and type of person (receptor) using the affected environment, based on assumed physical characteristics, behavior, and the predicted concentrations of substances in the environment;
- Combination of doses from the separate routes of exposure (such as inhalation of vapor or ingestion of water) for each substance and type of receptor, and evaluation of the total risk associated with the total dose by considering the toxicological information reported for the various substance.

Before discussing the AIR model and an example application, it is appropriate to briefly discuss the environment into which incinerator emissions are released.

EXISTING ENVIRONMENT

Individuals are exposed to a vast number of chemicals both of anthropogenic origin, such as automobile exhaust and industrial emissions and non-anthropogenic origin, such as particulates and combustion products from forest fires. The AIR model permits the calculation of the overall exposure both from background levels of chemicals (i.e., other than those derived from incineration) and incinerator emissions.

The background exposure can be estimated (1) from background concentrations of chemicals in air, soil, water, and foodstuffs (e.g. produce, beef and milk), and (2) by assessing chemical emissions from non-incineration sources in the proximate area.

Ideally, the background concentrations used in the assessment of a particular incinerator should be those measured in the proximate area prior to the commencement of incineration. Alternatively, data collected in a similar area distant enough not to be influenced by incinerator emissions could also be used.

Important non-incinerator emission sources, i.e., sources which emit chemicals similar to municipal incinerators, include road traffic, lead refining industries and paint manufacturing facilities. Data reported for local and regional studies, supplemented where necessary by literature values reported for other areas and countries, were used to characterize background levels.

THE AIR MODEL

The AIR model provides for a long-term analysis of the risks from both inhalation and ingestion pathways over an exposure period of 70 years. To estimate long-term effects, the Industrial Source Complex (ISC) model (long-term version) is employed. The AIR model is flexible and provides for the examination of incineration options which incorporate different combinations of existing and proposed designs.

Five groups of pollutants are considered in AIR: acid gases, metals, chlorinated hydrocarbons (PCBs, chlorophenols, chlorobenzenes), dioxins/furans and polyaromatic hydrocarbons (PAHs). Although some monitoring data may be available for existing incinerators, emission estimates are also typically based on literature values.

For a probabilistic analysis of uncertainty, AIR allows the investigator to use a distribution of emission estimates which, for example, might include a minimum, mode ("best estimate") and a maximum value. Furthermore, distributions of background concentrations of chemicals in air, water, soil, milk, produce, fish and meat can be used to assess the contribution that background levels make to total risk.

Direct and indirect long-term effects of incinerator emissions are characterized by developing a comprehensive suite of exposure pathways. The AIR model estimates risk for a reference adult and reference child who live in one of two types of residences (single-story house or apartment building). The reference adult is assumed to be a man between 20 and 39 years of age, weighing 70 kg, breathing 23 m^3 of air per day, and consuming 0.6 kg of produce and 2 L of water per day. The child is 2-3 years old, weighs 10 kg, breaths 5 m^3 of air per day, and consumes 0.3 kg of produce and 1.0 L of water per day.

The AIR model consists of control and component modules. Control modules interface with appropriate input data and control the performance of the component modules. Component modules, in turn, determine the environmental fate and receptor uptake of chemicals through different media. Individual component modules address air concentrations, inhalation, fish/water concentrations, soil concentrations, plant uptake, animal uptake, ingestion, dose and risk calculations (see Fig. 1).

The AIR concentration modules calculate annual average air concentrations. First, dilution factors are calculated for the location of each receptor by using the ISC long-term model. The AIR Dispersion Module calculates average air concentrations of chemicals at various elevations and distances from multiple sources on the basis of the estimated dilution factors and emission rates.

Brief comments are provided below on the pathways modules, the exposure calculation and the risk calculation.

Exposure Pathways

The pathways of receptor exposures from incinerator stack emissions include inhalation of dust or vapors, direct ingestion of dirt or dust, ingestion of plants grown locally in contaminated soil, ingestion of drinking water from an adjacent water body, and consumption of sport fish, meat and milk. The various pathways considered in the model are presented in Fig. 1.

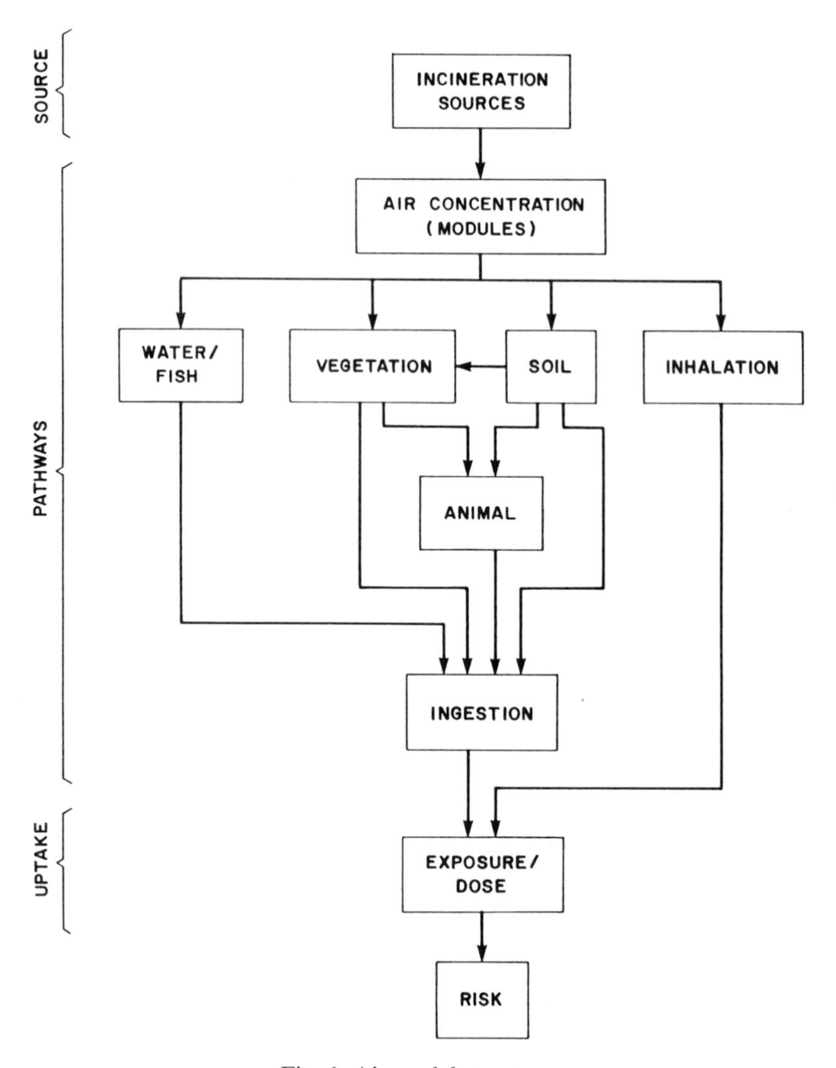

Fig. 1. Air model structure.

Inhalation. Exposures occur continuously from the inhalation of total suspended particulate matter (TSP) and gases in the air. They are estimated from the amount of air breathed and the calculated concentrations of TSP matter and gases both outdoors and indoors. Inhalation exposure algorithms take account of different activity patterns in the winter and summer for both the adult and child receptors. Indoor TSP concentrations are assumed to be 75% of outdoor concentrations.

Soil and Dirt. The concentration of a chemical in soil (C_s) is estimated assuming a steady state balance of atmospheric deposition and removal via biodegradation and leaching of chemicals into the soil profile[1]:

$$C_s = \frac{N_{\text{total}} \cdot [1 - e^{-k_{st} \cdot t}]}{D_{\text{soil}} \cdot Z \cdot k_{st}} + C_{sb} \tag{1}$$

where

C_s = concentration of chemical in soil (g/g)
N_{total} = ground-level deposition rate ($g/m^2/d$)
D_{soil} = soil bulk density (g/m^3)
Z = mixing depth (m)
k_{st} = total rate constant for environmental losses of the chemicals from soil (1/d)
t = time during which deposition occurs (d)
C_{sb} = background concentration in soil (g/g).

Ingestion of Dirt and Dust. Exposures by direct ingestion stem from the inadvertent or deliberate ingestion of dirt and dust. This pathway is particularly relevant to young children who may eat foreign material such as dirt and frequently put their fingers in their mouths. The adults may transfer dirt and dust from their hands to their mouths through activities such as eating or smoking after gardening, for example.

Produce. Uptake by plants generally is considered to occur in three ways: uptake through the root system, deposition of solid particles on leaves, and uptake of vapors through leaf pores. Uptake of vapors is considered to be of minor importance and, therefore, is not considered in the module.

Uptake through the root system is thought to be more important for highly soluble substances and for root crops such as carrots. Deposition of particulate matter on leaves is thought to be more important for less volatile chemicals and for leafy plants such as lettuce. The estimation of deposition is usually based on particle deposition velocities, duration of deposition, and processes, such as rainfall, which remove deposited matter from plant surfaces.

The total uptake of a chemical by plants, i.e., root uptake and foliar deposition, is estimated from[1]

$$C_{pl} = C_a U_p + C_{sl} B_v \tag{2}$$

where

C_{pl} = concentration of chemical in local plants (g/kg dry)
C_a = concentration of chemical in air ($\mu g/m^3$)
C_{sl} = concentration of chemical in soil (g/g)
B_v = transfer factor for soil to plants (g/kg dry)
U_p = plant deposition (g/kg dry).

Exposures resulting from the ingestion of produce, namely locally grown fruits and vegetables, are considered in the model. For the scenario in which the receptor lives in a single story house, some of the produce is assumed to come from an on-site garden. In the apartment building scenario the receptor is assumed to consume no local foods. The chemical level in the food is assumed to be that of background levels.

The amounts and types of produce that people might consume is influenced by the size of the garden, the yields of the crops grown, and the preferences of the receptors. Information from surveys of household garden sizes, yield, and other factors such as food preferences is used when available.

Water. Surface water deposition of chemicals is calculated by estimating wet and dry deposition and dissolution in rainfall. A simple mass-balance relation is used to estimate the order of magnitude of the concentration in the receptor lake, i.e., Lake Ontario in the current example. Deposition to the lake surface is offset by flushing from the lake and removal to sediment. In a report on dioxin in the environment, the ingestion of sport fish caught in Lake Ontario was identified as a potentially important pathway.[2] To calculate concentrations in fish flesh, bioconcentration factors are applied to chemical concentrations in the lake:

$$C_{fl} = C_w \cdot K_b \tag{3}$$

where

C_{fl} = the concentration of the chemical in Lake Ontario fish (g/g)
C_w = the concentration of a chemical in lake water (g/m^3)
K_b = the bioconcentration factor (m^3/g).

If a water body adjacent to an incinerator is being used as a drinking water supply, there is also a potential for exposure through this pathway. In the AIR model, the receptor is assumed to consume all his water from the adjacent lake (i.e., Lake Ontario).

Beef and Milk. The deposition of chemicals onto pastures and grasslands, accumulation of chemicals in beef and milk fat from cattle, and ingestion of contaminated beef and dairy products can be a significant pathway of human exposure for dioxin.[3] A similar observation applies to other chemicals.

In the animal uptake model, the transport of a chemical from ingested forage and grains to beef and milk cattle is estimated. The estimation is based upon the quantity of vegetation consumed, the estimated concentration of chemical in grains and grasses and retention factors.[4]

$$C_{bl} = F_b \cdot (Q_b \cdot C_{gl} \cdot CF) \tag{4}$$

$$C_{ml} = F_m \cdot (Q_m \cdot C_{gl} \cdot CF) \tag{5}$$

where

C_{bl} = concentration of the chemical in beef raised locally (g/kg)
C_{ml} = concentration of the chemical in milk from local dairy cattle (g/kg)
F_b = fraction of the chemical consumed each day which is transported and retained in beef (d/kg)
F_m = fraction of the chemical consumed each day which is transported and retained in milk (d/kg)
Q_b = quantity of non-leafy vegetation (hay, mixed grains, corn silage) eaten by beef cattle each day (kg wet/d)
Q_m = quantity of non-leafy vegetation (hay, mixed grains, corn silage) eaten by milk cows each day (kg wet/d)
C_{gl} = estimated concentration of chemical in grains and grasses (g/kg dry)
CF = conversion factor for dry to wet weight (kg dry/kg wet).

Soil adhering to forage is also a potential source of chemicals. For example, according to Simmonds *et al.*,[5] soil can contribute up to 0.4% of the dry matter consumed by cows and up to 20% of the intake by sheep.

Exposure and Dose

Given the concentrations of chemicals in the various exposure media, the rates of inhalation and ingestion are calculated by estimating consumption patterns and where appropriate activity levels. Different consumption rates are applied for the adult and child receptors, and in the case of household gardens for single-story houses and apartments. Final doses are calculated by adjusting exposure (via inhalation or ingestion) for pollutant bioavailability.

All of the algorithms used in this module consist of a common set of factors and share the following structure:

$$I = Q \cdot C \tag{6}$$

where

I = amount of chemical ingested/inhaled (g/d)
Q = quantity of foodstuff ingested or air breathed (kg/d or m^3/d)
C = concentration of chemical ingested/inhaled (g/kg or g/m^3).

The total dose of a receptor receives is a function of the exposure, the bioavailability of the chemical, and the receptor's body weight:

$$D_t = (I_{ig} \cdot B_{ig} + I_{ih} \cdot B_{ih})/B_w \tag{7}$$

where

D_t = total individual dose (g/kg/d)
B_{ig} = bioavailability factor for ingestion (g/g)
B_{ih} = bioavailability factor for inhalation (g/g)
B_w = receptor's body weight (kg).

Risk

The risks from both carcinogenic and non-carcinogenic chemicals are calculated using Relative Margin of Safety (RMOS) values. The RMOS is the ratio of the calculated dose to the Reference Dose (RFD) or the Risk Specific Dose (RSD). A RMOS value greater than 1 indicates estimated exposure levels greater than the reference exposure level and potentially unacceptable hazards to health. RMOS values between 0.1 and 1 would indicate a situation of some potential concern, although not necessarily unacceptable hazard to health. They identify situations warranting additional assessment of emission levels, exposure parameters and health criteria.

For cancer initiating agents (i.e., those without an accepted NOAEL), the RMOS was calculated as the ratio of the estimated dose to the RSD. The RSD is estimated according to EPA procedures using a linear multi-stage extrapolation model. For non-carcinogens, it is derived from the RFD, which is calculated by applying a safety factor to the NOAEL as recommended by the EPA. Generally, RSD and RFD values published by regulatory agencies are used. However, when published values are not available, appropriate values are calculated. In some cases, quantitative structure-activity relations are used. In all cases, the worst case scenario is assumed.

RMOS Values were determined for both adult and child receptors and for single-story residences and apartments. Since incinerator emissions would expose a person to several chemicals simultaneously, the effects of combined exposures must be evaluated. To accomplish this, the chemicals likely to cause similar health effects were grouped together into the following categories: acid gases, metals, dioxins/furans, chlorinated hydrocarbons (PCBs, chlorobenzenes and chlorophenols), and PAHs. The RMOS values for chemicals in each grouping were added to assess the potential hazard increment from simultaneous exposures to several chemicals with similar biological activities.

In AIR, individual cancer risk and annual cancer incidence in population can also be calculated with or without the contributions of background sources.

Probabilistic Approach

The AIR model incorporates a probabilistic approach based on Monte Carlo simulation for the analysis of uncertainty in risk estimation. By taking random samples of values from the distributions of various input parameters and subsequently making numerous model runs, it is possible to produce a distribution of "effects," i.e., risk estimates. This approach allows presentation of descriptive statistics such as mean risk values and the confidence interval, about the mean risk.

EXAMPLE APPLICATION

The Source

The Commissioners Street Incinerator is located approximately 1 km from Lake Ontario (see Fig. 2). The incinerator was constructed in 1953; new furnaces were installed in 1974/75. On August 1st 1988, the incinerator was ordered closed by Metro Toronto Council as a result of public pressure over perceived health risks.

The Incinerator is a single-stage, mass-burn, refractory facility with three units. A spray tower and an electrostatic precipitator are used to control atmospheric emissions. The Commissioners Street Incinerator stack is about 137 m tall. The exhaust gas temperature is 270°C and the exit velocity approximately 28 m/s.

The nominal design capacity is 820 tonnes/day while the actual feed rate has averaged 400 tonnes/day over the past two years. The actual daily feed rate may fluctuate considerably from the annual average. Each furnace operates approximately 60% of the year.

Measured emission rates obtained in three sampling programs for metals, PCBs, dioxins, furans and hydrogen chloride were employed in the modeling calculations. Emission rates for chemicals not measured in the sampling programs were estimated from the National Incinerator Testing and Evaluation Program (NITEP) studies carried out on other Canadian incinerator facilities and literature values including risk assessments of other incinerators. Table 1 shows the emission rates for the measured substances and the estimates for the remaining chemicals considered in this study. It was assumed that the emissions presented in Table 1 occur 365 days a year. Hence, the estimated exposure will tend to be an overestimate.

Background

In addition to the Commissioners Street Incinerator, several other sources of chemical emissions affect the local air quality. They include a nearby Sewage Sludge incinerator, manufacturing facilities, lead refining industries and road traffic.

Actual local air quality observations include contributions to each pollutant from all sources. These data excluding data from an area immediately proximate to a local source were considered to provide background air quality data for long-term average evaluations of total dose and risk. Similarly, local data or water quality soil and food contamination levels were also incorporated in the analysis where available.

Results

The results of the risk assessment for the Commissioners Street Incinerator are summarized in terms of RMOS values (for an adult) by chemical group in Figs. 3 and 4, background included and background excluded, respectively.

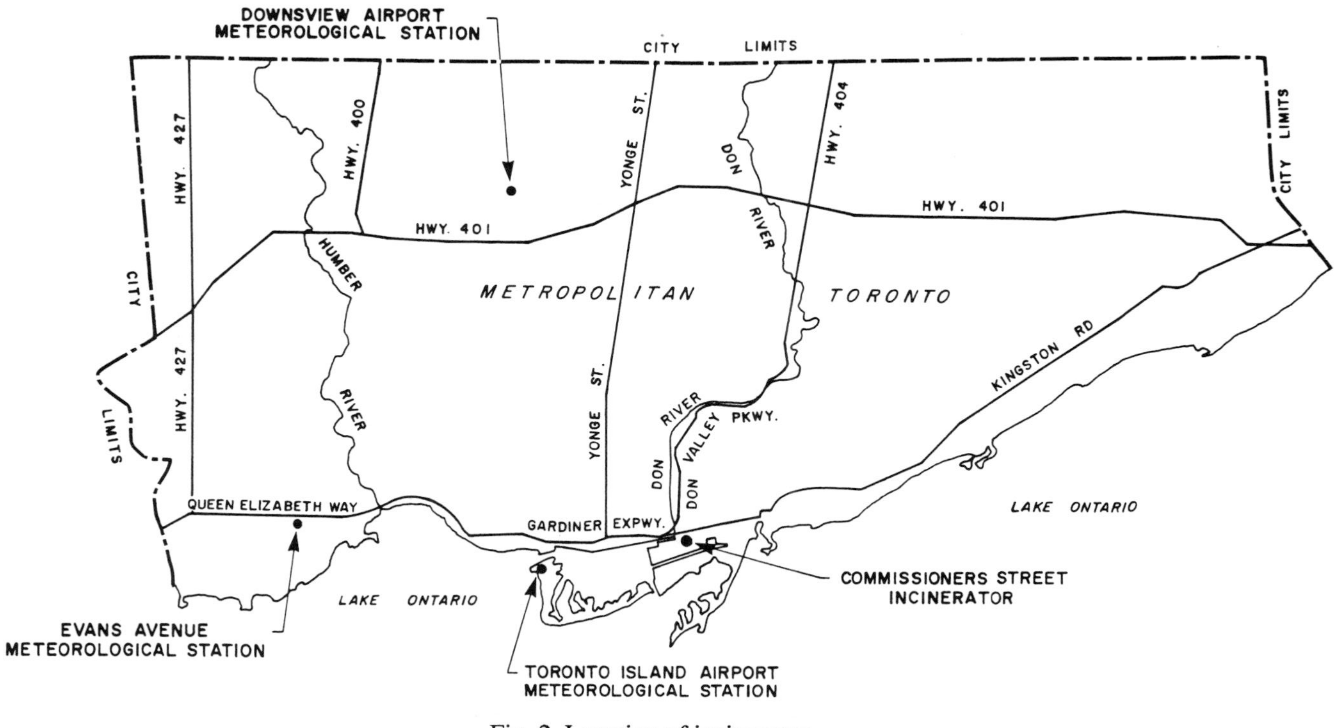

Fig. 2. Location of incinerator.

Table 1. Emission Rates for the Commissioners Incinerator

Chemical	Nominal Emission Rates (g/s)
Inorganics:	
sulfur dioxide	0.36
nitric oxides	0.17
hydrogen chloride	17.8
hydrogen fluoride	0.073 g/s
arsenic	3.63×10^{-3}
beryllium	5×10^{-5}
lead	0.342
cadmium	1.06×10^{-2}
nickel	1.3×10^{-3}
chromium	2.7×10^{-3}
mercury	1.35×10^{-2}
Particulates:	
Total Suspended Particulate	12.9
Organics:	
polychlorinated dibenzo-p-dioxins:	
T4CDD	5.1×10^{-6}
P5CDD	6.8×10^{-6}
H6CDD	3.1×10^{-5}
H7CDD	3.4×10^{-5}
08CDD	8.6×10^{-5}
polychlorinated dibenzofurans:	
T4CDF	1.8×10^{-6}
P5CDF	1.4×10^{-5}
H6CDF	2.9×10^{-5}
H7CDF	1.9×10^{-5}
08CDF	5.7×10^{-5}
polychlorinated biphenyls	5.4×10^{-5}
chlorobenzenes	3.8×10^{-4}
chlorophenols	9.0×10^{-4}
polycyclic aromatic hydrocarbons:	
naphthalene	5.7×10^{-5}
acenaphthene	3.4×10^{-6}
phenanthrene	7.0×10^{-5}
acenaphthylene	3.1×10^{-6}
fluorene	1.5×10^{-5}
anthracene	2.6×10^{-5}
fluoranthene	1.7×10^{-5}
pyrene	1.3×10^{-5}
chrysene	6.0×10^{-7}
benzo(a)anthracene	5.6×10^{-6}
benzo(b)fluoranthene	0
benzo(a)pyrene	7.5×10^{-7}
dibenz(a,h)anthracene	2.7×10^{-7}
Total PAH	2.2×10^{-4}

Notes: TSP and metals are based in 1988 measurements. SO_x and NO_x emissions are based on earlier test results and other emissions are based on literature values especially NITEP.[6]

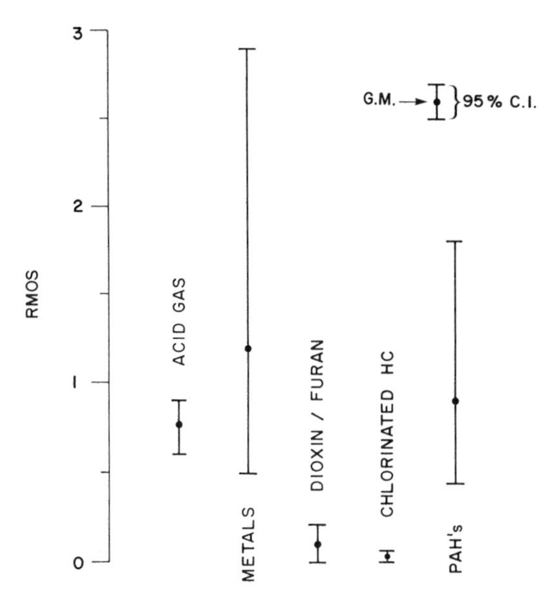

Fig. 3. Estimated RMOS values including background exposures.

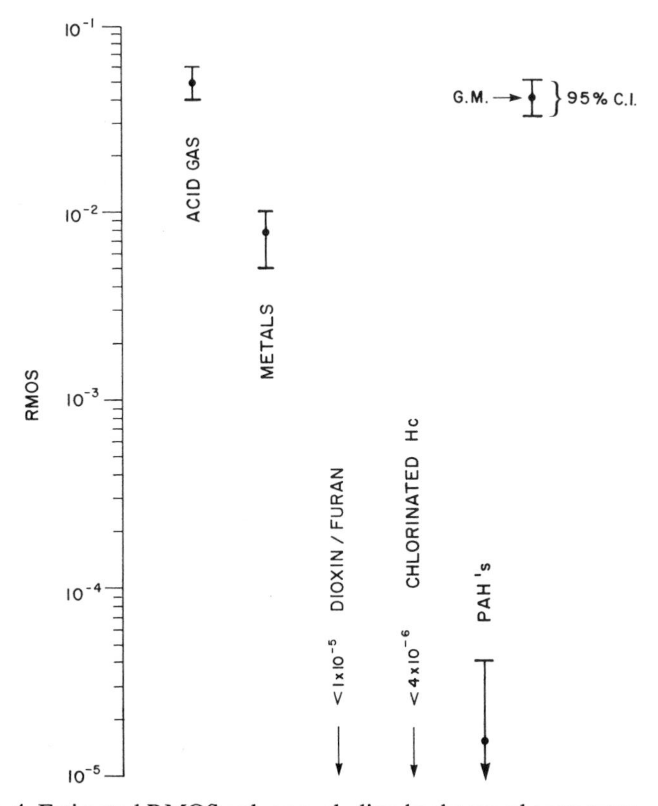

Fig. 4. Estimated RMOS values excluding background exposures.

Modeling to date indicates that, compared to "background" contributions, incinerator emissions are minor contributors to the overall receptor exposures. When "background" contributions are included, the RMOS values estimated for acid gases, metals and PAH's all potentially exceed 1. This suggests that further effort is required to define background contributions and to better examine whether or not background levels are associated with potential health risks. If background exposures are excluded (Fig. 4), none of the predicted RMOS values exceed 0.1, even at the upper 95% confidence level.

Table 2 shows percent contributions from each pathway to the maximum receptor's dose due to lead and dioxin (TCDD). The estimated total dosages, including background, are also shown. The data are self-explanatory and demonstrate that indirect pathways of exposure, e.g., via soil and foodstuff, must be considered if a proper analysis is to be provided.

DISCUSSION

In recent years, numerous risk assessments have been conducted on municipal waste and sewage sludge incinerators. In the following sections, key aspects of the different approaches employed in several of these risk assessments are presented. The risks predicted for the different facilities are strongly dependent on the particular features of each facility and the site at which each facility is located. Thus the following brief reviews focus on the study method or study approach as opposed to the predicted risks which are reported in the various studies.

California Air Pollution Control District

The California Air Pollution Control Districts have prepared a reference manual which outlines a step-by-step approach to estimating and assessing the public health impacts of individual sources of toxic chemicals released in the air during normal operation.[7] The manual, however, does not provide a comprehensive method for calculating air emissions or exposure pathways analysis.

The assessment process described involves five separate analyses: estimation of emissions rates, estimation of ambient concentrations using dispersion modeling, definition of impacted population and estimation of exposure levels (due to inhalation), evaluation of contributions from pathways other than inhalation, and evaluation of total health impact.

The manual outlines both procedures for screening assessments in which initial (conservative) simplifying assumptions are used to evaluate releases and exposure as well as procedures for a more formal risk assessment. Certain relevant features of the latter process are noted below.

The CAPCD manual does not provide a comprehensive method for calculating air emissions. It does, however, outline a process which includes the use of available data on air emission factors, published reviews or summaries of other assessments and source testing data.

According to the CAPCD manual, a formal assessment requires the applicant to use an appropriate air quality model to predict the air concentrations associated with a particular air emission rate. The CAPCD identify U.S. EPA models for possible use in an assessment. The actual model to be used in a particular application depends on various factors, including averaging time required for the analysis (e.g., hourly or seasonal), the location of the site in an urban or a rural setting and the need for a single or multiple source assessment.

Table 2. Average Percent Distribution

Pathway	Lead	Dioxin (T4CDD)
Inhalation	47	0.9
Water	8	7×10^{-4}
Soil	0.7	32
Beef/Milk	0	24
Fish	3	0.7
Produce	41	6
Dust	0.7	36
Total %	100	100

*Based on average results from 100 simulations. The total dose was calculated in units of μg/kg body weight per day and incorporates bioavailability factors. The actual total dose for lead and T4CDD are 0.492 and 0.203×10^{-5}, respectively.

The CAPCD identifies a number of non-inhalation pathways which may require consideration, including, among others, ingestion of soil containing deposited chemicals, ingestion of crops affected by deposition and translocated contaminants and ingestion of surface water contaminated by deposited pollutants.

The health risk assessment procedure described by CAPCD considers both cancer and non-cancer risks. The manual adopts unit risk values developed either by U.S. EPA's Carcinogen Assessment group or by the California Department of Health Services (DHS). The CAPCD notes that the unit risk values presented in the manual are health protective, that is the actual excess cancer risks are not likely to be higher than those estimated using the manual. For non-carcinogens, the CAPCD manual recommends the ratio of the calculated exposure (or dose) to an acceptable exposure level as a measure of the acceptability. The method proposed by CAPCD for non-carcinogens was employed in the present study for both non-carcinogens and carcinogens.

The manual also indicates that risk assessments should include an analysis of both incremental and cumulative exposure and discussion of the significance of background exposures.

U.S. Environmental Protection Agency

In 1987, Radian Corp.[8] performed an analysis of potential human health risks from and environmental effects of pollutants emitted from municipal waste incinerators for the U.S. Environmental Protection Agency (EPA). The report was prepared in support of a regulatory program on municipal waste combustion emissions under the U.S. EPA Clean Air Act.

In the analysis, the quantitative cancer risk assessment was restricted to direct inhalation of organic and metal emissions. For chlorinated dibenzo-P-dioxins (CDDs) and dibenzofurans (CDFs), a method based on toxic equivalency factors (TEF) was used to convert emissions of a mixture of CDD and CDF congeners to an equivalent quantity of the most toxic compound in the class, 2,3,7,8-TCDD.

Limited analysis of indirect exposure pathways, e.g., ingestion and dermal absorption, was performed to estimate the importance of these exposures relative to direct inhalation. Potentially worst-case assumptions were used to evaluate the contribution to total exposure. U.S. EPA considers it premature to produce quantitative risk results for indirect exposure pathways at this time. However, a quantitative evaluation of the exposure from indirect pathways is currently being conducted by the Oak Ridge National Laboratory for the U.S. EPA. The evaluation includes the deposition of chemicals onto soil and plants and the subsequent uptake of chemicals by plants.

Comparisons indicate that for close to point sources (at 0.20 km), HEM produces concentration estimates over 100 times higher than those produced by the ISC-LT model. Concentration estimates at 20 km downwind are of the same magnitude; the ISC-LT code estimates are slightly higher. Analyses indicate that HEM is totally insensitive even to large changes in stack gas temperature. These results seem to indicate that there may be a problem with the HEM method for calculation of plume rise or with its implementation.

City of Toronto

In 1987 CanTox Inc.[9] prepared a report for the City of Toronto Department of Public Health entitled, "Potential Health Hazard Assessment of Three City of Toronto Incinerator Facilities." The report provided an in-depth analysis of the risks associated with the operation of three incinerators in the City of Toronto: Commissioners Street Incinerator, the Main Treatment Plant Sewage Sludge Incinerator, and a generic facility employing Best Available Technology (BAT).

In the study emissions of combined dioxins/furans, PCB, lead and suspended particulate matter were assessed. A major assumption employed in this risk assessment was that all of the dioxin and furans emitted were 2,3,7,8-TCDD, the most toxic congener. This assumption leads to overestimates of the potential effects of the incinerator emissions.

A model prescribed by Ontario Regulation 308[10] was used in the risk assessment. This model does not predict adequately ambient pollutant concentrations resulting from incinerator emissions because of its restrictions on stability classes and wind speeds. In the study, concentrations were calculated for only stability class C and mean wind speeds. No annual or seasonal statistical wind summaries (STAR data sets) were employed. In the risk assessment, no reference is made to background exposure from the ingestion of water or food or the inhalation of ambient air or the use of uncertainty analysis. The CanTox report identifies several sources of uncertainty and suggests that these sources be considered, but did not evaluate them.

Of the models reviewed, the AIR model has the most complete suite of exposure pathways. In addition, it is the only model which directly permits Monte Carlo analysis of uncertainty about the risk estimates.

REFERENCES

1. Environ Corp., Site Assessment, Phase 4B: Risk Assessment, prepared for the Ontario Waste Management Corporation (OWMC), January 1988.
2. Ministry of the Environment (MOE), Scientific Criteria Document for Standard Development No 4-84, Polychlorinated Dibenzo-Dioxins (PCDD) and Polychlorinated Dibenzofurans (PCDF), September 1986.

3. C. C. Travis and H. A. Hattemer-Frey, Human Exposure to 2,3,7,8-TCDD, *Chemosphere* **12**:2331-2342 (1987).
4. G. Holton, C. Little, F. O'Donnell, E. Etner, and C. Travis, Initial Atmospheric Dispersion Modelling in Support of the Multiple-Site Incineration Study, ORNL/TM-8181, Oak Ridge National Laboratory, Oak Ridge, TN (1981).
5. J. R. Simmonds, G. S. Linsley, and J. A. Jones, A General Model for the Transfer of Radioactive Materials in Terrestrial Food Chains, Harwell, National Radiological Protection Board, NRPB-R89 (1979).
6. National Incinerator Testing & Evaluation Program (NITEP), P.E.I. Testing Program, June 1985.
7. California Air Pollution Control Districts (CAPCD), Interagency Working Group, Volume 1, Toxic Air Pollutant Source Assessment Manual for California Air Pollution Control District Permits (1987).
8. Radian Corp., Municipal Waste Combustion Study, Assessment of Health Risks Associated with Municipal Waste Combustion Emissions, prepared for U.S. Environmental Protection Agency, September 1987.
9. CanTox Inc., Potential Health Hazard Assessment of Three City of Toronto Incinerator Facilities, prepared for the Department of Public Health, City of Toronto, October 1987.
10. Ministry of the Environment (MOE), Environmental Protection Act, Regulation 308 (1984).

Organizational Factors in Reliability Models

M. Elisabeth Paté-Cornell
Stanford University
Stanford, CA

ABSTRACT

Probabilistic Risk Analysis (PRA) points to technical malfunctions and human errors that can lead to system failure. Integration of an analysis of a process for the lifetime of the system and of the organization that manufactures or operates it allows identification of the management roots of some of these failures. Information, incentives, procedures, and resource constraints are key elements of decisions made at each stage. In this paper, it is proposed to assess the probability that errors occur during the lifetime of the different components, the probability of error detection given the procedures of quality control, and the effects of uncorrected errors on the reliability of elements and of the system altogether. Three particular circumstances that affect reliability are discussed here: communication and degradation of incomplete information as it travels through an organization, conflicts of objectives (and corner cutting) on the critical path, and difficulties of learning in high-visibility organizations. An example drawn from work done for NASA is used as an illustration.

KEYWORDS: Reliability, organizations, management, probability, failure

INTRODUCTION

Risk reduction for complex systems, such as the space shuttle or nuclear power plants, can involve modifications of the technology or improvements of the organization. Under distributed decision making, problems involving communication as well as consistency of rules, incentives, and safety factors can become critical.

The object of this paper is to present a general method designed to incorporate organizational aspects in classical reliability models and, in particular, the probabilistic risk analysis (PRA) framework. The approach is logical and Bayesian. It includes (1) an analysis of the industrial process to identify basic problems and their probability per time unit or per operation; (2) an organizational analysis to assess the probability that organizational procedures and incentives allow problems to surface in time for corrective actions; (3) a probabilistic risk analysis of the physical system; and (4) an integration model that allows the assessment of various risk management strategies under different scenarios. Three effects are of particular interest: the difficulties of learning in high-visibility organizations, the pressures on the critical path, and deterioration of information in the communication process. The management of the tiles of the space shuttle by NASA and its contractors is used here as an illustrative example.

Risk Analysis, Edited by C. Zervos
Plenum Press, New York, 1991

GENERALIZATION OF PRA MODELS

Reliability Problems Under Distributed Decision Making

Complex systems, like nuclear power plants or dams, require a high level of reliability and, therefore, a disciplined approach to risk management. Options to strengthen the system can include technical changes, such as the introduction of redundancies, or organizational modifications, such as new channels of communication. Risk management decisions (about design, construction, manufacturing, or operations) are generally made under constraints of cost, time, or personnel efforts. The quantification of the overall risk, the relative contribution of the possible failure modes, and an estimation of the costs of risk reduction measures can help the management allocate resources so as to obtain maximum reliability for a given expenditure. Risk quantification is also important for measures that could have a negative as well as positive effect on system safety: a new channel of communication may not be perfectly reliable and one may want to check that the possibility of its failure does not increase the risk more than its normal operation reduces it.

Under distributed decision making, when several groups and organizations are in charge of different subtasks or subsystems, problems of incentives and communications can affect the reliability of the overall system.[1] Traditions and rules may also vary and there may not be any consistency in the safety levels obtained by the different groups. The use of safety factors in engineering gives no indication about actual failure probabilities: some groups may be much more conservative than others, and a "safety factor of two" may not imply the same failure probability in different subsystems. Therefore this approach gives no indication about the additional level of safety obtained by a marginal reliability investment in each part of the operation. Also, the communication of information may not be adequate for an informed centralized decision. When information is passed along in the organization, it may be subjected to omission or distortion.

Probabilistic Risk Analysis (PRA) provides a way of measuring the system safety and the relative contribution of each subsystem to the overall failure risk.[2] PRA involves two phases: a logical phase, in which the different failure modes (or conjunctions of events leading to failure) are identified, and a probabilistic phase, in which probabilities of basic events are assessed and combined to obtain an overall failure probability.[3] In particular, this second phase allows treatment of external events that do not necessarily lead to failure per se but decrease the reliability of the system. It also allows treatment of failure dependencies among the subsystems.

The classical PRA framework, however, is not designed to include explicitly organizational failure (such as failure to observe signals of deterioration) which, in turn, may lead to system failures. Yet, for the physical system to fail, one of the failure modes has to occur, and the consequences of organizational failures clearly depend on how they affect the technical system. The purpose of the work presented here is the extension of classical reliability models to include organizational failures. For a given system operating under distributed decision making, the idea is, first, to identify these potential organizational problems by examining the industrial process, and second, to assess their probabilities given the structure, the procedures, and the culture of the organization. Their consequences are then estimated by linking them to the failure modes of the physical system. The final objective is to identify desirable changes in the organization and to assess their effects on the system's reliability.

The approach is quantitative and Bayesian, based on a logical and probabilistic analysis of events. It is therefore "forward looking" and specific to the considered situation rather than a statistical study of comparable organizations. The probabilities are derived from statistical time series when they exist, and from experts' judgments when needed. There may be some practical difficulties in the assessment of probabilities of human behavior and of changes in these behaviors caused by organizational modifications. The problem, however, is similar to the classical PRA problem of assessing human errors. This admittedly imperfect information can be nonetheless valuable when it is properly encoded and logically combined.[4,5] Sensitivity analysis and explicit treatment of analytical uncertainties allow the analysts to represent the experts' level of confidence in their assessment of subjective probabilities.

The method is to construct a logical and probabilistic integration model that describes the link between the production (or operation) process, organizational procedures, and PRA (see Fig. 1). This integration model provides a measure of system reliability under specific circumstances. It can be extended to account for the variation over time of the different probabilities involved (e.g., deterioration phenomena, system upgrading, learning and identification of new signals), and also of the evolution of the organization according to the circumstances (e.g., crisis situation). One can then proceed to a normative evaluation of the risk reduction that can be expected from proposed changes (technical or organizational).

System Reliability in Organizations and Industrial Management

Behavioral decision research provides descriptive results regarding decision making mechanisms for individuals and for groups. Individual decision characteristics include, for example, biases in judgments under uncertainty[6] and sensitivity to ambiguity in information regarding risks.[7] Research on organizational decision making emphasizes the departure from the rational model,[8] the mechanisms of organizational decisions,[9,10] the organization's attitude towards risk and risk taking,[11] and the effect of ambiguity in the information.[12]

For a survey of the organizational literature related to performance reliability, a key source of information is a memorandum by Scott.[13] This survey is articulated around the conceptual scheme developed by Leavitt and includes works regarding goals, social structure (formal and informal), participants, technology, environment, and contingency predictions, i.e., the different two-way links between technology, structure, participants, and the environment. Some recent work has focused on characteristics of high-reliability organizations, in particular their ethnography,[14] the effect of design,[15] and the organizational culture.[16]

A recent paper by Arueti and Okrent[17] presents an attempt to quantify the link between management characteristics and system safety in the nuclear power industry. Yet there is little in the literature about quantifying in stochastic terms the effects of organizations on system reliability. There is considerable work, however, on performance and effectiveness measurements in which one can include the quantification of systems' safety.[18] This work can be divided into two types of approaches: empirical, for example, Scott's measurement of performance,[19] and "forward looking," for example, Cameron's use of fault tree analysis for organizations.[20]

The relevant literature in project management includes, in particular, the analysis of engineering failures in which organizational failures and their technical consequences are identified and described.[21,22] In the field of manufacturing and process control, one can find a more global approach to quality control than the simple analysis of statistics and test problems, for example, the work of Miller and Strong[23,24] on the analysis of engineering processes.

Integration of Organizational Effects in Reliability Models

For a given engineering system (or operation) formed of different parts, subsystems or tasks, the approach is to use a stochastic model for the integration of reliability and organizational features. This model is based on the identification of the operations to be performed, the availability of the required information, and the incentives for action

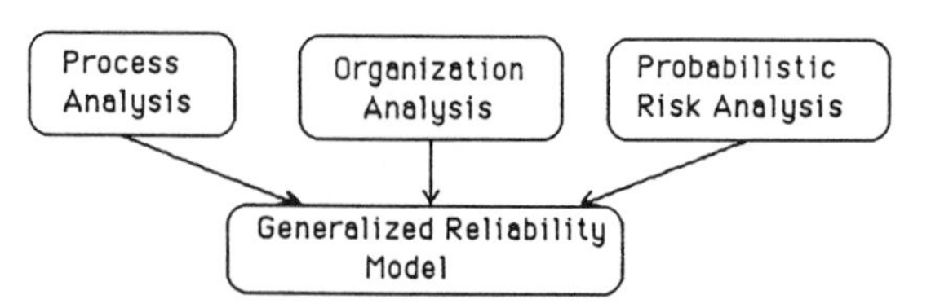

Fig. 1. Inputs to the generalized reliability model.

provided to groups and individuals, formally or informally, by customs and circumstances. The method of integration of these different aspects into a reliability model is based on three preliminary (descriptive) analyses: process analysis, organizational analysis, and PRA.

The process analysis involves an assessment of the successive tasks to be performed in the different phases of the life cycle of a product or an operating system: design, manufacturing, operation, and retirement. Operations of inspection and maintenance are a critical part of the process. Potential problems in each phase are identified, and their base rates (or probabilities per operations or time unit) are evaluated. These include, for instance, errors associated with inspection and maintenance. For the case of the tiles of the space shuttle, Fig. 2 gives an illustration of the elements of the process analysis.

Given the occurrence of a process problem, the organizational analysis allows an assessment of the probability that it will surface as a signal before it causes a system failure. The procedures and the structure of the organization involved in the processing and the communication of these signals are analyzed as "organizational filters" to compute the probability of missing or irrelevant signals (errors of type 1 and type 2). The first step is to identify the filters. The second step is to relate the signals to the failures of different engineering functions (systems failure modes) and to the failure probability of the overall system. In recent work, it was shown, for example, how a policy of maintenance on schedule or on demand affects the probability of defects.[25] Some of the key issues in the assessment of the probabilities of organizational failures are the following: how the information deteriorates as it is passed along through the different layers of the organization; how time pressures due, for example, to the position of a group on the critical path or in a full-blown crisis situation affect the incentives to detect and address problems; how the organization learns in high-visibility situations given a system of rewards for performance and of penalties for delays, failures, or cost overruns. The approval of a particular subsystem through inspections and board review can be represented by a GO/NO GO signal, sometimes modified by qualifiers (GO BUT). The question is to know how this GO signal is passed along through the sequence of organizational filters. Figure 3 illustrates, for the case of the tiles of the space shuttle, the principle of the analysis of the GO signal as the different parts are approved by the several technical groups and review boards, first through the phases of design, manufacturing, and installation (below the grey line), then through the cycle of flights including usage, inspection, maintenance, and approval. The question is then: what does the review board look for, what problems are likely to be addressed, and which ones will be generally ignored under different circumstances?

The object of the PRA phase is to compute the probability of failure, i.e., that the loads to which the system will be subjected are greater than its capacity. There are, in general, uncertainties about both. The design and management of a system affect its capacity to absorb loads. The purpose of risk management is to anticipate unusual levels of loads and to ensure that they do not exceed the capacity. Two key questions are therefore: what are the extreme values of the loads and their probabilities of occurrence? and what is the capacity under normal conditions (determined by the safety factors) and under

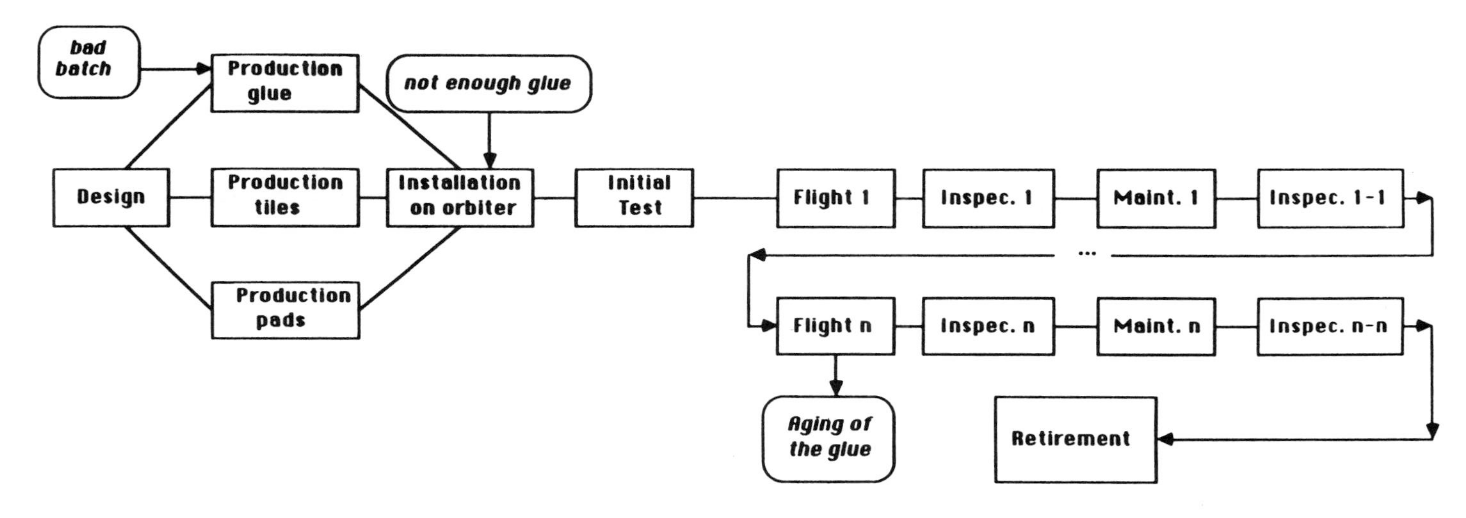

Fig. 2. Structure of the industrial process analysis for the TPS of the space shuttle.

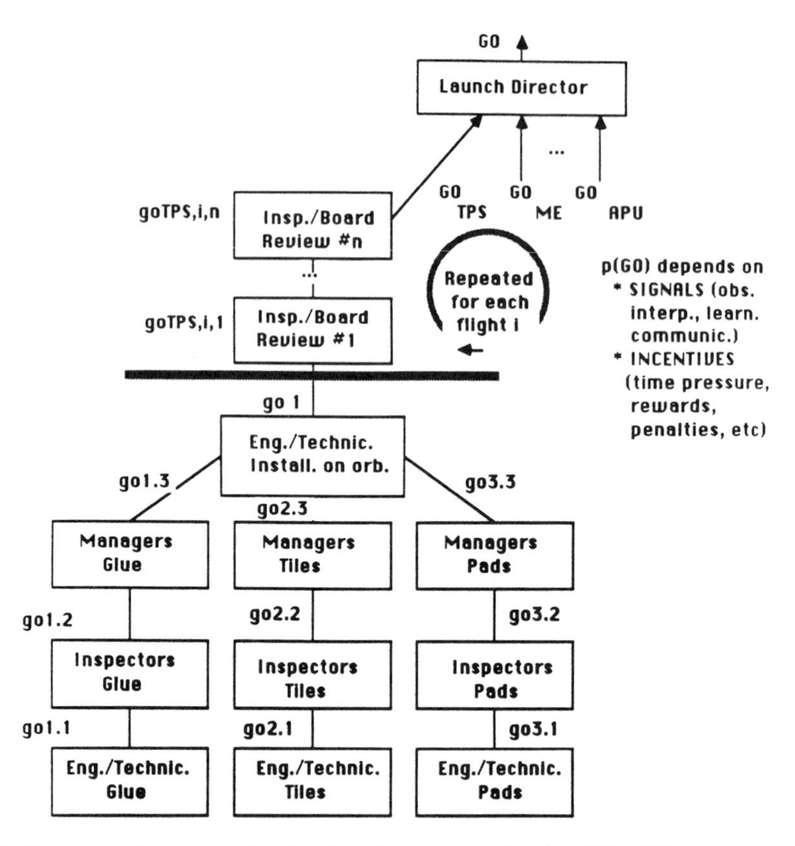

Fig. 3. Structure of the organizational review process for the TPS of the space shuttle.

unfavorable conditions when the capacity is reduced by processing problems that were not detected and corrected in time.

The integration model is based on an event tree gathering results from the first three phases. It allows identification of the scenarios leading to system failure and computation of their probabilities. The model represented here is a snapshot of a given situation characterized by probabilities of the different events. These probabilities and, therefore, the overall failure probability actually vary with time. The variations include updating of failure probabilities for the different subsystems; "debugging" and design improvements as problems are identified and corrected; occurrence of new problems caused by the corrections of old ones; internal variations of the system's capacity: deterioration and aging, or on the contrary, internal settling that increases the capacity; changes in the rate of human errors due to better training or increased experience, or on the contrary, increase in the probability of error due to pressures, crisis situations, lack of sleep, or cognitive error in the interpretation of a signal. Figure 4 represents the structure of the integration model for the Thermal Protection System of the space shuttle, mainly the tiles, whose main components are the tiles themselves, the bonding ("glue"), and the "pads" (located between the tiles and the aluminum skin) whose role is to compensate for deformations of the orbiter's surface due to temperature differentials.

NASA and the Management of the Thermal Protection System of the Space Shuttle

NASA presents some interesting features that influence its mode of operations and thus the reliability of its space systems. It is a high-visibility organization, uncertain about

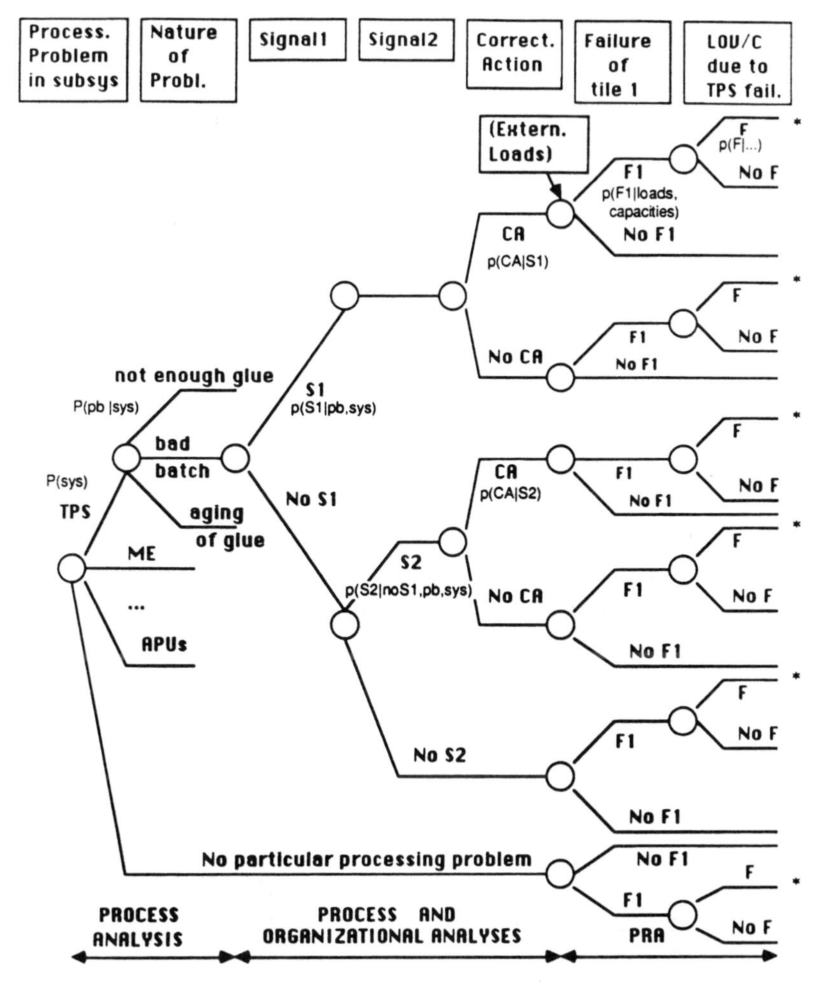

Fig. 4. Generalized reliability model (integration) for the TPS of the space shuttle.

its funding and, therefore, driven by public relations. It is fragmented in two ways: geographically among space centers and operationally among space programs. It has evolved from a "can-do" organization to a bureaucracy in which the influence of technicians and engineers has markedly decreased since the Apollo days.

Since the early 1960's, NASA has decided against probabilistic risk analysis in order to avoid the issue of "how safe is safe enough" in what is generally recognized as a high-risk operation. However, following the Challenger accident and deluged with a list of potential corrections with little information about priorities, NASA has been advised by the Slay Commission[26] to complement its qualitative method of identification of the failure modes by quantifying their probabilities and their dependencies. A current objective is clearly to increase the effectiveness of the organization by setting priorities among the technical problems to be addressed. Yet, as the Rogers Commission[27] pointed out, it is clear that some of NASA's technical problems cannot be resolved simply by design modifications because their roots are organizational. The fragmentation of the organization, the apparent buffering between engineers and managers and the divergence of their risk perceptions, problems of leadership, difficulties in learning and the absence of usable trend records, all are factors that have contributed heavily to the vulnerability of the shuttle operation.

The Thermal Protection System provides a practical example of the coupling between technical and organizational problems. It is a complex system made of black and white tiles (24,000 on the orbiter Discovery), reinforced carbon-carbon in the hottest zones, thermal blankets in cold zones, and flexible insulation. The TPS can fail in two ways: debonding and burn-through. It is subjected to a set of external loads, some of them predictable (e.g., vibrations), some of them random like the impact of debris or unexpected peaks of temperature under abnormal re-entry conditions. Important features of the PRA for the tiles are the high failure dependencies from tile to tile and the coupling between failure risk for the TPS and failure risk for the subsystems located directly under the skin.

The management of the TPS presents many of the organizational characteristics that are relevant to our study. First, it involves several organizations and contractors in different places (Rockwell, Lockheed, and NASA, both at Kennedy Space Center and Johnson Space Center). Second, the TPS inspection and maintenance procedures are extremely labor intensive and time consuming and are often on the critical path to the next launch. The training and the dedication of the personnel involved between flights is critical, yet they are presently at the lower end of the pay scale at the space centers. The current procedure virtually ignores the problems posed by the aging of the bond, relies mostly on maintenance on demand, and involves a mass of documents that are hardly accessible. Furthermore, the procedure does not involve any notion of priority among the TPS elements with respect to other critical systems.

Currently a new method to automate the inspection of the tiles is being implemented. The most important aspect of this method is that it greatly simplifies the current tasks of observing, communicating, storing, and retrieving information concerning the current state of the tiles and their past performance. At the same time it increases the reliability of the inspection and maintenance operations. By accelerating the process, automation also takes the tiles off the critical path to launch. The inspection and maintenance of another system obviously finds itself on the critical path, but this shift may reduce the time gaps to launch among the different orbiter's subsystems. The gain in reliability for the overall Space Transportation System (STS) from this automation is a function of the initial contribution of the TPS to the overall failure risk and of the gains made in TPS reliability. Recent work at Stanford University involves the development of a PRA for the TPS and its extension to include organizational features affecting its reliability and, therefore, the reliability of the orbiter.

THREE RELEVANT ORGANIZATIONAL EFFECTS

Communication and Degradation of the GO Signal

The "GO signal" reflects the approval of a given technical group regarding the reliability of a subsystem for a particular task (e.g., installation or maintenance). It reflects two things: an assessment by the group of the reliability of the subsystem and a value judgment that this reliability level is sufficient. The group therefore makes a choice of GO, NO GO, or GO (NO GO) with restrictions and qualifiers, then sends the message through organizational channels. It may be correctly communicated or distorted, or communications may fail entirely.

Communication Failures. The communications of information may fail, either completely or partially, for several reasons.

- Appropriate communication channels may simply not exist.

- The existing channels may not work due to accidental slip, or impractical procedures or deliberate refusal to pass on information.
- The signal may be ignored because of previous false alerts (the cry wolf effect).
- The signal may be distorted because incentives create biases towards optimistic reports (or, perhaps, pessimistic ones depending on the incentive system).
- The organization may not be equipped (in its procedures or its culture) to communicate properly imperfect information and uncertainty. Therefore, qualifiers may be dropped in the process.

Signals: Relevance and Reliability. The organization's problem is to identify and communicate signals that are relevant and reliable. Organizational filters may be such that some important signals are missed while irrelevant ones overload and confuse the system. The goal is to link these filter effects first to the probability of the different failure modes and second to the overall system failure probability in order to establish which pieces of information are most critical. The method is thus:

1. to identify the filters through a study of the organization's procedures,
2. to relate the occurrence and observation of the signals to the performance of engineering functions, and
3. to use PRA to relate the frequencies of the failure modes to the overall system reliability.

A key issue in the study of signals and filters is to determine how the organization or the group decides that it has a problem.

The Engineer Dilemma. In many engineering problems, the first level of signal communication leading to a decision can be represented as a game between engineers and management. The engineers can either say "GO" or "NO GO"; in either case, their judgment can either be supported or overruled by the managers. Initially the engineers, having all the incentives to claim "NO GO" even for minor problems (so that they are "covered" in case of failure), may be overruled by management. Assuming, however, that the probability of failure is small, if this happens repeatedly, the engineers will quickly lose credibility. For the management, an alternative is to support the NO GO. In this case, the engineers still cannot "prove" that they are right but have the opportunity to correct the problem. After a while, however, the incentive system will induce the engineers to say GO most of the time, incur a low risk of failure, and develop an image of performance. As Feynman[28] correctly pointed out in his investigation of the Challenger accident, it is not uncommon for engineers to be put in a position to "prove" that the NO GO is justified and that the system will fail, which is impossible by definition.

Cascading Biases in Report. The phenomenon described above may lead to over-optimism in reports and, therefore, to a degradation of the signal as it "travels" through the organization. Decoding of these exaggerations may occur from one level to the next when the individuals involved know each other or can communicate directly. Even then, the quality of the communication depends on the medium used. When the message is passed along through several organizational layers, the decision maker uses information generated several steps away. He may not then be in a position to "decode" it and to compensate for optimistic biases. In fact, in some cases he may even prefer an optimistic message if it simplifies his decision. There are in such cases incentives for a cascade of optimistic reports. This analysis may hold for organizations whose goal is to generate a "positive product" and thus for whom negative information goes counter to performance measures. In other organizations or groups whose goals is to actually generate signals of defects, the reverse phenomenon may be observed because incentives and performance definition may encourage pessimistic reports.

In this cascade of communication errors, one may detect not only clear type 1 and type 2 errors (false negatives and false positives) but also a degradation of information similar to what happens in the game of "telephone"; for example, the loss of qualifiers and the loss of context. A "GO BUT" may gradually be transformed into a "GO" without the initial restrictions. These qualifiers and, in particular, descriptions of uncertainties may be vulnerable to the "softness" of the information supporting them. This means that an engineer's "hunch" may be more quickly dropped in the communication chain than the results of a statistical analysis. It is also clear from the literature that the quality of the communication and the completeness of the message may depend on the communication medium (e.g., face to face, paper, telephone, or teleconference).

This cascade of distortions in the treatment of information has interesting implications for organizational design and the span of control problems[29] that results from a trade-off between the number of layers and the branching factor. If a small number of people report to the same manager, he may pay more attention to what they say, and, in particular, to NO GO signals that he rarely sees. On the other hand, the multiplicity of layers increases the distortion of the messages. If, on the contrary, there are only few layers and many people report to a single manager, he may have a better opportunity to make an informed synthesis, and the information is subjected to a smaller number of communication distortions. On the other hand, he may be more tempted to ignore negative information among the larger number of positive messages that he may receive: the NO GO signal, being more frequent, may be more easily ignored.

Relevance of the Theory to the Generalized Reliability Model. In our integration model, the degradation of the GO signal influences the probability that signals of processing problems will be detected and that the system monitoring will be reflected, in the PRA phase, by the system's capacity, given the nature of the initial processing problem and the effectiveness of corrective actions.

The Critical Path Theory

Most engineering groups facing safety issues are caught in a conflict of objectives: safety versus costs or safety versus schedule pressures. When the costs are a constraint, the form of the contract is critical. A cost-plus contract relieves the pressure on the contractant, whereas a fixed-cost contract may bring sharp constraints and incentives to cut corners when money has been overspent. In cases where there is a conflict between safety and time, the following theory is proposed.

- At any given time, the pressure is greater for the group whose system is on the critical path to production or operation. Furthermore, this pressure is an increasing function of the time by which the group on the critical path delays the whole process. This delay is equal to the difference of times to production or operation for the group g currently on the critical path, and for the next group g' that would come to be on the critical path if the current "long pole" were to be removed. In optimization terms, the pressure on group g is an increasing function of the shadow variable of the constraint that this group represents with respect to the objective to "minimize time to operation."

- For the groups that are not on the critical path, the pressure is lower than for group g. Yet there is always a threat that, because of unexpected delays, they may end up on the critical path and become "the long pole." The members of such a group g'' generally know who is the current long pole, but not necessarily who are the other groups in between. The potential pressure for group g″ is thus a function of the perceived slack or time to spare before they become the binding constraint.

In manufacturing or operation situations, being on the critical path and subjected to time pressure can be stimulating up to a point. Soon, however, the group on the critical path may be subjected to strong incentives to cut corners (in particular, if they came to be in this position due to unexpected delays) and to alter technical judgments of what constitutes a sufficient level of safety. The consequences of this slipping of standards depend on the criticality of engineering function that they manage.

This theory, if it is correct, has important implications for the monitoring of complex systems. Having identified through PRA the level of criticality of each of the subsystems, one can decide to check first the critical subsystems that have been at some point on the critical path: they are more likely to have been subjected to "the vicious circle of urgency"[30] in which pressures to get the job done faster create incentives to cut corners and increase the probability of failure later. This hypothesis, however, cannot be generalized to design situations because under pressures, when engineers are forced to do a quick design, they may tend to be more conservative rather than to take chances. This is because a large part of the design time is spent refining the design to save materials and reduce costs later.

Relevance of the Theory to the Generalized Reliability Model. In the integration model, the critical-path theory influences the probability that a processing problem occurs in a given subsystem. When one considers the dynamics of reliability and looks for the possibility of drifting of standards under time constraints, the theory implies that this drifting is more likely to have occurred for subsystems on the critical path.

Learning in High-Visibility Organizations

High-visibility organizations, in particular those like NASA that are driven by public relations to obtain external funding, are subjected to several internal and external phenomena that prevent them from assessing clearly their own performance and learning from past or current experiences. Feedback, when it finally comes, can be brutal and destructive for the organization because it may be unprepared for a setback if it has lived too long in an illusion of super-performance.

Internal Drifting and Performance Illusions. One of the internal effects of public relations designed for external consumption can be the drifting apart of managers and engineers within the organization. The role of the managers in charge of public relations is to convince the environment (e.g., public, Congress, or potential donors) of the quality and the safety of the product that they are trying to sell or promote. They may start exaggerating the system's performance, but in the end they may come to believe their own story. The engineers or the manufacturing people, on the other hand, may be more in touch with actual performances and characteristics of the system, but they may not be heard when they raise questions about quality or safety because their message disturbs the promotion efforts.

This buffering between managers and engineers can result in the phenomenon documented by Feynman[28,31]: the managers of one of the shuttle's sub-contractors were persuaded, after the Challenger accident, that the probability of failure of their subsystem was in the order of $10E^{-5}$ per launch operation, while the engineers of the same company agreed (in a secret ballot) that the risk was in the order of $10E^{-2}$. The engineers, however, have a partial view of the problem because they are working only on one part of the system. Therefore, in isolation they may not be in a position to make judgments as to what constitutes optimal safety levels given the global resource constraints, the characteristics of other subsystems and the multiple interfaces. Unfortunately, managers, who could have a more global view of the situation, may end up fooling themselves and acting as if they believed, without questioning it, the message that they have to deliver to keep the money flowing.

Learning Difficulties in High-Visibility Organizations. High-visibility organizations who manage a generally reliable system have difficulties learning from experience, for at least three reasons: the necessity to deliver an image of performance and confidence, the temptation to believe the message delivered when it satisfies the organizational goal and pride (for example, "zero risk"), and the power of preconceived ideas. If the probability of failure is low enough and the number of trials small enough, it is unlikely that a given manager will be proven wrong.

In situations where the organization is perceived as successful, high visibility reinforces the tendency to overconfidence: signals of malfunction the repeated erosion of the O-rings in the solid rocket boosters of the space shuttle are ignored or downplayed. If no serious malfunction occurs, there is even a reinforcement of the belief that it was "right" to ignore the signals. It is particularly difficult, in success situations, to interpret and learn from the occurrence of initiating events that were compensated by proper functioning of the corrective mechanisms.[32] The natural tendency is to emphasize the adequacy of the correction rather than the near-miss aspect of the event. Bayesian analysis allows separate updating of the initiating event probability and of the likelihood of the correction.[33] The difficulty, from the organizational perspective, is to identify the near-miss as a signal of a potential problem worthy of attention rather than a reinforcement of the preconceived idea that nothing can go wrong.

In situations where a high-visibility organization is perceived as failing, the incentives are so great to rebuild an image of safe performance that it can drown itself in a deluge of unsorted signals about potential problems to be addressed. Unless the organization adopts a systematic way of setting priorities, it may appear to be in a situation where nothing seems to be going right because every signal of a potential problem is perceived as a reinforcement of the failure image. One way of setting priorities is to assess the probability of the different failure modes and of conditional probabilities of signals given the occurrence of each failure mode. Then, considering the costs of corrections, one wants to invest resources where they will maximize the reduction of the overall risk accounting for the possibility of observation errors. The transition from a situation of success to a situation of failure can be very quick (one failure may suffice). It can be accelerated by the temptation to shift policy from "GO if proven safe" to "GO unless proven unsafe." By contrast, the transition from an image of failure to an image of success is generally much slower because it requires rebuilding a record of safety. This transition, however, is probably quicker if the public image of the product is positive (e.g., the space program), whereas it is much more difficult if the product is considered negatively (e.g., nuclear power plants).

It is, therefore, important to determine how a given organization decides that it has a problem and how quickly and effectively it can respond. Some responses can be simple adjustments; other situations require a quick shift to a crisis management mode. In high-visibility situations, this shift may be particularly difficult if it implies admitting mistakes. In this case, there may be strong incentives to cover up. This shift also requires that the structure of the organization be adaptable to prompt, informed, and immediately implementable decisions. The operations' reliability obviously depends on the organization's ability to take corrective actions in major crises situations.

Therefore, one way to improve performance and safety may be to identify a prior set of signals that may otherwise be ignored in periods of euphoria or overlooked in periods of panic and to plan for corrective actions given the lead time required to avoid major problems.[34] PRA can be an important tool to assess the relative probability of the different failure modes and, therefore, to set priorities for response to the multiple signals that can be observed. A system of observation, trend analysis, storage, and retrieval of information may be set up to provide perspective about problems' frequencies and consequences. Such a system may compensate for some of the effects of high visibility, for example, the incentives to ignore important problems when they may not have immediate effects and to rush into action when a minor problem has become visible. It is essential, in particular, to ensure that major information reaches decision makers who may otherwise find themselves disconnected from the parts of the organization that provide the technical expertise.

Relevance to the Generalized Reliability Model. In the integration model, learning is a critical element of the variations over time of the failure probabilities. Learning capabilities allow the organization to detect new processing problems, to identify precursors or signals indicative of these problems, to assess the probability that these signals are actually observed and the probabilities of type 1 and type 2 errors, and in general, to update failure probabilities in the light of experience, including near-misses. Bayesian updating accounts for the success or failure of each successive operation. At the same time, the parameters can be adjusted for the variations of the system's internal parameters such as aging or correction of flaws. This kind of logical reasoning allows the separation of fundamental (or epistemic) uncertainty about the system's parameters, which can be reduced with experience and proper updating, and observational (or aleatory) uncertainty which remains part of every new "experiment" even if the parameters are fully known. This use of logic and probability may thus prevent short organizational experiences from transforming quickly into illusions of guaranteed success or unavoidable failure.

CONCLUSION

The study presented here is part of a long term project whose goal is to link organizations and system safety in probabilistic terms. The proposed generalized reliability model includes processing errors and the probability that organizational procedures will detect and correct them. In its dynamic form, the model also addresses the long term modification of the failure probability through learning and improvement of organizational mechanisms. The application to the NASA problem emphasizes, in particular, the effects of high visibility and of the difficulties of communications and conflicting agendas in distributed decision making.

ACKNOWLEDGMENT

Several researchers at Stanford and at Carnegie Mellon have contributed to the generation of ideas presented here: James March, Baruch Fischhoff, Steven Miller, Granger Morgan, and Thierry Weil. We thank them for stimulating discussions.

REFERENCES

1. B. Fischhoff and S. Johnson, The Possibility of Distributed Decision Making, Workshop on Political-Military Decision Making, The Hoover Institution, Stanford University (1986).
2. E. J. Henley and H. Kumamoto, *Reliability Engineering and Risk Assessment.* Prentice Hall Inc., Englewood Cliffs, New Jersey (1981).
3. M. E. Paté-Cornell, Fault Trees vs. Event Trees in Reliability Analysis, *Risk Analysis* **4(3)** (1984).
4. U. S. Nuclear Regulatory Commission, *Handbook of Human Reliability*, NUREG/CR-1278, Washington, DC (1980).

5. D. E. Allen, Human Error and Structural Practice, Proceedings of a Workshop on Modeling Human Error in Structural Design and Construction, Ann Arbor, Michigan, June 1986.
6. D. Kahneman, P. Slovic, and A. Tversky, *Judgment Under Uncertainty: Heuristics and Biases*, Cambridge University Press, Cambridge, U.K. (1982).
7. H. J. Einhorn and R. M. Hogarth, Ambiguity and Uncertainty in Probabilistic Inference, *Psychological Review* **92(4)**:433-461 (October 1985).
8. J. G. March and H. A. Simon, *Organizations*, John Wiley & Sons, NY (1958).
9. J. G. March, Footnotes to Organizational Change, *Administrative Science Quarterly* **26**:563-577 (1981).
10. J. G. March, Decisions in Organizations and Theories of Choice, in *Perspectives on Organization Design and Behavior*, Andrew H. Van De Ven and William F. Joyce, eds., pp. 205-244. Wiley, New York (1981).
11. J. G. March and Z. Shapira. Managerial Perspectives on Risk and Risk Taking, Unpublished paper, Stanford University (1986).
12. J. G. March, Ambiguity and Accounting: The Elusive Link Between Information and Decision Making, Unpublished paper, Stanford University (1986).
13. W. R. Scott, Reliability in Organizations, Memo to the Berkeley Project on High Reliability Organizations, Department of Sociology, Stanford (August 1987).
14. T. R. La Porte, High Reliability Organization Project, University of California, Berkeley (1988).
15. A. Y. Lewin, Issues in the Design of High Reliability Organizations, Presentation at the 2nd U.S. Japan Workshop on Risk Assessment and Risk Management, Osaka, Japan (October 1987).
16. K. E. Weick, Organizational Culture as a Sources of High Reliability, *California Management Review* (Winter 1987).
17. S. Arueti and D. Okrent, Combining Objective and Subjective Techniques for Assessing Quality Management, Proceedings of SMiRT 1987, Lausann, Switzerland (September 1987).
18. A. Y. Lewin and J. W. Minton, Determining Organizational Effectiveness: Another Look, and an Agenda for Research, *Management Science* **32(5)**: 514-538 (May 1986).
19. W. R. Scott, Effectiveness of Organizational Effectiveness Studies, in *New Perspectives on Organizational Effectiveness*, Paul S. Goodman and J. M. Pennings, eds., Jossey-Bass, San Francisco, CA (1977).
20. K. S. Cameron, *The Effectiveness of Ineffectiveness*, JAI Press Inc. (1984).
21. R. E. Melchers, Examination of Published Cases of Structural Failure, Transactions of The Institution of Engineers of Australia, *CE 22* **3**:222-230 (1980).
22. C. Perrow, *Normal Accidents*, Basic Books, New York, NY (1984).
23. S. M. Miller and D. M. Strong, A Model for Evaluating the Performance of Operational Level Information Handling Activities, Proceedings of the Seventh International Conference on Information Systems, San Diego, California, December 1986.
24. D. M. Strong, Design and Evaluation of Information Handling Processes, Carnegie Mellon University (1988).
25. M. E. Paté-Cornell, H. L. Lee, and G. Tagaras, Warnings of Malfunction: The Decision to Inspect and Maintain Production Processes on Schedule or on Demand, *Management Science* **33(10)**:1277-1290 (October 1987).
26. National Research Council, Committee on Shuttle Criticality Review and Hazard Analysis Audit, Post Challenger Evaluation of Space Shuttle Risk Assessment and Management, National Academy Press (January 1988).
27. Report of the Presidential Commission on the Space Shuttle Challenger Accident, Washington, DC (1986).
28. R. P. Feynman, Personal Observations of Reliability of Shuttle, Appendix F to the Presidential Commission Report on the Space Shuttle Challenger Accident (1986).
29. J. R. Galbraith, *Organization Design*, Addison-Wesley Pub., Reading, MA (1977).

30. T. Weil and V. Rigal, Les pannes dans l'industrie, Ecole Nationale Supericure de Mines, Paris, France (June 1984).
31. R. P. Feynman, An Outsider's Insider View of The Challenger Enquiry, *Physics Today*, pp. 26-37, February, 1988.
32. S. Plous, Biased Assimilation of Technological Breakdowns, Unpublished Manuscript, Department of Psychology, Stanford University, CA (1988).
33. G. A. Tinsley and S. Kaplan, On Using Information Contained in Near-miss and Precursor Events by Means of Bayes' Theorem, Pickard, Lowe and Garrick, Inc., Newport Beach, CA (1988).
34. M. E. Paté-Cornell, Warning Systems in Risk Management, *Risk Analysis* **5(2)**:223-234 (1986).

Risk-Cost Tradeoff Analysis of Oil vs. Coal Fuels for Power Generation

Lawrence B. Gratt
IWG Corp.
San Diego, CA

Gregory S. Kowalczyk
Northeast Utilities Service Company
Hartford, CT

ABSTRACT

This study examines the economic requirements and health consequences of converting an electrical power generating unit from oil to coal combustion at the West Springfield, MA Generating Station. Three alternative coal combustion emission control technologies are investigated: electrostatic precipitator, fabric filter, and Venturi scrubber. Health risks are evaluated for excess lifetime cancers for arsenic, beryllium, cadmium, chromium^{+6}, formaldehyde and polycyclic organic material (POM) using the Air Emission Risk Assessment Model (AERAM). Emissions and resulting ambient concentrations are determined for copper, mercury, manganese, lead and nickel. Two residual fuel oils representing a nominal and extreme case for pollutant emissions were considered along with two coal fuels representing a "clean coal" and a nominal bituminous coal. Capital costs for control systems and conversion to coal in addition to the changes in annual operating costs were considered in the economic tradeoffs. Values were assigned to the cost of an excess cancer and differential costs between oil and coal in order to reach break-even conditions for fuel switching. Based on the scenarios for the West Springfield Plant and fuel characteristics, the cancer risk results are comparable for the types of fuels considered, with the tradeoffs dependent on the economics of fuel price differentials.

KEYWORDS: Coal-fired power plant, oil-fired power plant, air emissions cancer risk

INTRODUCTION

The use of fossil fuel for the generation of electricity produces a variety of atmospheric pollutants. Two of the most commonly used fossil fuels are coal and oil. Several factors determine which fuel is chosen. They may include cost and availability of the fuel, proximity of the fuel source, permitting and licensing considerations, and environmental impacts. Historically, coal-fired power plants were generally utilized in the mid-west while the New England and mid-Atlantic states have emphasized oil combustion. Over the past decade this has changed somewhat as high oil prices encouraged some east coast utilities to convert to coal. Oil prices have now become comparable to coal prices.

Risk Analysis, Edited by C. Zervos
Plenum Press, New York, 1991

Should they begin a rapid escalation relative to coal, however, utilities may once again consider conversion.

Fuel price is the most important factor in a decision for conversion of an established plant. However, it is important for the electric power industry to understand not only the health risks to the public associated with each fuel, but also how to manage these risks. Conversion plans, then, need take into account cost of conversion, differences in pollutant levels in each fuel, differences in abatement equipment and differences in fuel costs.

This is study investigates the risk-cost tradeoffs of a fuel conversion from oil to coal using the Electric Power Research Institute's (EPRI) Air Emissions Risk Assessment Model (AERAM) at Northeast Utilities' (NU) West Springfield Unit #3 power plant in West Springfield, Massachusetts. In the early 1980's this plant was targeted for coal conversion which never materialized. If coal conversion becomes an issue in the future, it may again be considered.

BACKGROUND

EPRI sponsored the development of AERAM, a computerized model for estimating human cancer risks associated with toxic air pollutants emitted from coal-fired power plants[1-3] to aid utility decision makers in the evaluation of power plant control strategies. AERAM is an integrated four-module FORTRAN computer program with each module addressing one of the four components of the risk analysis process: pollutant emission, atmospheric dispersion, population exposure, and health risk estimation. The AERAM methodology has been fully described previously.[4,5] Briefly, the first part of the program uses fuel properties, power plant operating parameters, and pollution control device efficiency to calculate the stack emission rates for pollutants of interest. The second part quantifies the pollutant dispersion from the stack emissions using EPA's Industrial Source Complex - Long Term (ISCLT) dispersion model to calculate ambient air concentrations.[6] The third part estimates population exposures using the modeled pollutant concentrations, demographic data, and breathing rates. The final part estimates cancer risk based on a unit risk factor or dose-response data from human exposure or animal studies.

NU was the first utility to apply AERAM to evaluate lung cancer risks from exposure to benzo(a)pyrene (BaP) and arsenic emitted by its coal-fired Mt. Tom power plant in Holyoke, Massachusetts.[4] This effort was subsequently extended to investigate the key sensitivities of the risk assessment process for inhalation of airborne emissions from power plants.[5]

METHODS

The location of the West Springfield Generating Station along with the study area used for this analysis is shown in Fig. 1. The plant consists of three oil-fired units with power produced primarily by the 111 MWe Unit #3. The conversion costs to coal, estimated to be $35 million, were based on escalation of a 1982 estimate. For this analysis, using oil the plant operates in a peak shaving mode with a load factor of 50%. For the conversion to coal it is assumed that the plant will be used in a base load mode with a load factor of 85%. Analysis inputs describing the plant and control efficiencies for the various options in the coal-fueled mode are summarized in Table 1.

Two fuels were considered for each case. The first was representative of what is expected to be used in the power plant. The second was selected to represent an extreme case of pollutant emissions based on available data.

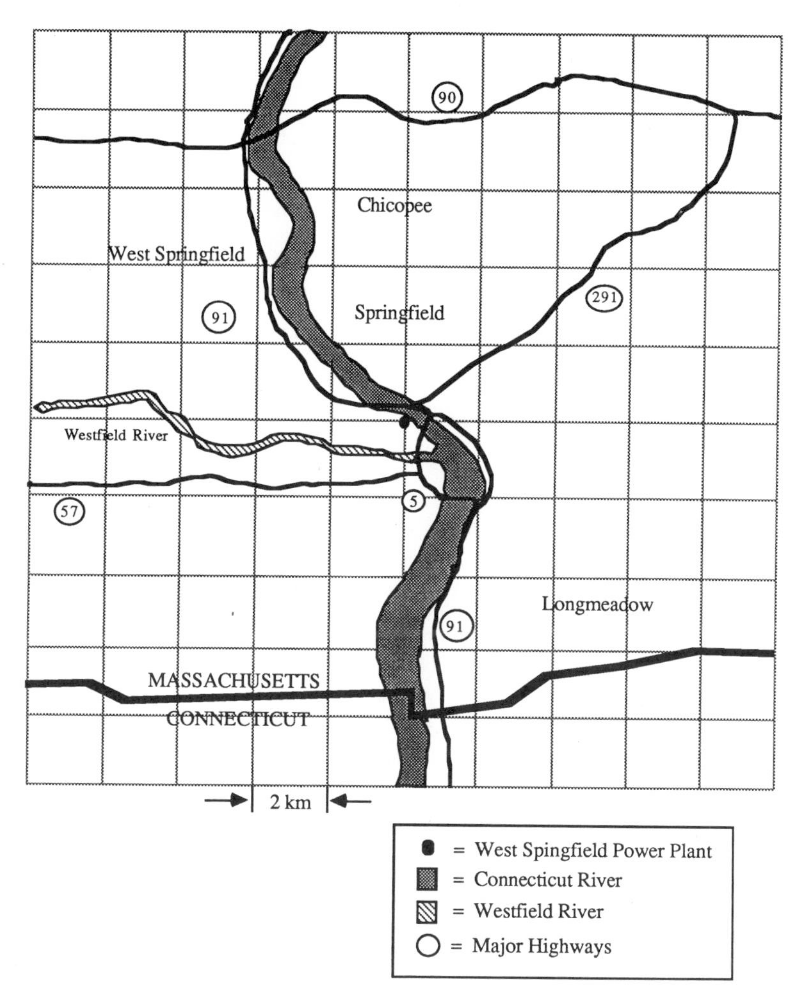

Fig. 1. West Springfield Power Plant analysis region (20 km × 20 km).

For coal-fired boilers three types of particulate emission controls were considered: electrostatic precipitator (ESP), fabric filtration (FF), and Venturi scrubbing (VS). ESP is the system most widely used by generating utilities. Fly ash particles are charged and guided by an electric field to a collector plate. Fabric filtration (FF) is gaining acceptability due to improved collection efficiency for particle sizes responsible for plume opacity. Scrubbers are not normally used for particulate control at power plants unless used for simultaneous gas removal. They are among the most efficient devices in removing particle sizes that cause plume opacity.

In the interest of brevity, only the results of intermediate calculations for ESP are shown in this paper. Table 2 presents the fuel data and the calculated elemental concentrations leading to the indicated emissions and corresponding ambient concentrations in the study area.

The ambient concentrations at 100 receptor locations were calculated using ISCLT with terrain elevations and the STAR meteorological data for Chicopee Falls, MA. An example of the resulting concentrations for arsenic is shown in Fig. 2.

Table 1. Summary of West Springfield Plant Parameters for Tradeoff Analysis

		Oil Cases		Coal Cases	
Fuel		Oil #1	Oil #2	Coal #1	Coal #2
Heating Value					
btu/gal		155,000	145,000		
btu/lb				14,300	13,000
Plant Heatrate, Btu/kwh		10,560	10,560	9,400	9,400
Plant Size, MWe		111	111	111	111
Load Factor		0.50	0.50	0.85	0.85
Stack Height, ft		220	220	220	220
Elevation, ft		70	70	70	70
Diameter, ft		13	13	13	13
Exit Temperature, deg F		300	300	300	300
Exit Velocity, ft/sec		55.1	55.1	55.1	55.1
Generated Power, kwh		4.86×10^8	4.86×10^8	8.27×10^8	8.27×10^8
Fuel Consumed,					
bbl/y		788,600	843,000	-	-
ton/y		-	-	271700	298800
Particle Size Classes		2	2	4	4
Lower Particle Size Cutoff Diameter, microns	1)	0	0	0.1	0.1
	2)	10	10	0.5	0.5
	3)	-	-	2.0	2.0
	4)	-	-	10	10
ESP Control Efficiency by Cutoff[a] Diameter	1)	-	-	0.985	0.985
	2)	-	-	0.96	0.96
	3)	-	-	0.99	0.99
	4)	-	-	0.998	0.998
FF Control Efficiency by Cutoff[b] Diameter	1)	-	-	0.998	0.998
	2)	-	-	0.995	0.995
	3)	-	-	0.997	0.997
	4)	-	-	0.998	0.998
VS Control Efficiency by Cutoff[c] Diameter	1)	-	-	0.70	0.70
	2)	-	-	0.95	0.95
	3)	-	-	0.998	0.998
	4)	-	-	0.99	0.99

a. ESP is Electrostic Precipitator Pollution Control
b. FF is Fabric Filter Pollution Control
c. VS is Venturi Scrubber Pollution Control

Using 1980 census data, the population at risk in the analysis region was estimated at 299,443 persons distributed into one hundred 4 sq. km exposure districts corresponding to the receptor locations.

The health hazard from the inhalation of particles depends on the concentration and size of the particles deposited in regions of the human lung. The respirable particles were considered to be in the range of 0.1 to 10 μm aerodynamic diameter. Respirable emissions used for calculating the cancer risk are given in Table 2.

For coal combustion emissions, arsenic is highly enriched on small particles. The mass of arsenic is primarily in the respirable range so the risk is only slightly reduced when only respirable particles are considered. Enrichment as a function of particle size has been considered for only arsenic from coal because of the paucity data for other elements. For oil

Table 2. Fuel Descriptions, Emissions and Calculated Ambient Concentration for the West Springfield Power Plant Conversion Tradeoff Analysis

Fuel	Pollutant	Content in Fuel[a] (ppm)	Total Emissions (lb/yr)	Respirable Emissions[b] (lb/yr)	Calculated Maximum Concentration (ug/m3)
Oil #1 (155,000 btu/gal)					
	Arsenic	0.36	97.5	48.8	2.24×10^{-5}
	Beryllium	0.08	21.7	10.8	4.98×10^{-6}
	Cadmium	0.3	81.3	40.6	1.87×10^{-5}
	Chromium(+6)	0.4	108	54.2	2.49×10^{-5}
	Formaldehyde		2090	1050	4.80×10^{-4}
	POM		43.4	21.7	9.96×10^{-6}
	Copper	5.3	1440	718	3.30×10^{-4}
	Mercury	0.06	16.3	8.1	3.73×10^{-6}
	Manganese	0.049	13.3	6.6	3.05×10^{-6}
	Lead	1	271	135	6.22×10^{-5}
	Nickel	24	6500	3250	1.49×10^{-3}
Oil #2 (145,000 btu/gal)					
	Arsenic	0.80	217	108	4.98×10^{-5}
	Beryllium	0.38	103	51.5	2.36×10^{-5}
	Cadmium	2.27	615	308	1.41×10^{-4}
	Chromium(+6)	5	1360	677	3.11×10^{-4}
	Formaldehyde		2090	1050	4.80×10^{-4}
	POM		117	58.3	2.68×10^{-5}
	Copper	79	21400	10700	4.92×10^{-3}
	Mercury	10	2710	1360	6.22×10^{-4}
	Manganese	27	7320	3660	1.68×10^{-3}
	Lead	2.4	650	325	1.49×10^{-4}
	Nickel	73	19800	9890	4.54×10^{-3}
Coal #1 (14,300 Btu/lb)			ESP Control System		
	Arsenic	8.8	85.3	83.7	6.19×10^{-5}
	Beryllium	0.69	3.71	3.43	2.69×10^{-6}
	Cadmium	0.8	4.30	3.98	3.12×10^{-6}
	Chromium(+6)	17	91.4	84.6	6.63×10^{-5}
	Formaldehyde		2.69	2.49	1.95×10^{-6}
	POM		0.59	0.55	4.29×10^{-7}
	Copper	8.3	44.6	41.3	3.24×10^{-5}
	Mercury	0.21	91.3	84.5	6.62×10^{-5}
	Manganese	12	64.5	59.7	4.68×10^{-5}
	Lead	5.1	27.4	25.4	1.99×10^{-5}
	Nickel	5.7	30.7	28.4	2.22×10^{-5}
Coal #2 (13,000 Btu/lb)			ESP Control System		
	Arsenic	20.3	197	193	1.43×10^{-4}
	Beryllium	5.6	30.1	27.9	2.19×10^{-5}
	Cadmium	25.5	137	127	9.95×10^{-5}
	Chromium(+6)	76	409	378	2.97×10^{-4}
	Formaldehyde		8.07	7.47	5.85×10^{-6}
	POM		1.77	1.64	1.29×10^{-6}
	Copper	53.4	287	266	2.08×10^{-4}
	Mercury	1	5.38	4.98	3.15×10^{-4}
	Manganese	300	1610	1490	1.17×10^{-3}
	Lead	45	242	224	1.76×10^{-4}
	Nickel	55.3	297	275	2.16×10^{-4}

a. Substance values from Reference 7 unless indicated otherwise.
Oil #1 ("clean" oil): Typical values for residual oil.
Oil #2 ("other" oil): Upper end of range values for residual oil.
Coal #1 ("clean" coal): Measured value for arsenic; others are mean values for bituminous coal.
Coal #2 ("nominal" coal): Mean for arsenic; most others two sigma above the mean.
b. Particles with diameters between 0.1 and 10 microns.

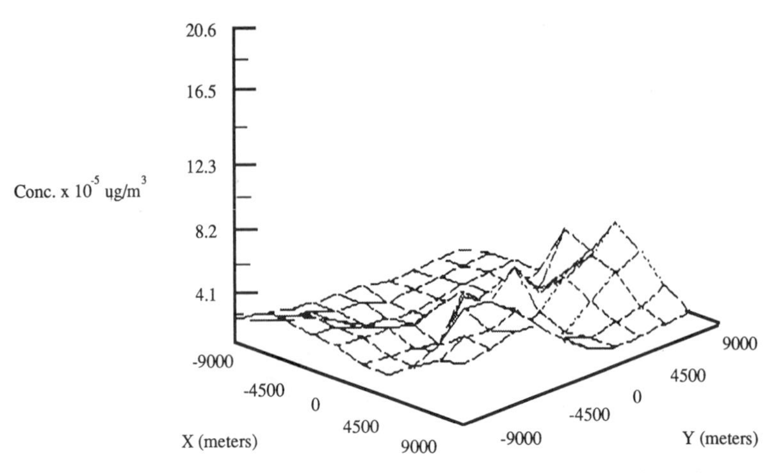

Fig. 2. Ambient concentrations for West Springfield arsenic emissions from coal #1.

combustion, two distinct particle sizes have been observed with about 50% of the mass of a pollutant on each side of a 10 μm diameter cutoff.

Arsenic, beryllium, cadmium, chromium, formaldehyde, and POM have been implicated as human carcinogens. The EPA unit risk factors[8] (plausible upper bounds on the risk for a lifetime exposure at 1 $\mu g/m^3$) were used for calculating the risk estimates which are summarized in Table 3.

The conversion to coal involves a significant capital investment that should be recovered from the use of a less expensive fuel. Accordingly, capital conversion costs were converted to yearly costs using a 10-year amortization and 12.5% interest rate. Based on the extrapolation of conversion studies performed in 1982, the 1988 estimated cost for conversion including the ESP particulate control system was $35 million.

Table 4 shows the conversion and control system costs used in the study. The tradeoff analysis range extends to fuel costs significantly above and below the current fuel prices ($15 per barrel for oil and $51 per ton of coal). The cost of a lifetime cancer is also considered for several values to establish the sensitivity with respect to this choice. The cost values are used to calculate the corresponding economic fuel switching points for oil to coal under the scenario conditions studied.

RESULTS

The calculated fuel switching points for the various conditions analyzed are presented in Table 5.

The conditions for fuel switching are based on the relative price of the fuels and the assigned cost of a cancer case. The cancer risk is very small in all cases. The "clean" fuels (Oil #1 and Coal #1) are comparable for the scenario analyzed with a resulting individual lifetime cancer risk of about 10^{-7}. These risks have been calculated using unit risk factors. The use of low-dose extrapolation models would result in much lower risk estimates.[9] For the extreme set of fuels the risks are about triple those of the clean fuels. The fuel switching decision for the clean fuels is driven by the fuel prices since risks are comparable. The differences provided by the different control technologies are not as important as the overall conversion cost required for the scenario analyzed; electrostatic precipitators appear to present the most economical option, followed closely by fabric filters.

Table 3. Excess Lifetime Cancer Risks for West Springfield Power Plant Conversion Tradeoff Analysis

Substance	Excess Lifetime Cancer Risk (per Capita)			
	Oil #1	Oil #2	Coal #1, ESP	Coal #2, ESP
Arsenic	4.0×10^{-8}	8.9×10^{-8}	8.9×10^{-8}	2.0×10^{-7}
Beryllium	1.5×10^{-9}	7.2×10^{-9}	6.6×10^{-10}	5.4×10^{-9}
Cadmium	1.4×10^{-8}	1.1×10^{-7}	1.9×10^{-9}	6.0×10^{-8}
Chromium(+6)	1.2×10^{-9}	1.5×10^{-8}	2.6×10^{-9}	1.2×10^{-8}
Formaldehyde	3.6×10^{-8}	3.6×10^{-8}	1.2×10^{-10}	3.5×10^{-10}
POM	7.0×10^{-9}	1.9×10^{-8}	2.4×10^{-10}	7.3×10^{-10}
Sum:	9.9×10^{-8}	2.7×10^{-7}	9.4×10^{-8}	2.8×10^{-7}
			Coal #1, FF	Coal #2, FF
Sum:			6.3×10^{-8}	1.9×10^{-7}
			Coal #1, VS	Coal #2, VS
Sum:			9.5×10^{-8}	2.9×10^{-7}

ESP is Electrostatic Precipitator
FF is Fabric Filter
VS is Venturi Scrubber

For oil at \$25/bbl, the switch to coal would require the price of coal to drop to about \$40/ton, significantly below current levels. The arbitrary dollar cost assigned to a cancer case has little impact on this result until this cost rises significantly above the \$10 million level. Fuel switching does not become attractive until oil prices increase to over \$30/bbl. Since the cancer cases are comparable for corresponding fuels, the cost associated with a cancer has a minimal impact on fuel switching decisions. Future oil and coal costs and the conversion costs are paramount for West Springfield fuel switching as opposed to the cancer risk costs or the conversion technology.

CONCLUSIONS AND RECOMMENDATIONS

A risk-cost tradeoff analysis for fuel conversion for the West Springfield Generating Station indicated that economic tradeoffs presented by the plant conversion and fuel costs are the dominant factors. Coal prices must have a significant price advantage over oil (\$40/ton of coal vs. \$25/bbl of oil for a projected period of 10 years) to facilitate fuel switching. The costs of cancer risks can become important as one compares "clean" fuels to other fuels, but the cancer risks were very small and comparable for analogous fuels. ESP control was the best economic choice for emission controls based on the rough cost estimates of this study.

The AERAM methodology has provided a useful and convenient means to support fuel tradeoffs for power plants that include the cost of health risk related to toxic air emissions.

ACKNOWLEDGEMENTS

This paper was based partially on work performed in support of the Electric Power Research Institute (Research Project 2141-2). This paper represents the views of the authors and does not necessarily reflect the views or policies of Northeast Utilities Service Company, IWG Corp., or the Electric Power Research Institute.

Table 4. West Springfield Coal Conversion and Control System Costs for Tradeoff Analysis

Control Technology	System Capital Cost ($/acfm)	Operating Cost ($/y/acfm)	Control System Capital Cost ($)	Plant Conversion Capital Cost ($)	Total Capital ($)	Yearly Capital Cost ($)	Control System Operation Annual Cost ($)
Electrostatic Precipitator	8.5	3	3,485,000	31,515,000	35,000,000	6,321,762	1,230,000
Fabric Filter	10	4.5	4,100,000	31,515,000	35,615,000	6,432,845	1,845,000
Venturi Scrubber	13	7.5	5,330,000	31,515,000	36,845,000	6,655,010	3,075,000

Size: 410,000 acfm (acfm is actual cubic feet per minute)
Interest Rate: 12.5%
Period: 10 y

Table 5. Fuel Switching Values for West Springfield Power Plant Conversion Tradeoff Analysis

Oil No.	Price ($/bbl)	Cancer Cost: $0 Coal #1	Cancer Cost: $0 Coal #2	$3,000,000 Coal #1	$3,000,000 Coal #2	$10,000,000 Coal #1	$10,000,000 Coal #2
		Electostatic Precipitator Control System					
1	15	15.75	14.32	15.73	14.87	15.69	16.15
1	20	30.26	27.51	30.25	28.06	30.21	29.35
1	25	44.78	40.71	44.76	41.26	44.72	42.54
1	30	59.30	53.91	59.28	54.46	59.24	55.74
1	35	73.81	67.10	73.79	67.65	73.75	68.94
1	40	88.33	80.30	88.31	80.85	88.27	82.13
2	15	18.75	17.05	18.16	17.08	16.80	17.16
2	20	34.27	31.15	33.68	31.19	32.31	31.26
2	25	49.78	45.26	49.20	45.29	47.83	45.37
2	30	65.30	59.37	64.72	59.40	63.35	59.48
2	35	80.82	73.47	80.23	73.51	78.87	73.58
2	40	96.34	87.58	95.75	87.61	94.38	87.69
		Fabric Filter Control System					
1	15	13.07	11.89	12.95	12.16	12.67	12.79
1	20	27.59	25.08	27.47	25.35	27.19	25.98
1	25	42.11	38.28	41.99	38.55	41.71	39.18
1	30	56.62	51.48	56.50	51.75	56.22	52.38
1	35	71.14	64.67	71.02	64.94	70.74	65.57
1	40	85.65	77.87	85.53	78.14	85.25	78.77
2	15	16.08	14.62	15.39	14.37	13.78	13.79
2	20	31.59	28.72	30.91	28.48	29.30	27.90
2	25	47.11	42.83	46.42	42.58	44.82	42.01
2	30	62.63	56.94	61.94	56.69	60.33	56.12
2	35	78.15	71.04	77.46	70.80	75.85	70.22
2	40	93.66	85.15	92.97	84.91	91.37	84.33
		Venturi Scrubber Control System					
1	15	7.73	7.03	7.72	7.59	7.69	8.90
1	20	22.24	20.22	22.23	20.78	22.20	22.09
1	25	36.76	33.42	36.75	33.98	36.72	35.29
1	30	51.28	46.62	51.26	47.18	51.23	48.49
1	35	65.79	59.81	65.78	60.38	65.75	61.68
1	40	80.31	73.01	80.29	73.57	80.26	74.88
2	15	10.73	9.76	10.15	9.80	8.79	9.90
2	20	26.25	23.86	25.67	23.91	24.31	24.01
2	25	41.77	37.97	41.18	38.02	39.83	38.12
2	30	57.28	52.08	56.70	52.12	55.34	52.23
2	35	72.80	66.18	72.22	66.23	70.86	66.33
2	40	88.32	80.29	87.73	80.34	86.38	80.44

Coal Fuel Switching Values ($/ton)

REFERENCES

1. Arthur D. Little, Inc., *Assessing the Health Risks of Airborne Carcinogens*, EPRI Research Project 1946-1, EA-4021, Electric Power Research Institute, Palo Alto, CA (1985).
2. Mindware Corporation, *Air Emissions Risk Assessment Model (AERAM)*, Programmer's Guide, (Draft), Columbus, OH (1987).
3. IWG Corp., *Air Emissions Risk Assessment Model (AERAM) Manager User's Guide* (Draft), San Diego, CA (1987).

4. G. S. Kowalczyk, L. B. Gratt and P. F. Ricci, An Air Emission Risk Assessment for Benzo(a)pyrene and Arsenic from the Mt. Tom Power Plant, *JAPCA* **37**:361-369 (1987).
5. G. S. Kowalczyk, L. B. Gratt, B. W. Perry and E. Yazdzik, Air Emission Risk Assessment Sensitivity Analysis for a Coal-Fired Power Plant, in (Advances in Risk Analysis), Vol. 7, pp. 165-174, J. J. Bonin and D. E. Stevenson, eds., Plenum Publishing Corp., NY (1989).
6. H. E. Cramer Co., Inc., *Industrial Source Complex (ISC) Dispersion Model User's Guide*, U.S. Environmental Protection Agency, Research Triangle Park, NC (1979).
7. R. C. Mead, B. K. Post, and G. W. Brooks, *Summary of Trace Emissions from and Recommendations of Risk Assessment Methodologies for Coal and Oil Combustion Sources*, Research Triangle Park, NC (July 1986).
8. U.S. Environmental Protection Agency, *Coal and Oil Combustion Study, Summary and Results, Office of Air Quality Planning and Standards*, Research Triangle Park, NC (1986).
9. B. W. Perry and L. B. Gratt, Multiple Low-Dose Extrapolation Models in Cancer Risk Assessment of Power Plant Air Emissions, Paper No. 87-41.6, 80th APCA Annual Meeting, NY (June 1987).

Analysis of Noncancer Health Risks Associated with Hazardous Air Pollutants

Timothy J. Mohin and David E. Guinnup
U.S. Environmental Protection Agency
Research Triangle Park, NC

ABSTRACT

Regulatory decisions made by the Environmental Protection Agency (EPA) concerning hazardous air pollutants (HAP) have been based primarily on quantitative assessments of cancer risk. Recently, however, more attention has been focused on effects other than cancer. The EPA has developed new methods to analyze the noncancer health risks associated with exposure to HAP. This paper discusses a newly developed method of analyzing short-term exposure to HAP and evaluating the public health risks resulting from these exposures. In the past, acute noncancer health effects were primarily analyzed on a screening basis. These analyses focused on the worst-case predicted ambient concentrations in comparison with health effects thresholds. Often several worst-case assumptions were factored into such analyses. When these analyses revealed an exceedance of the threshold (as was often the case) the degree of uncertainty was an unacceptable basis for regulatory decision making. The method presented herein represents a substantial improvement in EPA's ability to analyze the effects of short-term exposure to HAP. Based on the expected exceedance methodology developed for the criteria pollutant program, this method has been adapted to estimate health risks associated with exposure to HAP in terms of expected exceedances of specified health effects thresholds.

KEYWORDS: Noncancer risks, epichlorohydrin, exceedance, threshold, air pollutants

INTRODUCTION

The United States Environmental Protection Agency's (EPA) Office of Air Quality Planning and Standards (OAQPS) is responsible for administering the hazardous air pollutant program under Sections 111 and 112 of the Clean Air Act (CAA). Section 112 of the CAA defines a hazardous air pollutant as "an air pollutant to which no ambient air quality standard is applicable and which in the judgment of the Administrator (of the EPA) causes, or contributes to, air pollution which may reasonably be anticipated to result in an increase in mortality or an increase in serious irreversible or incapacitating reversible illness."[1]

The EPA's hazardous air pollutant program has relied primarily on risk assessments for regulatory decisions. In the recent past, the bulk of risk assessment activity has been focused on cancer as the health endpoint of concern. While cancer still remains very much a concern to the EPA, risk assessment for noncancer health endpoints has recently gained importance. As a result of this broadening of the focus of risk assessments for hazardous air pollutants there have been several advancements in the techniques used to assess both exposure and risk for potentially hazardous air pollutants. This paper describes a new methodology for analyzing exposure to hazardous air pollutants and discusses the possible ramifications for the regulatory process.

BACKGROUND

Epichlorohydrin (CAS 106-89-8) is one of the compounds recently analyzed by the OAQPS as a potentially hazardous air pollutant. Assessment of the public health risks associated with epichlorohydrin is described here only as an example of the exposure assessment technique. Epichlorohydrin is used in a variety of industrial processes. The major use is as a constituent of epoxy resins and glycerol.[2]

Assessment of epichlorohydrin as a potentially hazardous air pollutant was initiated in 1983 primarily due to concerns regarding its carcinogenic potential. Epichlorohydrin has been classified as a group B2 carcinogen according to EPA's guidelines for carcinogen risk assessment.[3] This categorization means that epichlorohydrin is regarded as a "probable human carcinogen" based on "sufficient" evidence in animals and "inadequate" evidence in humans.[3]

The animal evidence for the carcinogenicity of epichlorohydrin includes nasal carcinomas in rats,[4] local sarcomas in mice,[5] and forestomach neoplasms in rats.[6] From the available data on the carcinogenicity of epichlorohydrin, a series of quantitative risk estimates were derived and used in combination with exposure estimates to develop quantitative estimates of the cancer risk to the public exposed to ambient concentrations of epichlorohydrin.

In addition to the cancer risk estimates discussed above, the regulatory analysis included a preliminary assessment of the potential for noncancer health endpoints resulting from exposure to ambient concentrations of epichlorohydrin. Exposure to epichlorohydrin has been associated with a number of adverse health effects other than cancer. Contact with epichlorohydrin is irritating to the skin and mucous membranes of animals and humans. Repeated exposure to epichlorohydrin vapors resulted in both kidney and liver damage in rodents.[7]

To evaluate the potential for general toxicity in populations exposed to epichlorohydrin requires determination of the "no observed effect level" (NOEL) or the "lowest observed effect level" (LOEL). The LOEL for acute exposure to epichlorohydrin was identified in a study from the Russian literature.[8] Although the study employed methods that may have confounded the results, it suggested that minor liver effects in rats occur following a four-hour exposure to 2 ppm epichlorohydrin in the air.

To evaluate the public health significance of the Russian findings it was necessary to estimate the maximum ambient concentration of epichlorohydrin over a four-hour averaging period and the number of people that would be potentially exposed to that concentration. The estimates were subsequently compared to the LOEL multiplied by an uncertainty factor. For epichlorohydrin, this analysis revealed that the short-term ambient concentrations of epichlorohydrin may exceed the LOEL from the Russian study.

Prior to this finding the EPA had published a Notice of Intent Not to Regulate Epichlorohydrin under the CAA.[9] This notice was based primarily on the risk of cancer and included only a screening analysis of the noncancer health risks. The finding that short-term epichlorohydrin concentrations may exceed the LOEL has prompted the EPA to reevaluate the public health significance of ambient concentrations of epichlorohydrin with a focus on short-term exposures and noncancer health effects. This reevaluation included improvements of both the health effects and exposure databases for epichlorohydrin.

Analysis of exposure to ambient concentrations of hazardous air pollutants over short time periods is a relatively new area of study. In the past, most exposure analyses for hazardous air pollutants focused on annual or lifetime exposures due to the emphasis on cancer as the primary health endpoint of concern. Estimating exposures over the shorter time periods associated with acute or subchronic health effects presents an array of new problems to the exposure analyst. The discussion below outlines a new methodology for estimating exposure over short time periods.

The noncancer risk assessment for epichlorohydrin was the first project to employ this methodology; it will be used an example case for discussion. The reader is cautioned, however, that the analysis of the health risks associated with short-term ambient concentrations of epichlorohydrin is not yet complete, and it is premature to draw any conclusions from the data.

METHODS

Estimating the risks associated with short-term ambient concentrations of hazardous air pollutants emitted from a specific source(s) requires simulation of the emission characteristics of the source, the downwind dispersion of the pollutant in the atmosphere, and the distribution of the human population in the vicinity of the source(s). This estimation process differs in focus from that associated with long-term (i.e., cancer) risk estimation in that the latter tends to be dominated by continuous releases whereas the former may be strongly dominated by finite-duration, intermittent releases. Typical methods for modeling continuous releases cannot be used for such intermittent releases.

In general, to estimate the noncancer risk associated with an industrial facility with a significant release (or releases), one must appropriately trigger each intermittent release (on and off) throughout the simulation period. Our approach involves using historical plant data to establish the frequency of "on" time for each release, and then uses a random simulator to turn each release on and off with the appropriate frequency. Hourly meteorological data from a nearby weather station are then used to model the atmospheric dispersion of whichever release or releases is deemed to be "on" during any given hour. Resulting hourly concentrations are calculated for receptor sites in the plant vicinity, and each concentration is compared to some specified threshold concentration which is associated with the specific health effect for which the risk is being estimated.

If the calculated hourly concentration value at a particular receptor site is greater than the threshold concentration, a threshold "exceedance" is recorded for that site during that hour. The calculation process is repeated over the course of a year's 'meteorological data and over the course of hundreds of years of possible release combinations. This results in the determination of average annual exceedance rates at each receptor site. Finally, the exceedance rates are multiplied by the number of people living at (or near) each receptor site to estimate the average annual "person-exceedances". This estimate provides an environmental or public health decision-maker with a measure of the risk of a certain health effect to the general population exposed to ambient concentrations of potentially hazardous air pollutants.

The analysis described herein assumes that the emission characteristics of the source(s) are established and that the source emission rate is constant during the pollutant release. The emission may be continuous or intermittent. In the latter case, the frequency of

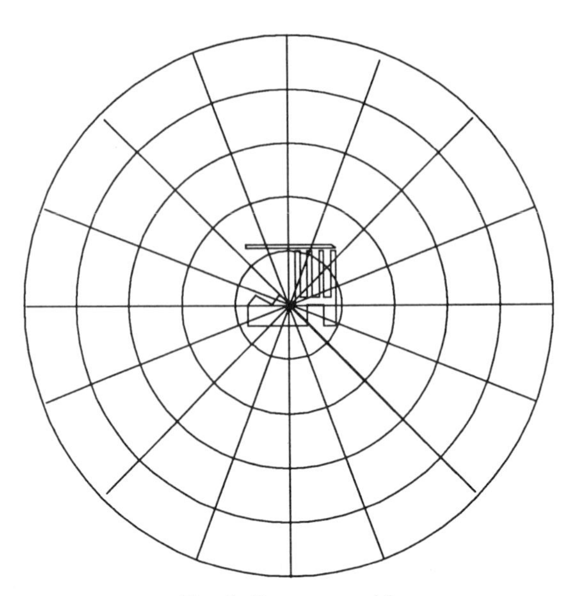

Fig. 1. Receptor grid.

the emission is known. Finally, each individual emission is assumed to occur independently of any other emission (i.e., randomly).

The analysis assumes that the subject for modeling is an industrial facility with one or more sources of a single pollutant. The object is to estimate the relative risk of a specific noncancer health effect to the population in the vicinity of the modeled facility.

Atmospheric dispersion of the pollutant from a source is modeled using the Industrial Source Complex–Short-Term (ISCST) model. Each intermittent source is modeled individually as if it were a continuous source, using its constant emission rate during release as its continuous emission rate. All continuous sources are modeled as a single source group (refer to the ISCST User's Guide[10] for the definition of ISCST source groups).

The emphasis in this analysis is placed upon short-term health effects. Accordingly, the ISCST dispersion model estimates one-hour average concentrations using one year of hourly meteorological data from the nearest reporting weather station. Concentrations are predicted for a 10-ring, 16 polar sector receptor grid which surrounds the plant (see Fig. 1), and the values of all concentrations (every receptor, for every hour of meteorological data) are stored in an output file (automatically created by ISCST). The computer program also generates a listing of the highest 50 concentration values estimated during the year along with their time and location of occurrence.

The task of estimating threshold concentration exceedances in the receptor grid resulting from various combinations of release events from the facility is completed using a modified version of the Expected Exceedances (ExEx) program, originally developed by Systems Applications, Inc. for the EPA.[11] This computer model, which was developed to assess short-term concentration threshold exceedances of sulfur dioxide (SO^2) in the vicinity of coal-fired power plants, incorporates a Monte Carlo simulation technique to randomly adjust SO^2 emission rates according to a specified log-normal distribution associated with the variability of total sulfur content in coal. The ExEx program reads

ISCST-predicted hourly concentrations for each source from the appropriate ISCST output file, adjusts the concentrations according to the Monte Carlo-selected sulfur content of the coal for each hour, and sums the concentration impacts from each source at each receptor.

In our version of ExEx, the ambient concentration predictions from each source modeled in the ISCST simulation are also read from the output file and summed, but the Monte Carlo simulator is used to randomly turn the intermittent sources either completely on or off according to their reported frequencies of occurrence. This modified version of ExEx differs from the original program in that the modified simulator uses a discrete distribution to turn the sources on and off instead of the original log-normal distribution. If a particular source is reported to be emitting about 20% of the hours in the year, the simulator will multiply receptor concentrations by 1.0 for 20% of the hours in the year and by 0.0 for the remaining 80% but randomly. In this way, the hourly ambient concentrations estimated for the combined contribution of all emissions at the plant result only from those sources which are determined to be emitting during that particular hour.

To achieve a model estimate which is representative, the Monte Carlo simulation process is carried out for a large number of "simulation years" and the hourly concentrations at each receptor are compared to a user-specified concentration threshold. If a particular threshold concentration is exceeded for a particular hour, a receptor-specific hourly exceedance counter is incremented by one. At the end of the simulation period, each exceedance counter is divided by the total number of simulation years to obtain the "annual expected exceedance rate" at each receptor. It should be noted that these expected exceedance rates reflect not only the likelihood that certain sources may be emitting at the same time, but also the likelihood that emissions may occur during adverse weather conditions.

In addition to concentration estimates which reflect the intermittent nature of a plant's operation, it is desirable to obtain an estimate of the size of the geographical area which might be affected by a "worst-case" incident at the facility. This requires a simulation to define the downwind area in which the ambient concentration exceeds a specific health effects threshold. To this end, our approach involves performing an initial dispersion simulation using ISCST to determine the highest ambient concentration resulting from the combination of all possible releases occurring simultaneously regardless of frequency.

The meteorological conditions that result in the maximum downwind concentration (listed in the printout of the 50 highest concentrations) associated with this worst-case emission event are identified and an additional ISCST simulation is performed only for this worst-case hour using a receptor grid which is focused on the downwind area. This technique estimates the highest concentration at each receptor for this worst-case hour, and the results are compared to a specified health effects concentration threshold (presumably the same one specified above) to determine which locations are exposed to concentrations above the threshold and which are not. The area defined by those receptors with concentrations which exceed the specified threshold is referred to as the "maximum impact area" for the specific concentration threshold.

To complete the analysis of risk resulting from the intermittent release of potentially hazardous air pollutants, it is necessary to estimate the population potentially affected by these releases. Outlined in the discussion above are the methods used to estimate the expected exceedances and the worst-case exceedances of concentrations associated with noncancer health effects. The population associated with these exceedances is estimated using data from the United States Census Bureau and an exposure model known as the Human Exposure Model (HEM). The HEM has long been used by the EPA to estimate exposure and risk resulting from long-term exposure to carcinogens in the ambient air. The HEM consists of both a dispersion model to predict ambient concentrations and an exposure model to predict the population exposed to the predicted ambient concentrations.

For this analysis the HEM has been modified to receive the annual expected exceedance rates from the ExEx model described above rather than the concentration estimates which it would normally receive. The HEM uses an extrapolation technique to apportion population data from the US census population centroids into the specific receptor grid used by the ExEx model. Finally, the receptor-specific population estimate is multiplied by the receptor-specific annual expected exceedance rate to arrive at the annual expected rate of "person-exceedances" for each receptor. These estimates can be summed to obtain the total annual person-exceedances rate for the modeled facility.

The population associated with the worst-case or maximum impact area for the threshold effect of concern is also estimated using US census data. However, the receptor grid used to define the maximum impact area is not easily matched to the population extrapolation model employed by the HEM. In order to estimate the population potentially exposed within the maximum impact area, the total number of people within a 10 kilometer (km) radius from the center of the modeled facility is estimated from the US census data and simply proportioned to the maximum impact area based on the ratio of the maximum impact area to the area within the 10 km radius. This technique provides a very crude estimate of the population potentially exposed to above-threshold concentrations resulting from a worst-case emission event. Although this technique is plagued by uncertainties, it provides a plausible upper bound estimate of the potential public health risk represented by the facility.

RESULTS

This section provides results from the application of the methods described above to a facility which produces epichlorohydrin. As was mentioned previously, the analysis on this chemical has not been completed; the results are provided simply to illustrate the method and a possible means for its interpretation.

Figure 2 shows in tabular form the spatial distribution of annual expected exceedance rates for the epichlorohydrin odor threshold in the vicinity of the modeled facility. Ring distances (in meters) are listed across the top, and radial directions (in degrees, clockwise from north) are listed along the left side. In this case, the facility boundary is a circle with a radius of 120m, the odor threshold concentration corresponds to an hourly average concentration of 0.06 ppm, and the ring distances are placed between 200m and 1.2 km from the center of the plant. The receptor with the highest number of annual expected exceedances is located 200m from the center of the plant in a north-northeasterly direction (22.5° clockwise from north), and the expected exceedance rate at this site is reported as 63.64 events per year. In other words, a concentration monitor located at this point would, on the average, be expected to record hourly concentrations above 0.06 ppm about 60 times per year, or a little over once a week. In addition, it can be seen from this table that one might expect to record hourly average concentrations in excess of 0.06 ppm as far away as 600m from the center of the facility, although this would occur rarely (about 2 or 3 times in 100 years).

The results from the maximum impact area simulation are shown in Fig. 3. Here, the receptor grid was placed between 190 and 210 degrees (about SSW) using the same ring distances with radials spaced at 2° intervals. Black circles indicate receptors with concentrations above 0.06 ppm and black diamonds indicate receptors below the threshold. The area enclosed in the maximum impact area, or "plume footprint," is about 10,000 m^2.

The exposure modeling results for the expected and maximum exceedance analyses are shown in Table 1. Using the methods described above, it was estimated that there are approximately 7180 total person-exceedances associated with this facility at the odor threshold of epichlorohydrin. This is not to say that 7180 people are annually exposed to

Radial directions	200m	250m	300m	400m	500m	600m	700m	1000m
N	9.38	5.82	4.13	1.07	0.00	0.00	0.00	0.00
NNE	63.64	38.73	27.33	6.05	0.00	0.00	0.00	0.00
NE	60.98	39.24	23.12	0.05	0.02	0.00	0.00	0.00
ENE	22.96	14.36	9.56	2.11	0.05	0.02	0.00	0.00
E	14.79	6.10	4.06	1.04	0.00	0.00	0.00	0.00
ESE	14.38	4.23	2.09	2.00	0.00	0.00	0.00	0.00
SE	17.27	10.09	10.00	4.00	0.00	0.00	0.00	0.00
SSE	6.11	5.03	3.03	1.00	0.00	0.00	0.00	0.00
S	8.14	5.06	5.02	0.00	0.00	0.00	0.00	0.00
SSW	36.22	33.09	21.04	6.02	2.02	0.00	0.00	0.00
SW	30.30	21.09	9.68	0.04	0.04	0.04	0.00	0.00
WSW	35.55	20.13	11.10	1.02	0.02	0.00	0.00	0.00
W	19.68	7.25	4.15	1.04	0.03	0.03	0.00	0.00
WNW	5.40	0.11	0.05	0.00	0.00	0.00	0.00	0.00
NW	2.67	0.29	0.09	0.00	0.00	0.00	0.00	0.00
NNW	6.53	2.19	2.08	0.00	0.00	0.00	0.00	0.00

Fig. 2. Annual expected exceedance rate by receptor.

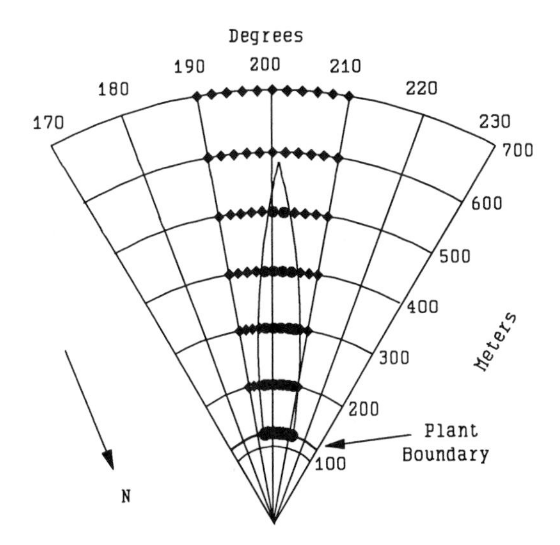

Fig. 3. Maximum plume impact area.

levels in excess of the odor threshold. Rather, this table represents the number of people exposed to levels exceeding the odor threshold multiplied by the expected number of times that threshold is exceeded annually.

Similarly, the maximum number of people potentially exposed at any one point in time to concentrations exceeding the odor threshold (i.e., the number of people within the

Table 1. Person Exceedances

Expected Exceedance Rate	Person-Exceedances
40 - 64	1.2
20 - 40	8.0
7 - 20	4.3
3 - 7	3970
1 - 3	1730
< 1	1470
Total	7180

maximum impact area) is estimated as 10. Again, this estimate is highly uncertain but provides a plausible upper bound estimate of exposure which might result from a worst-case emission event.

CONCLUSIONS

The assessment of short-term noncancer public health risks resulting from exposure to potentially hazardous air pollutants is a rapidly growing area of interest in the federal, state and local regulatory agencies. In the past, the focus of public health risk assessments for potentially hazardous air pollutants emphasized carcinogenicity as the primary endpoint of concern. This focus on carcinogenicity can be traced to the long-standing non-threshold assumption for the cancer endpoint. Although it is debatable as to whether public health thresholds for noncancer effects can be adequately defined, the bulk of the risk assessment efforts for effects other than cancer have employed some threshold for the onset of the effect of concern. Using the assumption of a definable threshold, the risk assessor must estimate the exposure (i.e., the number of individuals exposed) at concentrations exceeding this threshold. The problem is compounded when the effects of interest are acute in nature. The exposure assessment must incorporate randomly occurring short-term emission events and randomly occurring meteorological conditions to estimate ambient concentration in the vicinity of the emissions source.

In addition, the estimate of ambient concentrations must be coupled with the number of people potentially exposed to the concentrations to estimate the public exposure to the pollutant of concern. Finally, the estimate of exposure must be translated into an estimate of risk in order to provide information of regulatory decision making.

The method described above addresses the problem of short-term noncancer risk assessment by employing Monte Carlo simulation techniques to model the randomly occurring emission events and meteorological conditions. It assumes that short-term noncancer risk is defined relative to the number of times the threshold for the effect of concern is exceeded. The estimate of risk resulting from this method (i.e., annual average person-exceedances) describes the number of times a specific threshold is exceeded and the cumulative population associated with those exceedances for an average year of both weather conditions and short-term emission events. This estimate provides decision makers with a quantitative sense of the aggregate population risk resulting from emissions of the pollutant of concern.

In addition to the estimate of annual average person-exceedances, a method of estimating maximum risk to exposed individuals is also described. While this method incorporates assumptions which lead to a great deal of uncertainty in the resulting estimates, it represents an improvement over methods which have been employed in the past to estimate maximum short-term health risks in that it defines an area where there is the greatest likelihood of exposure to concentrations above the specified health effects threshold.

The methods described in this paper will not eliminate the uncertainties associated with short-term noncancer risk assessment for potentially hazardous air pollutants. These methods, however, do serve to reduce these uncertainties and hopefully provide better estimates of public health risks to support regulatory decision making concerning potentially hazardous air pollutants.

REFERENCES

1. Statutes-at-large, Clean Air Act Amendments of 1977, PL 95-95, August 7, 1977, Stat 91-685 (1977).
2. U. S. Environmental Protection Agency, Health assessment document for chloroform, EPA report no. EPA/600/8-84/004f, U.S. Environmental Protection Agency, Research Triangle Park, NC (1984).
3. U. S. Environmental Protection Agency, Guidelines for Carcinogen Risk Assessment, *Federal Register* **51(185)**:33992-34054 (1986).
4. S. Laskin *et al.*, Inhalation Carcinogenicity of Epichlorohydrin in Noninbred Spraugue-Dawley Rats, *J. Natl. Cancer Inst.* **65**:751-755 (1980).
5. B. L. Van Duuren *et al.*, Carcinogenic Activity of Alkylating Agents, *J. Natl. Cancer Inst..* **53**:695-700 (1974).
6. G. J. Van Esch, Induction of Preneoplastic Lesions in the Forestomach of Rats After Oral Administration of 1-Cloro-2,3-Epoxypropane, preliminary report no. 627805-005 (1982).
7. A. P. Fomin, Biological Effect of Epichlorohydrin and Its Hygienic Significance as an Atmospheric Pollutant, *Gig. Sanit.* **31**:357-363 (1966).
8. N. I. Shumskaya, N. M. Karamzina, and M. Y. Savina, Evaluating the Sensitivity of Integral and Specific Parameters in Acute Epichlorohydrin Intoxication, *Toksikol. Nov. Prom. Khim. Veshchestv.* **12**:33-44 (1971).
9. U. S. Environmental Protection Agency, Assessment of Epichlorohydrin as a Potentially Toxic Air Pollutant, *Federal Register* **50**:24575 (1985).
10. U. S. Environmental Protection Agency, *Industrial Source Complex – Short Term User's Guide*, EPA-450/4-88-002a and b, Environmental Protection Agency, Research Triangle Park, NC (1988).
11. Systems Applications, Inc., *User's Guide to the Expected Exceedances System*, EPA contract 68-02-4352 report (1988).

A Bayesian Approach to Import Sample Selection[a]

Richard A. Williams, Jr. and Robert N. Brown
Food and Drug Administration
Washington, DC

ABSTRACT

With over one million lots of imported food entering the U.S. each year, the Food and Drug Administration is able to sample only about 6% of these lots to determine if the food violates U.S. laws. To make the best possible use of scarce inspection resources, a Bayesian decision model for sampling imported food lots is proposed. The consequences of a violative lot being imported and consumed involve consumer health, consumer non-health and producer consequences. These consequences are integrated with the prior probabilities of each food lot being violative to generate the social utility of sampling. The social utilities are then ranked by the severity and costs of inspection and are used to prioritize sampling. Adaptive filters may smooth the daily variation in the prior probability of a lot being violative. To counteract game-playing importers, a simple weighted randomization scheme is superimposed upon the ranked utilities.

KEYWORDS: Food, imports, sampling, decision analysis, Bayesian

INTRODUCTION

A recurring decision problem is to choose a small subset of items to sample or inspect from among a large number of items in a cost-effective manner. Examples of this general class of constrained large-scale monitoring problems include decisions concerning which toxic chemicals to test, which income tax returns to audit, which potentially unsafe workplaces to investigate, which waste sites to investigate, which criminal cases and leads to pursue, which cars to sample for contraband at the border, and finally, which imported food lots to sample. Currently, FDA only samples about six percent of all imported lots of food.

With over one million lots coming into the U.S. each year, the sampling choice is critical for the purposes of protecting the public's health and pocketbook from violative products.

This paper proposes a model which could assist decision makers in the daily routine of choosing among food lots to sample and analyze for violations of acts enforced by the FDA. The proposed model is a Bayesian with social utilities and a random component to

---

a. The work described in this paper is the responsibility of the authors only and does not reflect official positions of the Food and Drug Administration.

Risk Analysis, Edited by C. Zervos
Plenum Press, New York, 1991

the sampling selection process to account for the dynamically changing and deliberate "game" aspects of regulatory sample selection.

The choice from among hundreds of lots to sample is currently made without an automated decision aid. Even with assistance from headquarters, the amount of information "screeners"[b] are asked to process is enormous. Without a well-specified model and decision aids to organize and integrate disparate pieces of information, heuristic decision making may evolve resulting in frequent misallocation of resources.[1]

This paper attempts to identify, illuminate and interrelate the major parameters that should be taken into account with respect to any decision sampling aid. It also suggests possible analytical solutions to selected technical problems within the suggested framework.

OBJECTIVE

The objective of the proposed model is to minimize the adverse social consequences of food import violations given limited government resources. Included in the adverse social consequences are *adverse expenditures* on imported food products by consumers. These are defined as post-purchase, societal costs including death, morbidity and fraud associated with consumption of imported products whether or not those costs are knowingly incurred. Costs may not be knowingly incurred when, for example, consumers mistakenly diagnose their symptoms as influenza instead of salmonella poisoning or are unaware of carcinogenic pesticides in their imported food. Yet this model assumes that these costs, despite consumers' unawareness, are real and should be factored into sampling decisions as part of FDA's mandate to protect the public.

PAST APPROACHES TO PRIORITIZING SAMPLING

An initial attempt to optimize the allocation of inspection resources was proposed by Bryan,[2] who investigated the problem of detecting foodborne pathogens in restaurant food. He identified three coefficients of risk of illness caused by food served in restaurants: (1) the food property risk coefficient; (2) the food operation risk coefficient; and (3) the average daily patrons risk coefficient.

The property coefficient is a measure of whether or not a food item could be a vehicle of pathogen transmission. It is determined either by the prior history of the food or by its innate characteristics. Evidence for this coefficient included: "physiochemical (e.g., pH, water activity, oxidation-reduction potential); biological (e.g., nutrient content), ecological (e.g., usual microfloral population and their source such as polluted waters and processing plant environment), and epidemiological (e.g., history as a vehicle for foodborne pathogens)" data.

The operations coefficient is the product of the probability that pathogens will survive certain food processing practices and the probability that before the food item is consumed the surviving pathogens will multiply in sufficient quantities to cause disease.

The average daily patrons coefficient is a measure of the number of persons served in each restaurant.

---

b. A screener is a person who reviews the paperwork of incoming lots and, with guidance from headquarters, chooses the lots to be sampled.

Although Bryan's approach lacked statistical sophistication, it was an important first step. A more formal approach to sampling was made by Weinstein,[3] who attempted to prioritize carcinogens for testing using modern decision theory to examine the expected value of a test. He assumed that the value of a test is a Bayesian function of the prior probability of a given potency state, the likelihood of a test result given the true state, the exposure-response relation, the magnitude of (potential) exposure change, the lag between the decision to undertake the study and its findings, and the lag between study findings and altered exposure. The resulting expected value divided by the cost of the test would give a cost-effectiveness ratio to be used to prioritize a carcinogenic testing.

MODEL

Assume that groups of (food) lots arrive in discrete time units (daily) and the "screener" is able to choose which lots will be sampled before they arrive. The "screener" makes a decision over all L lots prior to the beginning of the day as to what will be sampled and it is assumed that all sampling and testing is completed each day. This latter assumption puts aside the multiple-day scheduling and constraint problem. A lot is assumed to be composed of a production run of one food from a single plant in a particular country. As a result of sampling, a lot is either in violation (non-compliance) or not (compliance) and is accordingly rejected or accepted.

The decision to sample or not is based on the utility of the action taken as a result of the test. The process of sampling a lot involves taking lab subsamples and testing them for conformance with specifications required by the FD&C Act or related acts enforced by the FDA. The utility from sampling a lot, ℓ, is initially defined as

$$U_\ell = \sum_{t=0}^{1} \sum_{s=0}^{1} \pi_s p_{ts} u_{ts} \qquad (1)$$

where

π_s is the prior probability of state s (s=1 when the sample does not comply and s=0 when it does);

u_{ts} is the consequence of a decision (or test result) t, given state s;

p_{ts} is the probability of a test outcome t, given the true state s.

Initially, the probability of a test outcome

t = 1 if positive, and
= 0 if negative

will also represent a *de facto* decision to reject the lot when there is a positive test result and accept the lot otherwise, however the test is structured. This is reasonable since lab tests are normally structured to accept or reject. However, acceptance criteria should be conditioned upon the degree of violation that, from a health standpoint, it is important to find. This connection between acceptance criteria and degree of violation is not trivial. The prior probabilities π_0 and π_1 and the operating characteristics of the test p_{ts} change with the expected violation.

A singularly important question one could ask about the present sampling choices (of foods) and tests is, "What is the risk level that is being tested for and is that level achieved by the present strategy?" That is, each state s is represented by the mean dose level that represents the section of the distribution of being "in" or "out" of violation. Each average dose level also has an implicit risk level attached to it; in fact, even the non-violative state will have some nonzero risk. Without some crude knowledge of the risk levels of each state, it is impossible to compare the utility of sampling various lots.

Having defined the utility from a policy of sampling, it is now necessary to define the utility from a policy of choosing not to sample a lot, the default policy, which, in this initial framework, is equivalent to accepting the lot. It is defined as:

$$U_\ell = \sum_{t=0}^{1} \sum_{s=0}^{1} \pi_s \bar{p}_{ts} \bar{u}_{ts} \ . \tag{2}$$

However,

$$\bar{p}_{11} = \bar{p}_{10} = 0$$

where p is the probability of a positive finding, which is equivalent to the probability of rejection and, by design, all lots not sampled are accepted. Furthermore,

$$\bar{p}_{00} = \bar{p}_{01} = 1$$

because, by default, all "tests" are negative and all lots are accepted. Thus Eq. (2) reduces to[c]

$$\bar{U}_\ell = \pi_0 \bar{u}_{00} + \pi_1 \bar{u}_{01} \ . \tag{3}$$

Subtracting Eq. (3) from Eq. (1) yields the utility difference between the policies of sampling and not sampling:

$$\tilde{U}_\ell = U_\ell - \bar{U}_\ell = \sum_{t=0}^{1} \sum_{s=0}^{1} \pi_s p_{ts} u_{ts} - \pi_0 \bar{u}_{00} - \pi_1 \bar{u}_{01} \ . \tag{4}$$

Although $\tilde{U}_\ell$ appears to be the utility of a policy of sampling for one violation per lot, in fact each imported lot could potentially be tested for all violations. Due to resource constraints, however, only one violation is typically tested. Furthermore, when a lot is found in violation of any law it is rejected making further testing (for other violations) superfluous. Because, typically, only one potential violation per lot is tested, prioritization of lots will be constrained in this model by consideration of the most significant violation in each lot, i.e., the potential violation that generates the highest $\tilde{U}_\ell$ per lot. Nevertheless, to choose the most significant potential violation within each lot, it is necessary to know the operating characteristics, p_{ts}, of the tests for every possible violation. In a deterministic approach such as the one initially proposed, this limiting strategy probably loses very little in generality. In the next section, the potential test results of all possible violations within each lot are utilized.

Denoting violations as v, (v= 1, 2, . V), each lot may potentially be in violation of some or all v. The net utility for testing a lot ℓ for the vth violation is denoted as $\tilde{U}_{\ell v}$. Before deciding which lots to sample it is necessary to pick for each lot some v = $\hat{v}$ such that

$$\tilde{U}_{\ell\hat{v}} \geq \forall\, \tilde{U}_{\ell v} \ \text{for possible violation, v.} \tag{5}$$

The utility for sampling a lot for $\hat{v}$ is

$$\tilde{U}_{\ell\hat{v}} \sum_{t=0}^{1} \sum_{s=0}^{1} \sum_{v=1}^{V} \left[\pi_{sv}\ p_{ts\hat{v}}\right] - \sum_{v=1}^{V} \left[\pi_{0v} \bar{u}_{00v} + \pi_1 \bar{u}_{01v}\right] \ . \tag{6}$$

---

c. Note that $\bar{u}_{00} \neq u_{00}$ and $\bar{u}_{01} \neq u_{01}$. The consequences are different because for $\bar{u}$ the product will not be held while it is being sampled. For u, the product is held for testing even though it is ultimately released.

It should be noted that the operating characteristics, $p_{ts\hat{v}}$, apply only to the chosen violation, $\hat{v}$, although the prior probability π_{sv} and the utility consequences u_{tsv} are related to every possible violation, v. As a consequence, the total net utility of sampling applies to the possibility of accepting or rejecting the lot with all of the potential violative substances that may be in it.

To make rational sampling decisions, the utility of sampling a lot must be compared with the cost of sampling, defined as $t_{\ell v}$ (e.g., the cost of sampling versus not sampling where the cost of not sampling is zero). The cost of sampling is the government (i.e., FDA) cost of taking samples, analyzing them and making decisions as a result of lab tests. The net utility of sampling per unit cost for each lot is now defined as

$$\frac{\tilde{U}_{\ell v}}{t_{\ell v}} \; .$$

At this point each lot has a primary violation for which it could be sampled (for which the utility of sampling is greatest over all possible violations) and a test cost for sampling for that violation. Because it is not possible to sample all incoming lots, even for only one violation, the lots may be initially prioritized by ranking them in decreasing order of net sampling utility per unit testing cost from the lot with the greatest (positive) net sampling utility to that with the least as follows:

$$\frac{\tilde{U}_{1\hat{v}}}{t_{1\hat{v}}} \geq \frac{\tilde{U}_{2\hat{v}}}{t_{2\hat{v}}} \geq \ldots \frac{\tilde{U}_{L\hat{v}}}{t_{L\hat{v}}} \tag{7}$$

where the $\hat{v}$ for each lot *may* be different. This ordering defines an associated ranking, $R_{\ell\hat{v}}$.

Next, let $\bar{T}$ be the fixed budget in the time period (daily) over which a group of lots will be considered for sampling. The budget may be a combination of labor and capital or a single factor in short supply consisting of, for example, lab time, equipment limits, inspector man-hours or testing costs. Utilizing the budget constraint with the ranked lots, an initial set of lots can be selected to sample as a subset, $r_{\lambda\hat{v}}$, of the initial ranking as:

$$r_{\lambda\hat{v}} \sqsubseteq R_{L\hat{v}}$$

for $\lambda < L$ where the lots $\ell = 1,2, ..,\lambda$ are chosen such that the following relationship holds:

$$\sum_{\ell=1}^{\lambda} t_{\ell\hat{v}} = \bar{T} \; .$$

In other words, the screener would sample the most "important" to the least "important" lots until the budget was exhausted for that time period.

RANDOM (SURVEILLANCE) SAMPLING

The outlined sampling strategy assumes that no "game" exists with respect to submission of entries. However, to the extent that information concerning the regulatory sampling strategy and the distribution of daily entries is known by importers, importers have potential incentives to avoid being selected for sampling. Incentives to avoid sampling arise when producers of imported products have allowed their manufacturing or distribution quality control to deteriorate through neglect or when they have added illegal additives or pesticides in their products. Furthermore, under any sampling plan, the probability of any one lot being sampled is necessarily low because of budget constraints. Under the sampling scheme suggested here, the most likely lot to be sampled, for instance, would be a large lot of inexpensive food, easily accessible to sampling yet difficult to recall, and in which there is a high prior probability of immediate lethal food poisoning (see next section). In this case, the importer may do one of several things to avoid detection: mislabel the product to indicate an expensive food; divide a large lot into smaller lots (with different "marks" indicating different production runs); or pack the food into hard-to-open containerized cargo packages and redirect its destination once admitted into the country.[d] Such behavior would characterize, for the most part, importers who did not rely on reputation with the government to avoid the expense of sampling at the border.[e] But even importers who do rely on reputation may, from time to time, be tempted to take advantage of a well-known but limited-reach, deterministic strategy and submit violative goods, particularly goods containing violations that are not apparent from their immediate effects (e.g., carcinogens). In short, a well-known regulatory sampling policy that is too limited could encourage chronic sloppiness even by reputable importers.

Because of such potential "game playing" behavior on the part of importers, it may be necessary to adopt a strategy that involves either secrecy, random selection or both. However, it is fairly easy for importers to observe which lots are sampled at any given port, and this is now done by game-playing importers. Thus, use of secret deterministic strategy can gradually become ineffective to some extent, leaving a randomized prioritization strategy to compensate. Randomized prioritization can be superimposed on and integrate with the previous deterministic strategy, and although it is expected that the probability of "purposeful" cheating would be factored into the prior probability of violation, a random strategy would add an additional component of uncertainty for potential violators to contend with.

Further, besides adding a component of uncertainty, a random selection strategy can provide information about prior probabilities which are constantly changing. By attaching some non-zero probability of being sampled to any particular lot, a randomized prioritization strategy provides some information about changes in distribution with time on virtually all imported products, even those sampled infrequently. This is important if products are in violation more often as a result of ignorance on the part of the manufacturer/importer, rather than as a result of a deliberate attempt to import a violative food undetected. A random strategy would detect some of the temporally changing "ignorance" violations, e.g., change in microbial count due to changes in temperature for a thermally processed food.

As one possible way to implement a random strategy, define

$$\hat{U}_{\ell\hat{v}} = \frac{\tilde{U}_{\ell\hat{v}}}{t_{\ell\hat{v}}}$$

with the weight for each lot ℓ characterized as:

$$\frac{\hat{U}^{\omega}_{\ell\hat{v}}}{\sum_{\ell=1}^{L} \hat{U}^{\omega}_{\ell\hat{v}}}$$

with $\omega = 1$ in the simplest case. These weights would then be used as components of a weighted "roulette wheel" that would "randomly" select, without replacement, the lots to be sampled. The weight, ω, could be utilized to alter the utility-oriented prioritization scheme, where, for instance, $\omega < 1$ would give greater weight to the lower priority lots. Thus, this strategy is actually a *weighted* random strategy with the lots originally chosen to sample, λ,

---

d. Often, if a food is in containerized cargo, FDA import officials will allow the product to continue into the country and sample it at the warehouse at which it will be opened.

e. Importers who do not rely on reputation are those who tend to import only infrequently.

now having the highest *probability* of being sampled, yet all lots having some probability of being sampled.

CONSEQUENCES

Let u_{tsv} represent the positive and negative consequences of a decision or test result t given the true state s for a violation v. They can be partitioned into consumer health consequences, consumer non-health consequences and producer consequences. Consumer health consequences, c_{tsv}^{h}, include morbidity and mortality that would result from a violative lot being consumed.

Consumer health consequences are a function of the dose of the offending ingredient (per serving), its potency and the morbidity and mortality consequence of ingesting that dose.[f] If the societal valuation of health costs for particular groups are weighted differently from the average population, then it involves a social welfare transfer and is beyond the scope of this paper.

Specifying a probable dose/response relationship for an offending ingredient and an associated violative dose may be the most difficult part of any food safety sampling model. For chemicals, which are particularly carcinogenic and teratogenic, it is difficult to predict "true" risk at low doses and a linear-at-low-dose model is often assumed. Another problem is the need to extrapolate animal results to humans using studies of low statistical power and confounding variables to predict dose/response relationships.[g]

Published estimates of risks for carcinogens are extremely conservative because of the inherent risk modeling difficulties. As a consequence, other things being equal, they tend to skew the decision framework toward sampling potentially carcinogenic chemicals rather than microbiological agents.

The problem of establishing a dose/response relationship for microbiological risks including bacterial pathogens (e.g., salmonella), viral agents (e.g., Norwalk virus) and parasitic agents (e.g., trichinella spiralis) is at least as difficult.[h] Generally, only limited attempts have been made. One attempt was to define a "minimal infectious dose" (MID) as "the probability (Q) that never in a lifetime will a member of a population be exposed at any one moment to sufficient numbers of infective units of a food-transmitted pathogen to incite disease."[4] In the model, Q depends on the exposed individuals' "age, nutritional status, and condition of the gastrointestinal tract as well as the attributes of the organism itself.[4] Thus, rather than a dose/response relation, the model estimates the minimum doses of various microbiological hazards that would make anyone sick; it is silent about responses to larger doses[5] which remain elusive and possibly may only be estimated empirically from past microbiological outbreaks.

---

f. It should be noted that carcinogenic dose/response is normally defined as a lifetime dose/response from ingestion of an average daily dose, e.g., a dose consumed for 365 days a year for 75 years. The risk level applied to carcinogens, e.g., 10^{-6}, does not apply to the actual risk in that particular lot unless you assume that by detecting and preventing one shipment, you have prevented a lifetime dose. The risk levels attached to microbiological hazards, on the other hand, would be the risk from a single serving.

g. Human studies in general will have lower statistical power than animal studies because of the factors that cannot be controlled for the number of samples, the dose, and a less than lifetime follow-up. To raise the power of the test for animal studies, one can always increase the number of studies, the doses and follow the animals over a lifetime.

h. For microbiological risk, the only type of concern here will be health risks as spoilage of foods which does not involve clinical health risks is not generally a consumer problem.

With a broad distribution of population sensitivities and risk characteristics (e.g., gastrointestinal conditions) some crude conclusions about dose/response relationships may be drawn from case studies.[i] A separate problem — determination of the dose at the time of consumption when it can be tested only at the point when food crosses the border — requires knowledge of microbial growth. There is a fairly large body of research on this subject.[4,6]

For microbial risks, the consumer dose corresponding to a particular health violation may frequently be measured only by proxy. For example, rather than reject a lot based upon the actual level of microbial contamination, current policy calls for rejection based on a combination of water activity and pH values which could give rise to growth conditions for microbial agents.

The consumer non-health consequences, c_t^c, include costs and benefits resulting from the product either being consumed or not consumed, depending on whether the product is found non-violative or violative, respectively.[j] If a product is rejected (not allowed to be imported), for example, consumers will not be allowed to purchase and consume the food, resulting in a societal loss.

Producer consequences, c_{ti}^p, are the consequences to producers of being sampled, i=1, or not being sampled, i=0, and being found violative or non-violative (t=1 or 0, respectively). These consequences include any costs of sampling the producer might be required to bear, including warehouse costs and costs of rejection such as product destruction, reconditioning, reshipping or devaluation (value of product decreased because the product may only be used for animal feed).[k] The consequences can now be specified as:

$$u_{tsvi} = \sum_{t=0}^{1} \sum_{s=0}^{1} \sum_{v=1}^{V} \sum_{i=0}^{1} \left[c_{tsv}^h + c_t^c + c_{ti}^p \right] . \tag{8}$$

The producer consequences will fall into a non-symmetrical matrix, and will depend on whether or not the product is sampled and whether or not the product is accepted or rejected (negative or positive outcome of the test). The matrix of utility outcomes with respect to the consequences then will depend on whether or not the product is to be sampled, i, whether the product is accepted or rejected, t, and the true state of the product, s.

The consequences for each possible outcome are:

$$\begin{aligned}
tsi &= 000 = c_{00v}^h + c_0^c + c_{00}^p \\
tsi &= 010 = c_{01v}^h + c_0^c + c_{00}^p \\
tsi &= 001 = c_{00v}^h + c_0^c + c_{01}^p \\
tsi &= 101 = c_{10v}^h + c_1^c + c_{11}^p \\
tsi &= 011 = c_{01v}^h + c_0^c + c_{01}^p \\
tsi &= 111 = c_{11v}^h + c_1^c + c_{11}^p
\end{aligned}$$

---

i. Outbreak data are recorded by the Center for Disease Control in Atlanta (Annual Summaries 1977–1982). Unfortunately, CDC records represent only a small fraction of actual outbreaks and the larger and more interesting outbreaks are considerably overrepresented.

j. Consumer consequences in this case are the consumer surplus that is accrued if the product is consumed (accepted) or loss of surplus if it is not allowed to be consumed (rejected).

k. There is some question as to whether or not any particular sampling strategy should take into account the portion of the costs that are borne by importers. It may, for example, be argued that only those costs that can be passed on to domestic consumers should be counted. This philosophy implicitly values resources not owned by the domestic country at zero which, if adopted by all countries, could severely limit international trade.

The utility of sampling a lot can now be rewritten to incorporate the consequence terms as:

$$\tilde{U}_{\ell\hat{\mathrm{v}}} \sum_{t=0}^{1} \sum_{s=0}^{1} \sum_{\mathrm{v}=1}^{\mathrm{V}} \left[\pi_{s\mathrm{v}} \, p_{ts\hat{\mathrm{v}}1} \left\{ c_{ts\mathrm{v}}^{h} + c_{t}^{c} + c_{t1}^{p} \right\} \right]$$

$$- \sum_{\mathrm{v}=1}^{\mathrm{V}} \left\{ \pi_{0\mathrm{v}} \left(c_{00\mathrm{v}}^{h} + c_{0}^{c} + c_{00}^{p} \right) + \pi_{1\mathrm{v}} \left(c_{01\mathrm{v}}^{h} + c_{0}^{c} + c_{00}^{p} \right) \right\} \tag{9}$$

where $p_{ts\hat{\mathrm{v}}i}$=0, if i=0 and t=1.

Two additional parameters need to be added to the utility framework to modify the consequences of a decision, the quantity of a food, X_{ℓ}, and the probability of recall, r. The consequences, as previously described, u_{tsvi}, are the consequences for consuming a violative substance in a single unit of food, in this case a serving size. A serving size is chosen as the individual unit as this is the smallest divisible unit which may cause a health effect, e.g., a case of salmonella. To account for the total impact of sampling and subsequent regulatory action on a lot, the total quantity of food must be included.

The probability of recall, r, will affect the utility consequences when a violative food is mistakenly not rejected. Although r is termed the "probability of recall," it is more generally defined as the average percentage of a lot that will be recalled (once the market has found the product to be violative) and not consumed. Generally, r will be affected by the immediacy of the effect (how quickly the violation is discovered), the severity of the effect (when immediately detectable), the type of distribution and recordkeeping of the lot, the average time between entry and final consumption (perishability) and the amount of publicity surrounding the outbreak. In general, the greater the consequences and ensuing publicity, the higher r will be.

The inclusion of r may severely affect the choice of lots to sample because r is sharply different for acute (microbiological) effects than for latent carcinogenic and teratogenic effects. Unlike an acute microbiological hazard, a carcinogenic pesticide, if undetected at the border, would most likely remain undetected, i.e., r would be zero. Thus, inclusion of the recall factor r allows for a more proper comparison and better relative ranking (and sampling frequency) of acute versus latent violations to ensure sufficient sampling of latent hazards.

Even with a high recall probability, however, latent hazards from chemicals may still not be sufficiently weighted to be sampled as much as they should. The problem is that chemical hazard risks accrue from thousands of doses over a lifetime. Microbiological risks, on the other hand, occur as a result of a single (violative) dose. Yet not only may a chemical hazard go undetected by consumers in a given lot if it is not sampled at the border; it may continue undetected in many subsequent lots. To account for this effect, the weights,

$$\frac{\tilde{U}_{\ell\hat{\mathrm{v}}}^{\omega}}{\sum_{\ell=1}^{L} \hat{U}_{\ell\hat{\mathrm{v}}}^{\omega}}$$

may be adjusted for latent hazards by lowering the ω's.

There are two possible ways the probability of recall could come into effect: if the product is not tested and is hazardous (t,s,i = 0,1,0), or if the product is tested and a false negative occurs (t,s,i = 0,1,1). Both of these possibilities would lead to acceptance of a hazardous product. With the inclusion of the two consequence modifiers, the utility for sampling can be respecified as:

$$\tilde{U}_{\ell \hat{v}} \sum_{t=0}^{1} \sum_{s=0}^{1} \sum_{v=1}^{V} \left(1 - r_{sv}\right) x_\ell \left[\pi_{sv}\, p_{ts\hat{v}1} \left\{c^h_{tsv} + c^c_t + c^p_{t1}\right\}\right]$$

$$- \left\{\pi_{0v}\, c^h_{00v} + c^c_0 + c^p_{00} + \pi_{1v}\, c^h_{01v} + c^c_0 + c^p_{00}\right\} \tag{10}$$

where $0 \leq r_{sv} \leq 1$, if s=1 and t=0 and $r_{sv} = 0$, otherwise. In other words, if the lot is violative and released, there is some probability that at least part of the lot will be recovered once the problem is discovered. In this case r_{sv} approaches 1 for acute hazards and r_{sv} approaches 0 for latent hazards that would never be detected.

PRIOR AND POSTERIOR PROBABILITY OF VIOLATION

The prior probability of a lot ℓ being in state s will be a function of the type of food it contains, how the food was processed and transported, the country and company it came from, the importer's reputation, the past sampling history of similar lots, and the existence of various state and local food safety regulatory mechanisms. Initially, these probabilities could be determined either by subjective estimates of experts taking into account the factors mentioned above or they could be estimated econometrically (e.g., logistic regression analysis) where data is available.[l]

Through use of Bayes formula, prior probabilities could be combined together with the current test results at time τ to compute a Bayesian posterior probability, $\pi_{sv,\tau+1}$. The general Bayesian formula for the posterior probability that the lot is violative is:

$$\hat{\pi}_1 = \frac{\pi_1 L_1(\text{data})}{\pi_1 L_1(\text{data}) + \pi_0 L_0(\text{data})}$$

where L_1(data) is the likelihood of the observed test results, 1, given that the overall lot is actually violative and L_0(data) is the corresponding likelihood of the observed test results given that the overall lot is actually nonviolative. (The posterior probability for the lot being nonviolative is computed similarly and is equal to $1 - \hat{\pi}_1$).

Technically, the posterior probability applies only to the lot which was actually tested, not to the next independent lot. Furthermore, an unexpected test result (e.g., a low prior probability of violation and a positive sample result) may cause a large jump in the posterior probability. Thus, the posterior probability is not a perfect substitute for the next prior probability. Unfortunately, there is no perfect answer as to how much weight to give the last test posterior relative to the previous test posteriors (i.e., all historical information) when determining the next prior probability.

One way to use historical information with current information is to use an adaptive (smoothing) filter. Such filters take an average of past test results to attempt to estimate the true underlying prior.

---

l. Other regulatory devices which assure import food quality include memoranda of understandings with other countries which establish good manufacturing practices, interagency agreements (whereby other agencies may be sampling and monitoring products of interest to the FDA), and inspections of foreign plants.

Use of adaptive filters should account for the problem of possible correlation of one lot with subsequent lots and a temporally changing production process. The next prior would then be computed by an adaptive filter as a weighted moving average of past information and an adjustment of the weights (over time). In particular, an adaptive filter should allow reasonable tracking of both rapidly changing as well as slowly drifting production processes. In addition, the structure of such smoothing filters would give decision makers a simple means of control over the weighting process, if necessary, to deal better with crisis sampling situations. A nonadaptive filter could be formulated as:

$$\pi_{sv,\tau+1} = \alpha_\tau \hat{\pi}_{sv,\tau+1} + (1-\alpha_\tau)\, \pi_{sv,\tau}$$

where $\pi_{sv,\tau}$ represents the cumulative historical prior (or cumulative posterior), $\hat{\pi}_{sv,\tau+1}$ represents the posterior from the latest sample, and $\pi_{sv,\tau+1}$ represents the weighted average of the two components that will be used as the prior probability for the next similar lot that is sampled. The weights, $\alpha_\tau (0 < \alpha_\tau < 1)$ are fixed for a nonadaptive filter. For an adaptive filter they will vary over time.

SUMMARY

A decision model has been proposed to aid in the optimal selection of imported foods to sample. The model utilizes Bayesian statistical decision theory to deterministically choose lots for sampling. Utility consequences are divided into consumer health, consumer non-health and producer consequences. A randomized decision process can be superimposed upon this deterministic decision process to allow for more efficient handling of problems associated with deliberate game playing by importers and "inadvertent" bad manufacturing processes. A random strategy would also guarantee that low priority lots are occasionally sampled along with the higher priority items so that the information data base on all products is continuously updated. The randomized process can be controlled to mimic the deterministic process to any desired degree of precision by adjusting the power weights on the net sampling utilities. To account for scarce regulatory resources, the utility from sampling is divided by sampling costs so that the decision to sample or not will be cost effective. A further refinement of this decision process integrates prior historical testing information along with current testing information to produce adaptive updates to the prior probability of violation that are used in future sampling decisions. Potentially, various types of "fuzzy" qualitative information can be integrated with actual test result data. Because of the routine nature of this kind of decision making, it is suggested that this type of model might be a precursor to an automated expert system that could be used as an aid to the import screening and sampling decision process.

REFERENCES

1. D. Kahneman and A. Tversky, *Judgments Under Uncertainty — Heuristics and Biasis*, Cambridge University Press (1982).
2. Frank Bryan, Foodborne Disease Risk Assessment of Foodservice Establishments in a Community, *Journal of Food Protection* **45(1)**:93-100 (1980).
3. Milton C. Weinstein, Cost-Effective Priorities for Cancer Prevention, *Science* **221** (1983).
4. T. A. Roberts and F. A. Skinner, *Food Microbiology-Advances and Prospects*, Academic Press, Inc., New York (1983).
5. F. F. Drion and D. A. Mossell, The Reliability of the Examination of the Foods, Processed for Safety, for Enteric Pathogens and Enterobacteriaceae: A Mathematical and Ecological Study, *Journal of Hygiene* **78**:301-324 (1977).
6. Jeffry M. Farber, Predictive Modeling of Food Deterioration and Safety, in *Foodborne Microorganisms and Their Toxins: Developing Methodology*, IFT Basic Symposium Series, Merle D. Pierson and Norman J. Stern, eds., Marcel Dekker, Inc. (1986).

Safety Factors and Residual Cancer Risks

C. Brignoli Gable, C. Kopral, and C. Zervos
U.S. Food and Drug Administration
Washington, DC

ABSTRACT

There are two basic approaches to risk assessment in the regulatory setting: the NOEL/SF approach and the acceptable risk approach. In determining the conditions of safe uses of chemicals, safety factors are used in every evaluation scheme except that concerning chemical carcinogens. There have been proposals, however, to use safety factors in the evaluation of some chemical carcinogens as well. We have used bioassay data and the residual risk concept to compare the safety factor and acceptable risk procedures in the risk assessment of carcinogens.

KEYWORDS: Risk, carcinogenesis, safety factors

THE FOUR COMPONENTS OF RISK ASSESSMENTS (NAS/NRC)

In 1983, the National Research Council (NRC) published a study of risk assessment methods and their institutional uses by the government to control and minimize the potential adverse effects of man-made and natural toxins.[1] The NRC committee that prepared the study identified four major steps in the risk assessment process. They are shown in Table 1.

In the NRC scheme, the ultimate goal of the risk assessment process is the last step, risk characterization, i.e., the derivation of one or more statistics that estimate the likely damage to health or the environment expected to result from exposure to a toxin. An example of such a statistic, used in this study, is the residual risk, RR, or the risk above background due to exposure.

DOSE/RESPONSE ASSESSMENT

Dose/Response assessment, the relationship between the response and the rate of exposure to a toxin, is a necessary step in risk characterization. As a consequence, the NRC committee devoted considerable time to examine this assessment and identified a number of knowledge gaps that make it difficult. The NRC committee recognized that the government uses two approaches to risk evaluation, depending on the type of toxin. They devoted most of their attention to the method used to assess risks from exposures to carcinogens. They placed little emphasis on the method used to estimate safe exposures to other types of toxins

Risk Analysis, Edited by C. Zervos
Plenum Press, New York, 1991

Table 1. The Four Components of Risk Assessment According to the NAS

1. Hazard identification
2. Dose-response assessment
3. Exposure assessment
4. Risk characterization

even though it has a long history of use. The purpose of this paper is to compare the two approaches. Therefore, it is necessary to put in focus the dichotomy in methods.

STATEMENT OF DICHOTOMY

In the regulatory community the two approaches to the choice of dose/response functions are known as the NOEL/SF[2] approach and the acceptable risk[3] approach. Briefly, the NOEL/SF approach, which is an acronym of the phrase No Observable Effect Level/Safety Factor, is based on the experimental determination of a maximum NOEL and the application of a safety factor to determine an Allowable Daily Intake (ADI). The acceptable risk approach is based on the determination of what is known as a Virtually Safe Level (VSL) of exposure. The VSL of exposure to a toxin is such that it engenders risks not expected to be higher than what has been decided as acceptable.

The notion of thresholds of chemical toxicity provided the connection between increasing recognition of delayed effects from long term, low level exposures to chemicals, and the need to change dose/effect functions.[4] In the last 30 years, the scientific community partitioned itself into those who accepted thresholds for every type of toxicity, carcinogenicity included, and those who accepted them for most types of toxicity, excepting carcinogenicity.

The NOEL/SF approach has been justified on the basis of theoretical population attribute (sensitivity) distributions rather than rigorous experimental identifications of toxicity thresholds.[5] The approach has seldom been validated with data showing toxicity thresholds, although the approach is applied to toxicants assumed to have thresholds, which excludes carcinogens.

THE ARGUMENTS FOR AND AGAINST

Threshold supporters argue that the NOEL/SF approach has served well, and should be extended to cover at least some classes of carcinogens.[6,7,8,9] Weisburger and Williams,[7] for instance, have proposed a risk assessment scheme that would separate carcinogens into genotoxic and epigenetic classes and treat the former as if they have no threshold and the latter as if they do.

Kaplan *et al.*[10] accepted the notion that there are thresholds of toxicity and studied the way they are currently used to set ADIs. Specifically, Kaplan *et al.* examined the fraction of individual thresholds in a population likely to fall below the ADI and how such fraction might vary with the intrinsic properties of toxicants. The authors reported how that fraction is likely to be affected by the fact that the NOEL/SF approach disregards the slope of the dose response curve. Zervos[11] has discussed the principal defects of the NOEL/SF approach.

Some efforts have been made to bridge the two approaches by studying their foundations and introducing various compromises. Proposals to extend the NOEL/SF approach to carcinogens have often been based on the notion of variable safety factors ranging from 1,000 to 50,000. For justification, such safety factors have usually been partitioned in ways that account for important aspects of risk such as interspecies and intraspecies variability, shape of the dose-response curve, severity of experimental outcome, nature of human exposure, and data quality defects.[9]

Gaylor[12] proposed a method that bridges the two approaches. He used a mathematical model (as in the acceptable risk approach) to estimate the dose corresponding to a one percent increased risk above control and then applied a safety factor to this estimated dose. He proposed the use of variable, data dictated, safety factors to ensure that an acceptable level of risk is unlikely to be exceeded.

Crump[2] employed a method similar to that of Gaylor and proposed that noncarcinogenic substances be regulated on the basis of what he called a benchmark dose (BD). Crump's method uses a mathematical model to fit the dose response curve down to a 10% incidence above background to obtain the BD which then replaces the NOEL in the calculation of the ADI (ADI = NOEL/SF). We shall use this approach combining both methodologies and call it the TD_{10}/SF method.

THE DATA

We used the Carcinogenic Potency Database (CPDB) of Gold *et al.*[13] summarizing the extensive literature on animal bioassays, including those done by the National Cancer Institute (NCI)/ National Toxicology Program (NTP).

The database provides information (a record) about each significant observation in each experiment, including species, strain, sex of test animal, route of administration, duration of dosing, dose levels in mg/kg body weight/day, duration of experiment, carcinogenic potency and its statistical significance, shape of the dose response curve, author's opinion as to carcinogenicity, and the literature citation.

In the CPDB, the TD_{50} is the measure of potency for a particular compound and is defined as the dose rate in mg/kg bw/day which, if administered chronically for the standard lifespan of the species, will halve the mortality corrected estimate of the animal's probability of remaining tumorless through this period. Peto *et al.*[14] described the statistical procedures for this index of carcinogenicity and applied the results to experiments on 975 compounds in 3500 studies.

Peto *et al.*[14] used certain conventions to calculate the TD_{50} values in the CPDB. They include establishing two years as the lifespan in rats and mice, counting all tumors, both fatal and incidental, adjusting for intermittent mortality, and correcting for termination of the study before two years. Portier and Hoel[15] discuss the sources of error in estimating the TD_{50}, particularly intermittent mortality. Dose conversion to mg/kg bw/day was based on the assumption of 100% absorption. Conversion standards for each sex/species include factors for daily food, water and air intake and average weight.

The following data were extracted for use from the CPDB:

- Rates of hepatocellular carcinoma in male (MMBHC) and female (MFBHC) b6c mice;

- Rates of lung adenocarcinoma and adenoma in male (MMLUX) and female (MFLUX) swa mice.

Exposure was restricted to oral routes (feed, gavage, water) and duration limited to greater than 60 weeks. Database entries were selected only if the *p*-value associated with a test of the slope of the dose-response curve being different from zero is less than .05.

Table 2 shows relevant statistics for the selected TD_{50} entries.

The Carcinogenesis Model

It was noted earlier that in order to estimate residual risks it is necessary to assume a model for chemical carcinogenesis. Carcinogenesis models have, of course, been the subject of discussions and debates for the last 25 years and no obvious science-based choice seems in sight. However, the many years of data collection, analysis and discussion have proven at least one point: experimental data from bioassays will not decide the question. Different substances have been shown to follow different models at least in the range of responses that are accessible experimentally.[16,17]

We have assumed the one hit dose response model for our analysis, primarily for convenience. To the extent possible, we examined whether the CPDB data we selected for analysis contradict this assumption.

The majority of database entries showing an increase in lung adenoma and adenocarcinoma came from bioassays with only two groups of animals, one exposed and one control. For hepatocellular carcinoma most of the studies we used had two or more dosage levels and thus could shed light on the shape of the dose response curve.

Using non-linear regression analysis techniques, we examined selected CPDB data records with more than two exposure groups for goodness of fit to the one hit model

$$p(d) = 1 - e^{-\alpha - \beta \cdot d} . \qquad (1)$$

Table 3 shows the values of the squared correlation coefficient, R^2, which is equal to the model sum of squares divided by the total sum of squares and therefore measures the amount of total variation accounted for by the model. Generally, we observed that either the fit was reasonable or that unexpectedly small incidence rates at the highest exposure rates, as in the case of 2,6-dichloro-p-phenylene diamine, were responsible for the failure to obtain a reasonable fit. We concluded that the data we selected for our calculations did not contradict the one-hit model.

Calculation of Tumorigenic Dose, TD_y

General toxicant bioassays are designed and conducted specifically so that a maximum NOEL is experimentally observed. Carcinogen bioassays are usually not. Thus to estimate the maximum residual risk using the safety factor method, it is necessary to find a way to use available carcinogenesis data to estimate a dose at the limit of detectability.

We adopted the approach suggested by Gaylor[12] and Crump,[2] i.e., using the available data and the one hit model to calculate a rate of exposure TD_{10} (tumorigenic dose 10%) for each compound. The TD_{10} is estimated to reduce by 10% the exposed animals' chance of remaining tumorless to the end of their standard lifetime. Given the cancer bioassay protocol currently in use, the TD_{10} should correspond closely with the limit of detection of the animal bioassay. We next divided each TD_{10} by a safety factor, SF, to yield the ADI.

Table 2. TD_{50} Statistics for Sex/Histology Groupings

TD_{50}	MMBHC	MMLUX	MFBHC	MFLUX
N	47	25	58	36
Mean	282.7	267.5	973.2	200.7
Std Dev	437.3	903.7	1671.9	414.8
Minimum	0.7	1.3	1.4	0.6
Maximum	2150.0	4530.0	7500.0	2170.0

MMBHC = hepatocellular carcinoma in male b6c mice.
MMLUX = lung adenoma and adenocarcinoma in male swa mice.
MFBHC = hepatocellular carcinoma in female b6c mice.
MFLUX = lung adenoma and adenocarcinoma in female swa mice.

Table 3. Goodness of Fit Statistic R^2 for Substances with Greater Than Three Exposure Levels

Substance	CAS #	R^2	Exposure Levels
2,3,7,8-p-Dichloro-dibenzo-p-dioxin (TCDD)	1746-01-6	0.95	4
		0.92	4
Carbazole	86-74-8	0.54	4
		0.95	4
4-4'-Oxydianiline	101-80-4	0.92	4
2,6-Dichloro-p-phenylene diamine	609-20-1	0.15	5
Dieldrin	60-57-1	0.44	4

A number of specific safety or uncertainty factors have been mentioned in discussions of a potential change to the safety factor approach for carcinogens. We have used SFs of 5,000 and 10,000 in our calculations. Using the one hit model, we estimate the probability of tumor corresponding to the ADI. This probability minus the background tumor incidence is the residual risk, RR.

Through the following algebraic manipulations we obtained a formula for β and RR that makes use of the TD_{50} and does not require direct fitting of the observed incidence data to the one hit model. An error may be introduced into our calculation of the RR because of the use of the TD_{50}. This error can be either positive or negative, depending on the background incidence, and on whether the TD_{50} is within the observed data range.[15]

Simple substitution of the appropriate *d* values in Eq. (1) yields:

$$\alpha = -\ln(1 - p(0)) \tag{2}$$

and

$$\beta = \frac{\ln 2}{\mathrm{TD}_{50}} , \tag{3}$$

the values of the one-hit model parameters expressed in terms of $p(0)$, i.e., probability of tumor at dose=0, and TD_{50}, both parameters given in the Gold database.

Our objective was to estimate, in terms of the same two parameters, the probability $p(TD_{10}/SF)$ of cancer at exposure levels equal to the TD_{10} divided by the safety factor. To do so it was necessary, first, to estimate the TD_{10} in terms of the same parameters.

Earlier it was noted that we assumed that the TD_{10} is the dose rate at the limit of detectability of the animal bioassay. Because others might wish to define that level differently, we derived a general formula for TD_y, a dose such that, compared to control animals, animals exposed to TD_y have $1 - y$ chance of remaining tumor free, where $0 < y < 1$. The formula is given by

$$\mathrm{TD}_y = -\frac{\mathrm{TD}_{50} \cdot \ln(1-y)}{\ln 2} . \tag{4}$$

Using the formula for TD_y, we obtain the following equation for TD_{10}:

$$\mathrm{TD}_{10} = -\frac{\mathrm{TD}_{50} \cdot \ln 0.9}{\ln 2} . \tag{5}$$

Next, we divide the TD_{10} by a safety factor, x, and use the model to obtain the probability of tumor corresponding to this dose,

$$p\left(\frac{\mathrm{TD}_{10}}{x}\right) = 1 - \left[(1-p(0)) \cdot (1-y)^{\left(\frac{1}{x}\right)}\right] . \tag{6}$$

The residual risk is given by

$$\mathrm{RR} = p\left(\frac{\mathrm{TD}_{10}}{x}\right) - p(0) . \tag{7}$$

Further details of this derivation are given in the appendix.

The Results/Conclusions

We have used Eq. (7) to calculate residual risks (RR). The calculated values are shown in Tables 4a, 4b, and 4c. The first two tables show minimum and maximum values for hepatocellular carcinoma. Table 4c shows average values for lung adenoma and adenocarcinoma.

Examination of these tables leads to the following conclusions:

a. For the 166 data base entries examined, the average RR values using the TD_{10}/SF approach is 19×10^{-6} for SF = 5,000 and 10×10^{-6} for SF = 10,000. This means that a SF of 10,000 applied to the TD_{10} still "allows" about 10 times the risk usually considered acceptable.

b. The calculated RR's remain relatively constant across compounds, as shown by the minimum and maximum values given in Tables 4a and b. For a particular model and safety factor, the TD_{10}/SF method therefore has the desirable property of being consistent.

Table 4a. The Residual Risk Values (RR × 10^{-6}) for Hepatocellular Carcinoma in b6c Male Mice

		Residual Risk			
		SF=10^4		SF=5×10^3	
Log(TD_{50})	N	Min	Max	Min	Max
-0	3	7	9	15	18
0-1	6	8	11	16	21
1-2	14	7	11	15	21
2-3	20	8	11	16	21
3-4	4	8	11	17	21

Table 4b. The Residual Risk Values (RR × 10^{-6}) for Hepatocellular Carcinoma in b6c Female Mice

		Residual Risk			
		SF=10^4		SF=5×10^3	
Log(TD_{50})	N	Min	Max	Min	Max
0-1	7	8	11	17	21
1-2	17	10	11	20	21
2-3	19	9	11	18	21
3-4	15	10	11	20	21

Table 4c. Mean Residual Risk (RR × 10^{-6}) as a Function Log(TD_{50}) for Lung Adenoma and Adenocarcinoma in Male and Female swa Mice

	Mean Residual Risk					
	MMLUX			MFLUX		
Log(TD_{50})	N	SF=5×10^3	SF=10^4	N	SF=5×10^3	SF=10^4
				1	21	11
0-1	6	18	9	6	17	9
1-2	13	19	9	16	19	9
2-3	5	18	9	11	19	9
3-4	1	20	10	2	20	10

c. Judging from these findings, it appears that a SF larger than those proposed (probably about 100,000) applied to the TD_{10} may be needed to ensure risks at or less than the currently used 10^{-6} risk standard.

d. Doubling the safety factor halves the value of the RR because of the approximate linearity of the one hit model at low dose. The TD_{10}/SF approach, as we have used it, is therefore essentially the same as linear extrapolation used with the acceptable risk approach.

e. Other dose response models could have been chosen which would not be linear at low dose. However, the particular mathematical model is not critical to the $ED_{10}(TD_{10})$/SF approach. The dose response curve is fit to the observed data to determine the TD_{10}. Below this dose level, one makes no assumption about the form of the dose response relationship. The TD_{10} is then divided by an appropriate SF. Because we wanted to estimate the magnitude of the risk associated with particular SFs, we assumed a model below the TD_{10}. Further study with different dose response models is required to compare the SFs needed to ensure an acceptable residual risk for carcinogens.

The essential difference between the TD_{10}/SF and the acceptable risk approach is that the former makes no assumption about the shape of the dose response curve below the TD_{10}. We acknowledge that assuming the one hit model below the TD_{10} is the same as linear extrapolation. However, the assumption of a model below the TD_{10} is not an inherent part of the TD_{10}/SF method. This distinction is one of its advantages. Another positive aspect is its ease of application. In contrast to the safety factor approach using the NOEL, the TD_{10}/SF procedure uses the observed data, taking into account sample size, to determine the TD_{10}. The TD_{10}, unlike the NOEL, does not have to be experimentally determined.

APPENDIX

Derivation Of Formulas

From our definition,

$$p(\mathrm{TD}_y) = 1-(1-y)\cdot(1-p(0))$$

and

$$1-p(\mathrm{TD}_y) = (1-y)\cdot(1-p(0)) .$$

From Eq. (1) we have

$$\mathrm{TD}_y = -\frac{\ln(1-p(\mathrm{TD}_y)) + \alpha}{\beta} .$$

If we substitute ln for α, β, and $1-p(\mathrm{TD}_y)$, we obtain

$$\mathrm{TD}_y = \frac{\ln[(1-y)\cdot(1-p(0))] - \ln(1-p(0))}{\frac{-\ln 2}{\mathrm{TD}_{50}}}$$

$$\mathrm{TD}_y = \frac{\ln(1-y) + \ln(1-p(0)) - \ln(1-p(0))}{\frac{-\ln 2}{\mathrm{TD}_{50}}}$$

$$\mathrm{TD}_y = \frac{\ln(1-y)\cdot\mathrm{TD}_{50}}{-\ln 2} .$$

And since we have chosen $y = 0.10$,

$$\mathrm{TD}_{10} = -\frac{\ln 0.9 \cdot \mathrm{TD}_{50}}{\ln 2} \ .$$

Calculation of Residual Risk

Next we divide the TD_y by a safety factor x and use the model to obtain the probability of cancer corresponding to this dose, $p(\mathrm{TD}_y/x)$.

Using Eq. (1) and substituting the appropriate expressions for all parameters we obtain

$$p\left(\frac{\mathrm{TD}_y}{x}\right) = 1 - e^{\ln(1-p(0)) + \frac{\ln 2 \cdot \ln(1-y) \cdot \mathrm{TD}_{50}}{\ln 2 \cdot \mathrm{TD}_{50} \cdot x}}$$

$$p\left(\frac{\mathrm{TD}_y}{x}\right) = 1 - e^{\ln(1-p(0)) + \ln(1-y)^{\frac{1}{x}}}$$

$$p\left(\frac{\mathrm{TD}_y}{x}\right) = 1 - \left[(1-p(0)) \cdot (1-y)^{\frac{1}{x}}\right] \ .$$

The residual risk is given by

$$RR = p\left(\frac{\mathrm{TD}_y}{x}\right) - p(0) \ .$$

REFERENCES

1. National Research Council, *Risk Assessment In The Federal Government: Managing the Process*, National Academy Press, Washington, DC (1983).
2. S. K. Crump, A New Method for Determining Allowable Daily Intakes, *Fund. Appl. Toxicol.* **4**:554-571 (1984).
3. N. Mantel and W. R. Bryan, "Safety" Testing of Carcinogenic Agents, *J. Nat. Cancer Inst.* **27**:455-470 (1961).
4. Public Citizen vs Frank Young, U.S. Court of Appeals for the District of Columbia, No 86-1548.
5. A. J. Lehman and O. G. Fitzhugh, 100-Fold Safety Margin, *Assoc. Food Drug Off. U.S. Q. Bull.* **18**:33-35 (1954).
6. B. S. Salsburg, Use of Statistics When Examining Lifetime Studies in Rodents to Detect Carcinogenicity, *J. Toxicol. Env. Health* **3**:611-628 (1977).
7. J. H. Weisburger and G. M. Williams, Carcinogen Testing: Current Problems and New Approaches, *Science* **214**:401-407 (1981).
8. F. C. Lu, Safety Assessment of Chemical With Threshold Effects, *Reg. Toxicol. Pharmacol.* **5**:460-464 (1985).
9. F. C. Lu, Toxicological Evaluation of Carcinogens and Non-Carcinogens: Pros and Cons of Different Approaches, *Reg. Toxicol. Pharmacol.* **3**:121-132 (1983).
10. N. Kaplan, D. Hoel, C. Portier, and M. Hogan, An Evaluation of the Safety Factor Approach in Risk Assessment, Banbury Report 26, Developmental Toxicology: Mechanisms and Risk, pp. 335-346, Cold Springs Harbor Laboratory (1987).

11. C. Zervos, Risk/Benefit Analysis: The Case of Food Additives, in *Developments in Food Science: The Frontiers of Flavor*, G. Charalambous, ed., pp. 555-573, Elsevier, Amsterdam (1987).
12. D. W. Gaylor, The Use of Safety Factors for Controlling Risk, *J. Toxicol. Environ. Health* **11**:329-336 (1983).
13. L. S. Gold, C. B. Sayer, R. Magaw, G. M. Backman, M. de Veciana, R. Levinson, N. K. Hooper, and B. N. A. Ames, Carcinogenic Potency Database of the Standardized Results of Animal Bioassays, *Environ. Health Perspect.* **58**:9-319 (1984).
14. R. Peto, M. C. Pike, L. Bernstein, L. S. Gold, and B. N. Ames, The TD_{50}: A Proposed General Convention for the Numerical Description of the Carcinogenic Potency of Chemical in Chronic Exposure Animal Experiments, *Environ. Health Perspect.* **58**:1-8 (1984).
15. C. J. Portier and D. G. Hoel, Issues Concerning the Estimation of the TD_{50}, *Risk Analysis* **7**:437-447 (1987).
16. Food Safety Council, Scientific Committee, Proposed System for Food Safety Assessment, pp. 137-160, Washington, DC (1980).
17. R. D. Bruce, W. W. Carlton, K. H. Ferber, D. H. Hughes, J. F. Quast, D. S. Salsburg, J. M. Smith, and D. Clayson, Re-examination of the ED_{01} Study, *Fundam. Appl. Toxicol.* **1**:27-128 (1981).

Risk Perception of Technologies: Observations from Mainland China

M. Peter Hoefer, Elayn Bernay, and S. Basheer Ahmed
Pace University
New York, NY

ABSTRACT

Earlier studies have attempted to measure differences in the perception of risk associated with certain technologies on an international scale. This study, aimed at the Peoples Republic of China (mainland China), is a continuation of those efforts.

A questionnaire, which had also been distributed in various business schools in the United States, Portugal and France, was presented to students at the University of International Business and Economics in Beijing. Students at this university are trained for positions with the Chinese Foreign Trade and must be proficient in a second language. The survey was conducted among students in the English Department, so no translation of the questionnaire was necessary.

The results in this paper are preliminary. Nevertheless, there are some striking comparisons and contrasts with the earlier studies. In particular, this is the first study which fails to detect a significant difference between the way men and women perceive risk associated with certain technologies.

KEYWORDS: Risk perception, technologies, international, China.

INTRODUCTION

This study is a continuation of work begun by Ahmed and Hoefer in 1985[1] which measured the perceived risk associated with new or developing technologies. Because of our unique situation, we sampled graduate students of business, mostly evening students, who worked either in, or near to, the financial district of downtown New York City. We felt that, because of the responsibilities and the maturity of the population sampled, the results of our study would be more a measure of the feelings of "mainstream" Americans (or, more specifically, New Yorkers) than other studies that relied upon full-time undergraduate students.

We followed up our initial study by extracting samples from other populations, most importantly from business schools in Portugal and France.[2,3,4] Different authors have provided studies that summarized risk perception in the areas of technology, as well as other fields, taken from other European countries.[5,6,7] The purpose of this paper was to sample a similar group of business students from the People's Republic of China. Earlier this year we received permission to distribute our questionnaire to a sample of 52 students training for positions with the Chinese Foreign Trade Commission at the University of International Business and Economics (UIBE) in Beijing, China. This school is especially appropriate since much of the instruction for these students is in English and is conducted by American, British, and Canadian professors; thus no translation of our questionnaire was necessary.

METHODOLOGY

A questionnaire was constructed with an 11 point scale, from 0 to 10. Questions were devised to elicit a responding individual's perception of the risk associated with the following technologies: nuclear power generation (NPG), robotics (R), genetic engineering (GE), space defense technology (SDT), information technology (IT), and nuclear weaponry (NW). The questionnaire was then validated according to accepted validation methods.[8] The end result, consisting of 58 questions, was initially distributed to business students in the United States, Portugal and France. In the spring of 1988 the same questionnaire was then administered to 52 randomly selected students at UIBE in Beijing, China. We selected this school for a number of reasons, among the most important being the school is a "business" school, which is consistent with our previous studies, and the major language of instruction for the students is English.

We next took the raw data, responses to the 58 questions by 52 students, and translated the data so that a response of "0" to a question indicated minimal perception of risk by the subject, and a response of "10" indicated maximal perception of risk by the subject. We next calculated the average (arithmetic mean) responses by technology and demographic group and performed appropriate *t*-tests and analyses of variance to search for significant differences among technologies and groups. Because of the uniqueness of the Chinese, after reviewing the individual questionnaires we decided that the demographic categories that had been used in the surveys of students in western democratic countries were not applicable to this population — most specifically household income and religion. However, in all the previous studies we had found differences of risk perception on the basis of sex, an applicable demographic for this population.

STATISTICAL RESULTS

Table 1 is a ranking of the technologies according to measured perceived risk, along with the average response to all questions in each technological area, by all the Chinese subjects.

A simple perusal of the data indicates many similarities with the previously cited perception studies performed in Western countries. The ranking of the technologies prefixed by the word nuclear at the top of the list is consistent with the data we gathered in the United States and Portugal, the difference being that these two Western countries ranked nuclear power generation first and nuclear weaponry second. The concern for nuclear power generation in third world nations is believed by some to be less than in the West, because studies such as that of Ahmed[9] have demonstrated a high correlation between electric power usage and some forms of economic prosperity. This certainly does not appear to be demonstrated here, because, in ranking at least, the China data is more similar to the American and Portuguese data than to the French data we gathered. The reason may be that much of the power in China is produced by coal, and this is true of Beijing in particular, where there is heavy air pollution.

What we found to be most striking, however, was in the sex demographic. In all the previous studies we cited, women consistently exhibited significantly more perception of

Table 1. Ranking of the Technologies According to Measured Perceived Risk

Technology	Score
(1) Nuclear weaponry (NW)	6.45
(2) Nuclear power generation (NPG)	5.92
(3) Robotics (R)	5.61
(4) Information technologies (IT)	5.11
(5) Space defense technology (SDT)	4.96
(6) Genetic engineering (GE)	3.08

Table 2. Results of Contrast between Men and Women to Risk Perception

	Men	Women
Nuclear weaponry (NW)	6.61	6.27
Nuclear power generation (NPG)	5.78	6.08
Robotics (R)	5.60	5.62
Information technologies (IT)	5.16	5.04
Space defense technology (SDT)	4.88	5.05
Genetic engineering (GE)	3.16	3.00

risk associated with technologies than men. The results contrasting men with women are exhibited in Table 2.

The ranking of technologies with the most perceived risk is similar for both sexes. The differences by sex were not statistically significant in any area. This being the case, Chinese men and women have much more similar risk perceptions associated with technologies than their Western counterparts.

CONCLUSION

The results presented here we believe are unique and important because of the role China plays in the world today. Concerning the perception of risk associated with modern technologies, our study has two important conclusions: (1) The Chinese (at least in our sample) do not perceive risk much differently than many Western nations, in general and (2) more specifically, it appears that there is no bifurcation in the perception of risk by the sexes as there has been observed in Western studies. Obviously, there could be flaws in any more definitive statements than we have made. In particular, a sample taken from a population of educated people may not be as representative of the Chinese people as it may be of a developed Western country.

REFERENCES

1. M. P. Hoefer and S. B. Ahmed, How a Business Community Perceives Risk in Modern Technologies, Working Paper #41, Center for Applied Research, Pace University, New York, NY (March 1985).
2. S. B. Ahmed and M. P. Hoefer, Public Perception of Risk in Developing Technologies: A Case Study of a Business Community in Manhattan, in *Advances*

in Risk Analysis, pp. 325-335, Vol. 5., L. Lave, ed., Plenum Publishing Corp., New York (1987).
3. M. P. Hoefer, S. B. Ahmed, E. K. Bernay, and C. DuSaire, Risk Perception of Technologies: The Perception of Similar Groups in Portugal and the United States, in *Advances in Risk Analysis*, pp. 251-258, Vol. 7, J. J. Bonin and D. E. Stevenson, eds., Plenum Publishing Corp., New York (1989).
4. M. P. Hoefer, E. K. Bernay, and S. B. Ahmed, Technological Risk Perception: The Perspective of University Business Students in the United States, Portugal and France, submitted for publication.
5. O. Renn, Attitudes Towards Nuclear Power: A Comparison Between Three Nations, Working Paper: International Institute for Applied Systems Analysis, WP-84-11, Laxenburg (Austria) (1984).
6. T. Englander, K. Farago, P. Slovik, and B. Fischoff, A Comparative Analysis of Risk Perception in Hungary and the United States, *Social Behavior* **I**:55-56 (1986).
7. B-M. Drottz and L. Sjoberg, Attitudes and Conceptions of Swedish Adolescents with Regard to Nuclear Power and Radioactive Wastes, paper presented at the 1987 Conference for the Society for Risk Analysis, Houston, TX (1987).
8. Fred Nichols Kerlinger, *Foundations of Behavioral Research; Educational and Psychological Enquiry*, Holt, Rinehart and Winston, New York (1964).
9. S. B. Ahmed, An Economic Relationship Between Electric Usage and The Gross National Product, paper presented at Los Alamos National Laboratory, Los Alamos, New Mexico (1984).

Differences in Risks of Commodity Chemical Versus Specialty Chemical Production Facilities

Robert E. Unsworth and James Cummings-Saxton
Industrial Economics, Inc.
Cambridge, MA

Frederick W. Talcott
U.S. Environmental Protection Agency
Washington, DC

ABSTRACT

This study examines potential differences in the risks posed by production of specialty chemicals compared with those posed by production of commodity chemicals. The motivating factor for this research is the structural shift of the U.S. chemical industry away from production of commodity chemicals and towards production of lower volume, higher margin specialty chemicals. Three hypothesis are examined: (1) specialty chemicals tend to be produced in areas of higher population density than locations where commodity chemicals are produced; (2) less is known about the toxic properties of specialty chemicals, as compared to commodity chemicals, but, where existing data indicate that specialty chemicals are relatively more toxic than commodities; and (3) chemical properties, plant configuration and process specific factors at specialty chemical production facilities may present a potential for a higher incidence of accidental releases as well as a relatively higher level of systematic releases than at commodity chemical facilities. The implications of the results on future regulatory policy are considered, especially for community emergency planning under SARA Title III.

KEYWORDS: Commodity chemicals, specialty chemicals

INTRODUCTION

This research summary is presented in four sections. The first section reviews factors driving the structural shift under way in the U.S. chemicals industry. In this section we present our definitions of commodity and specialty chemicals. The second section presents a summary of the three hypotheses tested in our research. The third section contains a brief description of the data sources and methodology used in performing this research. The final section summarizes some of the conclusions of our work. Methodologies and results presented in this paper represent part of the work IEc has performed in analyzing this topic. Final results, complete documentation, and a full discussion of limitations to the analysis will be published at a later date.

Structural Shift in the Industry

A structural shift is occurring in the U.S. chemicals industry. Chemical firms increasingly are focusing research efforts and capital investment on the production of specialty chemicals, as opposed to their traditional focus on commodity petrochemicals. This structural shift is driven by both demand and supply factors. High technology industries, such as the electronics industry, are demanding new, high performance specialty chemicals. As the pace of technological advance quickens, so will the demand for new specification chemicals. In addition, energy rich nations, such as Saudi Arabia and Mexico, hold material cost advantages in the production of commodity chemicals. As technological know-how to produce commodity chemicals is transferred to these nations in the form of modern, highly efficient production facilities, U.S. commodity chemical producers are, on average, not recapitalizing, and thus, U.S. commodity chemical production facilities have remained comparatively older and less efficient. Many U.S. chemical producers have opted to focus their efforts on the production of high value-added, high margin specialty chemicals instead.

Definitions

Specialty chemicals are high value added, low production volume chemicals. Users of specialty chemicals typically differentiate on the basis of manufacturer, often requesting that the manufactured product meet unique specifications or properties. Examples include engineering thermoplastics, industrial and institutional cleaners, and electronic chemicals. Specialty chemicals represent 92 percent of the total number of unique chemical products produced in the U.S.

Commodity chemicals are chemicals produced in high volume, to composition specifications. Purchasers of commodity chemicals differentiate between producers based on product price rather than product quality. Thus, commodity chemicals are generally undifferentiated and fungible. Examples include ethylene, ammonia and methanol. Commodity chemicals represent 99 percent of the total volume of chemicals produced annually in the U.S.

In performing the research outlined in this summary, IEc adopted working definitions of commodity and specialty chemicals. We define commodity chemicals as those chemicals priced less than or equal to one dollar per pound and produced nationally in quantities greater than 50 million pounds per year. Specialty chemicals are defined as those chemicals that are priced at greater than two dollars per pound and produced nationally in quantities less than 10 million pounds per year. Figure 1 displays schematically our working definitions of commodity and specialty chemicals.

In addition, IEc developed working definitions of commodity and specialty chemical production facilities. Commodity chemical production facilities are those that produce at least 75 percent commodity chemicals by volume. Specialty chemical facilities are those that produce at least 75 percent specialty chemicals by volume. These definitions were implemented using U.S. International Trade Commission (ITC) Data and the 1979 TSCA Inventory. All facilities fitting neither of these definitions are classified as "other".

RESEARCH HYPOTHESES

Three hypotheses were examined.

1. Specialty chemical production facilities are, on average, located in areas of higher population density than commodity chemical production facilities.

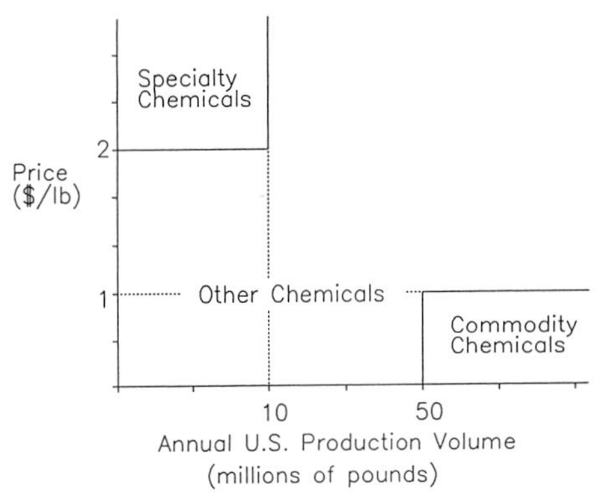

Fig. 1. Categorization of chemicals.

2. Less is known about the toxicity of specialty chemicals as compared to commodity chemicals; and, where data are available, analysis indicates that specialty chemicals are, on average, more toxic.

3. The characteristics of specialty chemical production facilities indicate an enhanced probability for an incidental release when compared to commodity chemical facilities.

METHODOLOGY

The methods used to test each of the above three hypotheses are summarized below.

Population Comparison

IEc utilized results from the 1979 TSCA Inventory and from the 1982 U.S. Census [accessed through EPA's Graphical Exposure Modeling System Atmospheric Modeling Subsystem, CENBAT procedure (GAMS CENBAT)] to compare populations surrounding samples of commodity and specialty chemical facilities. All facilities reported in the TSCA Inventory were coded as commodity, specialty or other, based on the definitions noted above. Systematic random samples of facilities were drawn from these populations. Facility locations were then determined, using both the reported facility ZIP Code, as well as the reported latitude and longitude coordinates. Population estimates for disks of various radii centered on the facility, up to 50 kilometers, were obtained through GAMS CENBAT. Additional data on daytime population changes in the locales of the sampled facilities were obtained from the Census Bureau's Journey-to-Work and Migration Statistics Branch.

Toxicity Comparison

IEc performed the toxicity analysis utilizing toxicity and regulatory guidance data published in the Registry of Toxic Effects of Chemical Substances (RTECS). Using the definitions discussed above, IEc classified over 1,000 chemicals as specialty or commodity. A subset of these chemicals (those for which the ITC reports valid CAS numbers) were researched in RTECS, from which toxicity and guidance data were obtained.

Using this information IEc performed a number of comparative analyses. First, commodity and specialty chemicals were compared by using appearance of the chemical in RTECS as a metric of availability of health effects information. Other metrics of availability of information (such as the number of toxicity citations per chemical in RTECS) were also computed.

IEc then examined the relative toxicity of specialty and commodity chemicals, using various measures of toxicity. For example, using results of LD_{50} studies on rats, where the route of administration was oral, IEc compared the predicted relative toxicity of commodity and specialty chemicals.

Last, IEc considered the existence of regulatory and/or guidance citations in RTECS as an indication of information availability. For those chemicals with reported regulatory and/or guidance levels, IEc quantitatively compared the values for the two samples.

Release Potential Comparison

IEc utilized knowledge of chemical process configurations and the U.S. EPA's Acute Hazardous Events Data Base (AHE/DB) compiled by IEc to develop profiles of the incidental release potential of commodity and specialty chemicals. The AHE/DB provides information on chemical release events, including parameters defining cause and location. Chemical properties, plant configuration, and process specific factors are expected to differ significantly between facilities producing commodity chemicals and those producing specialty chemicals. IEc developed sets of assumptions concerning "typical" commodity and specialty chemical facilities, focusing on parameters available in the AHE/DB. This methodology allowed IEc to test the hypothesis: specialty chemicals demonstrate a higher probability of incidental releases than commodity chemicals. In addition, IEc considered the magnitude of health effects from predicted releases of specialty chemicals as compared to predicted releases of commodity chemicals.

RESULTS

Examples of the results obtained from the tests of each of the hypotheses are summarized below.

Population Comparison

Utilizing the methods summarized above, IEc compared the average populations of geographic areas containing specialty and commodity chemical production facilities. Figure 2 shows a sample of the results. For all disks of radius greater than one-half kilometer, we reject the null hypothesis of no difference in the average population surrounding commodity and specialty chemical production facilities, i.e., we are confident at the 99.5 percent level that true differences in the size of the populations exist. These results remained consistent when either rings or disks were used, for any radial distance up to 50 kilometers. They also remained consistent whether reported ZIP Codes or latitude/longitude pairs were used to locate facilities.

Information provided by the U.S. Census Bureau's Journey-to-Work and Migration Statistics Branch allowed IEc to include daytime shifts in population when comparing the relative sizes of populations in the geographic areas of the two types of production facilities. Daytime population shifts are of importance, since many release events will occur during working hours. But, the Census reports residential or nighttime populations, which may vary significantly from daytime populations due to commuting. Inclusion of daytime population shifts in the population analysis had no significant effect on the results, i.e., results remained consistent after daytime population shifts were taken into account.

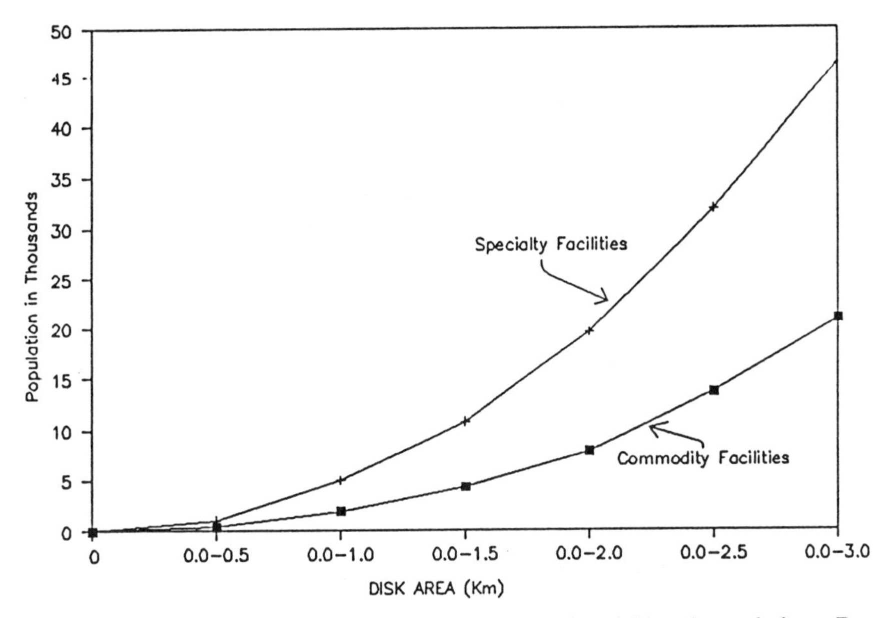

Fig. 2. Commodity and specialty facilities: comparison of local populations. Based on commodity and specialty chemical facility samples of 48 and 45, respectively.

Toxicity Comparison

Four separate sets of data analyses were performed in assessing the availability of information on toxicity of commodity and specialty chemicals, and in comparing their relative toxicity. For example, IEc compared the frequency of occurrence of toxic effects data in RTECS for the two types of chemicals. As is shown in Fig. 3, five to seven times as many studies are reported in RTECS for commodity chemicals as for specialty chemicals. This result remains consistent across effect categories (i.e., RTECS reports the results of an average of 3.5 mutagenicity studies for each commodity chemical, but less-than one study of this type for each specialty chemical).

Second, IEc compared the average toxicity of commodity and specialty chemicals, using a variety of metrics. For example, the normalized distributions of oral LD_{50} values in rats for commodity and specialty chemicals are shown in Fig. 4. The average LD_{50} value for commodity chemicals is 2,512 mg/kg; for specialty chemicals is 912 mg/kg. Given the means and variances of the two samples, we can reject the null hypothesis of no difference between the two populations at the 99 percent confidence level and state that specialty chemicals are, on average, more toxic than commodity chemicals. Similar results were obtained across a variety of species, routes of administration, and end points.

Although it can be demonstrated that statistical differences in the means of such metrics as LD_{50} values exist when comparing commodity and specialty chemicals, questions as to the existence of differences of biological significance remain. Many toxicologists look for "order-of-magnitude" differences or use other rules of thumb when comparing the toxicities of individual chemicals or groups of chemicals. There are many factors that support such beliefs. They include, but are not limited to, the inherent uncertainty present in any toxicological study; the difficulties of abstracting results from animal studies for use in drawing conclusions concerning predicted human health effects; and reporting errors in, and omissions of, data in RTECS. While we cannot state conclusively that biological differences exist, on average, between these two types of

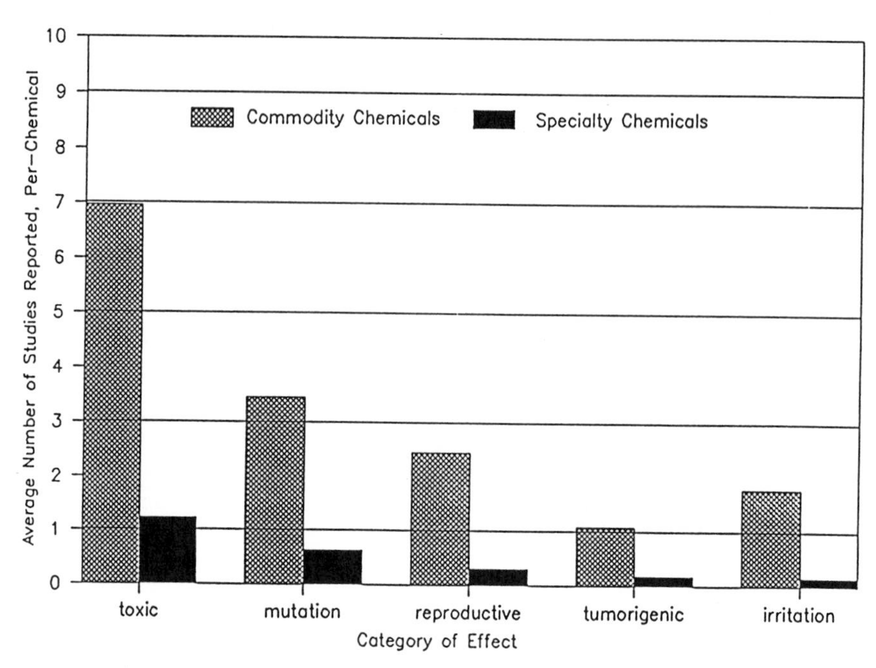

Fig. 3. Frequency of toxic effects data in RTECS: comparison of commodity and specialty chemicals. Analysis included 113 commodity chemicals and 923 specialty chemicals.

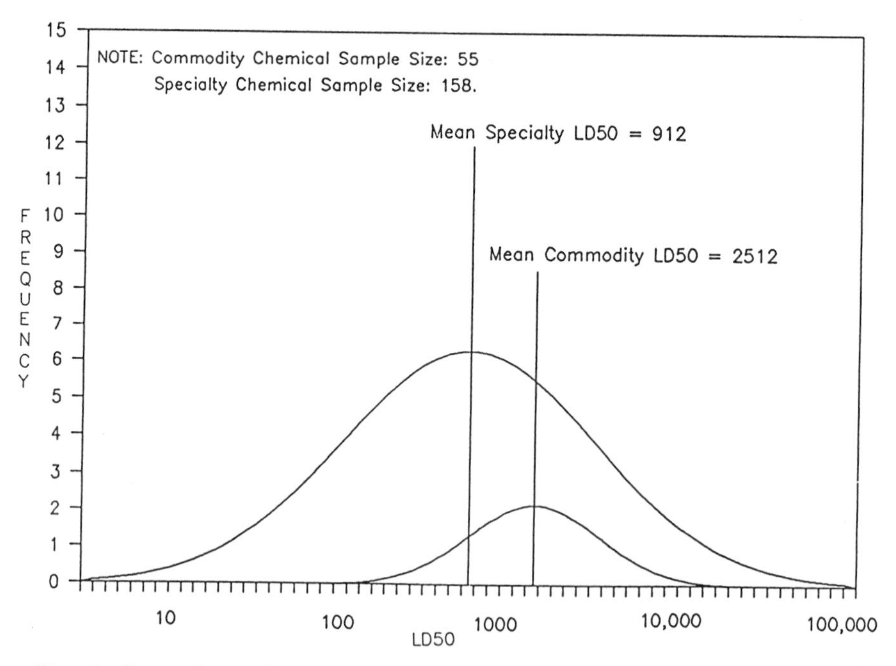

Fig. 4. Comparison of commodity and specialty chemical LD_{50} values. Based on studies with test species rat, dose administered orally.

chemicals, we are confident in reporting that there are indications to support that hypothesis.

IEc also compared the frequency of regulatory or guidance citations in RTECS for the two types of chemicals. As is shown in Fig. 5, for a number of regulatory guidance categories, more information is available from RTECS for commodity chemicals than for specialty chemicals. The first set of bars represents the frequency of chemicals with no citations in RTECS. Of all specialty chemicals 60 percent have no regulatory guidance citations in RTECS. The next three sets of bars represent guidance levels currently addressed by the regulated community [American Conference of Governmental Industrial Hygienists (ACGIH); Mine Safety and Health Administration (MSHA); and Occupational Safety and Health Administration (OSHA)]. For example, 60 percent of the commodity chemicals included in the analysis have a guidance level set by OSHA, while the same can be said for less than 10 percent of specialty chemicals. The last two columns represent sources of data that are likely to be used in setting future guidance or regulatory levels (data available from the EPA Genetox program and the International Agency for Research on Cancer (IARC) Cancer Review program). Again, RTECS is more likely to report information for commodity chemicals than for specialty chemicals.

Fourth, IEc considered reported ACGIH, MSHA and OSHA guidance levels for the two types of chemicals. In all cases the average guidance level for specialty chemicals is less than the average guidance level for commodity chemicals, by two or more orders of magnitude (Fig. 6). Since lower guidance levels (expressed generally in parts per million) indicate higher predicted toxicity, the hypothesis that specialty chemicals are more toxic than commodity chemicals is supported.

Release Potential Comparison

IEc is still in the initial stages of research into the release potential differences. Using profiles of specialty and commodity chemical facilities developed according to the methods

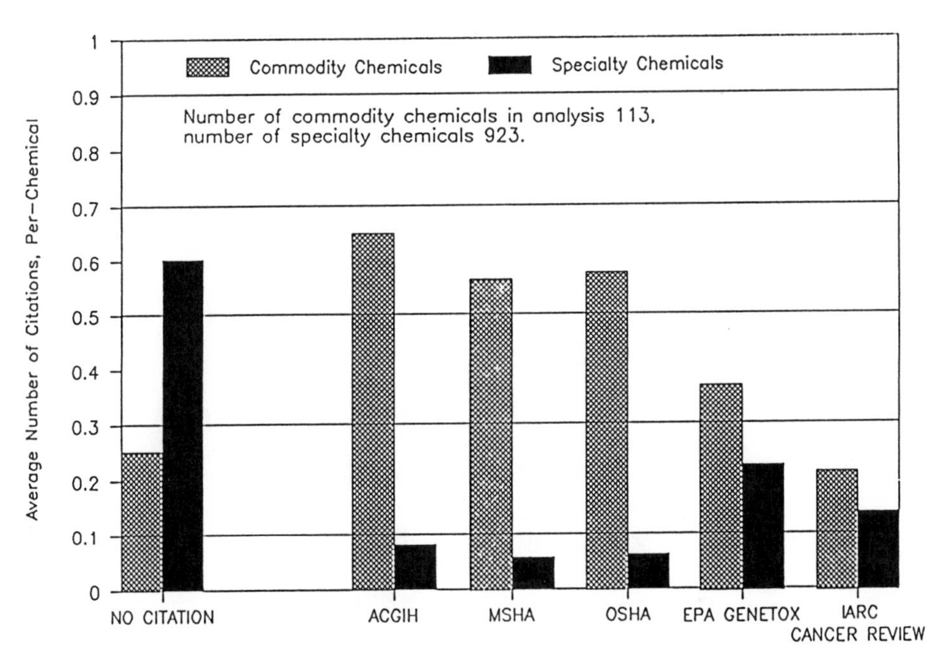

Fig. 5. Frequency of guidance citations in RTECS: comparison of commodity and specialty chemicals.

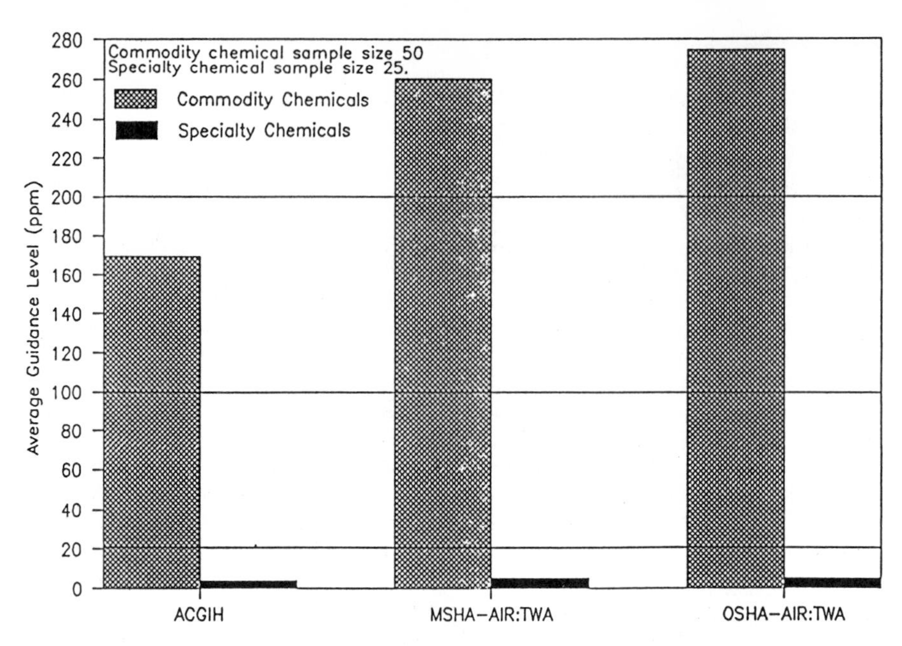

Fig. 6. Comparison of guidance levels from RTECS for commodity and specialty chemicals.

described above and information contained in EPA's AHE/DB, IEc assessed the predicted frequency and magnitude of acutely hazardous releases of both specialty and commodity chemicals. Initial results of this comparison indicate differences of the correct sign, but of insignificant magnitude. For example, since specialty chemical facilities are assumed to produce small volumes of a large number of chemicals, it can be assumed that more production steps at specialty facilities involve operator intervention as compared to commodity facilities. Thus, more events involving specialty chemicals are expected to include a "spill" than are those involving commodity chemicals (as opposed to events involving fires and/or explosions, for example). But, using data from the AHE/DB, IEc

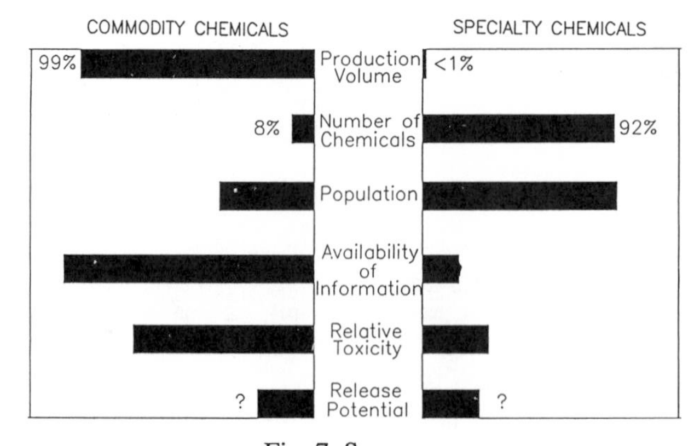

Fig. 7. Summary.

found that, while 78.6 percent of events involving specialty chemicals included spills, the same could be said for 65.5 percent of events involving commodity chemicals. While this difference is of the correct sign—more spill events would be predicted at specialty facilities, and thus, more events involving specialty chemicals involve spills—the magnitude is not great enough to allow rejection of a null hypothesis of no true difference. Research in this area is continuing.

CONCLUSIONS

Figure 7 shows graphically a summary of the conclusions of this paper. Commodity chemicals represent 99 percent of the volume of chemicals produced in the U.S. annually. Correctly, regulatory efforts to date have focused on these chemicals. But the role of specialty chemicals in the U.S. chemical industry is growing. Already 92 percent of all unique chemicals produced in the U.S. can be classified as specialty chemicals. These chemicals are produced at facilities located in more densely populated areas; less is known about their toxicity, and where information is available, indications are that specialty chemicals are more toxic than commodity chemicals; and the profiles of specialty chemical production facilities and processes are hypothesized to indicate a higher potential for incidental and continuous releases than those of commodity chemical production facilities.

Acceptable Risk in Regulation: The Impact of Recent Court Decisions on Public Policy for Risk Management

Chauncey Starr and Chris Whipple
Electric Power Research Institute
Palo Alto, CA

ABSTRACT

The Court of Appeals, DC Circuit, has ruled that the consideration of costs by regulatory agencies in their decisions of whether or not to regulate is inconsistent with the relevant law in two important recent cases. As a consequence of these decisions, the EPA and NRC are required to base their policies and standards on acceptable risks levels rather than on the costs of risk reductions. These decisions are leading agencies toward policies involving increasingly explicit definitions of acceptable risk. This paper describes the significance of these judicial decisions for regulatory decision making and their implications for risk analysis and offers suggestions on how to approach the definition of acceptable risk. The effect on regulation of these changes also is discussed.

KEYWORDS: Vinyl chloride decision, Court of Appeals, DC Circuit, NRC backfit rule, acceptable risk, Clean Air Act Section 112

INTRODUCTION

In two important recent cases, one concerning vinyl chloride regulation by EPA,[1] the other the Nuclear Regulatory Commission's Backfit Rule,[2] the Court of Appeals, DC Circuit, has found the use of cost-effectiveness analysis by regulatory agencies in their decisions of whether or not to regulate to be inconsistent with the relevant law. A consequence of these decisions is that health and safety regulatory agencies are being pushed to determine actions on the basis of acceptable risks levels rather than on cost grounds. These decisions, as well as the Supreme Court's benzene decision concerning the need by OSHA to establish that a significant risk exists prior to regulation, are leading agencies toward policies involving increasingly explicit definitions of acceptable risk.

INTERPRETATION OF THE JUDICIAL DECISIONS

The vinyl chloride decision most clearly describes the principles that lie behind these two decisions of the D.C. Court. We will therefore use it for our further discussion. That decision focused on the intent of Congressional Acts and the methodology for regulatory decisions on setting emission standards for non-threshold carcinogenic pollutants to protect public health with an ample margin of safety. The D.C. Court review establishes the following concepts.

1. Safety is judgmental.
2. Verifiable safe levels do not exist and are unlikely to be established.
3. Elimination of risk is not required (i.e., zero levels are not mandated).
4. A safe level is one which may reasonably be anticipated to result in a health risk acceptable in the world in which we live (i.e. a comparative societal benefit/risk basis).
5. A safe level should be inferred from scientific data and expert opinion, and thus will contain uncertainty.
6. Feasibility, either technical or economic, is not a basis for setting a safe level (i.e., best available technology is not relevant to the safe level).
7. Regulatory standards may be more stringent than a safe level to provide a margin of safety against uncertainties. The societal benefits of such reductions should be consistent with technical and economic feasibility (i.e., cost-effectiveness analysis is relevant).

A schematic interpretation of the full discussion of the D.C. Court is shown in Fig. 1. The judgmental nature of the regulatory decision arises from the fact that experientially determined public health effects are generally associated with high levels of hazard exposure, and the regulatory targets are always below such levels. The extrapolation from the experiential range to the low level regulatory range is always hypothetical and speculative, with the uncertainty becoming large when the extrapolation leads to hazard reductions of ten or more, as is the usual case with such logarithmic scale variables.

The key point is that a "safe" or acceptable public risk level must be defined by the regulatory agency under Step 1. The further provision of an adequate margin of safety, Step 2, then results in regulatory standards below this safe level. The two D.C. Court decisions emphasize that costs should not be considered in establishing the safe level, but costs may be considered in determining a feasible margin of safety in the regulatory standard.

Implicit in the vinyl chloride decision is a basic perception of the nature of public health risks in our society that arise from involuntary exposure to a hazard, as follows.

1. The existence of such a hazard should not necessarily lead to significant harm to any specific individual (i.e., it is a probability issue).
2. It is publicly unacceptable for specific individuals to be involuntarily exposed to a hazard which has a probability approaching certainty of substantial harm (e.g., death). Thus, no level of specific death is socially acceptable as a regulatory target. Such a causative hazard is "unsafe."
3. Conversely, when the hazard arises from a socially useful activity, a low probability of distributed harm to the general public has been and is societally acceptable. Thus, a regulatory "safe" level of health risk exists for each hazard.
4. The regulatory task is establishing for each hazard, first, a safe level which meets the above criteria, and second an additional margin of safety for the uncertainties involved. The safe risk level should be consistent with the commonly accepted risks in the society in which we live (i.e., a comparative risk-benefit criterion). The additional margin of safety provided in the regulatory target should be a reasonable balance of the economic costs and the health benefits of extending the margin.

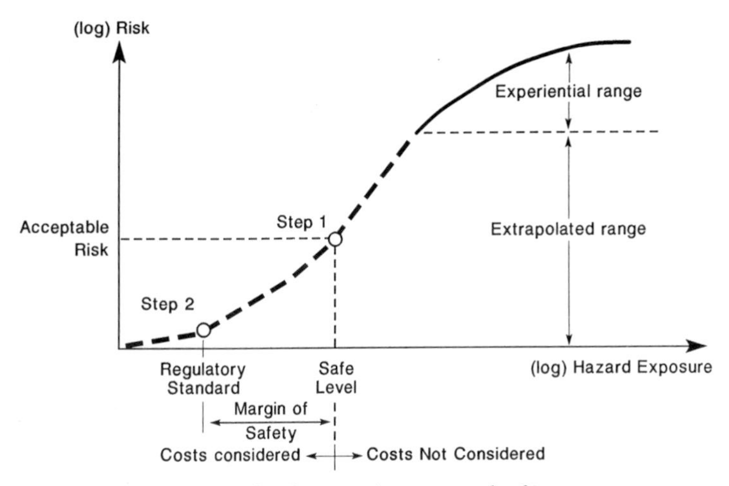

Fig. 1. Setting regulatory standards.

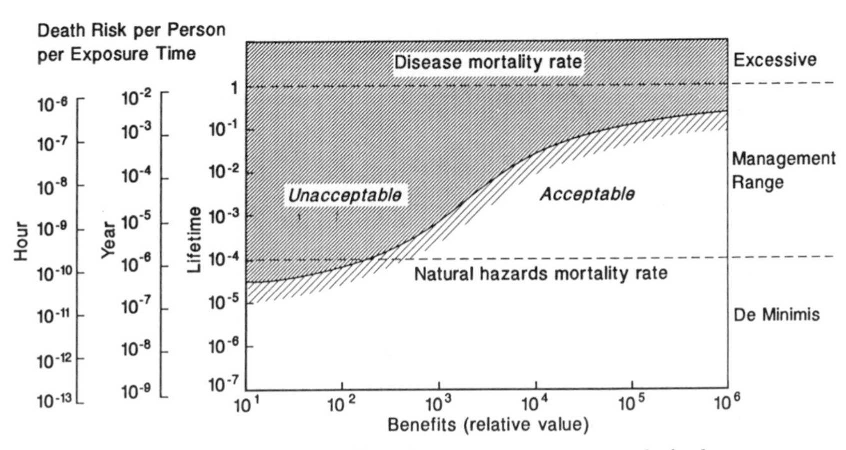

Fig. 2. Benefit-risk pattern of involuntary exposure to technical systems.

The subject of comparative public risk has been voluminously addressed in the risk analysis literature. The early papers of C. Starr[3,4] suggested the basic hypothesis, illustrated in Fig. 2, which is generally inherent in most comparative risk discussions of involuntary public exposure. The proposed principles are few.

1. No society is risk free.
2. Nature alone imposes a public risk minimum of about 10^{-6} per person per year (or 10^{-4} death per hour per million) from such unavoidable causes as lightning and weather extremes.
3. Risks approaching the high level of the normal public death rate of about 10^{-2} per person per year (or 1 death per hour per million) are considered excessive.
4. A hypothetical curve, such as shown in Fig. 2, is suggested to separate the domains of public acceptability and unacceptability. The key variables are the risk per unit time of exposure to the hazard and the benefits derived from the activity creating the hazard.

The pragmatic process of comparative public risk analysis for establishing "safe" and "regulatory" levels for any hazard is, of course, both complex and judgmental. Nevertheless, the risk analysis studies of the past two decades contain many examples of reasonable outcomes adequate for regulatory purposes.

IMPLEMENTATION OF THE JUDICIALLY MANDATED GUIDELINES

The Acceptable Safe Level

1. The basic determination is that of a "safe level" which meets the criterion of a health risk "acceptable in the world in which we live."
2. In "the world in which we live," there are mixed views on the acceptability of public health risks. Individual concerns may be determined by personal health issues and benefit-risk perceptions. Societal concerns may be based on measurements of real risks, on total population exposures, and on the social values of the activity creating the hazard.
3. Every society evolves a roughly reasonable allocation of societal resources to protect public health.
4. Minimizing the total risk exposure of the public requires a distribution of these resources such that the expenditure on each risk reduction is equally effective (i.e., a Pareto optimality). For example, very high expenditures on insignificant risks reduce the remaining resources available to mitigate significant risks. This is why a difference between risk reality and public perception may lead to a political misallocation of resources and a reduction in public health.
5. Social acceptability of risks is the outcome of a complex balance of the societal benefits derived from an activity and the societal risks. These are both tangible (measurable and visible) and intangible (cultural and psychological). The result of such a relationship is illustrated in Fig. 2.
6. Regulatory agencies thus must arrive at "safe level" determinations by a comparative risk analysis based on the existing levels of societal acceptability for present involuntary public health risks.
7. Absolute risk targets, such as one in a million per lifetime, have been used by regulatory agencies as a de minimis level. This target is about two orders of magnitude less than the minimal risk from natural events such as lightning or storms.
8. Comparative risk analysis involves a complex of societal goals, alternative modes of achieving each goal, their associated risks, the distribution of risk demographically and temporally. The associated societal benefits are equally complex. Nevertheless, it is feasible for professional judgment to establish domains of benefits and risks within orders of magnitude. In view of the basic uncertainties in all such projections, such quantitative domains may be adequate for regulatory purposes.
9. The Acceptable Safe Level is thus a judgmental choice of a health risk acceptable in the world in which we live.

Travis *et al.*[5] suggest that the past history of regulatory decisions on environmental carcinogens provides an empirical guide to acceptable risk levels. He points out that individual lifetime risks above 10^{-3} have all been regulated, and that large population lifetime risks above 10^{-4} have been regulated. The perception that the regulatory process is implicitly more concerned with large group exposures than with a relatively small number of individuals is probably correct. It may also reflect an evaluation that a broad societal benefit from the use of a substance might justify a somewhat higher risk exposure for a small fraction of the population.

Travis also suggests that these population based numbers be explicitly adopted as maximum "safe" levels of exposure. It is interesting that the 10^{-4} lifetime risk is also the natural hazards mortality rate (Fig. 2). This may just be a coincidence, or it may be that regulatory agencies have sought a defensible common de minimis level for all carcinogen exposures and have avoided the complexities of adjusting regulatory levels for the societal benefits associated with use.

The Margin of Safety

1. Regulatory targets usually are set more tightly than the "acceptable safe level" to accommodate the uncertainties in the management of the risk. The effectiveness of any risk management approach can only be estimated if new and only roughly measured if in use. Thus, if the "acceptable safe level" is not to be exceeded, a margin of safety is desired for regulatory purposes.
2. The risk management alternatives for minimizing the potential risks arising from any hazard usually have varying feasibilities, including social, political, and economic constraints.
3. The margin of safety provided by a risk management approach depends on the magnitude of the societal investment allocated to it. Considering the total social resources available for reducing public health risks, the allocation to any one risk should depend on the relative social importance of providing a margin of safety against the specific hazard involved. Again, this is a judgmental decision.
4. The chosen risk management approach should provide the maximum margin of safety for a reasonable societal investment. Given equal feasibility for social and political implementation, the economic cost of a risk management alternative determines the margin of safety that can be provided.
5. Thus, in the narrowest sense, the economic benefit/cost analysis that has been used in choosing among risk management alternatives has a useful role in the ultimate provision of a margin of safety.

COST-EFFECTIVENESS VERSUS COST-BENEFIT FRAMEWORKS

Cost-effectiveness analysis refers to comparison of cost and benefit at the margin; in the context of risk management, cost-effectiveness often describes the ratio of cost of a risk reduction to the degree of reduction, i.e., dollars per unit of harm averted. In contrast, cost-benefit analysis refers to the comparison of the social benefits from an activity or investment with its social costs. An example illustrates the difference: whether the social benefits of a new dam are worth its cost is a cost-benefit issue; whether a dam should be 60 or 65 feet high, where the higher dam is safer but more expensive, is a cost-effectiveness question.

As noted above, a central feature of the vinyl chloride and NRC backfit decisions is that cost-effectiveness analysis is not permitted in the initial decision of whether or not to regulate. The regulator must judge whether the activity at issue is safe without considering the costs of incremental controls on the risks involved. For exposures or activities judged unsafe, risk reductions are required regardless of their cost; for activities judged to be safe, further safety improvements (i.e., the margin of safety) can be required or not depending on cost as well as other factors.

The major point of the vinyl chloride decision is that cost-effectiveness analysis cannot be used to judge safety. What is less clear is how to make a judgment of whether or not an activity is safe. The court's decision requires the administrator to "decide what risks are acceptable in the world in which we live," and notes that few people would consider driving a car or breathing city air to be unsafe.

These examples—driving a car and breathing city air—shed light on what the court means by safe in the world in which we live. From a risk analyst's perspective, the risk from driving a car is much higher than most other risks; it is implausible that risks this high would be accepted in most other contexts. It clearly follows that what the court means by "decide what risks are acceptable in the world in which we live" is to consider whether something is safe based on the social significance of the activity as a whole. In its use of risks of driving a car as an example, the court seems to be indicating that judgments of safety or acceptability of risk cannot be made in an abstract, context-free way. It seems apparent that the court recognizes that the social importance of an activity or technology, including its benefits, is an appropriate consideration in determining an acceptable level of risk; activities with risks as great as those from driving a car would probably not be acceptable if they were socially unimportant.

Three of the four approaches proposed by EPA for benzene regulation are abstract and context-free; these proposed safe levels are (1) a societal risk of less than one per year, (2) individual risks of less than 10^{-4} per lifetime, or (3) individual risks of less than 10^{-6} per lifetime. The final EPA approach is to consider what is safe on a case-by-case basis. Only this last approach is consistent with the logic of the vinyl chloride decision.

The vinyl chloride decision permits consideration of benefits but not of cost-effectiveness in risk control when it comes to the determination of acceptable risk. However, the distinction between cost-benefit and cost-effectiveness frameworks is insufficiently distinct for regulatory agencies to develop a clear policy based on the court's ruling. A series of examples will indicate the potential confusion.

Here is an easy example. EPA discovers a carcinogenic compound in the air arising from chlorination of drinking water. Exposures and risks are estimated to be small in comparison to the risks that would be associated with bacteria in nonchlorinated drinking water. Just as the court noted that "breathing city air" is not considered an unsafe activity by most people, these exposures are judged acceptable in view of the social value of chlorination. Consistent with the terms of the vinyl chloride decision, EPA declares the risk to be acceptable, and looks for cost-effective exposure reduction opportunities to increase the margin of safety.

As another easy example, emissions of carcinogenic compounds are found to be associated with production of a certain type of paint. Emission controls are technically feasible although expensive; if implemented, paint costs would increase by 50%. Following the vinyl chloride decision, EPA does not consider the cost or technical feasibility of emission control and decides that present emissions pose an unacceptably high risk.

Here is a harder example, as above, emissions of carcinogenic compounds are found to be associated with production of a certain type of paint. Emission controls are technically feasible although expensive; if implemented, the cost of domestically manufactured paint would increase to well above that of imported paint. Were EPA to find that the emissions pose unacceptable risks, thousands of U.S. jobs would be lost as domestic manufacturers shut down. EPA's mandate is uncertain.

The guidance from Congress, as interpreted in the vinyl chloride case, requires protection of public health without consideration of cost; however, some consideration of benefit is permitted. If the jobs are considered to be an important social benefit that justifies acceptance of a moderate degree of risk, then EPA might argue that the ongoing emissions are acceptable. But if the loss of U.S. jobs as a consequence of regulation is viewed as a cost, it is not an admissible consideration (because costs are not legitimately considered in decisions for this class of pollutants). Depending on one's viewpoint, loss of domestic jobs is an incremental cost of reducing emissions or the loss of valued social benefits. Whichever interpretation EPA takes, the issue would likely be returned to the courts for clarification.

The point these examples are meant to convey is that it is difficult to draw a clear distinction between cost-effective and cost-benefit perspectives. While the court has indicated that a marginal or incremental cost cannot be considered in judging whether an activity is safe, the court has also found that it is appropriate for EPA to consider the social context of the decision, which presumably includes such things as social benefits from the activity, including employment. The way in which EPA evaluates an activity in context, i.e., "in the world in which we live," without considering control opportunities and their costs is unclear and has yet to be determined.

EFFECT OF THE VINYL CHLORIDE DECISION ON RISK ANALYSIS

The vinyl chloride decision addresses scientific uncertainty in the following way: "Congress, however, recognized in Section 112 that the determination of what is 'safe' will always be marked by scientific uncertainty and thus exhorted the Administrator to set emission standards that will provide an 'ample margin' of safety. This language permits the Administrator to take into account scientific uncertainty and to use expert discretion to determine what action should be taken in light of that uncertainty. ... In determining what is an 'ample margin' the Administrator may, and perhaps must, take into account the inherent limitations of risk assessment and the limited scientific knowledge of the effects of exposure to carcinogens at various levels, and may therefore decide to set the level below that previously determined to be 'safe'."

The obvious interpretation of the court's decision is that "safety" is judged comparatively (i.e., "decide what risks are acceptable in the world in which we live") using central or best estimates of risk, and that, subsequently, the uncertainty in the risk estimate is considered in determining an "ample margin" of safety. The decision reflects the view that it is not appropriate to use pessimistic or worst-case risk estimates for comparison to everyday risks to determine if emissions will lead to an unacceptable risk; it also recognizes the relevance of uncertainty to the final regulatory decision through the "ample margin" of safety requirement.

This approach apparently requires the agency to conduct risk assessments that provide both central (or unbiased) estimates of risk along with descriptions of the uncertainties in those estimates. It may be that the conventional assumptions of risk assessment for carcinogens that lead to a "plausible upper bound" risk estimate[6] will be suitable for describing the uncertainties in risk to some degree; it is apparent that these upper bounds cannot be simultaneously used as unbiased estimates of risk.

It seems apparent that risk analysts will be asked to tell more than they know about cancer risks. Many plausible assumptions and models can be use to estimate risk, but there is no known way to determine which assumptions and models are correct. Given this situation, it is difficult to define what is meant by an unbiased or central estimate of risk.

A likely consequence of this situation is the reexamination of the assumptions used to estimate risk. Whether a scientific consensus can be obtained for assumptions and models appropriate for unbiased or best estimates of risk in contrast to those used to provide plausible upper bounds is not yet certain.

While there has been a continuing trend towards reducing overly pessimistic risk estimates, there are some sound steps that can be taken to move risk assessment towards a more explicit effort to estimate risks as accurately as possible. One important area is the careful analysis of data for carcinogens where there are both human and animal data. For substances where human studies are available for risk assessment and, consequently, where animal studies are not likely to affect risk estimates (e.g., radon), it is still important to conduct animal studies. Analysis and experiments designed to test and calibrate our systems for risk assessment through interspecies comparisons are needed.

Finally, by separating consideration of the level of risk from carcinogenic emissions from consideration of the uncertainties in those risks, the vinyl chloride decision enhances the importance of the conceptual separation between risk assessment and risk management. This raises another issue for risk analysts: investigation of the limits and consequences, both positive and negative, of increasing this separation.

FINAL COMMENTS

The court's decision in the two cases discussed here reflect a new step to balance equity and economic concerns in risk management. The prohibition against cost considerations in the determination of whether a safe level exists for carcinogenic emissions or nuclear power plant operations reflects the view of the Congress that individual members of the public have a right to be free from significant, involuntarily imposed risks. Conversely, the obvious social value in considering both technical and economic characteristics of techniques for reducing risk is also permitted once a minimal level of safety has been achieved. The practical implementation of the approach outlined by the court is still to be developed; it remains to be seen how thinking and policies at the EPA will respond to the need to make repeated decisions about what is safe.

REFERENCES

1. Petition for Review of an Order of the Environmental Protection Agency, Decided July 28, 1987, U.S. Court of Appeals, D.C. Circuit, No. 85-1150.
2. Petition for Review of Orders at the Nuclear Regulatory Commission, Decided August 4, 1987, U.S. Court of Appeals, D.C. Circuit, No. 85-1757 and No. 86-1219.
3. C. Starr, Social Benefit versus Technological Risk, *Science* **166**:1232 (1969).
4. C. Starr, National Academy of Engineering Colloquium, Perspectives on Benefit-Risk Decision Making, p. 17, April 26, 1971.
5. C. C. Travis and H. A. Hattemer-Frey, Determining an Acceptable Level of Risk, *Environ. Sci. Technol.* **22**:873 (1987).
6. E. L. Anderson and the Carcinogen Assessment Group of the U.S. Environmental Protection Agency, Quantitative Approaches in Use to Assess Cancer Risk, *Risk Analysis* **3**:277-295 (1983).

Risk Assessment of Mixtures: A Model Based on Mechanisms of Action and Interaction[a]

M. A. Clevenger
U.S. Environmental Protection Agency
Washington, DC

R. M. Putzrath and S. L. Brown
ENVIRON Corp.
Washington, DC

M. E. Ginevan
RiskFocus
Springfield, VA

C. T. DeRosa and M. M. Mumtaz
U.S. Environmental Protection Agency
Cincinnati, OH

ABSTRACT

Approaches to assess risks from mixtures include curve-fitting to observed responses of whole mixtures, combining risks from each chemical based on toxic endpoint, or predicting responses based on mechanisms of interaction. Using the latter approach, the interaction of mixed-function oxidase (MFO) metabolism of the substrate hexobarbital (HB) and the MFO modulator piperonyl butoxide (PBO) was modeled, based on relationships between dose, elimination rate, and duration of pharmacological effect. This model estimates a bioequivalence factor to convert doses of PBO+HB to an equivalent dose of HB. This modeling approach has considerable utility for predicting risks from complex mixtures. Experiments can be performed to derive bioequivalence factors for other MFO interactions that can use the same model to predict type and extent of interaction. The model has been incorporated as one option in a larger decision-tree approach predicting interactions among constituents of mixtures.

KEYWORDS: Mixtures, interaction, hexobarbital, piperonyl butoxide, mixed-function oxidase, risk assessment

---

a. The views in this paper are those of the authors and do not necessarily reflect the views or policies of the U.S. Environmental Protection Agency. The U.S. government has the right to retain a nonexclusive royalty-free license in and to any copyright covering this paper.

INTRODUCTION

The U.S. Environmental Protection Agency (EPA) has developed guidelines to deal with the assessment of risk from chemical mixtures of carcinogenic and noncarcinogenic chemicals.[1] For noncarcinogenic chemicals, the guidelines suggest using a hazard index (HI) procedure, which involves the summation of ratios of the estimated exposure level to the reference dose (RfD) for each component of a mixture. The HI procedure is based on the assumption that the components act by the same mechanism but do not interact. Chemical interactions may occur, however, between some mixture components under certain conditions of exposure (e.g., within a certain range or ratio of doses). The EPA guidelines allow for incorporation of quantifiable interactions where appropriate. This provision allows the opportunity to develop techniques to deal with chemical interactions in instances where adequate information is available.

There are several ways in which two or more chemicals can interact. For example, mixture components may interact chemically or physically by competing for a receptor site, by cooperative binding at a receptor site, by altering responsiveness or potentiating a toxicological effect, or by inducing or inhibiting metabolizing enzymes.

Toxicological interactions are generally classified by the observed effects. Thus, the classification of additivity, synergy, antagonism, and independence of action are operational definitions that result from observed effects in a given system within a given range of doses.

Interactions may also be described according to the involved biological site. As described first by Veldstra[2] and later by Murphy,[3] there are three biological sites of interaction: sites of action, sites of activation, and sites of loss.

This study focuses on the development of models based on the underlying biological mechanism of interaction. For each site and mechanism, certain fundamental parameters describe the nature of the interaction (e.g., receptor binding affinity, degree of enzyme induction). Once a model is tested and validated, the parameters of the model might become the basis for estimating interactions for different sets of chemicals having the same mechanism.

The nature of an interaction may change with changes in dose and relative proportions of the components of the mixture. Thus, it is necessary to know where in the dose-response relationship those changes occur in order to predict the effects of a mixture. Further, in constructing models to describe interactions, it is desirable to generate dose-response surfaces that may be examined for "critical loci," or regions at which the interaction changes from, for example, additivity to synergy.

This study involves the development of a mathematical modeling approach that is potentially useful for predicting quantitatively the interaction between modulators and substrates of the mixed-function oxidase (MFO) enzyme system. The relatively uncomplicated interaction of the drug hexobarbital (HB) with the MFO modulator piperonyl butoxide (PBO) was examined. HB induces hypnosis (sleeping) when blood concentration reaches a critical or threshold level. The parent compound is the active form of the drug, and HB is metabolized solely by the MFO enzyme system to inactive metabolites. Hexobarbital-induced sleep time (HST) has been used extensively as a measure of *in vivo* MFO induction and inhibition.

PBO is a substrate of the MFO system that can also induce or inhibit the metabolism of other substrates. PBO has no pharmacological hypnotic effect but has the potential to alter hexobarbital sleep time by altering the rate of HB metabolism. In this study, the MFO inhibitory effect of PBO on HST was modeled as an example of a chemical interaction at the site of loss.

METHODS

Biological Data

The data used to develop the model were derived from Kamienski and Murphy.[4] Briefly, a single dose of HB alone or combinations of HB and PBO were administered intraperitoneally to male mice, and duration of HST was measured. The HB/PBO combinations were given sequentially as follows: (a) a single dose of PBO (6.25 to 500 mg/kg) was administered either 30 minutes or 48 hours prior to a single dose of 125 mg/kg of HB, or (b) a single dose of 100 mg/kg of PBO was given 30 minutes or 48 hours prior to a single dose of 50 or 75 mg/kg of HB. PBO given 30 minutes prior to HB resulted in prolongation of HST, whereas PBO given 48 hours prior to HB resulted in reduction of HST. This time-dependent effect reflects the bimodal action of PBO on MFO activity. The data chosen for the modeling exercise were that which described the interaction between HB and PBO during the MFO inhibitory phase.

Interaction Model

The derivation of the equations and assumptions of the model are described in detail in Appendix A.

RESULTS

A model was developed to describe the interaction between the MFO substrate, hexobarbital, and an inhibitor of the MFO system, piperonyl butoxide (PBO). Knowledge about the biological site and mechanism of interaction of these chemicals was the starting point for the model. The MFO inhibitory action of PBO involves a competitive interaction for the MFO enzyme system. Thus, the site of interaction between HB and PBO is at the site of metabolism of HB, and the consequence is a decrease in the rate of metabolism of HB to inactive metabolites. The rate of elimination of HB does likewise decrease, since HB is excreted primarily as metabolites.

As shown in Appendix A, the basis for the model is a generalized equation that relates dose, elimination rate, and duration of effect. The equation takes the form of

$$\ln C_m = \ln C_o - KT \,, \tag{A}$$

which rearranges to

$$T = 1/K \cdot (\ln C_o - \ln C_m) \,, \tag{B}$$

where K is the elimination rate constant, C_o is the initial blood concentration, and C_m is the minimum effect blood level.

According to Eq. (A), the duration, T, of the effect is a linear function of the log of concentration; if the initial concentration is proportional to the administered dose, the relationship between sleep time and the log of the HB dose also should be linear. Figure 1 shows this relationship using the data of Kamienski and Murphy.[4] The slope of the relationship is $1/K$, and a change in the elimination rate constant (K) will affect both the slope and intercept of the relationship. With competitive inhibition by PBO, the rate of

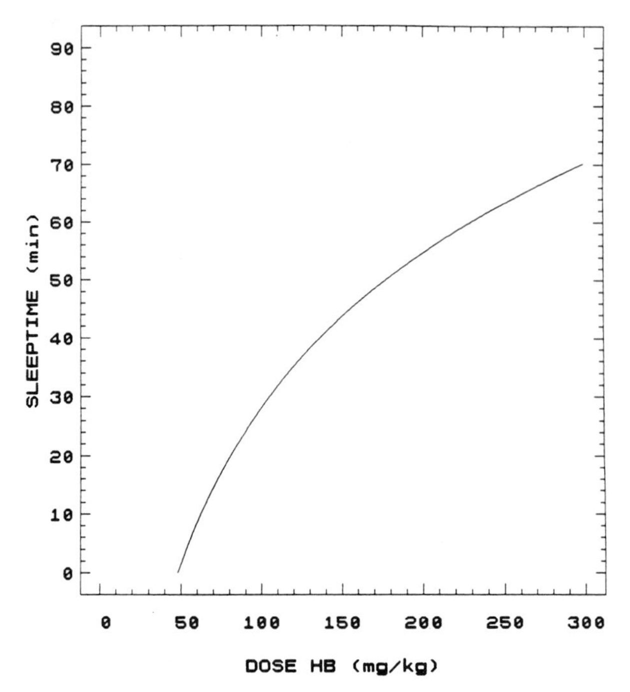

Fig. 1. Hexobarbital sleep time as a function of dose. No piperonyl butoxide administered.

elimination of HB should be proportional to the relative blood concentration of HB (C_1) and PBO (C_2). Appendix A shows that this relationship can be modeled as:

$$K' = K \cdot \frac{C_1}{C_1 + Z \cdot C_2} , \tag{C}$$

where Z is a "bioequivalence constant" that converts blood concentration of PBO to equivalent blood concentration of HB, and K is the rate of elimination of HB without competitive inhibition. The constants K and Z can be determined from the data of Kamienski and Murphy[4] showing the relationship of sleep time to dose of PBO for a constant dose of HB and the relationship of sleep time to dose of HB for a fixed dose of PBO, as detailed in Appendix A. The bioequivalence constant was obtained from the data plotted in Fig. 2, which shows the relationship of sleep time to dose of PBO for a constant dose of HB. If the parameters are substituted into Eq. (B) with K' replacing K, the resulting relationship of sleep time to the dose of HB and PBO is

$$T = \left(1 + \frac{9 \cdot \mathrm{PBO}}{\mathrm{HB}}\right) \cdot 46 \cdot \ln\left(\frac{\mathrm{HB}}{48}\right) . \tag{D}$$

In Eq. (D) above, HB and PBO are the administered doses (mg/kg) of the two substances.

For Eq. (D) to hold, PBO must be administered before HB; furthermore, the dose of HB must exceed the threshold of 48 mg/kg for the animal to fall asleep at all. Sleep time is a relatively simple function of the two dose variables and can be represented in terms of a dose-response surface in those two dimensions. The result is presented in Fig. 3. The line showing zero response at HB = 48 mg/kg for all doses of PBO is the minimum dose

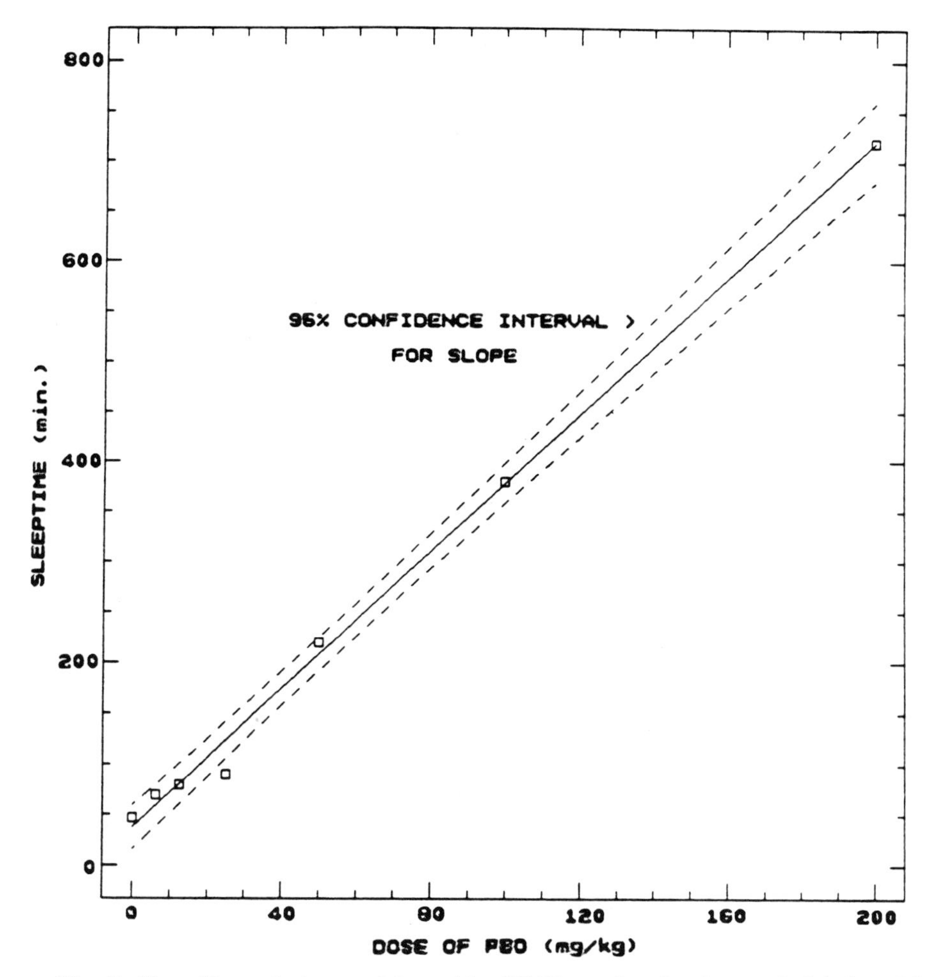

Fig. 2. The effect of piperonyl butoxide (PBO) on the sleeping period induced by hexobarbital (HB). Data are for a fixed dose of 125 mg/kg HB.

required for sleeping and represents one "critical locus" of the surface. Also, a maximum of sleep time occurs for a finite dose of HB (about 300 minutes for about 150 mg/kg HB if the dose of PBO is 100 mg/kg, for example). This phenomenon occurs because the dose of HB eventually overcomes the high bioequivalence factor for PBO. The locus of these maxima is another "critical locus." These predictions of the model provide an interesting avenue for future experimental confirmation. Clearly, the bioequivalence factor is one of the critical factors in developing a risk assessment procedure for chemical interactions mediated by the MFO system.

DISCUSSION

The modeling exercise presented provides a quantitative description of the data on HB-PBO interaction. It both explains all of the qualitative features of the data and provides a good quantitative fit, as can be verified by examining the data points shown in Fig. 3. Where adequate data exist, this type of modeling approach has considerable utility for conducting risk assessments for chemical mixtures. Although sleeping time is not ordinarily considered a toxic effect, Eq. (A) is applicable to pharmacological or toxicological

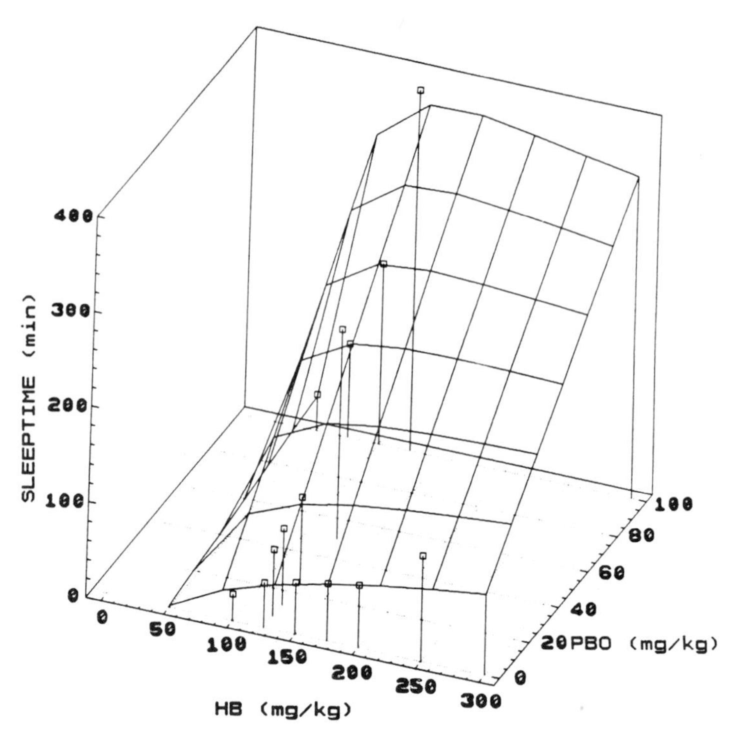

Fig. 3. Dose-response surface for the interaction of hexobarbital (HB) and piperonyl butoxide (PBO). Data points (rectangles on sticks) are from Kamienski and Murphy.[4]

endpoints other than the return to a normal state of wakefulness. For example, it can be applied to any physiologic parameter if expressed as a percent above or below normal values. Equations have also been developed to deal with repeated exposures.[5] Therefore, Eq. (C) can be applied to pairs of chemicals in which one is a MFO inducer (i.e., a substitute for PBO) and the other is a toxic parent compound metabolized by the MFO system (i.e., a substitute for HB). The bioequivalence factor in Eq. (C) can be determined by pharmacological experiments and the rate constant K by toxicological observations entailing only the toxic substance; the dose-response surface could be predicted without resort to a specific experiment designed to measure interaction.

With knowledge about the involvement of mixture components with the MFO system (be it an inducer, inhibitor, or substrate), the interaction between MFO-active chemicals can be predicted. At this time, only a qualitative prediction is possible in most instances, but as illustrated with hexobarbital and piperonyl butoxide, a quantitative model may be developed with appropriate data.

Presented in Fig. 4 is a decision flow diagram that can be used to categorize or define the involvement of mixture components with the MFO system. Shown in the inset is a matrix which predicts the interaction between chemicals falling into the four categories defined in Fig. 4. The flow diagram deals only with two chemical interactions. The decision tree does not address the situation in which an inducer or inhibitor is also a substrate altering its own metabolism. Such a situation would resemble a three-chemical interaction. Techniques should be developed to incorporate such multi-component interactions into models for risk assessment. Potential interactions at other sites (e.g., receptor) are not considered, and it is assumed that MFO metabolism is the only biotransformation pathway for the substrate. The interaction predicted in the matrix is assumed to hold only over a

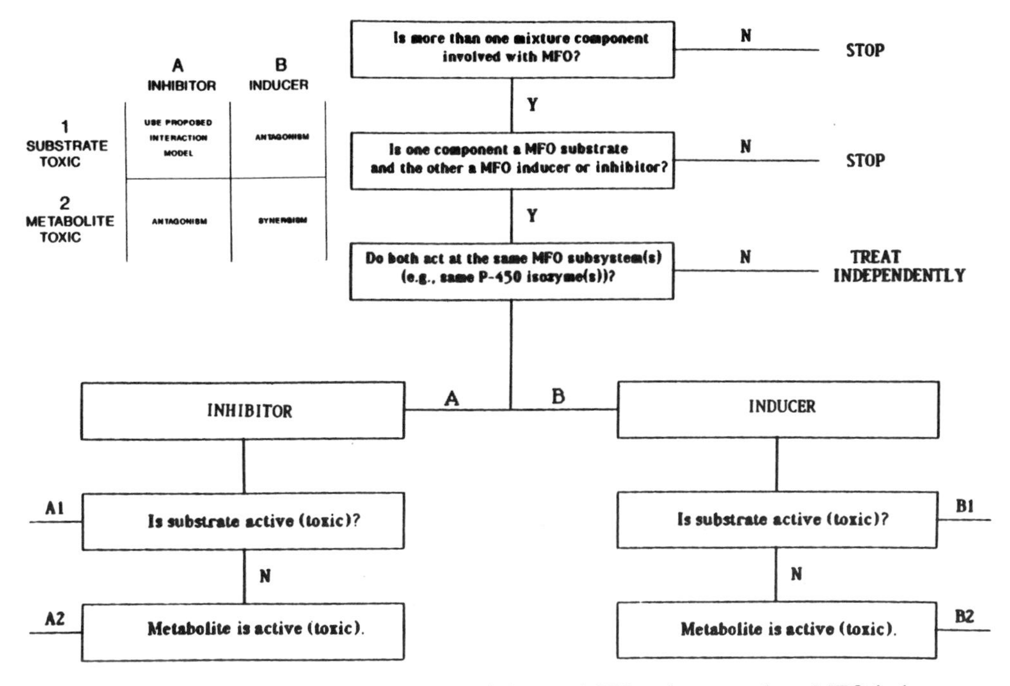

Fig. 4. Assessment of mixtures containing an MFO subtrate and an MFO inducer or inhibitor.

finite dose range. At low doses for both constituents, the interaction may be indistinguishable from additivity, whereas at very high doses, other interactions may come into play.

To use the decision flow diagram, it must first be determined if more than one mixture component is involved with the MFO system. If not, a different criterion must be used to determine if the components interact. If more than one component is involved, it is necessary to determine if the components are substrates, inducers, or inhibitors. If an inducer or inhibitor influences its own metabolism through its induction/inhibition action, the situation resembles a three-chemical interaction, and therefore cannot be addressed in this decision tree. If both chemicals act strictly as inducers or inhibitors, no interaction is expected. If one component is a substrate and the other an inducer or inhibitor, it must be determined whether the two chemicals act at the same MFO subsystem, for example the PB-inducible cytochrome P-450 isozyme. If the answer is no, the chemicals would be expected to act independently. If the answer is yes, the next step is to classify the one component as an inducer or an inhibitor (A or B) then to classify the substrate with respect to the relative activity of the parent compound and the metabolite (1 or 2).

This decision tree for interactions at the MFO system may be incorporated as a branch of a larger decision tree that also includes branches for other types of interactions as well as branches for independent effects and dose additivity (the hazard index approach).

APPENDIX A

Levy and coworkers[5,6] have described the mathematical relationship between dose, elimination rate, and duration of pharmacological effect of drugs. For a given chemical, the time necessary to decrease an initial body content to the minimum effective level can be calculated by rearranging the exponential expression for first order elimination as follows:

$$\ln C_m = \ln C_o - KT \ , \quad \text{(A)}$$

rearranged to

$$T = (1/K) \cdot (\ln C_o - \ln C_m) \ , \quad \text{(B)}$$

where K is the first order rate constant of drug elimination, T is the duration of the drug effect, C_m is the minimum blood concentration in the blood, and C_o is the initial blood concentration.

According to Eq. (B), a plot of T versus log dose should be linear, C_m can be calculated from the y-intercept, and K is equal to 1/slope. For Eqs. (A) and (B) to hold, the following assumptions are necessary:

1. The parent compound is the active form.
2. Biotransformation products are inactive.
3. Intensity of activity at any given time is a function of drug in the body at that time.
4. A minimum body drug content is necessary to elicit a measurable effect.
5. The drug is eliminated from the body by an exponential (first-order) process.
6. Absorption is instantaneous.

Most of these assumptions are applicable to the pharmacokinetics of HB. The parent compound is the active form, and its metabolites are inactive.[7] HB is not extensively stored in any extravascular tissues, and HB blood concentration closely correlates with duration of HST.[7] It has been shown that HB is eliminated by a first-order process over a range of doses.[8] To simplify the model, the assumption was made that distribution from intraperitoneal administration is instantaneous and that absorption is 100%. It has been demonstrated that the duration of HST is quite similar with intraperitoneal and intravenous administration.[8] It was shown by Noordhoeck[8] that hexobarbital-induced sleeping time, T, increase linearly with the logarithm of dose, $\ln(D)$, of hexobarbital in excess of some threshold dose, D_o. That is:

$$T = k \cdot \ln(D/D_o) \ , \quad \text{(A-1)}$$

where k is a coefficient relating sleep time to log dose. Figure 1 shows the relationship using data from Kamienski and Murphy.[4]

It was also shown by Noordhoeck[8] that the concentration of HB in the blood at awakening, C_{tw}, is approximately a constant and that removal of HB from the blood is fit by an approximately exponential decay function:

$$C_t = C_o \cdot \exp - Kt, \quad \text{(A-2)}$$

where C_t is the HB blood concentration at time t after HB administration, C_o is the HB blood level immediately after HB administration, and K is an exponential decay constant. Sleep time can be derived from Eq. (A-2) as follows:

$$\ln C_{tw} = \ln C_o - KT \ , \quad \text{(A-3)}$$

where C_{tw} is the concentration of HB in the blood at awakening, C_o and K are defined as in Eq. (A-2), and T is defined as in Eq. (A-1). Rearrangement of Eq. (A-3) yields:

$$T = (1/K) \cdot (\ln C_o - \ln C_{tw}) . \tag{A-4}$$

Equation (A-4) looks much like Eq. (A-1) with $1/K$ replacing k and $(\ln C_o - \ln C_{tw})$ replacing $\ln D$. It can also be shown that:

$$C_o = M \cdot D . \tag{A-5}$$

That is, the initial concentration in the blood is a linear function of dose. This relationship is assumed to hold with intraperitoneal administration. Thus Eq. (A-4) can be rewritten as:

$$T = (1/K) \cdot (\ln D + \ln M - \ln C_{tw}) \tag{A-6}$$

or

$$T = (1/K) \cdot (\ln D - \ln C_{tw} + \ln M) .$$

That is

$$K_1 = 1/K , \tag{A-7}$$

and

$$T > 0 \text{ if } (M \cdot D)/C_{tw} > 1 \tag{A-8}$$

or if

$$D > C_{tw}/M .$$

Note that M is a "nuisance" parameter in the mathematical sense. That is, it is not necessary to know the value of M because it does not effect the slope estimate $(1/K)$.

Equations (A-1) through (A-8) can be used to define the action of an inhibitor qualitatively. Decreasing the value of k makes the slope of the dose-response function steeper for a given dose of inhibitor, and lengthens sleep time for a given value of D. It is also apparent that the value of k, the slope of sleep time on dose, is exactly equivalent to the reciprocal of K, the exponential decay constant for blood concentration of HB. The remaining issue is development of a function:

$$K' = F(\text{PBO}) , \tag{A-9}$$

which relates the rate of elimination of HB to the dose of PBO received. If it is assumed that the rate of elimination of HB is proportional to the relative blood concentrations of HB (C_1) and PBO (C_2) then,

$$K' = K \cdot \frac{C_1}{C_1 + Z \cdot C_2} , \tag{A-10}$$

where Z is a "bioequivalence constant" that converts blood concentration of PBO to blood concentration of HB, and K is the rate of elimination of "pure" HB. Because it is thought that the primary mechanism by which PBO increases sleep time is competitive inhibition, this assumption is probably a reasonable approximation of reality. If the dose of HB is fixed, the equation relating sleep time to PBO dose [from Eq. (A-4)] is given by

$$T = \frac{C_1 + Z \cdot C_2}{C_1} \cdot \frac{1}{K} \cdot \left(\ln C_o - \ln C_{tw}\right) ,$$

or

$$T = \left(1 + \frac{Z \cdot C_2}{C_1}\right) \cdot \frac{1}{K} \cdot \left(\ln C_o - \ln C_{tw}\right) . \tag{A-11}$$

For a fixed concentration of HB (C_1), all terms except C_2 are constants. If X is defined as the constant:

$$X = \frac{1}{K} \cdot \left(\ln C_o - \ln C_{tw}\right) , \tag{A-12}$$

then Eq. (A-11) simplifies to

$$T = X + \frac{Z \cdot X}{C_1} \cdot C_2 . \tag{A-13}$$

The first prediction of the preceding equation is that sleep time for a fixed dose of HB should be a linear function of PBO dose with intercept X and slope $(Z \cdot X)/C_1$.

Kamienski and Murphy[4] provide data to validate the model. Mice were administered 0 to 200 mg/kg of PBO thirty minutes prior to a dose of 125 mg/kg of HB, and duration of sleep time was measured. These data are plotted in Fig. 2. The strong linear trend in sleep time with dose of PBO is obvious. As noted, the dose of HB was 125 mg/kg. The baseline sleep time, X, is 47 minutes and the regression slope, K_1, is 3.41 minutes of sleep time per mg/kg PBO. The bioequivalence constant, Z, can be obtained from

$$Z = K_1 \cdot \frac{C_1}{X} . \tag{A-14}$$

Thus Z is calculated to be 9.07, i.e., one unit of PBO is equal to about 9 units of HB, in terms of competitive inhibition. The accuracy of this prediction can be checked using data from Kamienski and Murphy.[4] The authors found that a dose of 50 mg/kg HB produced a sleep time of 30 minutes if given 1 hour after a dose of 100 mg/kg PBO, but that a dose of 105 mg/kg HB was required if no PBO was given. The effect of the PBO dose on K is easily calculated using Eq. (A-10). K' is calculated as follows:

$$K' = \frac{50}{50 + 9 \cdot 100} \cdot K , \tag{A-15}$$

or

$$K' = 0.05 \cdot K .$$

This implies that one hour after administration of 100 mg/kg PBO, a given dose of HB above C_{tw}/M is 20 times more effective, on a log scale, than the same dose of HB with no PBO given. Kamienski and Murphy[4] found that 105 mg/kg HB was necessary to produce a sleep time of 30 minutes in animals not treated with PBO, but in animals pretreated with 100 mg/kg PBO the same sleep time was induced by a dose of 50 mg/kg HB. It can be estimated from the data of Kamienski and Murphy[4] that the dose of HB that just induces some sleeping is C_{tw}/M or 48 mg/kg. This information permits a second data-based estimate of the relative potencies of HB with and without PBO. First, because the same sleep time was induced in both circumstances, from Eq. (A-4):

$$\begin{aligned} T &= \frac{1}{K} \cdot \left(\ln 105 - \ln 48\right) \\ &= \frac{1}{K'} \cdot \left(\ln 50 - \ln 48\right) , \end{aligned} \tag{A-16}$$

or

$$\frac{K'}{K} = \frac{\ln 50 - \ln 48}{\ln 105 - \ln 48} = 0.052 \ . \tag{A-17}$$

This value is in good agreement with that obtained with Eq. (A-15), but it must be noted that K'/K is rather sensitive to the value of MC_{tw}. For example, if C_{tw}/M was about 45 mg/kg rather than 48 mg/kg, Eq. (A-16) would yield a K'/K ratio of 0.12. When all of the above information is combined, the relationship of sleep time to the doses of HB and PBO is as shown in the following equation:

$$T = \left\{1 + \frac{9 \cdot \text{PBO}}{\text{HB}}\right\} \cdot 46 \cdot \ln\frac{\text{HB}}{48} \ . \tag{A-18}$$

This equation is plotted as a dose-response surface in Fig. 3.

ACKNOWLEDGEMENTS

The authors would like to thank Drs. Robert G. Tardiff and Duncan Turnbull for their useful review of the manuscript and Towanda Spencer and Greg Chandler for typing it. This work was partially funded by EPA contract No. 68-01-7090.

REFERENCES

1. U.S. Environmental Protection Agency (USEPA), Guidelines for the Health Risk Assessment of Chemical Mixtures, *CFR* **51(185)**:34014-34024 (1986).
2. H. Veldstra, Synergism and Potentiation with Special Reference to the Combination of Structural Analogues, *Pharmacol. Rev.* **8**:339-387 (1956).
3. S. D. Murphy, General Principles in the Assessment of Toxicity of Chemical Mixtures, *Environ. Health Perspect.* **48**:141-144 (1983).
4. F. X. Kamienski and S. D. Murphy, Biphasic Effects of Methylenedioxyphenyl Synergists on the Action of Hexobarbital and Organophosphate Insecticides in Mice, *Toxicol. Appl. Pharmacol.* **18**:883-894 (1971).
5. G. Levy, Kinetics of Pharmacologic Effect, *Clin. Pharmacol. Therap.* **7**:362-372 (1966).
6. G. Levy and E. Nelson, Theoretical Relationship between Dose, Elimination Rate, and Duration of Pharmacologic Effect of Drugs, *J. Pharm. Sci.* **54**:812 (1965).
7. M. T. Bush and W. L. Weller, Metabolic Fate of Hexobarbital (HB), in *Drug Metabolism Reviews*, Vol. 1, pp. 249-290, J. J. DiCarlo, ed., Marcel Dekker, Inc., New York (1973).
8. J. Noordhoek, Pharmacokinetics and Dose-Sleeping time Lines of Hexobarbital in Mice, *Eur. J. Pharmacol.* **3**:242-250 (1968).

Sensitive and Hypersusceptible Populations: Risk Assessment Considerations for Exposure to Single Chemicals or Chemical Mixtures

B. C. Seidman and S. L. Brown
ENVIRON Corp.
Washington, DC

C. T. DeRosa and M. M. Mumtaz
U.S. Environmental Protection Agency
Cincinnati, OH

ABSTRACT

Dose-response curves of human effects to a single chemical may be normally distributed or bimodal. Those individuals falling at the lower end of the normal curve or within the lower mode of the range of doses are termed, by convention, "hypersusceptibles." Where adequate human dose-response data have been available, environmental standards have been proposed and/or set to protect not only the general population but hypersusceptible groups as well. Lead, nitrate, and carbon monoxide are three such examples. Wherever quantitative human data are sparse, human reference doses are extrapolated from animal "No Observed Effect Levels" or "Lowest Observed Effect Levels" by use of safety factors. The accuracy of this approach is unknown and the uncertainty may be compounded when applied to a situation involving exposures to chemical mixtures with constituents which either act independently or synergistically. The analyst should therefore be aware of the possible consequences of the distribution of susceptibility for individual components of chemical mixtures and the nature of the interactions of these components.

KEYWORDS: Hypersusceptibility, chemical interactions, chemical mixtures, toxicity, hazard index

INTRODUCTION

The terms "sensitivity" and "hypersusceptibility" describe states in which individuals respond to chemicals at doses that fail to produce a response in most of the population (Fig. 1). Whereas "sensitive" individuals respond at the low end of a normal dose-response distribution of the general population, "hypersusceptibles" respond at doses significantly lower than those that produce no response in the most sensitive individuals in the general population. Although the terms "sensitivity" and "hypersusceptibility" are often used interchangeably, each represents a different biological circumstance and will be treated as a separate phenomenon in this discussion. An individual may respond in a sensitive or

Risk Analysis, Edited by C. Zervos
Plenum Press, New York, 1991

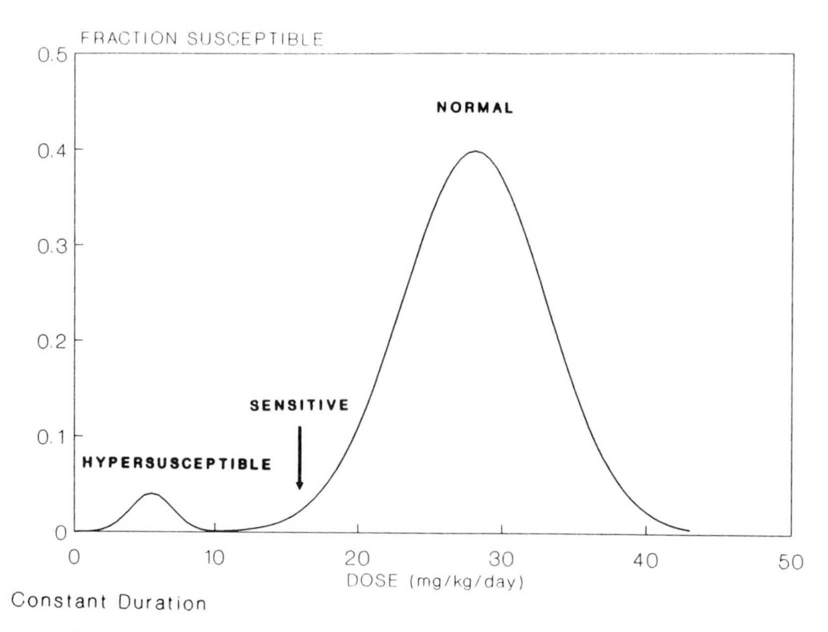

Fig. 1. Hypothetical distributions of sensitivity and hypersusceptibility (dose versus fraction susceptible).

hypersusceptible fashion to a single chemical or a group of chemically related or unrelated compounds. The purpose of EPA's Reference Dose (RfD) is to protect the general population (including sensitive individuals, but not necessarily hypersusceptibles) from potential adverse effects due to exposure to single compounds; EPA's use of the Hazard Index (HI), on the other hand, is for the purpose of protecting public health (again, including that of sensitive individuals but not necessarily hypersusceptibles) from potential adverse effects due to exposure to chemical *mixtures*. We have critically examined the applicability of these regulatory risk assessment and risk management approaches for sensitive individuals and hypersusceptibles.

EXAMPLES OF SENSITIVITY AND HYPERSUSCEPTIBILITY

Factors predisposing individuals to sensitive responses to pollutants include developmental processes, existing disease, prior exposure to a particular chemical (or chemical class or group which acts mechanistically in a similar manner), nutritional deficiencies and smoking and alcohol consumption (Table 1). Genetic factors can render certain individuals hypersusceptible to individual chemicals or chemical mixtures. The following review is organized to a large extent according to Calabrese' treatment of this topic,[1] and much of the following discussion has been drawn from this source.

Developmental Processes

Three groups are believed to be predisposed to sensitivity solely by virtue of their age or reproductive status: neonates, young children, and pregnant women. The unborn and infants less than 2-3 months of age, for example, do not possess fully developed enzymatic detoxification systems, limiting metabolic conversion and excretion of certain toxic substances. Young children are particularly at risk of toxicity associated with the ingestion of heavy metals due to increased gastrointestinal absorption of these compounds. Iron and calcium-deficient pregnant women are at an increased risk of experiencing the toxic effects of cadmium, manganese, and lead.

Table 1. Examples of Sensitivity and Hypersusceptibility

Sensitivity	Hypersusceptibility
Developmental Processes • neonates • young children • pregnant women	Genetic Disorders • sickle cell anemia • thalassemia • glucose-6-phosphate-dehydrogenase deficiency • immunologic sensitivities
Existing Disease • chronic heart and lung disease	
Other • prior exposure • nutritional deficiencies • smoking and alcohol consumption	

Existing Disease

Individuals with chronic heart and lung disease have been shown to be extraordinarily susceptible to some environmental compounds. Sulfur dioxide may exacerbate chronic pulmonary disease, and some compounds (e.g., carbon monoxide and nitrates) may place stress upon the heart by making it work harder to compensate for the reduction in the blood's oxygen carrying capacity.

Other

Some individuals may be predisposed to the toxic effects of certain environmental agents for other reasons discussed below.

Prior exposure to certain agents, such as occupational exposure, might sufficiently increase an individual's body burden of a given compound and predispose him or her to adverse effects from relatively small increases in dose. If for example, an individual were exposed to lead in the workplace, the apparent dose of lead necessary to induce toxic effects from ambient exposures (i.e. community air, and water) would likely be less than that of most in the general population.

Nutritional deficiencies may exacerbate toxic effects of environmental exposures. For instance, low dietary calcium can reduce the dose necessary for the induction of lead toxicity.[2]

Smoking and alcohol consumption may also predispose individuals to the adverse effects of pollutants. Smoking not only acts synergistically with asbestos exposure in the induction of lung cancer[3] but also interferes with lung clearance mechanisms, rendering the exposed individual particularly susceptible to additional chemical insults. Similarly, alcohol acts in a synergistic manner with other chemicals, such as carbon tetrachloride and other halogenated hydrocarbons, thereby increasing the likelihood of an individual developing liver disease.[4]

Genetic Disorders

Genetic disorders, such as the red blood cell disorders sickle cell anemia, thalassemia, and glucose-6-phosphate-dehydrogenase deficiency (G-6-P-D-D), all predispose affected individuals to the toxic effects of certain environmental exposures, sometimes to the extent of rendering them hypersusceptible. Individuals with sickle cell anemia and thalassemia produce an aberrant hemoglobin molecule, resulting in a decreased capacity of the blood to carry oxygen. Carbon monoxide, which has a higher affinity for oxygen than hemoglobin would be expected to place physiologic stress on those expressing sickle cell anemia and thalassemia. G-6-P-D-D individuals, unlike those with sickle cell anemia and thalassemia, do not produce abnormal hemoglobin; however, the red blood cells of this group are unusually sensitive to the lytic action of various drugs and chemicals such as primaquine and napthalene.[5] Immunological sensitivities appear to be genetically determined in many cases. These predisposing conditions may cause some individuals to respond at very low doses of such environmental agents as isocyanate. Such groups might have an increased risk of developing asthma, an allergy-related disorder.

REFERENCE DOSE (RfD) VALUES AND SENSITIVE AND HYPERSUSCEPTIBLE GROUPS

Background

In an attempt to estimate a level of toxicant exposure that would not be expected to cause adverse effects in a general population of humans, including those who might be especially sensitive, a reference dose (RfD) value is generated. When human data from sensitive subpopulations are available and adequate, they are used for the derivation of an RfD in either a quantitative or qualitative fashion. (To our knowlege, RfDs have not been derived from human hypersusceptible populations.) In the absence of adequate human data, animal data from laboratory studies are used. RfDs are extrapolated from animal No Observed Effect Levels (NOELs), No Observed Adverse Effect Levels (NOAELs) or Lowest Observed Adverse Effect Levels (LOAELs) using uncertainty (or safety) factors. For instance, a 10-fold factor is included to account for the variation in human sensitivity (intraspecies variability).[6] The use of such factors creates an uncertainty in itself; the derived RfDs might be overprotective (i.e., too conservative) or might be underprotective of some individuals. Given that sensitive persons fall at the low end of the dose-response curve (and are therefore closer to the threshold) and that RfDs are often derived from animal data and not from data from sensitive (or hypersusceptible) human populations, sensitive and hypersusceptible groups are at greatest risk of being affected by uncertainties associated with safety factors.

How Powerful Are Uncertainty (Safety) Factors?

Uncertainty factors are not derived from data, but are *a priori* estimations of the ranges of variation in extrapolations involved in determining an RfD. Weil[7] reported dose-response analyses for 490 tests of acute lethality in rats for single oral doses of toxic substances. Using log-dose versus probit response, he generated a frequency distribution of probit slopes (the number of standard deviations per 10-fold change in dose). Over 90% of the slopes were between 2 and 20, with a median of about 8. Dourson and Stara[8] interpreted this information as supporting the adequacy of a 10-fold uncertainty factor in adjusting for intraspecies variability. Whether this conclusion would also hold for less severe endpoints and longer exposure periods, however, is unknown. For instance, the intraspecies variability of subacute, subchronic or chronic LOAELs, NOAELs or NOELs were not examined. Also, the goodness-of-fit of the probit regressions is unknown. Additionally, variability among laboratory animals (in this case, rats) would be expected to be lower than in humans due to homogeneity of species and strain (genetic homogeneity), age, exposures, and nutrition. One would anticipate human populations to be far more diverse with respect to all these factors.

In spite of the drawbacks of this analysis, its conclusions were supported by Hattis *et al.*,[9] who indicated that inter-individual variability in the processing of various drugs among normal, healthy humans (based upon three factors related to such variability) was within a 10-fold range for essentially all chemicals studied. The three factors were elimination half-time, peak concentration in blood, and area under the plasma concentration versus time curve. According to their log-probit analysis, less than one-hundredth of one percent (10^{-4}) of a population would show parameter values more than 10 times lower than the median value. However, the authors acknowledged that their analysis was limited in that the parameters considered were "only components" of human sensitivity to toxins, and variability relating to exposure and response (such as that due to disease states or other predisposing conditions) was not taken into account.

Sensitive and Hypersusceptible Groups and Chemical Mixtures

EPA's approach to the assessment of chemical mixtures and their potential toxicity involves the hazard index (HI). The HI is described as follows:

$$HI = E_1/RL_1 + E_2/RL_2 + ... + E_i/RL_i ,$$

where E_i is the exposure level for the ith toxicant and RL_i is the acceptable level of exposure for the ith toxicant.

For mixtures of noncarcinogens, the acceptable or reference level (RL) of exposure is determined separately for each individual component of the mixture. The RL may correspond to an agency RfD or may be derived in a similar manner. The level of exposure (E) to each component is then divided by its RL and those ratios summed to determine the HI value. If the value of the HI exceeds 1, exposure to the mixture is considered to be of concern in the same way that exposure to an individual chemical is of concern if exposure to it exceeds its RfD. The EPA however notes in its guidelines, "the hazard index does not define dose-response relationships, and its numerical value should not be construed to be a direct estimate of risk."[10]

The HI approach assumes that the chemicals in a mixture contribute to the toxic effect in an additive manner and act on the same organ and by the same mechanism and differ only in their relative potency. EPA advises that for compounds in a mixture which have dissimilar effects the HI approach should be used only if dose addition for the effects of concern is scientifically justifiable.[10] The guidelines also present mathematical models for estimating response when interaction among components of the mixtures occurs (i.e., potentiation, synergism, or inhibition), but note that the data requirements for fitting such models are extensive and not likely to exist for most chemical mixtures.

For substances acting on the same organ by the same mechanism (dose additivity), the HI approach yields exactly the same level of protection for the mixture as the RfDs provide for the individual components. Whenever the ratios of dose to RfD add up to 1, the organ would be affected to the same degree, independent of which substances contributed what shares. Exactly the same individuals would be affected as if exposed to only one substance at its RfD; if each Rfd were adequately protective, the HI approach would be equivalently protective.

What is the significance of sensitive or hypersusceptible groups for the assessment of a mixture if we were assured all of the RfDs for its components were individually protective of these groups? We have identified two situations which the HI approach does not address; both involve components with independent actions. If the actions of individual components are independent, the HI approach can be either underprotective or overprotective depending on the details of the distribution of susceptibilities. Consider first the situation in which a mixture consists of two substances, each of which follows a typical log-normal distribution of susceptibilities with sensitive subpopulations falling at the low end of the dose-response curve. The dose-response relationships at low doses would follow the shape shown in Fig. 2, which appears as a straight line if plotted as log dose versus probit response. The response plotted is for probit slope = 1, which is among the smallest seen in animal toxicology experiments and corresponds to the greatest divergence in susceptibility. The RfD for each substance is shown as corresponding to a 10^{-3} response rate. The HI approach (dose additivity) predicts that the total response for exposure to 0.5 RfD each of both substances would also be 10^{-3}. But one can see that the responses predicted from Fig. 2 would be approximately 0.35×10^{-3} each; with *response* additivity, the total risk would be 0.7×10^{-3}, and for this hypothetical mixture the HI approach would be more protective than necessary. In this case, the degree of conservatism is only a factor of 1/0.7 or about 1.4. If we had chosen a smaller risk as defining the RfD, this factor would have been slightly larger (about 2 for RfD = 10^{-5} risk, for example). The factor is also larger for larger probit slopes (about 4 for slope = 2, for example). Finally, the degree of conservatism would also increase as more substances were included in the HI (although not when one dominated the risk assessment). For example, the factor is about 3 when three chemicals each appear at 1/3 the RfD. In summary, if the susceptible population is simply the tail of an approximately log-normal distribution of susceptibilities (i.e., is a sensitive subpopulation), the HI approach will usually be overprotective, possibly substantially so.

The opposite result—underprotection by the HI approach—can sometimes occur when the chemicals act independently on distinct and different hypersusceptible groups. Figure 3 shows a hypothetical distribution of susceptibilities in response to a single chemical that is approximately log-normal for most people but includes a hypersusceptible group with mean susceptibility well below that of the "normals." The relative peak sizes of the two "modes" of the distribution are exaggerated in the figure, but could be drawn to include approximately 0.1% of the population in the hypersusceptible group. An RfD anywhere within a large range of values between the two modes will be essentially equally protective. Now suppose there were two substances in a mixture and no person belonged to both susceptible groups (Fig. 4). If the population were exposed to 0.5 RfD of each substance, if the gap between the modes were sufficiently wide, and if the RfD had been set near the fringes of the "normal" distribution as shown, halving the exposure might still leave all of the hypersusceptibles affected for each chemical. With risk additivity, the total risk would be 2×10^{-3}, which would be unacceptable according to the presumed rules for setting RfDs.

Policy Considerations

How do we ensure that the health of all members of society will be protected? The issue of sensitivity and hypersusceptibility forces a policy decision. Social resources are limited and the possibility exists that there will always be some fraction of the population which will respond adversely to a compound or mixture, regardless of the dose. Should policy makers establish a number, analogous to *de minimis* risk associated with cancer policy?

CONCLUSIONS

Some individuals respond to chemical exposures at doses much lower or after much shorter periods of exposure than the general population. Children, pregnant women, individuals suffering from certain genetic disorders or heart and lung disease, those previously exposed, the nutritionally deficient, or those with a history of smoking are all unusually susceptible to the toxic effects of certain environmental compounds. EPA

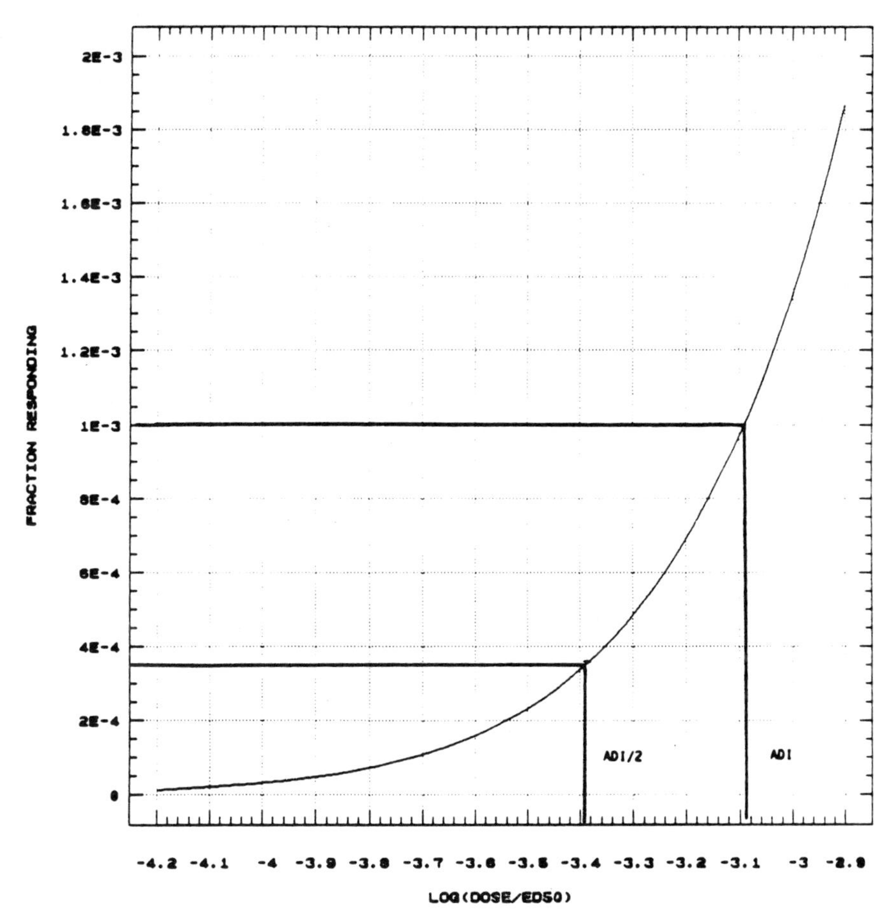

Fig. 2. Low-dose portion of a log-probit dose-response relationship. Exposure to 0.5 RfD for each of two components of a mixture yields a risk 0.7 times that of exposure to the RfD for one substance.

attempts to protect susceptible groups with RfD and HI determinations for exposure to individual chemicals and chemical mixtures, respectively.

We have discussed the RfD and HI and their associated uncertainties and illustrated the potential for their over- or underprotection of sensitive or hypersusceptible groups. Based on two hypothetical examples, we suggested that the HI approach may be overprotective for sensitive groups but underprotective for hypersusceptibles. Policy considerations for protection of sensitive groups and hypersusceptibles have also been raised. These considerations are unrelated to the scientific aspects of detection and protection of sensitive and hypersusceptible groups. The ultimate question we are faced with is: Given limited resources, what percent of individuals are we willing to underprotect?

ACKNOWLEDGMENTS

The authors wish to acknowledge Dr. Carl Schulz for his helpful comments on this manuscript.

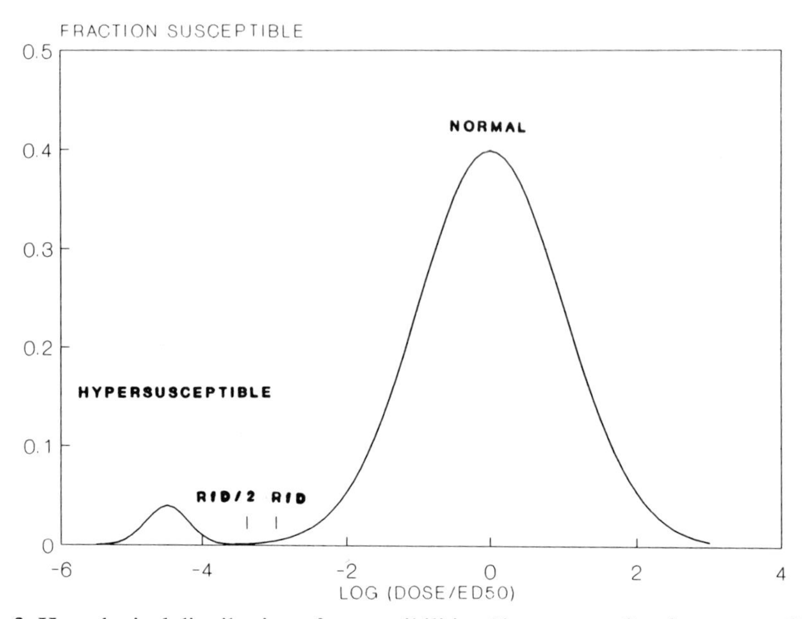

Fig. 3. Hypothetical distribution of susceptibilities (dose versus fraction susceptible).

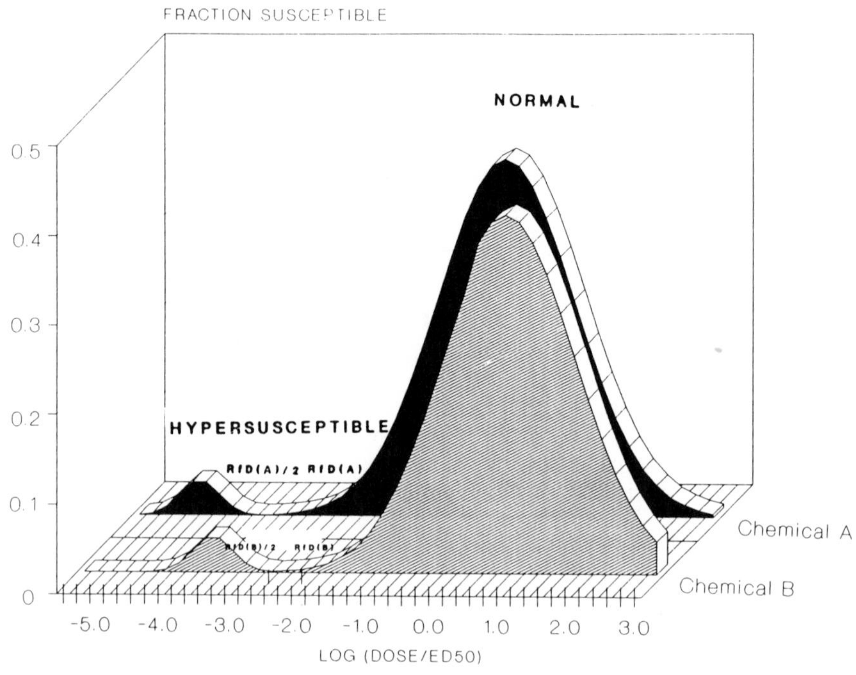

Fig. 4. Bimodal susceptibility to the toxic effects of each of two chemicals in a mixture.

REFERENCES

1. E. J. Calabrese, *Pollutants and High-Risk Groups: The Biological Basic of Increased Human Susceptibility to Environmental and Occupational Pollutants*, John Wiley and Sons, New York (1978).
2. K. R. Mahaffey, Nutritional Factors in Lead Poisoning, *Nutr. Rev.* **39**:353-362 (1981).
3. U.S. Department of Health, Education and Welfare (USHEW), The Health Consequences of Smoking, Washington, DC (1971).
4. G. L. Plaa, *Toxic Reponses of the Liver, in Toxicology: The Basic Science of Poisons*, 2nd ed., J. Doull, D. C. Klaaseen, and M. O. Amdur, eds., Macmillan Publishing Co., New York (1980).
5. E. Beutler, Glucose-6-Phosphate Dehydrogenase Deficiency, in *The Metabolic Basis of Inherited Disease*, pp. 1629-1653, J. B. Stanbury, J. B. Wyngaarden, D. S. Fredrickson, J. C. Goldstein, and M. S. Brown, eds. (1983).
6. U.S. Environmental Protection Agency (USEPA), Approaches to Risk Assessment for Mutliple Chemical Exposures, Report No. EPA-600/9-84-008 (March 1984).
7. C. S. Weil, Statistics vs Safety Factors and Scientific Judgment in the Evaluation of Safety for Man, *Toxicol. Appl. Pharmacol.* **21**:454-463 (1972).
8. M. L. Dourson and J. F. Stara, Regulatory History and Experimental Support of Uncertainty (Safety) Factors, *Reg. Tox. and Pharm.* **3**:238-244 (1983).
9. D. Hattis, L. Erdreich and M. Ballew, Human Variability to Toxic Chemicals—A Preliminary Analysis of Pharmokinetic Data from Normal Volunteers, *Risk Analysis* **7**:415-426 (1987).
10. U.S. Environmental Protection Agency (USEPA), Guidelines for the Health Risk Assessment of Chemical Mixtures, *CFR* **51(185)**:34014-34024 (1986).

Quantitative Cancer Dose-Response Modeling for All Ages

R. L. Sielken, Jr.
Sielken, Inc.
Bryan, TX

ABSTRACT

New dose-response modeling tools with expanded capabilities are emerging. Quantitative cancer dose-response modeling can reflect (1) the time-dependent progress of the biological events associated with cancer and (2) the way in which the risks of cancer change with time during the course of a lifetime. This modeling can be facilitated by a user-friendly personal computer software system called GEN.T. By explicitly considering each time in a lifetime, the cancer dose-response models can be made to reflect time- or age-dependent changes in exposure levels, pharmacokinetic processes, normal cell population sizes, proliferation of non-normal cells, cancer defense mechanisms, susceptibilities, and background dose levels. GEN.T can be used to determine the quantitative impacts on risk characterizations of these factors, their functional representations, and the use of biologically-based dose-response models, physiologically-based pharmacokinetic modeling, biologically effective doses, and interindividual (intraspecies) variation in susceptibility and background exposure. New decision-analysis-based techniques are also emerging. These techniques provide a means of considering and presenting multiple biological possibilities and a means of evaluating sources of uncertainty.

Several examples in terms of the carcinogenicity of chloroform are included.

KEYWORDS: Decision analysis, risk assessment, computer software, weight of evidence, age dependence, susceptibility, biologically effective dose, decision tree, chloroform

INTRODUCTION

The primary purpose of cancer dose-response models is to quantify the relationship between the exposure to a suspected carcinogen and the frequency and timing of occurrences of a specified carcinogenic response. It is not to answer the question "Is this chemical carcinogenic?" The older dose-response models, e.g., probit, logit, Weibull, multihit, and multistage, are overly simplistic, probabilistic representations of complex biological phenomena. They are not detailed biological models.

Overly simplistic representations of complex biological phenomena are not the answer to high-to-low-dose extrapolation. There are several examples where the older models have similar fits to the dose-response data at the experimental doses (which are

Risk Analysis, Edited by C. Zervos
Plenum Press, New York, 1991

relatively high) but yield very dissimilar risk predictions at lower doses. Extrapolations from high to low dose call for biologically-based models as do extrapolations from one exposure route to another, one exposure pattern over time to another, and one species to another.

General Tool, GEN.T, is a computer software system designed to help incorporate biologically-based dose-response extrapolation techniques into quantitative cancer risk assessments. It was developed by the author for such purposes. It is user-friendly and has been designed for IBM-compatible personal computers.

GEN.T helps incorporate time and age dependence, physiology, carcinogenic mechanism, and variation among individuals into cancer dose-response extrapolations.

Human carcinogenic effects depend on three factors: (1) the biologically effective dose, (2) the probability of a specified carcinogenic response for a given biologically effective dose, and (3) the proportions of the exposed population receiving particular biologically effective doses.

QUANTITATIVE CANCER DOSE-RESPONSE MODELING

Biologically Effective Dose

The dose scale used for dose-response modeling is critical. For instance, in inhalation studies the dose could be represented in terms of (a) the chemical's concentration in the air, (b) the amount of chemical inhaled, (c) the amount of the chemical or its active metabolite reaching the target tissue, or (d) the net amount of cancer related activity at the target site, e.g., the amount of DNA adducts formed and not repaired or the amount of cell regeneration. In general terms, these four representations correspond respectively to (a) the administered dose, (b) an intermediate dose, (c) the delivered dose, and (d) the biologically effective dose. Each representation is a better scale for dose-response modeling than its predecessor. Biologically, the most relevant measure of exposure is the biologically effective dose.

The biologically effective dose is a representation of the exposure in terms of a dose scale based on the delivered dose (e.g., a physiologically based pharmacokinetic model of the absorption, delivery, metabolism, and elimination of chemicals) as well as research on cell turnover rates, repair mechanisms, immune system responses, etc.

Administered doses can be time dependent. Even in controlled animal experiments the administered dose level may not be the same throughout the duration of the experiment. For example, in the course of the NCI[1] chloroform gavage studies on rats and mice, the exposure level (mg/kg body wt/day) was changed at least once and often twice. In the chloroform drinking water study on rats,[2] the administered dose level (mg/kg/day) was changed continually.

The delivered dose is a function of the administered dose. Which particular function depends on the chemical and the route of administration. In the simplest cases the delivered dose can be equal or proportional to the administered dose. In some other cases pharmacokinetics may imply a known mathematical relationship between the delivered dose and the administered dose. Still in other cases the only available information may be observed or pharmacokinetic model values of the delivered dose for particular values of the administered dose. Usually, the functional relationship between delivered and administered dose cannot be inferred from the tumor counts in a chronic bioassay. Rather it is determined from additional research such as physiologically-based pharmacokinetic modeling.

GEN.T accepts any of the types of descriptions illustrated in Fig. 1 of the delivered dose as a function of the administered dose.

The biologically effective dose is a function of the delivered dose. In GEN.T it is possible for the biologically effective dose to be specified by the user to be equal to the delivered dose. But GEN.T can also handle biologically effective doses determined by more complex functional relationships. Susceptibility can influence the functional relationship between the biologically effective and the delivered doses. Susceptibility can reflect the factors which either amplify or diminish the normal delivery process in some individuals. In such instances a specific individual's delivered dose would be equal to the average person's delivered dose multiplied by the individual's susceptibility. Such might be the case if "susceptibility" reflects the rate of production of a metabolite which is also the carcinogen.

Susceptibility can also reflect cell defense mechanisms, DNA repair, immune system responses, etc. These processes may make the biologically effective dose a "hockey stick" shaped function of the delivered dose. In this context susceptibility assumes the role of a "susceptibility frontier." The susceptibility frontier is the individual's dose corresponding to the transition from substantially lowered carcinogenic effectiveness to the dose region where the mechanisms resisting or suppressing carcinogenesis are overwhelmed. The user of GEN.T can specify the shape of the "hockey stick" by specifying the relationship between the biologically effective and the delivered doses for delivered doses below the susceptibility frontier (Fig. 2). Usually, the particular form of the chemical specific functional relationship between biologically effective and delivered doses (or biologically effective and administered doses) would not be inferred from the tumor counts in a chronic animal bioassay. Rather it must be determined from supplemental research such as research in cell biology, molecular biology, immunology, DNA adduct formation, etc.

Combining Time and Age Dependence, Physiology, Carcinogenic Mechanism, and Interindividual Variation Data

A graphical overview of the way GEN.T combines physiology, carcinogenic mechanism, and interindividual variation data into cancer dose-response extrapolations is given in Fig. 3. The overall process begins with consideration of the biologically effective dose in animals which depends on animal physiology, the animal delivered dose, and the role of animal susceptibility. The animal delivered dose depends on the animal administered dose, animal background dose, and possibly animal susceptibility. Background dose is the dose of the chemical received from any source other than the administered dose.

Once the biologically effective dose has been determined in animals, the observed cancer incidences in chronic animal bioassays can be compared to those doses and a dose-response model estimated based on the biologically effective dose scale.

GEN.T can utilize several forms for the individualized dose-response model relating the probability of cancer to the biologically effective dose. The user can specify an older quantal response model (probit, logit, Weibull, multihit, or multistage) or a time-to-response generalization of the multistage model (multistage-Weibull, Weibull-Weibull, Hartley-Sielken, generalized Hartley-Sielken or Armitage-Doll). The Armitage-Doll time-to-response model allows each stage in the multistage process to be explicitly considered and allows either one or two of the transition rates from stage to stage to be dependent on age and/or biologically effective dose. The user may also specify a particular form of the two-stage growth model which can include cell proliferation.[3-7]

In light of the continuing research on dose-response models and the chemical specific nature of dose-response relationships, it certainly seems appropriate for regulatory agencies to adopt a flexible perspective on dose-response modeling. The 1986 EPA *Guidelines for Carcinogen Risk Assessment*[8] takes a step in that direction when it stating: "When

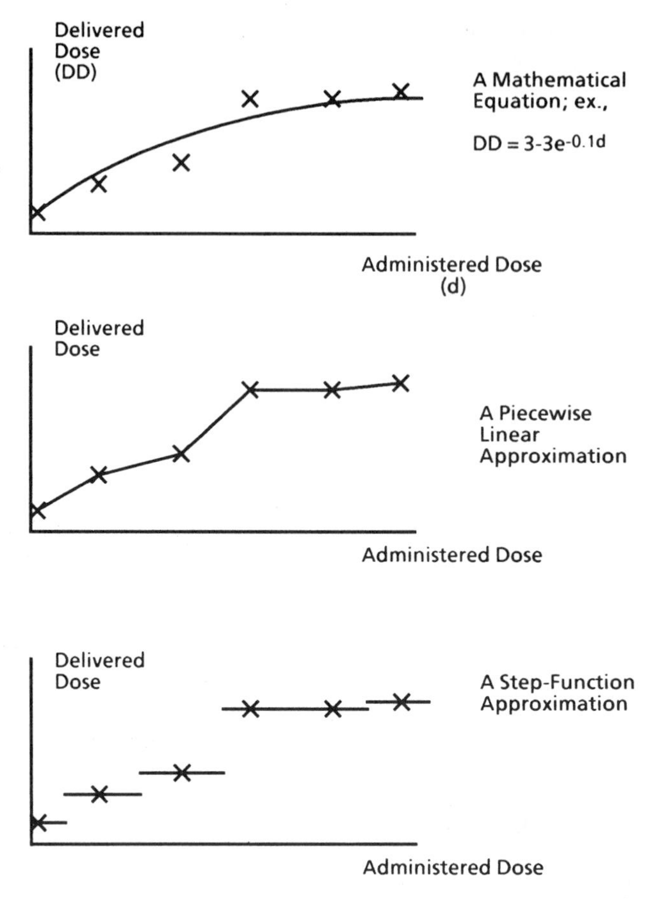

Fig. 1. GEN.T accepts any of these types of descriptions of the delivered dose as a function of the administered dose.

pharmacokinetic or metabolism data are available, or when other substantial evidence on the mechanistic aspects of the carcinogenesis process exists, a low-dose extrapolation model other than the linearized multistage procedure might be considered more appropriate on biological grounds."

Time-to-response and two-stage growth models correctly treat the cancer development as a biological process that evolves in time. For example, in the two-stage growth model the number of normal stem cells is affected by the stem cell proliferation rate which is allowed to be dependent on age and/or the biologically effective dose. The number of normal stem cells is also affected by the transition rate of normal stem cells to intermediate (initiated) cells. This transition rate can depend on age and/or the biologically effective dose. The number of intermediate cells is affected by the rate of intermediate cell proliferation and the rate of transition of intermediate cells to malignant cells. Either or both of these rates can be age and/or dose-dependent. The number of malignant cells arising per unit time determines the probability of a specified carcinogenic response by a particular time for a given biologically effective dose. The biologically effective dose is a function of administered dose, background dose, and susceptibility — all of which may be time dependent.

Because the time-to-response and growth models correspond to real biological phenomena, it is possible to identify a correspondence between a chemical's suspected

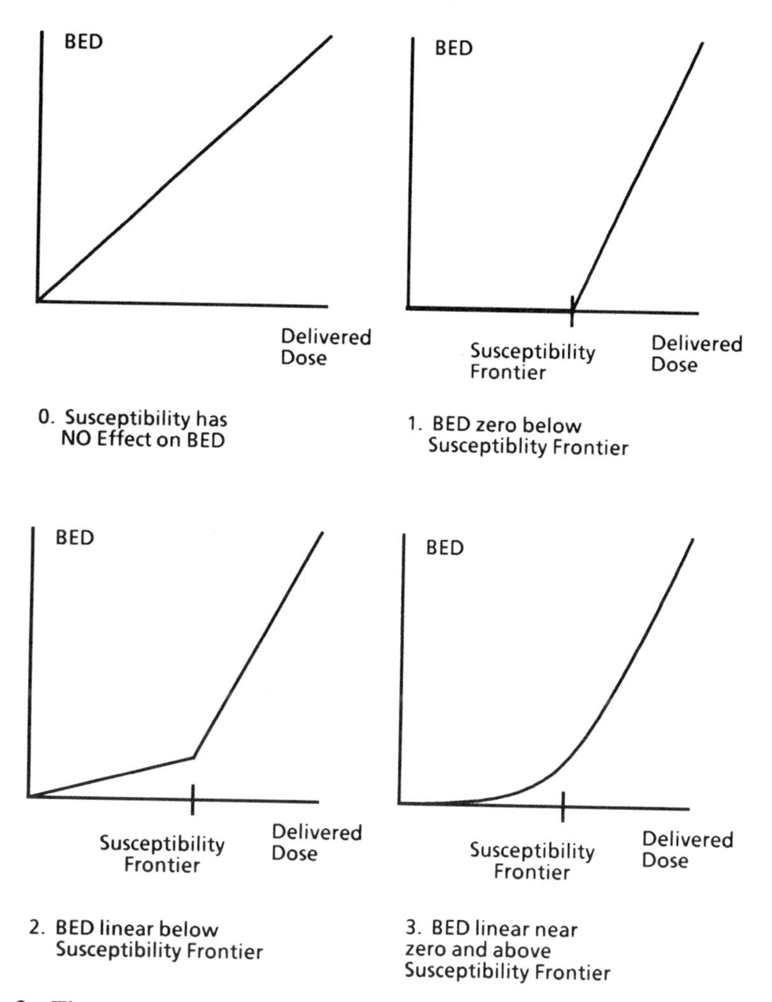

Fig. 2. The user can specify the relationship between susceptibility and the biologically effective dose (BED).

carcinogenic mechanism and the components (parameters) of the model which ought to be functions of the biologically effective dose.

Relative to older models, time-dependent models of dose-response relationships based on biologically effective rates of exposure are usually much more justified biologically. In addition, they make more extensive use of the qualitative and quantitative information gathered by biologist and toxicologist.

Extrapolation from the Experimental Situation to the Inference Situation

As noted in the EPA Guidelines,[8] interspecies extrapolation is not a simple task: "Low-dose risk estimates derived from laboratory animal data extrapolated to humans are complicated by a variety of factors that differ among species and potentially affect the response to carcinogens. Included among these factors are differences between humans and experimental test animals with respect to life span, body size, genetic variability, population homogeneity, existence of concurrent disease, pharmacokinetic effects such as metabolism and excretion patterns and the exposure regimen." Modeling with biologically defined components allows the identified differences between species, exposure routes, exposure

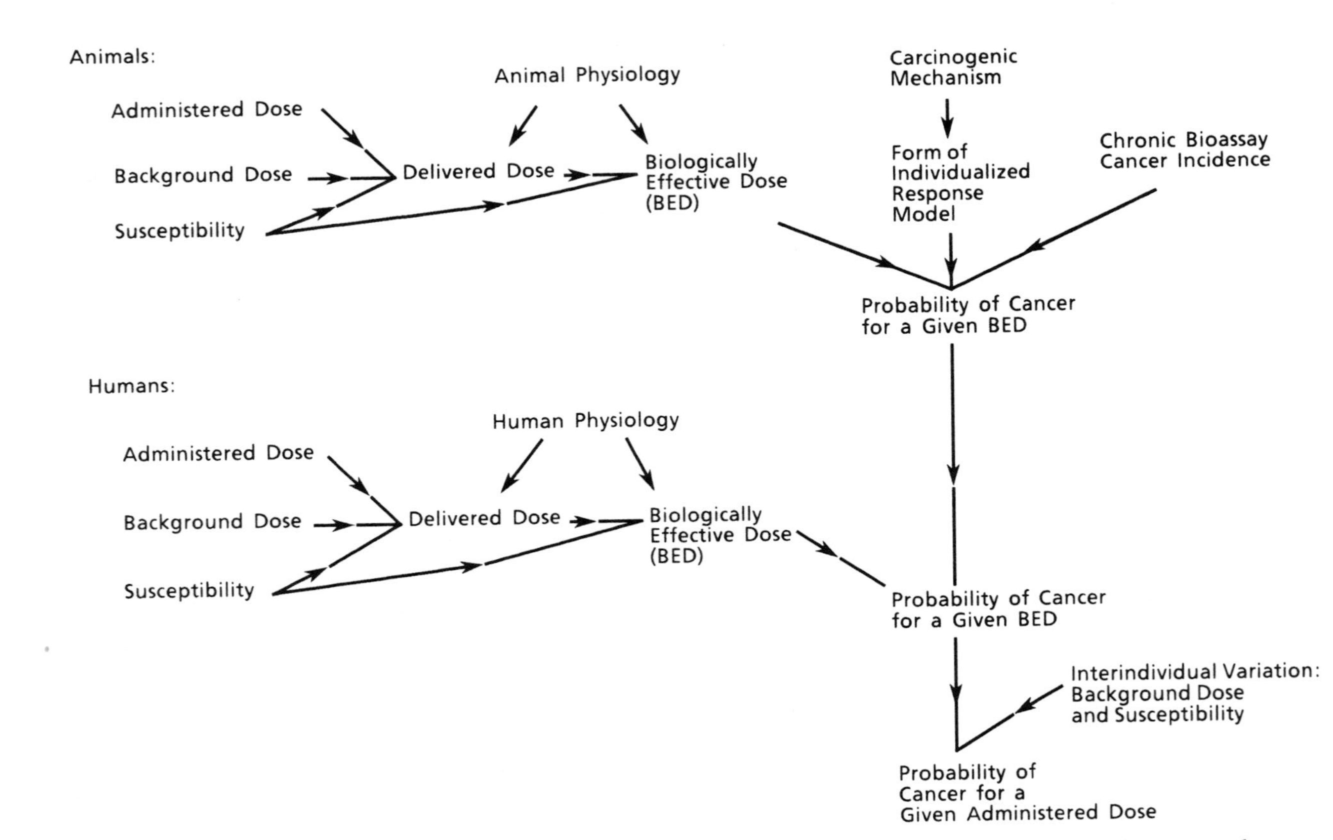

Fig. 3. Combining physiology, carcinogenic mechanism, and interindividual variation in cancer dose response extrapolations.

time frames, etc. to be explicitly incorporated into extrapolations. In particular, as shown in Fig. 3, when a prediction is to be made for humans, it is the human delivery process, and the human susceptibility (not their animal counterparts) that are used to calculate the human biologically effective dose. The human and animal biologically effective doses refer to the same biological phenomenon, e.g., DNA adduct formation, cell proliferation etc. However, the functional relationship between the biologically effective dose and its components (administered dose, background dose, and susceptibility) can be different for animals and humans. Therefore, the human biologically effective dose is determined on the basis of human evidence.

GEN.T enables the user to represent the human administered dose as an age-dependent variable instead of as a single number, e.g., a lifetime average dose. This capability is useful when, for example, soil ingestion is the route of administration in humans and the amount of such ingestion (and hence the administered dose level) is highly age-dependent. The same capability is also useful when the exposed population contains individuals whose exposures begin in different years and at different ages.

The background dose can also be age-dependent in GEN.T. This is important if secondary sources of exposure change over time.

In GEN.T the delivered dose can derive from the administered and the background doses. This would be appropriate if the two delivery processes were independent. In other cases the delivered dose can correspond to a delivery process acting on the sum of the administered dose and the background dose. This would be appropriate if the two doses were additive, i.e., delivered by the same process. The delivery processes can all be age-dependent if necessary.

GEN.T also accepts age-dependent human susceptibilities.

Once the human biologically effective dose has been quantified, the human probability of cancer can be determined by combining the human biologically effective dose with the animal-based model for the probability of cancer for given biologically effective doses. Thus, the relationship between animal cancer incidence and biologically effective dose is used to model cancer probability as a function of biologically effective dose, but the biologically effective dose entered into that model is determined from human data. Adjustments can be made to the probability model to rescale time from an animal lifespan to a human lifespan. Similar adjustments for pharmacodynamic differences are possible but their appropriateness and magnitude have been very much debated especially when well-founded biologically effective dose scales are being used.

Interindividual Variation

If individuals in an exposed population with the same administered dose do not have the same biologically effective dose because of individual differences in background dose and/or susceptibility, some additional quantitative risk assessment steps must be taken to reflect this interindividual variation. GEN.T can describe the cancer probability for individuals with specific susceptibility values and/or background dose values — for example, a median susceptibility value that exceeds 50% of the population's susceptibility values, or a high susceptibility value that exceeds 95% of the population's susceptibility values. GEN.T can also describe the average cancer risk for a group of individuals — for example, the entire population or the subpopulation of more susceptible individuals. The capability to reflect differences in background dose and susceptibility may be increasingly useful as regulatory concern shifts from hypothetical worst case situations to more realistic characterizations of the exposed population. The 1986 EPA Guidelines[8] reflect the concern for individual differences in susceptibility and background exposure: "Subpopulations with heightened susceptibility (either because of exposure or predisposition) should, when possible, be identified."

RISK QUANTIFICATIONS INCLUDING TIME

Risk can be quantified in several ways. Two chemicals can have the same probability of a specified response at a reference time late in a lifetime but have very different probabilities earlier. The mean response free period is the expected amount of time within a specified period that an individual would be free from a specified response (e.g., the number of years in a 70 year lifespan without a tumor). Such cancer free times quantify risk on the time scale and supplement "added risk" and "extra risk" calculations which quantify risk on the probability scale. The EPA Guidelines[8] suggest an openness to the use of time-to-response models, namely: "When longitudinal data on tumor development are available, time-to-tumor models may be used." Unfortunately, the use of such models to provide supplemental characterizations of risk on the time scale has not been realized.

USE OF DECISION ANALYSIS TECHNIQUES

Introduction

Risk management decisions benefit from comprehensive presentations of the available information. However, current quantitative cancer risk assessments focus on only a small portion of the available evidence. Current quantitative risk assessment procedures focus on one animal data set, one interspecies extrapolation procedure, one simplistic mathematical dose-response model, one risk dimension (frequency of cancer, ignoring age at occurrence), the most susceptible individual, one upper bound (ignoring estimates and the lower bound), and one bounding procedure.

New decision-analysis based techniques provide a means of presenting the implications of all of the available information as well as a means of identifying critical factors and directing research. Decision analysis (1) incorporates all available sources of information, (2) displays the risk quantification for each combination of possibilities, and (3) identifies the factors having the greater impact on the quantitative cancer risk assessment.

A Decision Analysis for Chloroform

The following decision analysis for chloroform exemplifies some of the decision analysis techniques and their utility. The five major components of the cancer dose-response assessment of chloroform are (1) the risk attribute, (2) the dose scale used for dose-response modeling, (3) the dose-response model, (4) the interspecies extrapolation procedure, and (5) the experimental data set. The exposure assessment combined with the dose-response assessment for risk characterization is also amenable to decision analyses but such analyses are not illustrated here.

Three risk attributes, (1) upper bound, (2) maximum likelihood estimate, and (3) lower bound, are considered for each risk description. (All bounds presented herein are based on experimental variability and the nonparametric bootstrap procedure.)

The available literature suggests three possible dose scales for dose-response modeling. The simplest possibility is (1) the administered dose scale, although it reflects no mechanistic information. More reflective measures of the biologically effective dose are (2) the amount of phosgene formation resulting from chloroform metabolism, and (3) the amount of cell regeneration caused by chloroform related cytotoxicity.

The literature suggesting that the carcinogenicity of chloroform may be related to the effects of phosgene formation includes the following information on the percentage of orally administered chloroform metabolized to carbon dioxide presumably via phosgene: (a) 85% in mice;[9] (b) 66% in rats;[9,10] and (c) 50% in humans.[11] This information suggests a biologically effective dose scale which is a species-specific percentage of the administered dose. (Changes in the percentages with the level of the administered dose could also be incorporated.)

Reitz et al.[12] reported that chloroform did not produce the type of genetic alterations associated with known genotoxic chemicals. Furthermore, they noted that carcinogenic doses of chloroform produced severe necrosis and increased cell regeneration at the sites where tumors developed in the mouse bioassays. Figure 4 indicates the observed cell regeneration data for the liver and kidney along with the corresponding fitted relationships between biologically effective dose and administered dose.

Four dose-response models are considered for use with each dose scale. The probit model corresponds to a lognormal distribution of individual cancer tolerances. The multistage model is one of the simplest mathematical representations of the multistage theory of cancer. The multistage-Weibull time-to-response model is a generalization of the multistage model which includes observations of time. The two-stage growth model is a generalization of the multistage-Weibull time-to-response model which includes the role of cell proliferation.

Three bases for interspecies extrapolation are considered. First, the dose scales used for dose-response modeling expressed on a body weight (bw) basis can be used for interspecies extrapolation of cancer probabilities. Second, Travis and White[13] found that the best regression estimate was that species had equivalent maximum tolerated doses when dose was expressed on a $(bw)^{3/4}$ basis. Finally, studies of metabolic rates within species have suggested $(bw)^{2/3}$ (i.e., approximately body surface area) as the appropriate basis for intraspecies scaling. The latter two candidates for interspecies extrapolation have arisen from studies based on administered not biologically effective dose.

Among the positive chronic animal bioassays of chloroform there are six data sets with sufficient data to perform quantitative dose-response modeling: (1) kidney adenoma or carcinoma in male Osborne-Mendel rats in the NCI[1] gavage study, (2) hepatocellular carcinoma in male B6C3F1 mice in the NCI[1] gavage study, (3) hepatocellular carcinoma in female B6C3F1 mice in the NCI[1] gavage study, (4) kidney tumors in male ICI mice in the Roe *et al.*[14] gavage study, (5) renal tubular cell adenoma or carcinoma in male Osborne-Mendel rats in the Jorgenson *et al.*[2] drinking water study, and (6) renal tubular cell adenoma or carcinoma in male Osborne-Mendel rats at the lowest three doses in the Jorgenson *et al.*[2] drinking water study.

A Decision Tree for Chloroform

The decision tree for chloroform shows the characterizations of the dose (mg/kg body wt/day) of chloroform corresponding to an added cancer probability of 1/100,000. Analogous decision trees can be constructed for other increments of risk. Alternatively, the decision tree can be expanded to include multiple measures of risk.

The chloroform decision tree has three major branches — one for each risk attribute, namely, lower bound, maximum likelihood estimate, and upper bound. The continuations of one of these three branches are shown in Fig. 5 which indicates the maximum likelihood estimates of the dose of chloroform corresponding to an added probability of 1/100,000 corresponding to every combination of possibilities for the remaining four decision factors (dose scale, dose-response model, interspecies extrapolation procedure, and experimental

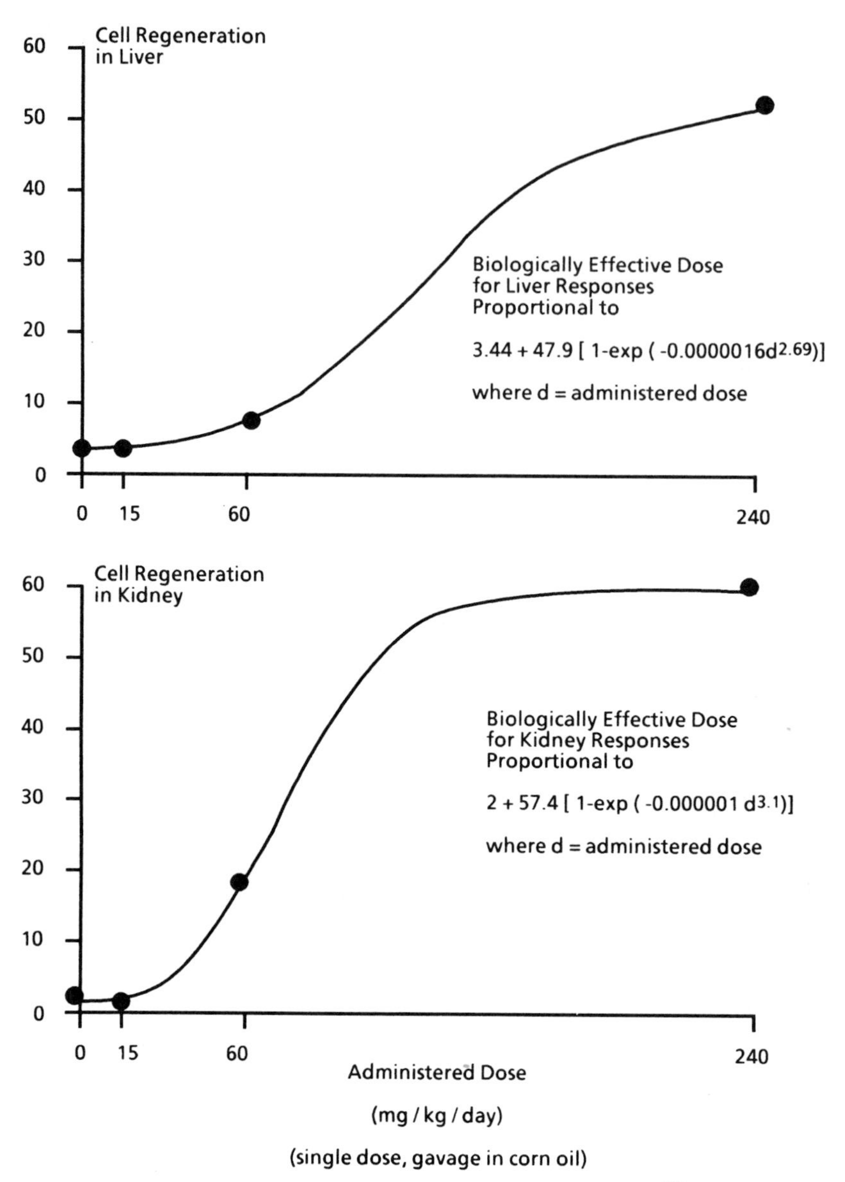

Fig. 4. Dose response data in male B6C3F1 mice.[12]

data set). The continuations of the branches for the upper and lower bounds were also evaluated but are not displayed herein.

A decision tree allows the risk manager or any concerned individual to identify the particular risk number corresponding to any specific combination of possibilities.

The relative frequencies and percentiles of the decision tree values for the dose with cancer risk increment of 1/100,000 can be determined. However, this summary may be too simplistic because not all possibilities in a decision tree are equally likely to represent the actual dose.

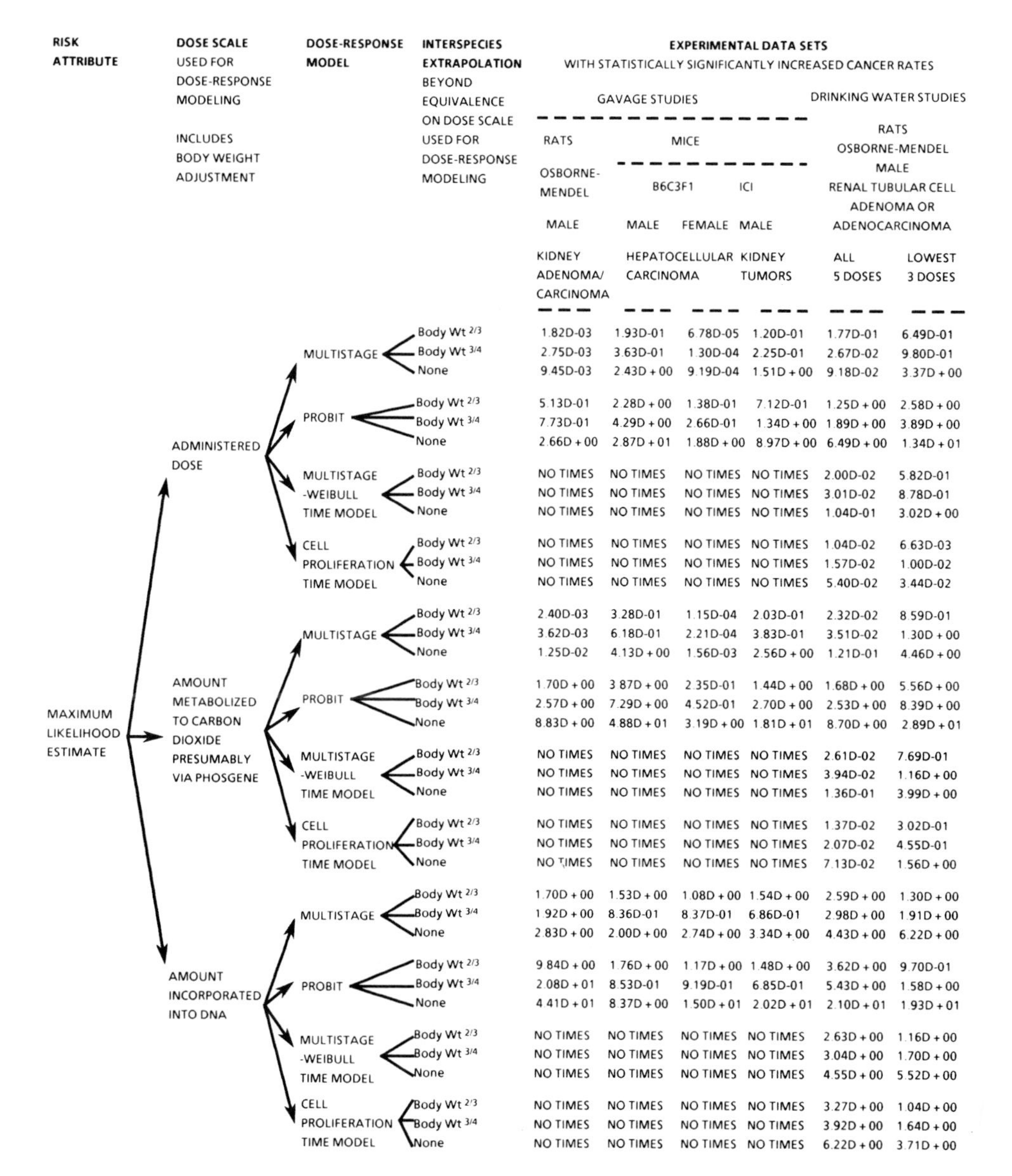

Risk attribute: MAXIMUM LIKELIHOOD ESTIMATE

EXPERIMENTAL DATA SETS WITH STATISTICALLY SIGNIFICANTLY INCREASED CANCER RATES

DOSE SCALE USED FOR DOSE-RESPONSE MODELING INCLUDES BODY WEIGHT ADJUSTMENT	DOSE-RESPONSE MODEL	INTERSPECIES EXTRAPOLATION BEYOND EQUIVALENCE ON DOSE SCALE USED FOR DOSE-RESPONSE MODELING	GAVAGE STUDIES: RATS, OSBORNE-MENDEL, MALE, KIDNEY ADENOMA/CARCINOMA	GAVAGE STUDIES: MICE, B6C3F1, MALE, HEPATOCELLULAR CARCINOMA	GAVAGE STUDIES: MICE, B6C3F1, FEMALE, HEPATOCELLULAR CARCINOMA	GAVAGE STUDIES: MICE, ICI, MALE, KIDNEY TUMORS	DRINKING WATER STUDIES: RATS, OSBORNE-MENDEL, MALE, RENAL TUBULAR CELL ADENOMA OR ADENOCARCINOMA, ALL 5 DOSES	DRINKING WATER STUDIES: RATS, OSBORNE-MENDEL, MALE, RENAL TUBULAR CELL ADENOMA OR ADENOCARCINOMA, LOWEST 3 DOSES
ADMINISTERED DOSE	MULTISTAGE	Body Wt $^{2/3}$	1.82D-03	1.93D-01	6.78D-05	1.20D-01	1.77D-01	6.49D-01
		Body Wt $^{3/4}$	2.75D-03	3.63D-01	1.30D-04	2.25D-01	2.67D-02	9.80D-01
		None	9.45D-03	2.43D+00	9.19D-04	1.51D+00	9.18D-02	3.37D+00
	PROBIT	Body Wt $^{2/3}$	5.13D-01	2.28D+00	1.38D-01	7.12D-01	1.25D+00	2.58D+00
		Body Wt $^{3/4}$	7.73D-01	4.29D+00	2.66D-01	1.34D+00	1.89D+00	3.89D+00
		None	2.66D+00	2.87D+01	1.88D+00	8.97D+00	6.49D+00	1.34D+01
	MULTISTAGE-WEIBULL TIME MODEL	Body Wt $^{2/3}$	NO TIMES	NO TIMES	NO TIMES	NO TIMES	2.00D-02	5.82D-01
		Body Wt $^{3/4}$	NO TIMES	NO TIMES	NO TIMES	NO TIMES	3.01D-02	8.78D-01
		None	NO TIMES	NO TIMES	NO TIMES	NO TIMES	1.04D-01	3.02D+00
	CELL PROLIFERATION TIME MODEL	Body Wt $^{2/3}$	NO TIMES	NO TIMES	NO TIMES	NO TIMES	1.04D-02	6.63D-03
		Body Wt $^{3/4}$	NO TIMES	NO TIMES	NO TIMES	NO TIMES	1.57D-02	1.00D-02
		None	NO TIMES	NO TIMES	NO TIMES	NO TIMES	5.40D-02	3.44D-02
AMOUNT METABOLIZED TO CARBON DIOXIDE PRESUMABLY VIA PHOSGENE	MULTISTAGE	Body Wt $^{2/3}$	2.40D-03	3.28D-01	1.15D-04	2.03D-01	2.32D-02	8.59D-01
		Body Wt $^{3/4}$	3.62D-03	6.18D-01	2.21D-04	3.83D-01	3.51D-02	1.30D+00
		None	1.25D-02	4.13D+00	1.56D-03	2.56D+00	1.21D-01	4.46D+00
	PROBIT	Body Wt $^{2/3}$	1.70D+00	3.87D+00	2.35D-01	1.44D+00	1.68D+00	5.56D+00
		Body Wt $^{3/4}$	2.57D+00	7.29D+00	4.52D-01	2.70D+00	2.53D+00	8.39D+00
		None	8.83D+00	4.88D+01	3.19D+00	1.81D+01	8.70D+00	2.89D+01
	MULTISTAGE-WEIBULL TIME MODEL	Body Wt $^{2/3}$	NO TIMES	NO TIMES	NO TIMES	NO TIMES	2.61D-02	7.69D-01
		Body Wt $^{3/4}$	NO TIMES	NO TIMES	NO TIMES	NO TIMES	3.94D-02	1.16D+00
		None	NO TIMES	NO TIMES	NO TIMES	NO TIMES	1.36D-01	3.99D+00
	CELL PROLIFERATION TIME MODEL	Body Wt $^{2/3}$	NO TIMES	NO TIMES	NO TIMES	NO TIMES	1.37D-02	3.02D-01
		Body Wt $^{3/4}$	NO TIMES	NO TIMES	NO TIMES	NO TIMES	2.07D-02	4.55D-01
		None	NO TIMES	NO TIMES	NO TIMES	NO TIMES	7.13D-02	1.56D+00
AMOUNT INCORPORATED INTO DNA	MULTISTAGE	Body Wt $^{2/3}$	1.70D+00	1.53D+00	1.08D+00	1.54D+00	2.59D+00	1.30D+00
		Body Wt $^{3/4}$	1.92D+00	8.36D-01	8.37D-01	6.86D-01	2.98D+00	1.91D+00
		None	2.83D+00	2.00D+00	2.74D+00	3.34D+00	4.43D+00	6.22D+00
	PROBIT	Body Wt $^{2/3}$	9.84D+00	1.76D+00	1.17D+00	1.48D+00	3.62D+00	9.70D-01
		Body Wt $^{3/4}$	2.08D+01	8.53D-01	9.19D-01	6.85D-01	5.43D+00	1.58D+00
		None	4.41D+01	8.37D+00	1.50D+01	2.02D+01	2.10D+01	1.93D+01
	MULTISTAGE-WEIBULL TIME MODEL	Body Wt $^{2/3}$	NO TIMES	NO TIMES	NO TIMES	NO TIMES	2.63D+00	1.16D+00
		Body Wt $^{3/4}$	NO TIMES	NO TIMES	NO TIMES	NO TIMES	3.04D+00	1.70D+00
		None	NO TIMES	NO TIMES	NO TIMES	NO TIMES	4.55D+00	5.52D+00
	CELL PROLIFERATION TIME MODEL	Body Wt $^{2/3}$	NO TIMES	NO TIMES	NO TIMES	NO TIMES	3.27D+00	1.04D+00
		Body Wt $^{3/4}$	NO TIMES	NO TIMES	NO TIMES	NO TIMES	3.92D+00	1.64D+00
		None	NO TIMES	NO TIMES	NO TIMES	NO TIMES	6.22D+00	3.71D+00

Fig. 5. Decision tree maximum likelihood estimates on the dose (mg/kg/day) of chloroform corresponding to an added cancer probability of 1/100,000.

Weighting the Decision Tree Characterizations

The characterizations in a decision tree can be weighted. The weights can reflect the scientific support for the characterizations. Although the determination of weights is not easy, weights can be determined using (1) objective measures of appropriateness (e.g., empirical or historical behavior), (2) evaluation of scientific credibility, (3) consensus evaluation, (4) expert opinions, etc. The assignment of weights should improve with experience.

The weights that have been chosen for discussion illustrate the nature and role of weights in a decision analysis of chloroform. They should still be illustrative even though they may be subjective.

The weights for the risk attributes are (1) 9/20 for the lower bound (95% lower limit on dose); (2) 9/20 for the maximum likelihood estimate; and (3) 2/20 for the upper bound (95% upper limit on dose). The total weight (1.0) is partitioned with 9/20 (45%) assigned to lower bounds, 9/20 (45%) assigned to maximum likelihood estimates, and 10% assigned to upper bounds. The weights (which always add up to 1.0) represent a division of emphasis or importance. Here lower bounds on the dose with an added cancer probability of 1/100,000 have been assigned greater emphasis because of their protective nature. The maximum likelihood estimates have been assigned equal emphasis because of their role as the most accurate estimate of the actual characteristic. The upper bounds on the dose have been assigned substantially less weight.

The weight for each attribute is subdivided among the possibilities for the other components in the cancer dose-response assessment. The weight given to an attribute is subdivided among the dose scales used in dose-response modeling with (1) 1/6 (17%) for using the administered dose scale; (2) 2/6 (33%) for using the amount of phosgene formation (i.e., the amount of chloroform metabolized to C02 presumably via phosgene); and (3) 3/6 (50%) for using the amount of cell regeneration (measured by the amount of radioactivity incorporated into DNA). Here, the weight is partitioned with greater weight being assigned to more biologically relevant dose scales.

The subdivision of emphasis among the dose-response models used for high-to-low-dose extrapolation is (1) 2/20 for the probit quantal response model; (2) 5/20 for the multistage quantal response model with at most three stages; (3) 6/20 for the multistage-Weibull time-to-response model with at most three stages; and (4) 7/20 for the cell-proliferation-based two-stage growth model where the model parameters are independent of time but the normal stem cell proliferation rate is dose dependent. The models founded on the multistage theory of cancer (2)-(4) have each been assigned greater weight than the probit model which is representative of the tolerance-based models. As the representations of the multistage theory of cancer include more information like time-to-response ((2) and (3)) and cell proliferation (3), they have received slightly greater weight.

The EPA Guidelines[8] imply that "If data and procedures become available, the Agency will provide 'most likely' or 'best' estimates of risk." The determination of such estimates calls not only for finding a model's best estimate but also for a measure of the appropriateness of the type of model. By weighting the dose-response models, the corresponding model maximum likelihood estimates (and bounds) have weights reflecting the probability that the underlying model is appropriate.

The partitioning of the emphasis by the method used for interspecies extrapolation need not necessarily be the same for all dose scales. In fact, as the dose scale incorporates more of the differences between species the remaining differences will be less. When the administered dose is the dose scale used for dose-response modeling, the weight is divided equally with (1) 4/12 for body weight equivalence, (2) 4/12 for $(bw)^{3/4}$ equivalence, and (3) 4/12 for $(bw)^{2/3}$ (i.e., surface area) equivalence. When the species differences in phosgene formation are accounted for and the dose scale used for dose-response modeling is the amount of phosgene formation, the weight is divided with (1) 8/12 for no further species extrapolation, (2) 2/12 for additional species extrapolation using $(bw)^{3/4}$ equivalence, and (3) 2/12 for additional species extrapolation using $(bw)^{2/3}$ equivalence. When cell regeneration is the basis for a more explicit biologically effective dose scale, the weight is divided with (1) 10/12 for no additional species extrapolation, (2) 1/12 for additional species extrapolation using $(bw)^{3/4}$ equivalence, and (3) 1/12 for additional species extrapolation using $(bw)^{2/3}$ equivalence.

The subdivision of emphasis among the experimental data sets gives almost all of the weight to the rodent studies; i.e., (1) 4/9 for mice, (2) 4/9 for rats, and (3) 1/9 for dogs. Each strain within a species receives equal weight as does each sex. Because of its greater similarity to the route of human exposure, a drinking water study gets twice the weight of an oral gavage study. Studies which are positive for carcinogenicity receive twice the weight of negative studies. (The weight for the Eschenbrenner and Miller[15] positive study on Strain A mice and the weight for the Rudali[16] positive study on NLC mice were transferred to the studies on B6C3F1 and ICI mice respectively because the former study reports lacked sufficient details for quantitative analysis.) The weights assigned to the chloroform experimental data sets are (1) 3/54 for kidney adenoma or carcinoma in male Osborne-Mendel rats in the NCI[1] gavage study, (2) 3/54 for hepatocellular carcinoma in male B6C3F1 mice in the NCI[1] gavage study, (3) 3/54 for hepatocellular carcinoma in female B6C3F1 mice in the NCI[1] gavage study, (4) 5/54 for kidney tumors in male ICI mice in the Roe *et al.*[14] gavage study, (5) 6/54 for renal tubular cell adenoma or carcinoma in male Osborne-Mendel rats in the Jorgenson et al.[2] drinking water study, and (6) a combined total of 34/54 for all of the negative studies (i.e., negative for a particular sex, strain, or species).

To display the emphasis corresponding to each particular dose characterization in the decision tree, the decision tree can be redrawn with the dose characterizations in Figs. 6 and 7 replaced by their respective weights. For example, in Fig. 6 the maximum likelihood estimate of the dose of chloroform corresponding to an added cancer probability of 1/100,000 is 0.136 when modeling is based on phosgene formation, the dose-response model is the multistage-Weibull model, no additional interspecies extrapolation is done, and the experimental data set corresponds to renal tubular cell adenoma or adenocarcinoma in male Osborne-Mendel rats at all 5 doses in the Jorgenson *et al.*[2] drinking water study. The weight of emphasis for this dose characterization is $(9/20) \times (2/6) \times (6/20) \times (4/6) \times (2/54) = 0.00111$ where (1) 9/20 is for the risk attribute being a maximum likelihood estimate, (2) 2/6 is for the dose scale used for dose-response modeling being based on phosgene formation, (3) 6/20 is for the dose-response model being the multistage-Weibull model, (4) 4/6 is for no additional interspecies extrapolation, and (5) 2/54 is for the experimental data set being renal tubular cell adenoma or adenocarcinoma in male Osborne-Mendel rats at all 5 doses in the Jorgenson *et al.*[2] drinking water study. The weight actually assigned to this dose characterization is 0.00204 which is 0.00111×1.84. If the time-to-response information had been available for the gavage studies, then there would have been no "unavailable" dose characterizations (e.g., "NO TIMES" in Fig. 5) and the above weight would have been 0.00111. These "unavailable" dose characterizations would have had approximately 45.5% of the total weight corresponding to the positive studies and each risk attribute. The weights for the "available" dose characterizations are amplified to preserve the total weight for the positive studies and each risk attribute. The 1.84 is the appropriate amplification factor because $100\% = (100\% - 45.5\%) \times 1.84$.

Analyzing a Weighted Decision Tree

A good summary of the weight of evidence concerning the dose of chloroform corresponding to an added cancer risk of 1/100,000 is the weighted frequencies of the decision tree values for this dose. Figure 6 shows the distribution of the weighted decision tree values. For example, only 3.1% (i.e., 0.2% + 0.7% + 2.2%) of the weight is on doses less than 0.01 mg/kg/day, 11.5% of the weight is on doses less than 1.0 mg/kg/day, and 63% of the weight is on data sets suggesting no significantly increased cancer risk at tested doses. The location of the percentiles of the weight of evidence is also shown; for example, 25% of the weight of evidence is on dose values less than approximately 4 mg/kg/day. Although single number summaries of risk are always less informative than more complete summaries, a single number such as a percentile from a weight-of-evidence analysis may provide a better basis for comparing chemicals than single numbers derived otherwise.

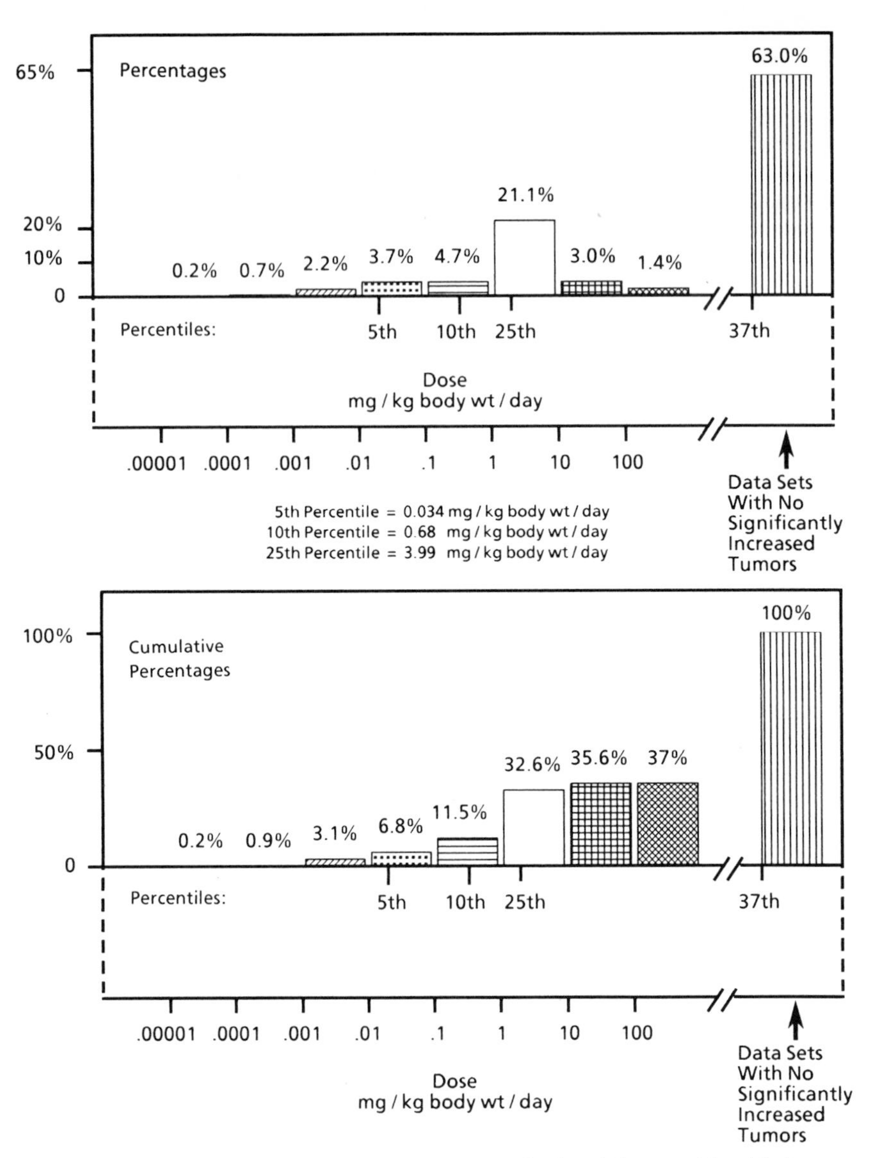

Fig. 6. Weighted frequencies of decision tree calculated doses with added cancer risk of 1/100,000.

The weight of evidence from only the positive carcinogenicity studies can also be summarized (Fig. 7). The dose characterization from these studies had a total of 37% of the weight. Of this 37% weight (1) 57% was on dose values between 1 and 10 mg/kg/day, (2) 95% was on dose values less than 44 mg/kg/day, (3) 50% was on dose values less than 2.7 mg/kg/day, (4) 10% was on dose values less than 0.01 mg/kg/day, and (5) 5% was on dose values less than 0.003 mg/kg/day.

The need to understand the uncertainty in quantitative cancer risk assessments is clearly reflected in the EPA Guidelines[8]: "An attempt should be made to assess the level of uncertainty... in a cancer risk assessment. This measure of uncertainty should be included in the risk characterization in order to provide the decisionmaker with a clear understanding of the impact of this uncertainty on any final quantitative risk estimate." The assessment of

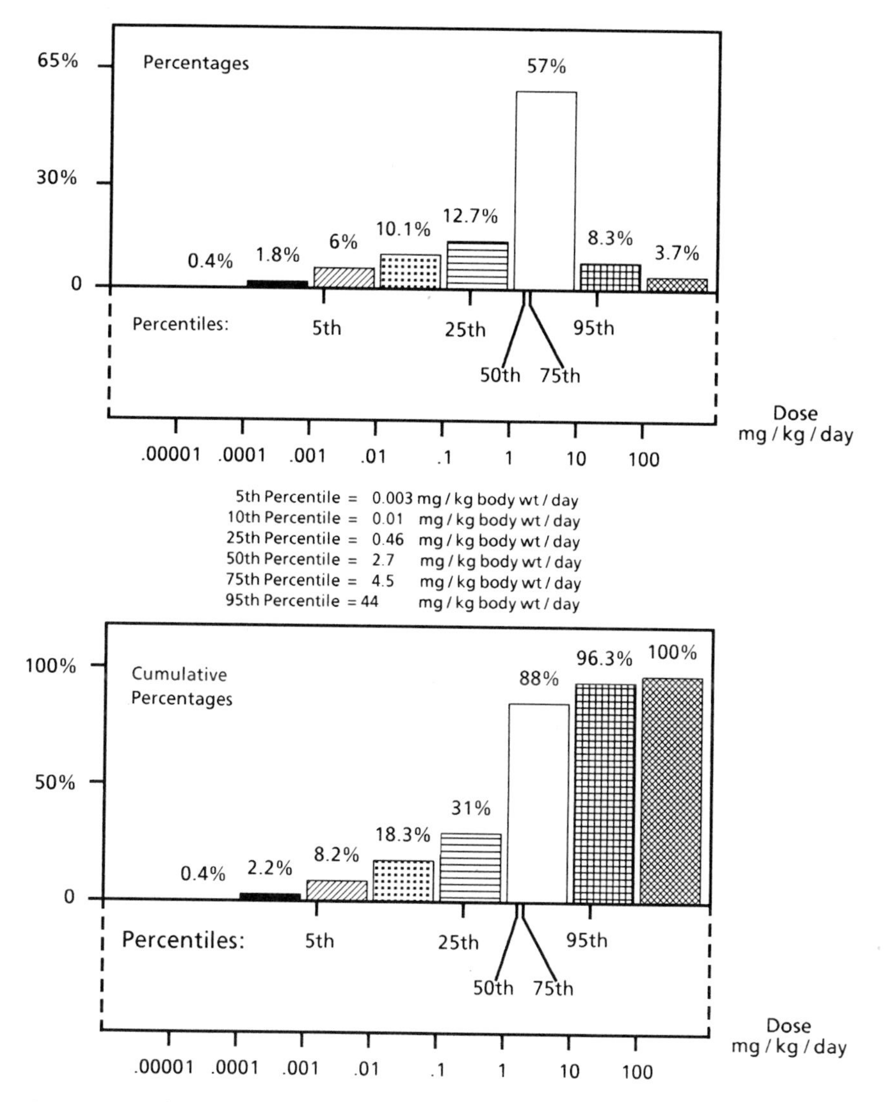

Fig. 7. Weighted frequencies of decision tree dose with added cancer risk of 1/100,000: percentages and percentiles among calculated doses for experimental data sets with significantly increased tumors.

this uncertainty is the objective of a decision analysis and its associated decision trees (e.g., Fig. 5) and weight of evidence evaluations (e.g., Figs. 6 and 7).

Relative Impacts of Different Components in a Decision

The decision analysis for chloroform includes five major components (1) risk attribute, (2) dose scale used for dose-response modeling, (3) dose-response model, (4) interspecies extrapolation, and (5) experimental data set. The relative impacts of the different possibilities within each of these components can be evaluated. Figures 8-12 illustrate such evaluations. For example, Fig. 9 indicates the weighted frequencies (distribution) in the decision tree of the dose (mg/kg/day) corresponding to an added cancer risk of 1/100,000 when each of the three possibilities for the dose scale is used for dose-response modeling. The distributions show the proportion of weight associated with dose

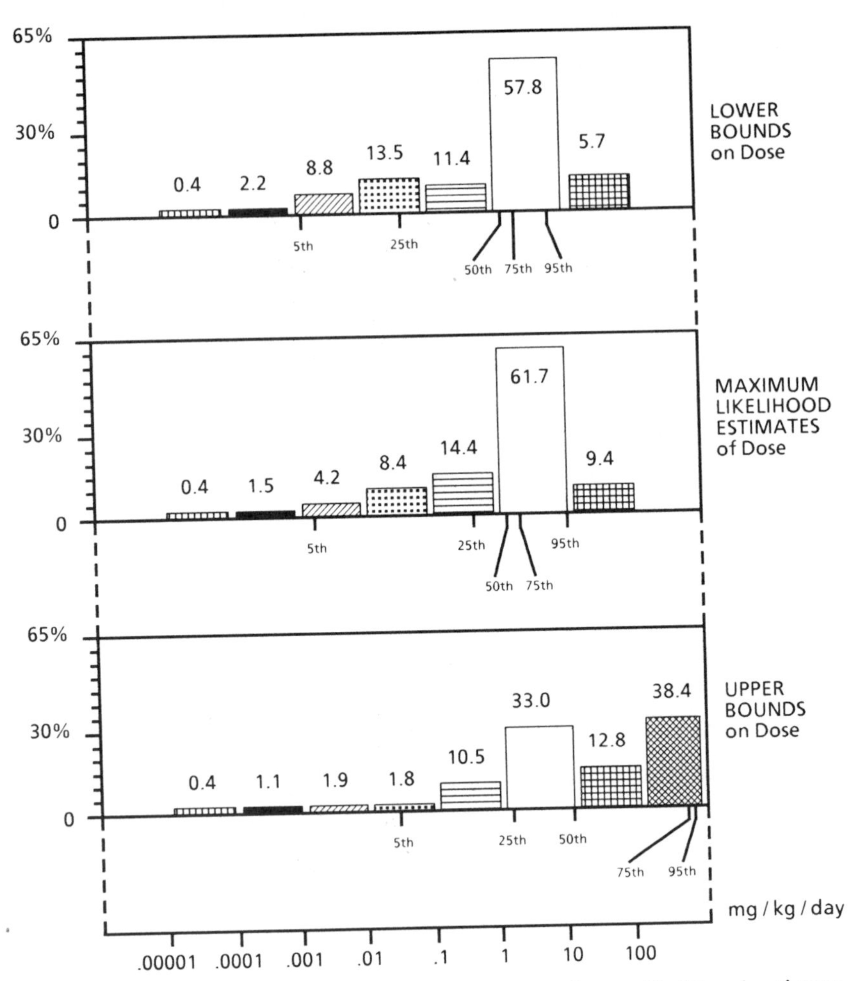

Fig. 8. Impact of risk attribute (lower bound, maximum likelihood estimate, upper bound) on calculation of dose with added cancer risk of 1/100,000.

values in specified intervals when only the positive carcinogenicity studies are considered. The significant differences between these three distributions indicate that the dose scale used for dose-response modeling has a substantial influence on the value obtained for the dose corresponding to an added cancer risk of 1/100,000. Knowledge of the relative impacts of the different components in a decision tree can help prioritize and direct research. For instance, research on the biologically effective dose scale for chloroform should receive a high priority.

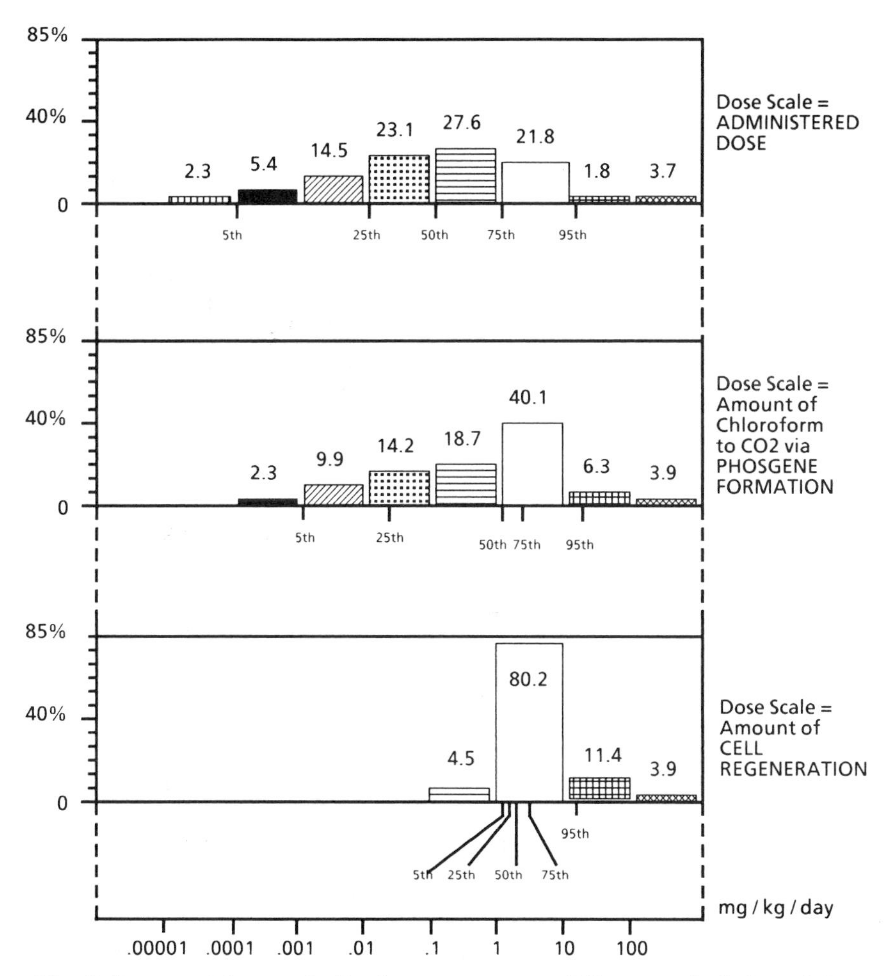

Fig. 9. Impact of dose scale for dose response modeling on calculation of dose with added cancer risk of 1/100,000.

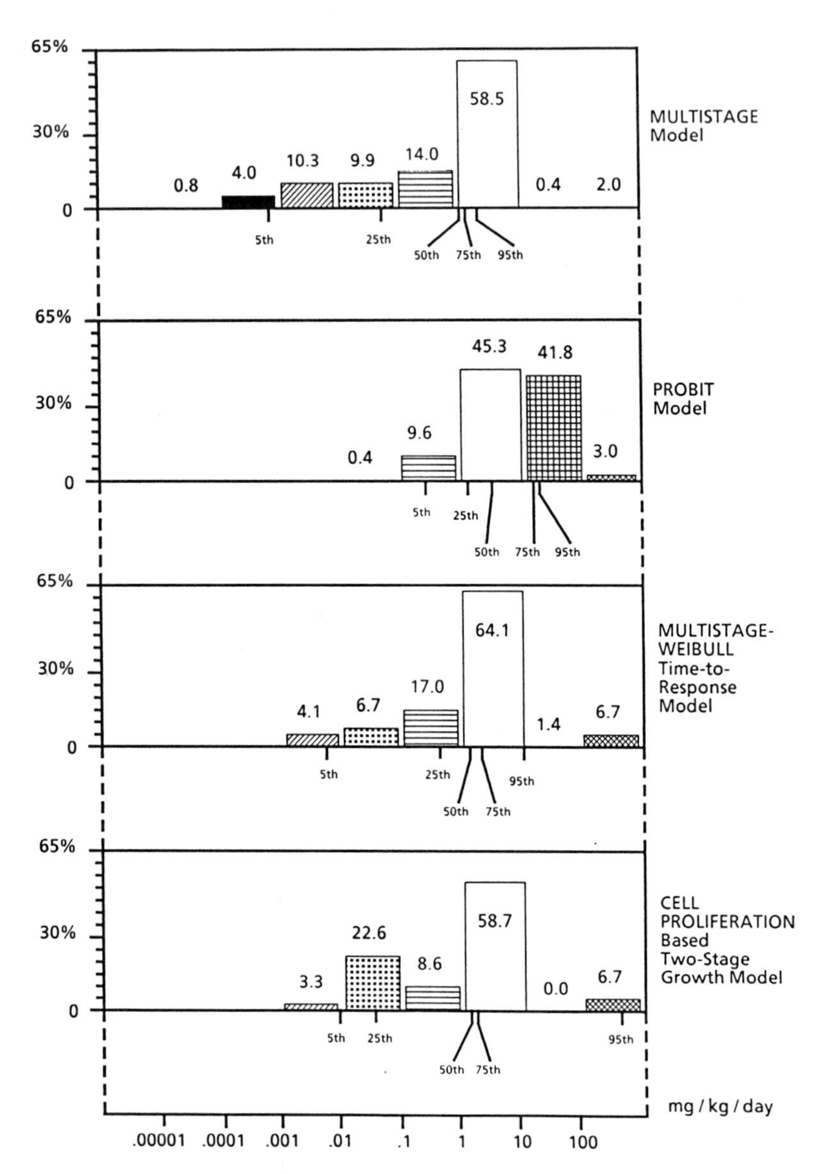

Fig. 10. Impact of dose response model on calculation of dose with added cancer risk of 1/100,000.

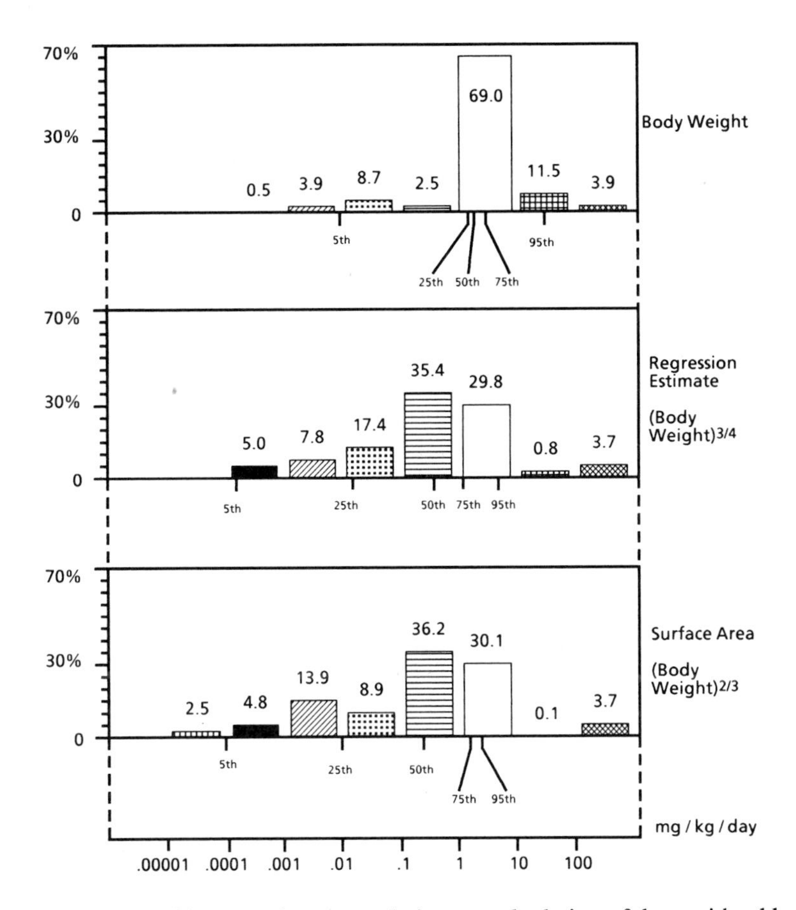

Fig. 11. Impact of interspecies extrapolation on calculation of dose with added cancer risk of 1/100,000.

REMARKS

Any reasonable evaluation or sensitivity analysis of the risk in an actual exposure situation ought to include the uncertainty in the techniques used to quantify the cancer risk. There are several sources of uncertainty in a quantitative cancer risk assessment. Decision analysis based techniques provide a means of identifying and presenting the uncertainty in cancer risk assessments and a means of identifying alternative or supplemental measures of cancer risk.

The new dose-response modeling tools and new decision-analysis-based techniques of presenting quantitative cancer risk assessments should encourage greater utilization of scientific information, stimulate and direct increased scientific research, and promote better decision making.

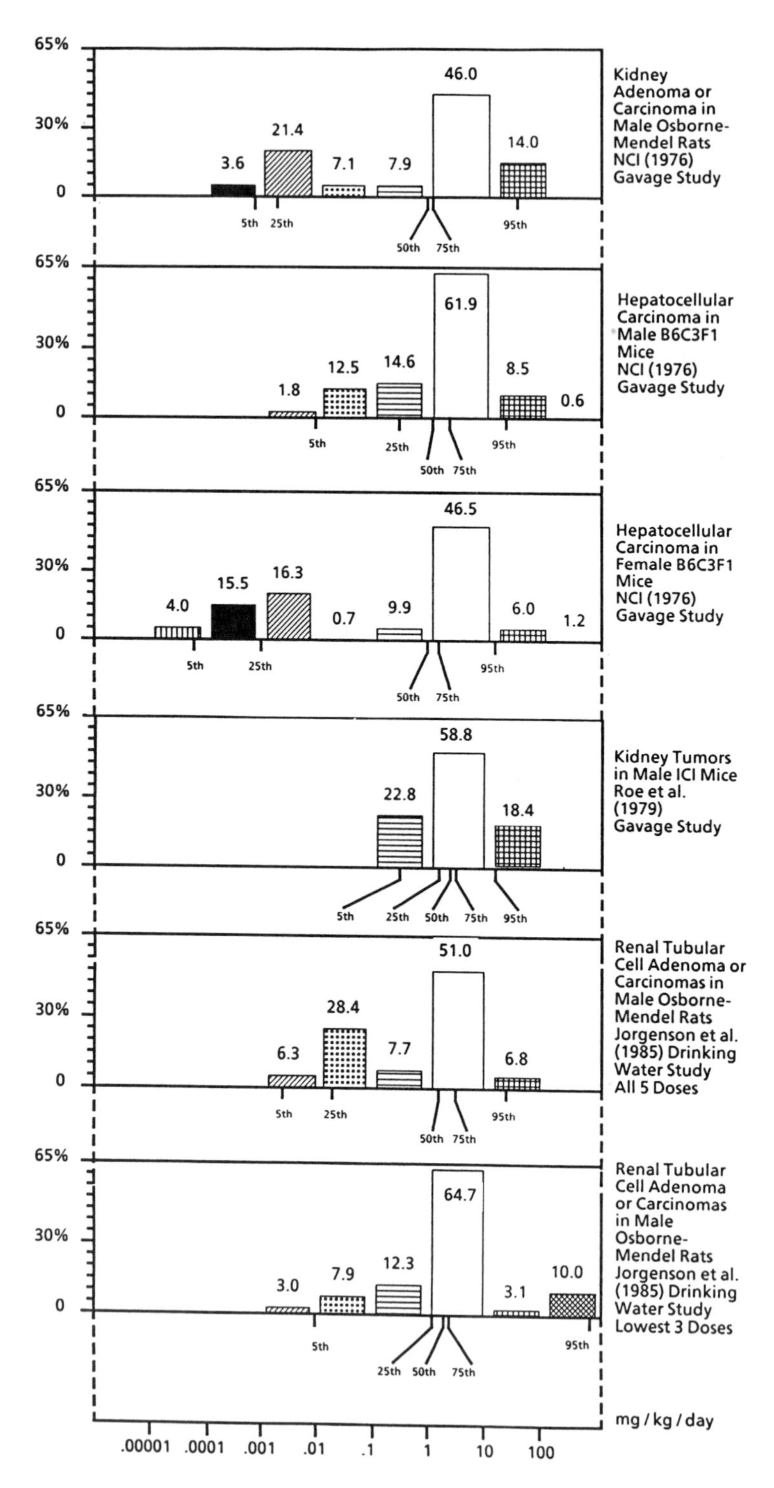

Fig. 12. Impact of experimental data set on calculation of dose with added cancer risk of 1/100,000.

REFERENCES

1. NCI (National Cancer Institute), Report on Carcinogenesis Bioassay of Chloroform, NTIS PB-264018 (1976).
2. T. A. Jorgenson, E. F. Meierhenry, C. J. Rushbrook *et al.*, Carcinogenicity of Chloroform in Drinking Water to Male Osborne-Mendel Rats and Female B6C3F1 Mice, *Fund. Appl. Toxicol.* **5(4)**:760-769 (1985).
3. S. H. Moolgavkar and D. J. Venzon, Two-Event Models for Carcinogenesis: Incidence Curves for Childhood and Adult Tumors, *Math. Biosci.* **47**:55-77 (1979).
4. S. H. Moolgavkar and A. G. Knudson, Jr., Mutation and Cancer: A Model for Human Carcinogenesis, *JNCI* **66**:1037-1052 (1981).
5. S. H. Moolgavkar, A. Dewanji, and D. J. Venzon, A Stochastic Two-Stage Model for Cancer Risk Assessment I: The Hazard Function and the Probability of Tumor, *Risk Analysis* **8(3)**:383-392 (1988).
6. L. B. Ellwein and S. M. Cohen, A Cellular Dynamics Model of Experimental Bladder Cancer: Analysis of Sodium Saccharin in the Rat, *Risk Analysis* **8**:215-221 (1988).
7. T. W. Thorslund, C. C. Brown, and G. Charnley, Biologically Motivated Cancer Risk Models, *Risk Analysis* **7**:109-119 (1987).
8. U.S. Environmental Protection Agency, Guidelines for Carcinogen Risk Assessment, *Federal Register* **51**:33992-34054 (1986).
9. D. M. Brown, P. F. Langley, D. Smith, and D. C. Taylor, Metabolism of Chloroform: I. The Metabolism of [14C] Chloroform by Different Species, *Xenobiotica* **3**:151-163 (1974).
10. E. S. Reynolds, R. J. Treinen, H. H. Farrish, and M. T. Moslen, Metabolism of [14C] Carbon Tetrachloride to Exhaled, Excreted and Bound Metabolites, *Biochemical Pharmacology* **33**:3363-3374 (1984).
11. B. J. Fry, T. Taylor, and D. F. Hathway, Pulmonary Elimination of Chloroform and Its Metabolite in Man, *Arch. Int. Pharmacodyn.* **196**:98-111 (1972).
12. R. H. Reitz, T. R. Fox, and J. F. Quast, Mechanistic Considerations for Carcinogenic Risk Estimation: Chloroform, *Environmental Health Perspectives* **46**:163-168 (1982).
13. C. C. Travis and R. K. White, Interspecific Scaling of Toxicity Data, *Risk Analysis* **8**:119-125 (1988).
14. F. J. C. Roe, A. A. K. Palmer, A. N. Worden, and N. J. Van Abbe, Safety Evaluation of Toothpaste Containing Chloroform: I. Long-Term Studies in Mice, *J. Environ. Toxicol.* **2**:799-819 (1979).
15. A. B. Eschenbrenner and E. Miller, Induction of Hepatomas in Mice by Repeated Oral Administration of Chloroform with Observations on Sex Differences, *JNCI* **5**:251-255 (1945a).
16. G. Rudali, Oncogenic Activity of Some Halogenated Hydrocarbons Used in Therapeutics, *UICC Monogr. Ser.* **7**:138-143 (1967).

Critical Item Ranking for the Space Shuttle Main Engine

Kurt Reinhardt
Rockwell International
Canoga Park, CA

ABSTRACT

After the Challenger tragedy, industry has performed intensive reanalysis of the space shuttle's Failure Modes and Effects Analysis. As a result of this effort, the associated Critical Items List for the space shuttle main engine has grown from fifty items to more than five hundred. Clearly, some type of prioritization was warranted to direct management attention to those items of greatest concern and aid them in allocating resources to address these items. Lack of data has made a pure probabilistic analysis unfeasible. This paper discusses the semi-quantitative analytical method used to ordinally rank the critical items. The approach uses a hierarchy of technical and failure history questions to generate a point score which, in turn, is used to rank the critical items. Results of these methods were compared with a delphi-style survey of in-house engineering experts. Spearman ranking correlation analysis was used to assess the agreement between the analytical method and the consensus of expert opinion. Some ties were encountered when the ranking was performed; this paper also discusses the three different methods considered for resolution of ties, and which method was finally selected.

KEYWORDS: Ranking, ordinal, space shuttle, prioritization, critical item, failure mode

INTRODUCTION

After the Challenger tragedy, Rocketdyne, the maker of the space shuttle main engine (SSME), issued a major revision to its Failure Mode and Effects Analysis and Critical Items List (FMEA/CIL). This revision increased the number of Critical Items for the SSME from less than one hundred to nearly five hundred. While more complete, this increase also had the effect of diminishing the attention paid to any one Critical Item. Since the purpose of the Critical Items List is to direct management attention to certain key failure modes, and to focus inspection and engineering efforts on those items which present the greatest potential hazards to mission safety, it seemed appropriate to devise a method for ranking the more than four hundred items. This would enhance management ability to optimize resources in addressing potential risks. This paper is an explanation of that ranking method and also describes a study comparing the method to a delphi-style survey.

Risk Analysis, Edited by C. Zervos
Plenum Press, New York, 1991

METHODOLOGY

Because of the unique and complex nature of the SSME, quantitative estimates of probabilities associated with many failure modes had such large uncertainties as to make them practically useless.

For this reason, the method employed for ranking Critical Items is semi-quantitative. It does not use theoretical or empirical probabilities to characterize risk, but instead tallies points from a questionnaire based on factors which influence failure initiation, propagation, consequence, and prevention.

The method ranks items on an ordinal scale, in contrast to a nominal, cardinal, or ratio scale. In plain terms, the method puts things in order of concern, but does not make any claim on the relative magnitude of adjacent items, or allow algebraic operations on ranked items, e.g., it cannot be said that an item ranked tenth is twice the concern of an item ranked twentieth.

To best understand how the system works, a simple analogy may be considered first. There is a carnival game in which a marble is dropped over an array of pins, and as the marble falls, it bounces off the pins and ultimately lands in a box, which corresponds to a prize (see Fig. 1).

In this analogy, the marble is a CIL Item, which passes through a hierarchy of questions (rows of pins) and lands in a box (final ranking).

By careful arrangement of the questions, we can ensure that the right-most box indicates the item of greatest concern, the box second from the right is of 2nd most concern, and so on.

This careful arrangement is accomplished by doing two things: putting the most important classes of questions in the top rows and having a negative response indicated by a turn to the right. In our case, we have determined four classes of questions:

1. worst case severity;
2. likelihood of initiation;
3. likelihood of propagation to worst case; and
4. protection.

This arrangement is shown schematically in Fig. 2.

It can be readily seen that if we have the most important class of question in the first row (severity of effect) and the second most important class of question (likelihood of initiation) in the second row, and so on, and if we answer in the negative (worst situation) for all questions, we will wind up in the right most bottom box, which would be the item of greatest concern. Similarly, if we responded in the positive at each level we would wind up in the left-most box in the bottom row. This would be the most benign situation possible. In most cases, responses are a mixture of positive and negative, resulting in the item being classified to one of the middle boxes.

The schematic shown in Fig. 2 is an illustrative simplification of the structure actually employed for ranking. In the actual system, there are five choices for severity of effect, three choices to characterize likelihood of propagation, three choices to characterize likelihood of initiation and seven types of protection responses. This results in a total of three hundred and fifteen possible final outcomes, or ranks. Figure 3 illustrates this scheme.

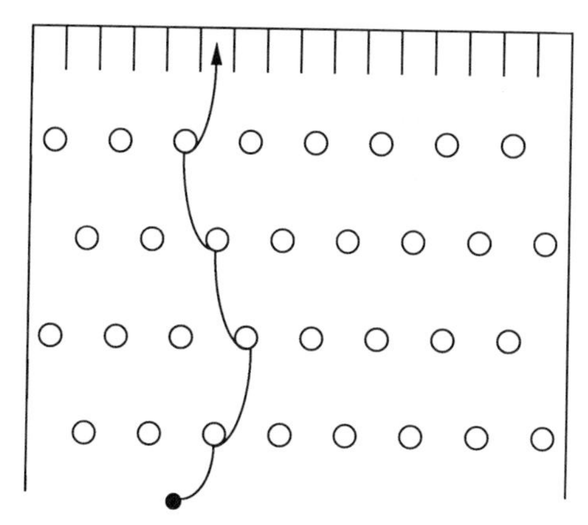

Fig. 1. Carnival game analogy.

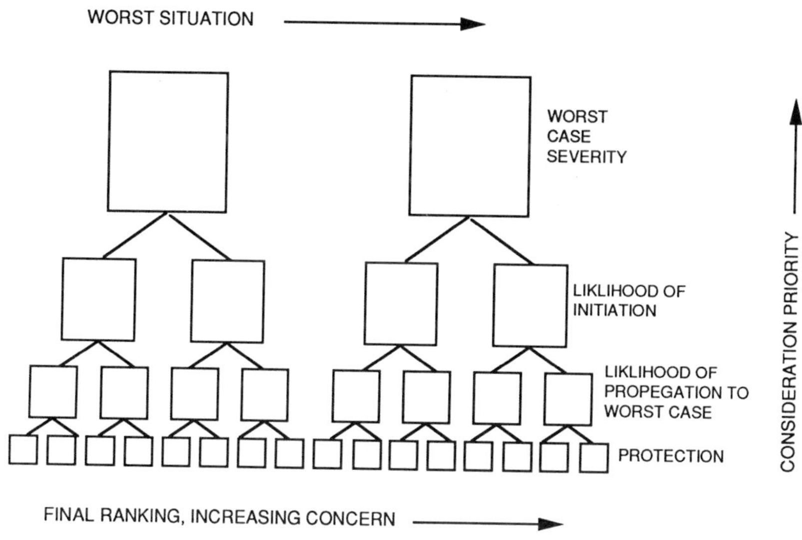

Fig. 2. Schematic representation of question hierarchy.

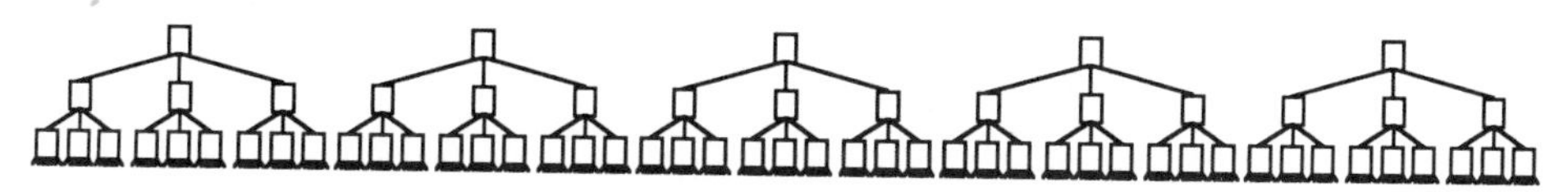

Fig. 3. Actual response options at hierarchy levels.

The choice of which response to give at each level is made by answering a questionnaire containing questions associated with issues at each level. These questionnaires appear in Appendix 1. Appendix 2 contains the ground rules established to aid in filling out the questionnaire.

Rather than arrive at the "Ranking Box" graphically each time, a formula was empirically derived to determine the ranking directly from questionnaire responses. In applying this formula, a point total is accumulated: the higher the total, the higher the level of concern. For example, heat exchanger rupture (FMEA item A150-01) accumulated 314 points and was ranked as being the CIL Item of greatest concern. This formula and example calculation is shown in Fig. 4.

Inherent in this method, as it has been presented, is the possibility of items tying for an ordinal ranking score, just as several marbles might fall in the same box in the carnival game. This is an expected and acceptable outcome. However, some benefit may be gained by applying an even finer level of discrimination, and a tie breaking method was established. This tie breaker further refines the list so that a ranking, from one to four hundred and seventeen with no ties can be listed.

EVALUATION OF THE METHOD

After development of the ranking method, it became desirable to evaluate the results, so that any necessary modifications to the method could be made. The obvious difficulty, of course, was lack of an objective standard by which to evaluate. Individuals differ in their beliefs of which items are of most concern.

Ultimately, a consensus of expert opinion was determined to be the best yardstick for comparison. Before the ranking of all items was completed, a small sample of eighteen critical items was randomly selected from a larger list of all combustion devices and turbomachinery CIL items. This list was sent under a cover letter to technical staff and management possessing in-depth knowledge of the engine system. They were asked to intuitively rank the items in order of concern. Their ranking responses formed a basis of comparison to the analytical method.

SUMMARY

By averaging the individual ranking of each respondent, a consensus ranking by the respondents was arrived at as follows:

CIL Item	Failure Mode
B400-03	HPOTP turbine blade structural failure
A150-01	HEX coil fracture/leakage
B200-22	HPFTP fuel leakage past lift-off seal
A700-04	OX preburner non-uniform fuel flow in inspection element
B200-23	HPFTP loss of balancing capability
B200-14	HPFTP fragmentation of volute liner
B200-03	HPFTP turbine bearing support bellows failure
B200-18	HPFTP loss of coolant to turbine inlet struts and turbine bearing support bellows
A200-03	Main injector blockage of one ASI passage
A330-03	MCC internal rupture at MCC/nozzle interface
A200-09	Main injector interpropellant plate cracks
A340-01	Nozzle, multiple internal tube fuel leaks
B200-01	HPFTP leakage past preburner G-5 seal
A050-01	Powerhead liner failure
B200-09	HPFTP pressure drop/flow distortion impellar
A600-01	Fuel preburner ASI fails to ignite
A330-05	MCC lee JGT blocked
B400-11	HPOTP inadequate preburner pump head rise

Criticality Ranking Computations

FMEA Item: A150-01

Rank = (X-1)(B*C*D) + (Y-1)(C*D) + (Z-1)(D) + (Q-1) +1

where:

Constants

(always these values in the equation)

A = # Classifications, top level (severity) = 5
B = # Classifications, 2nd level (initiation) = 3
C = # Classifications, 3rd level (propagation) = 3
D = # Classifications, 4th level (protection) = 7

Variables

(dependent on questionnaire responses)

X = 5 = Loss of vehicle
Y = 3 = Initiation possible
Z = 3 = Propagation possible
Q = 6 = Test/inspection

RANK = 4*63 + 2*21 + 2*7 + 5+1 = 314

NOTE: Rankings range from 1 to 315, 315 indicating greatest concern.

Fig. 4. Computation of final ranking.

While there were some large differences from one individual to another, overall agreement was good, with an average standard deviation in ranking of 3.61.

Table 1 shows individual responses and the method ranking.

Analysis of this data shows good agreement between the method and the consensus. To summarize:

1. The method never gives a response more extreme (either high or low) than any respondent at any time.
2. The method falls out of 1 sigma limits on only 4 occasions.
3. The method exhibits strong correlation with the consensus and agrees with the consensus more closely than nine of the eleven respondents.

Table 1. How Experts Ranked the Selected Failure Modes

		Respondents												
CIL #	Method Ranking	#1	#2	#3	#4	#5	#6	#7	#8	#9	#10	#11	Mean	Std Dev
B400-03	2 :	2	1	1	2	1	3	1	11	3	1	1 :	2.45	2.87
A150-01	1 :	1	2	3	1	9	1	2	13	6	2	2 :	3.82	3.83
B200-22	5 :	4	7	6	6	5	4	3	3	8	10	12 :	6.18	1.88
A700-04	4 :	13	3	11	3	2	2	6	14	12	9	8 :	7.55	4.57
B200-23	6 :	6	4	5	10	4	8	14	7	5	17	3 :	7.55	2.98
B200-14	11 :	9	6	14	5	14	14	5	5	4	5	11 :	8.36	3.93
B200-03	12 :	10	9	7	12	8	7	7	8	1	14	9 :	8.36	2.76
B200-18	7 :	5	10	9	11	3	15	16	2	2	12	10 :	8.64	4.85
A200-03	9 :	7	5	18	9	6	12	8	12	7	8	4 :	8.73	3.68
A330-03	8 :	3	8	15	8	10	5	12	16	15	4	7 :	9.36	4.22
A200-09	3 :	14	11	2	15	12	11	9	6	9	11	6 :	9.64	3.60
A340-01	16 :	15	16	16	4	17	6	4	1	13	15	17 :	11.27	5.70
B200-01	15 :	16	17	4	13	7	10	15	4	16	13	13 :	11.64	4.70
A050-01	13 :	18	18	13	14	13	13	10	10	11	3	5 :	11.64	3.13
B200-09	14 :	11	13	10	17	11	9	13	9	17	16	15 :	12.82	2.81
A600-01	10 :	8	12	12	16	16	17	18	15	14	7	16 :	13.73	2.82
A330-05	18 :	17	15	17	7	18	16	11	17	10	6	18 :	13.82	3.51
B400-11	17 :	12	14	8	18	15	18	17	18	18	18	14 :	15.45	3.13

DISCUSSION

Three approaches were used to assess how well the method performed with respect to the consensus of expert opinion: (1) comparison to the range, (2) comparison to the standard deviation, and associated binomial probability, and (3) Spearman rank correlation coefficient.

Comparison to the Range

The simplest check to perform was simply to compare the method response to the range of ranking responses given for each CIL item. There was no case in which the method gave a ranking either higher than the highest or lower than the lowest respondent ranking. In two cases the method did tie with the outer range response: CIL Item A150-01, which the method ranked first along with three other respondents, and A330-05, which the method ranked 18th along with one other respondent (mean response was 13.82). The results are shown graphically in Fig. 5.

Comparison to the Standard Deviation, and Associated Binomial Probability

A more sophisticated analysis was performed by comparing the method response with the standard deviation of each ranking. Considered this way, there are four items (B200-03, A200-09, A600-01, and A330-05) which are more than one standard deviation away from the mean response. This information is shown graphically in Fig. 6.

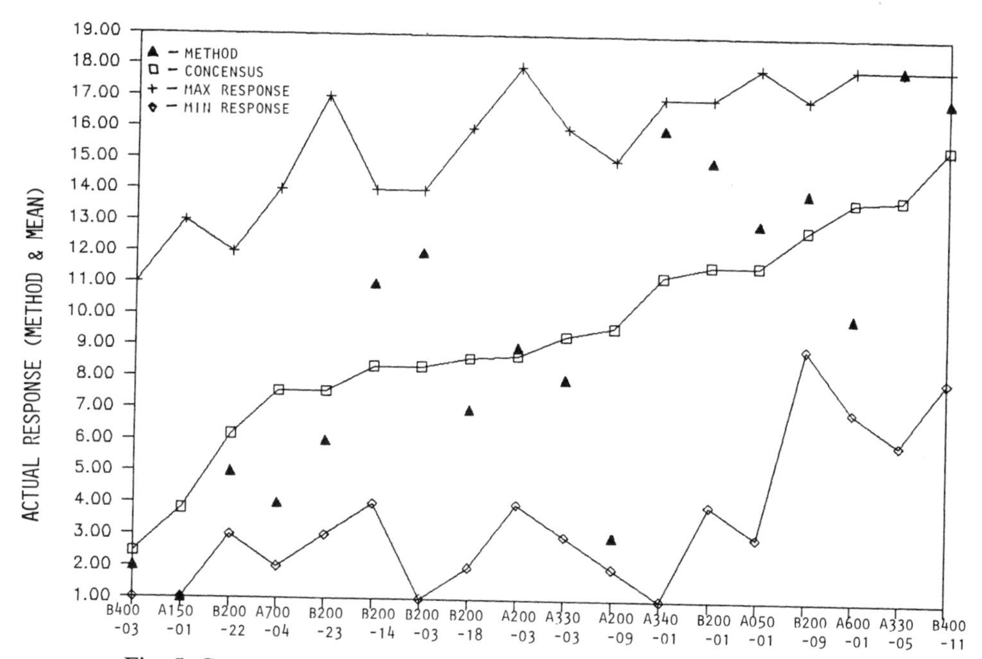

Fig. 5. Consensus (average) response with max/min of expert's responses.

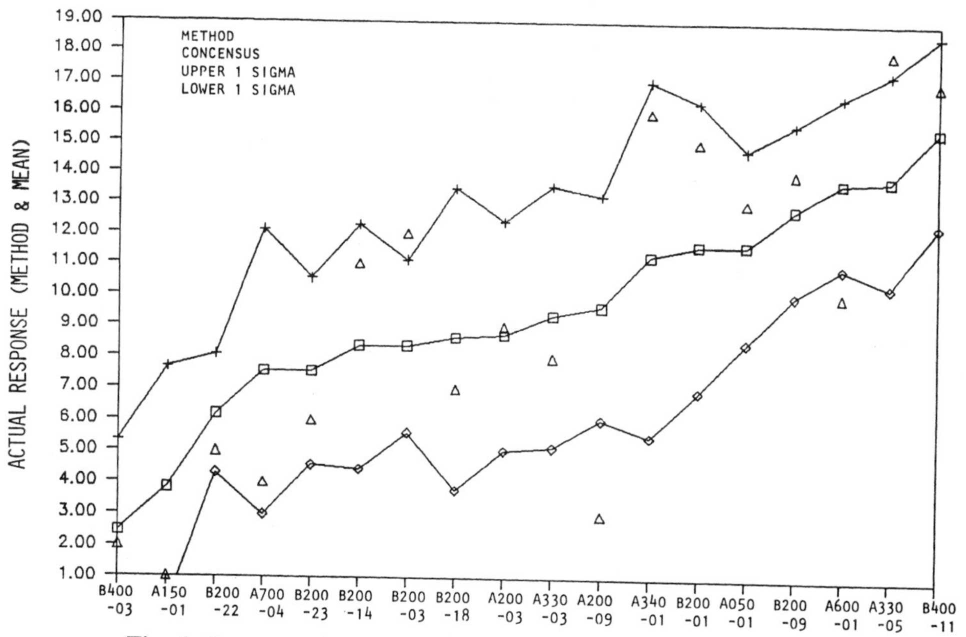

Fig. 6. Consensus (average) response with 1 σ of expert's responses.

If we consider that in a normally distributed population, 68% of the population falls within 1 standard deviation from the mean, then the chances of four or fewer of eighteen falling outside 1 is 0.269. This means that if our method was distributed in the same way as the consensus, we would have a 74% chance of seeing more points fall outside the limits than we actually did. (This result is arrived at using the binominal distribution with P=0.68.)

The only item which the method ranked more than one and a half standard deviations from the mean was A200-09. The method ranked it 3rd out of the eighteen items sampled, while its ranking by the group was 11th. The most likely reason for this disparity is that while it is generally accepted that interpropellant plate cracks are self-limiting, it does constitute an initiating event which is observed frequently and is therefore rated highly by the method.

Spearman Rank Correlation Coefficient

Finally the Spearman rank correlation coefficient was calculated for the data. This coefficient, r_s is a measure of the linear relationship between two variables, in this case rank by group and by method and is given by

$$r_s = 1 - \frac{6 \cdot \sum_{i=1} d^2}{n(n^2 - 1)}$$

where d is the difference between the ranks assigned to x and y, and n is the number of pairs of data.

Our calculated r_s=0.72. The critical value for testing the null hypothesis, that the rank correlation coefficient is zero, against the alternative hypotheses, that it is greater than zero, with $p = 0.005$ and n=18, is 0.625. Thus, we reject the null hypothesis and conclude that a positive correlation does exist, with only a 0.005 probability of making this claim when it is actually false. It is with noting that only two respondents had a greater r_s value, i.e., only two respondents predicted the group's wisdom better than the method.

CONCLUSION

All analysis performed demonstrates that the method is a credible means of performing critical item ranking; the results indicate a high correlation with the expert consensus, and that the consensus itself has a significant positive slope.

While agreement with expert opinion is encouraging, mere parroting (i.e., repeating without understanding) of conventional wisdom does nothing to gain insight into possibly unnoticed weaknesses in the system. Given that the method is credible, then perhaps it's systematic application can give new insight thinking on some issues. Bearing this in mind, it is clearly important to delve into the reasons certain items appear high on the list when they are generally held to be benign.

APPENDIX 1

Hierarchical Questionnaires for Ranking

A. Severity of Fully Propagated Event

Enter CIL Number : :

5. Loss of Vehicle
4. Engine Shutdown
3. Hydraulic Lockup
2. Loss of Readline
1. Degradation of Mission

Please Enter the Severity for this CIL Item

: :

B. Likelihood of Initiating Event

Design Confidence

F 1. Design safety factor. The design safety factor is less than adequate.

F 2. Design complexity. The design is considered complex.

F 3. Static versus dynamic functions. The item is dynamic.

F 4. Operating environments. Hardware is exposed or sensitive to high temperatures, high pressure, high stress, etc.

F 5. Contamination. Failure mode is dependent on contamination.

F 6. Failure causes. There are multiple failure causes for the CIL item.

Failure History

F (x2) 7. Initiating event observed.

F (x3) 8. Initiating event observed frequently.

F 9. Initiating event observed, but hardware subsequently modified.

The Value of Y in the Ranking Criteria Formula Is Determined by the Following:

Number of True Stmts.	Value of Y	Likelihood
5+	3	Possible
3 - 4	2	Unlikely
0 - 2	1	Very Unlikely

APPENDIX 2

Groundrules for Answering Questionnaires

C.I.R.A. Groundrules

*	High Pressure:	ΔP Across Item > 50 PSI.
*	Complex:	Any mechanical assembly which contains moving parts, has a regulating or compensating function, is non-steady state, or is pressure assisted, or any electronic assembly which uses logic or has non-steady state circuitry, or any device which mixes or ignites propellants.
*	Design Complexity:	Is relative to the causal element, not the functional FMEA item.
*	Dynamic:	Rotating hardware or rotating hardware interface.
*	Inspection and Test:	Field only. In-house and acceptance testing and inspection do not count.
*	Reaction Time:	May be with reference to computer or human. If a redline limit exists and is referenced in the FMEA, reaction time is said to exist.
*	Fully Propagated Effect:	For single point failure.
*	Factor of Safety:	Adequate, unless covered by D.A.R.
*	Dependent on Mission Phase:	If failure effect can occur during start-up, mainstage, and cutoff, the effect is not dependent on mission phase.
*	Worst Case:	Test experience demonstrating credibility that initiating event can propagate to worst case; actual catastrophic event not necessary.
*	Reduced Power Level:	Scored same as hydraulic lockup.
*	Contamination:	Cannot be inspected for; contamination which induces fracture not considered.
*	Leak Testing:	For failures dependent on crack propagation, leak testing is not an inspection/test.
*	Each CIL Item:	Consider worst effect at the worst time.
*	Manufacturing Defects:	All hardware is assumed to be as designed, and free of defects.

Risk Assessment and Risk Management for an Experimental Nuclear Waste Processing Facility

Daniel A. Reny, D. P. Mackowiac, and R. M. Stallman
Idaho National Engineering Laboratory
Idaho Falls, ID

ABSTRACT

This paper describes the application of probabilistic risk assessment (PRA) and risk management to an experimental nuclear waste processing facility. The Process Experimental Pilot Plant (PREPP) utilizes an incineration process to prepare the waste for final storage at the Waste Isolation Pilot Plant (WIPP). The PRA goes beyond the normal scope of risk to the general public. The scope includes the management risks associated with personnel injury or exposure, major equipment damage or extensive plant downtime, and potential onsite releases and facility contamination. These risks, which are more likely to occur, have significant consequences and are of equal concern to the operation and management of the facility. The initial PRA will provide input to optimize the facility design and operational safety. The PRA model will then be contained within a risk management system. The risk management system will provide continuing input to the operation and management of the facility. The expected result of this effort is a better managed and operated facility, which reduces risk not only to the operators and management but to the general public as well.

KEYWORDS: Probabilistic risk assessment (PRA), risk management, waste, incineration, nuclear, Process Experimental Pilot Plant (PREPP)

INTRODUCTION

The purpose of this paper is to describe the application of probabilistic risk assessment (PRA) techniques and risk management to an experimental nuclear waste processing facility. The PRocess Experimental Pilot Plant (PREPP) is an experimental Transuranic[1] (TRU) waste processing facility. The facility is located at the Idaho National Engineering Laboratory (INEL). PREPP is owned by the U.S. Department of Energy and operated under contract by EG&G Idaho, Inc.

The PREPP facility is built and operational and is currently undergoing preoperational testing and development prior to TRU processing. Preoperational testing includes testing the design efficiency requirements of the incineration process and supporting functions. Further developments include modifications for shielding and confinement control and other requirements.

The PREPP process will accept TRU waste in various solid forms and prepares the waste for permanent storage at the Waste Isolation Pilot Plant (WIPP). PREPP uses an incineration process combined with cement grouting solidification to prepare the waste to meet the WIPP storage criteria.

Any time a facility handles radioactive material of this type there are inherent hazards. The TRU waste that will be processed by the PREPP facility will not be in quantities large enough nor will the process possess the potential to form a significant hazard or threat to the general public. In general the potential for offsite consequences is much less than the potential for onsite consequences. The inherent hazards are for the most part generally limited to the facility and the operating personnel.

The risks to management associated with personnel injury or exposure, major equipment damage or extensive plant downtime, and potential onsite releases and facility contamination form the major portion of the risks of operating the facility. Management is equally concerned with managing the onsite risks and ensuring the prevention of offsite risks. The management and prevention of onsite operating risks will lead to a lower potential for offsite consequences. This produces a better managed and operated facility with reduced risk not only to the operators and management but also to the general public.

FACILITY DESCRIPTION

The PREPP facility will accept transuranic contaminated waste for processing to meet the WIPP permanent storage criteria, which require the waste to be converted to an essentially stable state solid. The PREPP process utilizes a high temperature incineration process and a solidification process. The PREPP process is shown in the simplified diagram of Fig. 1.

The waste enters the PREPP facility in containers which may be steel drums or box containers. The containers are transported to an opening and verification chamber for inspection as necessary. The containers are put into an industrial shredder. The shredded material is then conveyed to the incinerator.

The incinerator is a two-stage system consisting of a rotary kiln stage and a secondary combustion chamber stage. The rotary kiln is a cylindrical kiln which rotates as it operates and transports the waste from one end to the other. The rotary kiln operates at approximately 1800°F. At the end of the rotary kiln the remaining solid waste is passed through a residue cooling step while the offgases are superheated to approximately 2100°F in the secondary combustion chamber. The offgases are then processed through an offgas scrubbing system where it is cooled, scrubbed, and filtered prior to release to the atmosphere.

The solid waste residue is put into a trommel where the ash is separated from the large pieces and stored. The large waste then is collected in a large glove box where the drum fill and grout process occurs. The large waste remains, along with ash and other waste remains from the offgas scrubbing effluent, are mixed with a cement and sand grout and poured into steel drums. The drums are then stored for curing and inspection before shipment to WIPP.

The PREPP facility is housed in a steel-lined building which utilizes negatively pressurized zones for confinement. The ventilating system creates a negative pressure on the innermost building zones so that all air leakage is from the outside to the inside. The inside air is then filtered through the offgas system or through the ventilating system HEPA filters before exhausting to the atmosphere. The waste material is confined to the innermost

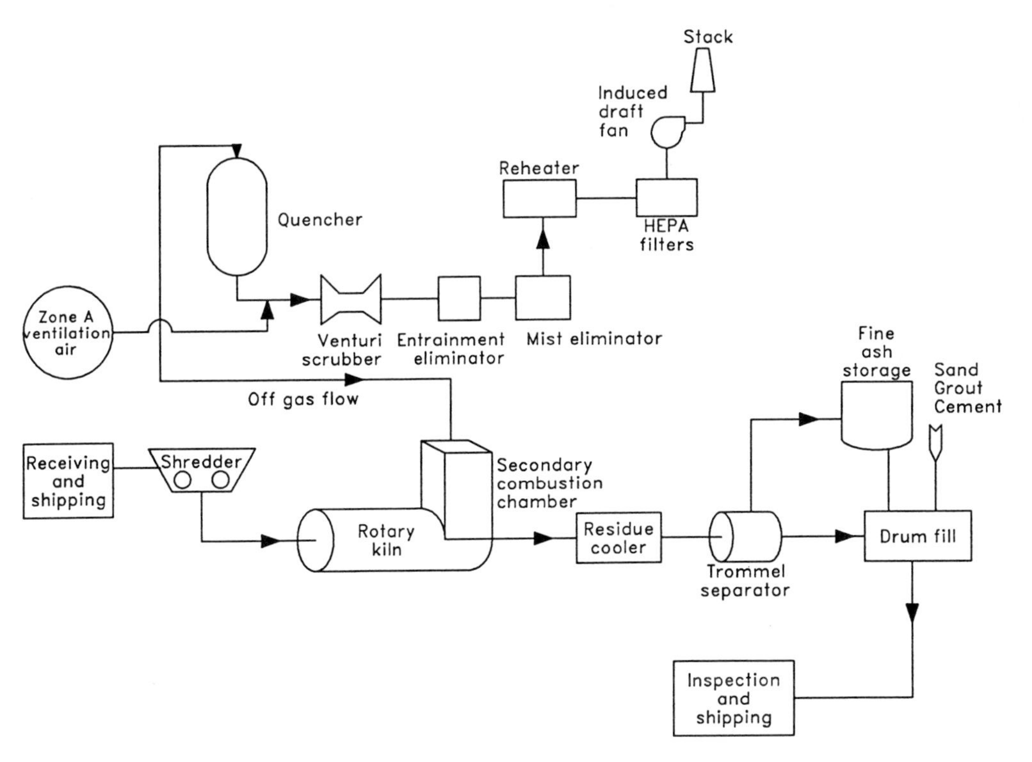

Fig. 1. Simplified PREPP flow diagram.

zones. Sealed rooms with doorlocks and other confinements are used to separate the innermost zones from the outer zones.

The PREPP operation is controlled with a combination of local control stations and a centralized control room. The entire process is monitored and under the control of the central control room, which allows each of the individual local control operations to function. The PREPP operation is basically a batch process with material being put into the process and controlled each step of the way.

OBJECTIVES

The PRA effort will serve two main objectives: (1) input to the decisionmaking process prior to TRU processing, and (2) a basis for risk assessment and management during TRU processing operations. The kinds of analyses and decisions the PRA will support prior to startup are safety analyses, safety reviews, design and modification tradeoffs, and ultimately a final measure of facility risk due to operations. The facility measures of risk and safety will be used to compare against applicable facility design and operating guidelines[1,2] for compliance with DOE safety and ALARA (as-low-as-reasonably-achievable) criteria.

During operation the PRA will form the basis of a risk management system used to monitor the performance of the facility, provide feedback for safety improvement, and provide risk based input to management decisions concerning safety of operations.

PRA APPLICATION

A Level 3 PRA[3] with limited external events analysis is being conducted. The analysis will be limited to internal events occurring onsite such as internal fires and internal floods due to pipe breaks. The externally occurring events such as earthquakes, tornadoes, and floods will be analyzed as a separate issue.

The PRA application was tailored to fit the needs of PREPP management. PREPP management defined the types of events and level of consequences that were considered unacceptable to PREPP operations. The PRA application is directed toward fulfilling these definitions.

Risk Assessment Criteria

The risk assessment top event definitions were developed according to management's intent to assess all risks (onsite and offsite) associated with the operation of the PREPP facility. The top event definitions for the risk analysis were defined in accordance with management's direction of what events and level of consequences were unacceptable to the PREPP operation. The management's perception of event and consequence acceptability is driven by a number of influences. Regardless of these influences, management's intent is to minimize risk and maximize safety within the technological and budgetary constraints of the PREPP facility. The risk assessment top event criteria are shown in Table 1.

As can be seen in Table 1, the risk assessment criterion goes beyond the normal scope of risk to the surrounding environment and general public. The risk assessment criterion includes risks from toxic material consequences, from normal industrial hazards, facility releases, and economic risks due to facility or major equipment damage. In conjunction with the onsite consequences, the assessment will also look at the potential for offsite releases.

Activity and Hazard Classification

The PREPP process activities are classified and categorized according to the process flow diagram of Fig. 2. The PREPP process activities are shown within the confinement zones (Zones A, B, and C) of the facility. Each process is screened for type of activity, potential hazards, and effects (consequences) as shown in Fig. 2. The preliminary hazards screening identifies the activities, types of hazards and potential consequences for further detailed analysis. The effects or consequences of the PREPP activities are screened according to the definitions in Table 2.

These consequence definitions are consistent with the risk assessment top event criteria shown in Table 1. The screening hazards analysis format is shown in Fig. 3. The form of Fig. 3 allows the identification and tracking of all hazards to completion.

Plant Damage State Analysis and Quantification

After identification and classification of all the PREPP process activities, a detailed analysis of each of these activities is performed. The analysis depends on the type of activity and hazard. The manual functions performed by operators during the front-end handling of waste material and back-end drum fill and grout operations are highly operator-action intensive. Therefore, these activities will receive a human actions task analysis to determine frequency and probability of errors or accidents. The automated control of the incineration process and all facility support systems required for confinement and operation will require a typical PRA event sequence analysis. The results of all the detailed analyses will be combined into plant damage states. Plant damage states are the Level 1 PRA results

Table 1. Risk Assessment Top Event Criteria

Onsite Consequences

- Personnel exposure (radiological or toxic) in excess of normally allowable limits.
- Severe bodily harm or fatal injury to personnel.
- Facility contamination or release of radioactive or toxic material outside of normal operating boundaries.
- Facility damage in excess of $1 million or 1 year plant downtime.

Offsite Consequences

- Offsite release of radioactive or toxic material to the surrounding environment.

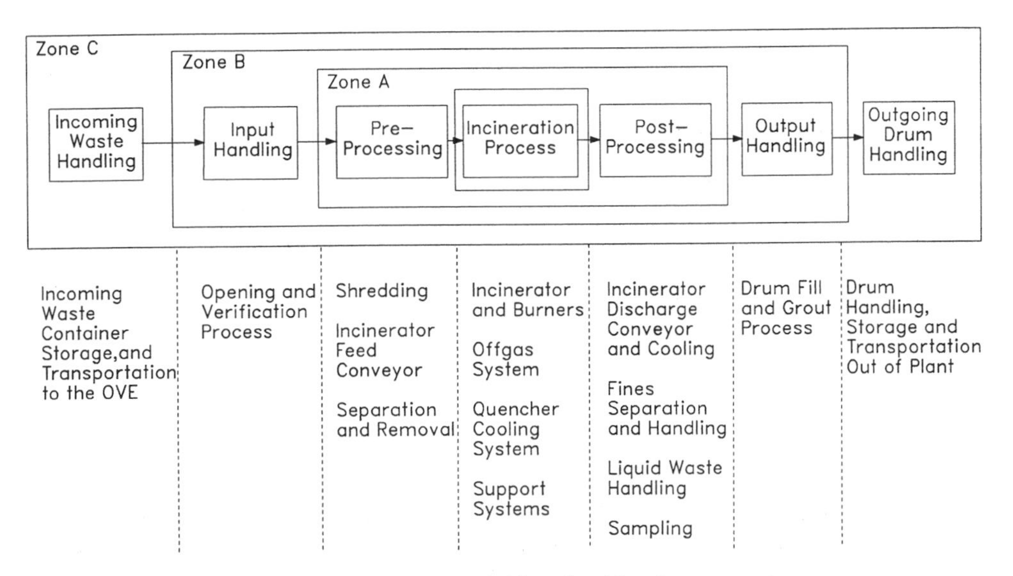

Fig. 2. Process activities classification.

which define the types of damage as a result of each event sequence, according to the defined top event criteria in Table 2.

Consequence Analysis

The PRA Levels 2 and 3 plant damage phenomenology and consequences will be accomplished for the plant damage states of Level 1. The Levels 2 and 3 analyses do not follow the typical types of defined analyses a reactor PRA would have. Instead, the expanded top event and consequence criterion and the unique nature of the PREPP facility require a blend of varying types of Levels 2 and 3 analyses.

For the onsite consequences, some plant damage states may require little or no phenomenological and consequence analysis, while some may require very extensive analysis. For example, some events may result in limited personnel injury, facility damage,

Table 2. Hazards Analysis Definitions

Injury:	Minor	No loss of work days.
	Major	Loss of work days.
	Severe	Severe injury or hospitalization.
	Fatal	Fatality potential.
Exposure: (Onsite)	Minor	Less than 100 mrem.
	Major	More than 100 mrem.
	Severe	More than 1 rem.
(Offsite)	Any exposure outside of PREPP boundaries.	
Contamination:	Minor	Confined to local area (1 or 2 rooms) within PREPP.
	Major	Unconfined within PREPP boundary (all rooms and areas).
	Severe	Outside of PREPP boundary but onsite.
	Catastrophic	Any release offsite.
Facility Damage:	Minor	Can be repaired within normal maintenance costs and time.
	Major	Above normal maintenance efforts but below $1 million and 1 year plant downtime.
	Severe	More than $1 million and 1 year plant down-time.
	Catastrophic	Permanent plant shutdown.

or contamination that may require only a limited response and consequences analysis. Other events may result in several plant damage states which require a detailed plant response analysis along with a consequences analysis to determine the degree and level of consequences.

Those event sequences leading to offsite releases and consequences will require typical Levels 2 and 3 analyses. Source terms[2] will be established along with plant response conditions. Release paths, environmental conditions, topology, and other factors will be utilized to determine offsite consequences.

PRA Results

The final PRA results will be ranked and reported by probability of occurrence and magnitude of consequence. The level of consequences will be grouped according to the management definitions of Table 1. Of course, all high consequence events will be evaluated for acceptability. In addition, the high probability-low consequences scenarios will also require evaluation as potential candidates for alternative analysis. Also to be reported are the results of the PRA at the various stages of input to the PRA Levels 1, 2, and 3 analyses.

Activity Description	Potential Hazards	Effects				Corrective Actions Minimizing Provisions	Frequency of Occurrence	Notes
		Injury	Exposure	Contam- ination	Equipment Damage			
Opening and Verification Process								
1 – Container Handling	Dropped Container	Major– Severe		Minor	Minor	Procedure 3.8		
2 – Opening and Verification	Unknown material – Combustibles – Flammables – Corrosives – Poisons – Carcinogens	Major– Fatal	Major– Severe			Procedure 3.10		

Fig. 3. Preliminary hazards analysis application.

RISK MANAGEMENT

Using the results of the PRA application, the risk attributes of the PREPP facility can be reported and ranked according to management's acceptability criteria. The risk attributes, being composed of probability of occurrence and magnitude of consequences, are then candidates for risk reduction by reducing either the probability of occurrence or magnitude of consequences.

Risk Management During Design and Development

The risk management efforts will affect the design and development phase of the PREPP facility. The PRA and risk management efforts will work in conjunction with PREPP management and safety to identify and define the appropriate operating safety and risk guidelines.[1,2] Once the guidelines are defined, the various facility designs and operations can be evaluated for compliance with the guidelines. The design and development tasks supported by the PRA and risk management effort are:

- Definition of critical safety functions and success criteria.
- Safety analysis report and plant safety review.
- Criticality safety analysis and review.
- Emergency response procedures and review.
- Systems reliability and availability.
- Plant operating and maintenance staff requirements for safety.
- Automated versus manual operations.
- Shielding and protective clothing requirements.

The PRA and risk management activities will provide valuable insight into plant success criteria, integrated plant operations, operational dependencies, and other insights from a risk standpoint that would not evolve from standard facility safety practices.

Risk Management During Operation

During operation of the facility a "living PRA" risk management system[4] is developed and utilized. The risk management system for PREPP is shown in Fig. 4. It will perform the following functions:

- Collect operational data and evaluate plant performance.
- Validate baseline plant risk model with operational plant performance data.
- Provide feedback to management about plant safety, risk performance and status.
- Propose and evaluate options for improvement.
- Evaluate any changes to plant equipment and operations for impact on plant safety and risk.

CONCLUSIONS

The risk assessment and risk management application of the PREPP facility is in support of management's policy of maximizing safety through identification and reduction of operating risks. The PRA provides a systematic way of identifying the facility safety

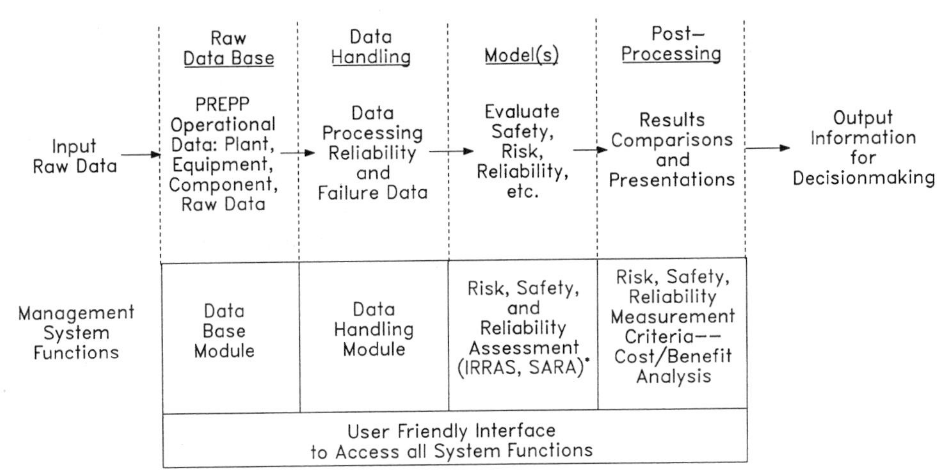

* Integrated Reliability and Risk Analysis System (IRRAS), System Analysis and Risk Assessment (SARA), computer programs developed for the U.S. Nuclear Regulatory Commission under DOE Contract No. DE-AC07-761D01570.

Fig. 4. Risk management system.

requirements and qualitatively and quantitatively analyzing and ranking the contributors to risk.

Risk management takes the results of the PRA and compares the results with established guidelines and levels of safety required for the facility. Where the results indicate that the risk or safety of the facility does not meet requirements and guidelines, then modifications and improvements can be made. The proposed modifications and improvements can be identified from the PRA results and evaluated for effectiveness with the PRA model.

A "living PRA" risk management system can be developed from the results of the PRA effort. The risk management system can track and monitor plant safety and risk and provide management with indications of plant risk and safety performance. Continuous monitoring and improvements will result in optimized facility safety and minimized risk to the operators and management of the facility as well as to the general public.

REFERENCES

1. W. J. Brynda *et al.*, *Nonreactor Nuclear Facilities: Standards and Criteria Guide*, DOE/TIC-11603-Rev. 1, DE87 009786 (September 1986).
2. J. C. Elder *et al.*, *A Guide to Radiological Accident Considerations for Siting and Design of DOE Nonreactor Nuclear Facilities*, LA-10294-MS, UC-41 (January 1986).
3. U.S. Nuclear Regulatory Commission (NRC), *PRA Procedures Guide*, NUREG/CR-2300 (January 1983).
4. D. L. Batt *et al.*, Organization of Risk Analysis Codes for Living Evaluations (ORACLE), *Probabilistic Safety Assessment and Risk Management PSA 87* **II**:698 (1987).

Cross-Entropy Estimation of Distributions Based on Scarce Data

Niels C. Lind
University of Waterloo
Waterloo, Ontario, Canada

Vicente Solana
National Research Council of Spain
Madrid, Spain

ABSTRACT

A method is described to estimate a random variable using fractiles as constraints. The fractiles are exactly known for random samples, whether small or large. The method minimizes the cross-entropy, or entropy relative to a reference distribution, which may be selected to minimize the cross-entropy of the sample data. The method is simple to implement and avoids several disadvantages of the methods presently in common use.

KEYWORDS: Cross-entropy, relative entropy, distribution, scarce data, estimation, information, fractile constraints

INTRODUCTION

Assigning a distribution or a quantile to a random variable is of fundamental importance in reliability and risk analysis, which are impossible without good statistical estimates of the basic random variables. In risk analysis the concern is directed at extreme and rare events. However, classical methods borrowed from the natural or social sciences are generally focused on the central portions of distributions, and they are not well suited to the task. Data are often scarce. There is a need for methods of estimation that are robust, justifiable by rational arguments, and oriented specifically towards extreme or rare events and sparse data.

Conventional statistical methods begin by assuming a particular distribution for the random variables. In risk analysis, such assumptions cannot generally be justified rationally. Moreover, as shown below, such assumptions contradict a fundamental property of random sampling, by which the sample elements are known fractiles in the distribution and provide strict constraints on the estimation. In recent years there has been a growing interest in nonparametric estimation, making less rigid assumptions about the distributions. Noteworthy among these are the methods of density estimation.[1] These methods, still under active research, apparently perform well when there is ample data.

Risk Analysis, Edited by C. Zervos
Plenum Press, New York, 1991

This paper uses instead another nonparametric approach, the minimum cross-entropy method.[2,3] This method is used in a new interpretation, in which the distribution is estimated from two inputs, namely the information, which here is in the form of fractile constraints, and a reference distribution. The reference distribution provides invariance of the entropy functional under transformation of variables and is essential for this reason. It is usually referred to as the "prior" distribution in the literature.[2-4] Unlike a Bayesian prior, it need not be prior in time to the data and it need not reflect prior knowledge about the distribution of the random variable[5] or any knowledge whatsoever.

Estimation is more difficult for continuous than discrete random variables. The events for which the probabilities are being sought have never occurred (this is an infinite set of events, namely the range of the continuous variable less the finite set of events observed; moreover, each such simple event has probability 0). The reference distribution provides an extension from the finite set of observed values to the uncountably infinite set of the sample space.

A general solution of the minimum cross-entropy problem with fractile constraints is presented, and it is shown that the resulting distribution piecewise is equal to the reference distribution scaled by a factor that is constant in between the prescribed fractiles. The estimated distribution, correspondingly, is piecewise a linear function of the reference distribution.

Some criteria for selection of the reference distribution are given from the perspective of minimizing the deviation from the reference distribution or, alternatively, minimizing the discontinuities in the density function that minimizes the cross-entropy.

BACKGROUND

A common approach to estimating the distribution of a random variable is first to postulate the distribution type and next to assign the parameters on the basis of the data. This is done by optimizing a function of the parameters and the data. In scientific work it is common then to test the postulate and accept the distribution (for the time being) if it cannot be rejected. In applications this step is often omitted — by necessity or by custom. This approach is appropriate when the data are homogeneous, i.e. obtained under reproducible laboratory conditions, in which case the hypothesized distribution may well be obviously suitable and replication of the distribution parameters is nearly assured for large samples.

Random variables that occur in nature, or in technology outside the laboratory, are of unknown type. Wind velocities are an example: extreme winds may arise in hurricanes with a frequency of occurrence that varies with location in a way different from ordinary cyclones. The probability of extreme winds is not related to the probability distribution of daily winds. Extreme winds may also be produced by tornadoes, which again are a different meteorological phenomenon. No simple mathematical distribution can reflect the distribution of a random variable that arises as a mixture of different random phenomena with various rates of occurrence.

The capacity of components or systems is important in risk analysis. Such capacities must be considered as mixtures of different distributions, for example specimens with and without gross error. Statistical analysis of distributions as mixtures of elementary distributions is computationally and conceptually complex.[6] Modern methods to estimate density functions and distributions are available; see Silverman[1] for a recent survey. These methods are quite demanding of data and perform best in the central portions of the distributions rather than the tails that are of paramount importance in reliability and risk analysis.

In summary, distribution assumptions can rarely be justified for variables that occur in the physical world. This is of little consequence when concern is with the common or the ordinary; you can always take samples large enough to show that at least the central portion of a distribution is sufficiently close to some assumed shape. Indeed, if evidence should accumulate to force us to reject our assumption, that same evidence readily suggests a new model. However, the matter is entirely different when the concern is with extreme or rare events, disastrous consequences or social responsibility. Any distribution assumption must, like any other assumption made under such circumstances, be defensible in rational discussion among knowledgeable persons. Any distribution assumption of simple form is suspect. It is best to avoid strong assumptions about distribution type in risk analysis; the distribution assumptions should be weak in the sense that they should have minimal influence on the final decision.

In conventional statistics there is another difficulty: estimation from a sample is often made indirectly, by way of the sample moments (mean, variance, skewness, etc.) only. Usually, the first n moments are used as estimators to calibrate the distribution if n parameters are to be determined. This would make good sense if the distribution type were known *a priori*. Indeed, many such procedures are optimal for the specific type. However, when the distribution type is uncertain, such methods fare less well. In reliability analysis they have been shown to lead to absurdities, and they perform poorly in many areas where their application is now standard procedure.[7] Since any sample of two or more elements permits the estimation of moments of any order, it might well be better to use more than n moments, or a different selection of moments, in the estimation of n parameters. Or, when it is important not to introduce unwarranted assumptions, it is best to avoid the use of moments altogether.

In the Bayesian approach the subjective aspect of probability is openly acknowledged. The emphasis is on accumulating information to update a subjective probability in a consistent manner. In Bayesian practice the distribution type is assumed, and its posterior parameters are calculated from prior parameters and the corresponding prior likelihood of the observations. It is common to make a further assumption, in using a conjugate prior, merely to simplify the calculations. When great or public risks are involved, this may be difficult to justify. Also, the private and arbitrary nature of subjective probability stands in the way of wide acceptance of the Bayesian approach in risk analysis. An alternative type of procedure, a variational approach based on the information-theoretical concept of entropy,[3,8] is to choose the distribution $q(x)$ that minimizes the Kullback-Leibler entropy functional

$$D(q,p) = \int_I q(x)[\log q(x) - \log p(x)]dx \ , \tag{1}$$

where the integration extends over all possible states of x, subject to constraints that reflect the information available about $q(x)$. $D(q,p)$ is invariant under monotonic mappings of x. This functional has since come to be known as the cross-entropy of $q(x)$ with respect to the density $p(x)$.[2,3]

The minimum cross-entropy method was derived on a firm axiomatic basis by Shore and Johnson[2,3] as an inference method in which the information is provided in the form of functional expectation constraints on $q(x)$. Kapur and Kesavan[4] more descriptively call $D(p,q)$ in Eq. (1) the "directed divergence" of the distribution $q(x)$ from $p(x)$. In this paper $D(q,p)$ is called the cross-entropy or the (directed) distance from p to q and the function $p(x)$ is called the reference distribution. The distribution $q(x)$ that minimizes $D(p,q)$ is here called the minimum cross-entropy distribution.

The role of $p(x)$ may resemble a Bayesian prior, but it is different in many respects since the processing and the results are quite different. Indeed, it may be given a very different interpretation altogether.[9] As will be shown in the following, minimum cross-entropy estimation with prescribed fractiles is robust and quite insensitive to assumptions about $p(x)$.

In entropy methods the available information is usually translated into moments before it is used, following the pattern established by Jaynes.[8] This is appropriate in contexts where the data are available in the form of moments. Thus, to select a model with p parameters, given a random sample, it is common to estimate the first p moments (or something equivalent) from a sample and use them as constraints in the extremization of the entropy. Analogous procedures are followed in classical statistics, where they are usually justified by known properties of optimality. But in entropy methods this approach has no comparable justification. It is natural to ask: why stop at exactly p moments assumed known, when sample moments of any order are available for the calculating? After all, an observation of x is at the same time an observation of x^2, x^3 and so on. A satisfactory answer to this question, basic to the theory of entropy methods of estimation, is not available. Since $p+1$ moments convey more information than p moments, the translation involves an arbitrary amount of information, invalidating the powerful claim that entropy methods introduce no bias.

A FUNDAMENTAL PROPERTY OF RANDOM SAMPLING

An exact and well known[10,11] property of random samples is of great importance when estimating the distribution of a continuous random variable of unknown type. Because the result contradicts conventional approaches, it is worth while to put the argument in detail here. We are given a random sample of size r, and we wish to assign a probability $Q(x_i)=\Pr\{x < x_i\}$, $i=1,...,r$, to the event that the next observation, x, falls in the interval below sample value x_i. This probability, associated with one future event is what Matheron[12] calls "monoscopic." We are not concerned with the ensemble of all such future or past events or both, the "panscopic." The monoscopic probability equals $i/(r+1)$ as can be seen from the following argument.

Consider the following experimental protocol. Experiment A: a sample of size $r+1$ is assembled as a collection of $r+1$ different real numbers. These elements are then rearranged in ascending sequence, S. Experiment B: one element of S is selected at random and labelled x. The remaining elements in S are labelled $x_1, x_2, ..., x_r$ in ascending order.

Since element x is selected at random in Experiment A, the probability Q_1 that it is the first number in sequence S equals the probability that it is element number i in sequence S, $i = 2, 3,..., r+1$. These events are all equally probable, and so $Q_i = i/(r+1)$ for all $i = 1,..., r+1$.[10] Denoting the probability that x is less than x_i by $Q(x_i)$, it follows that

$$Q_X(x_i) = \frac{i}{(r+1)}, \qquad i = 1, 2, ..., r \quad . \tag{2}$$

This result is independent of the distribution of the numbers in Experiment A. Indeed, it doesn't matter whether a parent distribution exists. In particular, the numbers may, but need not, be realizations of a random variable. Equation (2) follows solely because the selection in Experiment B is random.

The constraints in Eq. (2) prescribe the fractiles at the random sample points for any process of estimation of a distribution when the only usable information is the sample S. Estimation on the basis of moments from random samples generally contradicts this exact and intrinsic property of random sampling.

Q_i are probabilities in the frequentist sense. On the other hand, $Q(x_i)$ in Eq. (2) are a decisionmaker's probabilities. Suppose that a person is offered a bet on the value of x given the set $\{x_1,...,x_r\}$. It is sensible to accept such a bet on the premise that the $Q(x_i)$ in Eq. (2)

are probabilities in the classical sense. Certainly the $Q(x_i)$ in Eq. (2) cannot be labelled subjectivist; they are objective in the sense that no one can rationally assign any different values. They are not Bayesian either; these probabilities are known *a priori.*

In the frequentist view the probabilities Q_i, i=1,...,r+1 are not influenced by any belief about the distribution of x, or whether such belief is adopted prior to sampling or after rearrangement. Moreover, they are not influenced by any knowledge about the distribution parameters. Thus, the elements in a random sample of size r of a random variable X are exactly the $i/(r+1)$-fractiles in the distribution of X. The result may be restated as the following Sample Rule:

Drawing an element at random (with replacement) from a population is equivalent to drawing an element at random from a random sample of the population.

When the type of the distribution is prescribed or selected *a priori*, the estimation generally produces different values of these fractiles. There are many situations where estimation by classical or Bayesian methods is appropriate, and there is a large literature available on these approaches. The remainder of this paper considers the situation that a random sample is available for a random variable of unknown distribution type and unknown moments, and it is desired to estimate, i.e., assign, a fractile (other than those of the sample) of a prescribed probability.

The set of r+1 equations in Eq. (2) concern the probabilities of a finite set of events, and so it is interesting to note that they can also be derived from the principle of maximum Shannon entropy, whose application gives directly that all events have equal probability, so that each has probability $1/(r+1)$. Cumulative summation gives Eq. (2).

MINIMIZING CROSS-ENTROPY FOR GIVEN FRACTILES

A finite or infinite domain, $I = [x_0, x_{r+1}]$, of the real numbers is partitioned into r+1 subintervals $I_0 = [x_0, x_1], I_1 = [x_1, x_2],..., I_r = [x_r, x_{r+1}]$. Given is a reference distribution $p(x)$ that is positive everywhere in I. Information about the random variable X is provided in the form of fractile pairs or quantile points $(x, Q(x_i))$, i=1, 2,..., r. By definition $Q(x_0)=0$ and $Q(x_{n+1})=1$. We seek a posterior distribution $q(x)$, with posterior distribution function $Q(x)$, that minimizes the cross-entropy functional (1) and satisfies the r+1 fractile constraints

$$Q(x_i) \quad = \quad \frac{i}{(r+1)} \ , \qquad\qquad i \ = \ 0,1,...,r \ . \tag{3}$$

Equivalent to Eq. (3) are the r+1 interval constraints

$$q_i \quad = \quad \int_I q(x)dx \quad = \quad Q(x_{i+1}) \ - \ Q(x_i) \quad = \quad \frac{1}{(r+1)} \ , \tag{4}$$

in which $q_i = Q_{i+1} - Q_i$.

This problem in the calculus of variations can be solved by the Lagrange multiplier method[3] if the constraints are rewritten as expectations of discontinuity functions.[13] The solution is in interval i:

$$q(x) \quad = \quad \frac{q_i}{p_i} p(x) \quad = \quad (p(x)/p_i)/(r+1) \ , \tag{5}$$

in which p_i is a constant analogous to q_i in Eq. (4). When $q(x)$ satisfies Eq. (5) the cross-entropy functional takes the minimum value

$$D_{\min} \quad = \quad -\frac{\log(1+r) + \log p_0 + \log p_i + ... + \log p_r}{(r+1)} \tag{6}$$

Equations (5) and (6) establish two important results concerning the influence of the reference distribution:

1. The minimum cross-energy distribution $q(x)$ is piecewise of the same form as the reference density function $p(x)$, but scaled individually over each interval between data points by the constant factor $1/p_i/(r+1)$.

2. The minimum value of the cross-entropy functional is a function of the r reference distribution values P_i. In particular it is functionally independent of the values assumed by the reference at any other point and it is not directly dependent on the reference density function $p(x)$.

The expression for the minimum value of the cross-entropy, Eq. (6), is analogous to the minimum cross-entropy for discrete distributions.[4,8] This, as is to be expected, corresponds to a set of $r+1$ possible events with reference probabilities p_i and minimum cross-entropy probabilities $1/(r+1)$.

The distribution function that minimizes the cross-entropy functional is, by integration of Eq. (6),

$$Q(x) = \{1+[P(x) - P_i]/p_i\}/(r+1), \; x_i < x < x_{i+1} \; . \tag{7}$$

Figure 1 shows an example. The random variable X has domain $I = (-1,1)$. A random sample — small (r=4) for clarity of illustration — is {3.71, 6.24, 4.25, 7.18}.

This gives the fractile constraints

$$(X,Q)_i = (3.71,.2), (4.25,.4), (6.24,.6), (7.18,.8).$$

The fractiles are plotted on a normal probability graph (Fig. 1) and, since it is judged appropriate for the data and the context, the reference distribution is selected to be of normal type. Also, for clarity of illustration two poorly fitting reference distributions $P_a(x)$ and $P_b(x)$ (shown with broken lines) are used. The figure shows the results, $Q_a(x)$ and $Q_b(x)$, of applying the cross-entropy formalism of Eq. (7).

SELECTION OF REFERENCE DISTRIBUTIONS

For a given random sample, application of the method of minimum cross-entropy yields an estimate of the distribution $q(x)$ as the transformation of an arbitrary reference distribution $p(x)$. Each reference distribution $p(x)$ generates a different and unique solution $q(x)$. In practice it is necessary to select a particular reference distribution $p(x)$ and it is desirable to have some criteria available for this selection. It is desirable that the choice can be defended rationally when the risk is an important one. Although $p(x)$ has no influence on the value of $q(x)$ at the fractiles, it generates the function of interpolation between fractiles and, what is more important for risk analysis, the function of extrapolation outside the range of fractiles $[x_1, x_r]$.

The selection of a reference distribution may be different in each individual case, but two possible kinds of criteria can be suggested for practical application, as described in the remainder of this paper. The first kind expresses that the reference distribution should be close in some sense to the resulting distribution. One such criterion uses the cross-entropy as a measure of distance, while another uses Euclidean distances in a probability plot. The second kind of criterion, only briefly discussed, aims to minimize the discontinuities of slope in the resulting distribution $Q(x)$ in the least squares sense.

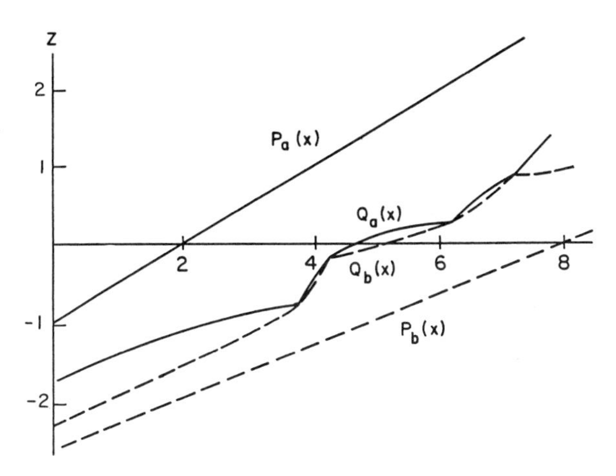

Fig. 1. An example of the distribution function that minimizes the cross-entropy functional.

MINIMIZING THE DISTANCE FROM *P*(*x*) TO *Q*(*x*)

The cross-entropy $D(p,q)$ is a semi-metric (i.e., it is not symmetrical in its arguments, and the triangle inequality does not generally hold true) and it can be interpreted as the directed distance from $p(x)$ to $q(x)$.[3] It therefore makes sense to choose $p(x)$ such as to minimize D_{min} in Eq. (6). The approach depends on whether, or how, the reference distribution is subject to constraints.

Within a linear transformation, the minimum cross-entropy, Eq. (6), may be written

$$D_{\min} = -\log p_1 - \log p_2 - \ldots - \log p_r \ . \tag{8}$$

Thus D_{min} is the sum of a convex function of the interval lengths p_i that are constrained to sum to 1. Therefore the p_i are all equal when an unconditioned reference distribution minimizes D_{min} to 0.

First consider the case that there are no constraints on the reference distribution. Equation (6) gives the minimum distance solution $p_i = q_i = 1/(r+1)$ and renders D_{min} equal to 0, which is the absolute minimum.

Thus, any distribution function $P(x)$ that contains all fractile points minimizes D_{min} to 0. This value is attained if $Q(x)$ is identically equal to $P(x)$. The posterior is indeterminate except at the fractiles. One may without the cross-entropy formalism choose $Q(x)$ directly as any suitable interpolation function between fractiles. Polynomial or spline transformations of appropriate distribution types are suitable for the purpose.

If the reference distribution type is given, in the sense that $P(x)$ is constrained to belong to a parametric family of distributions, then the approach depends on the number of parameters (degrees of freedom) in the expression for $P(x)$. Minimizing D_{min} in Eq. (6), expressed as a function of these parameters, gives $P(x)$ and hence p_i. Then $q(x)$ is found from Eq. (5). This is a standard problem in nonlinear programming. Closed form solution is rarely possible.

TWO-PARAMETRIC APPROXIMATE SOLUTIONS

Equation (8) suggests that the graph of $P(x)$ in the present conditioned case should pass close to all fractile points. Several convenient approximate solutions may be based on this observation. It is common in applications to choose the reference distribution from a class P_0 generated from a particular prototype distribution $P_0(x)$ by a linear transformation of x in which probabilities are preserved:

$$P(x) = P_0(z),\ z = \frac{x-a}{b}, \tag{9}$$

$$p(x) = \frac{p_0(z)}{b} \tag{10}$$

Here, a is the location parameter and b is the scale parameter. The uniform, normal, lognormal, Gumbel and Weibull distribution types are examples. All distributions of class P_0 plot as the straight line $z = a+bx$ on a graph of $z = P_0^{-1}(P(x))$ vs. x. When a random sample $\{x_i\}$ of size r is plotted as the points $(x_i, P_0^{-1}(i/(r+1))$ in such a graph, these points should nearly lie on a straight line. This permits visual verification that the distribution may belong to the class and allows easy determination of the parameters, a as the intercept on the abscissa and b as the reciprocal of the slope.

If the sample points in the graph are acceptably close to a straight line, this line may be used as reference distribution. Then the slope $q(x)$ will everywhere be almost equal to $p(x)$, and will be almost constant in the representation of the graph so that $Q(x)$ is nearly composed of straight line segments connecting the sample points. When the domain is finite this polygon is a reasonable approximation that is determined directly from the sample independent of the reference distribution. Where the domain extends to infinity, the reference distribution has considerable influence on $Q(x)$. Then it may be reasonable to determine $P(x)$ by least squares fit to the sample.

If the sample points are not acceptably close to a straight line, the graph will suggest a more suitable family P_0.

MINIMIZING DISCONTINUITIES IN DENSITY

The density functions of the distributions of minimum cross-entropy are in general discontinuous at the points x_i, $i = 1,..., r$, partitioning I. The jump in $q(x)$ at $x = x_i$ is

$$s_i = \left(\frac{q_i}{p_i}\ \frac{q_{i-1}}{p_{i-1}}\right) \cdot p(x_i), \quad i = 1, ..., r\ . \tag{11}$$

The sum of the squares of such jumps is uniquely determined by $p(x)$. For a given sample there is a unique value S_m of the sum of the squares of the jumps associated with any distribution $p(x)$. This can be considered as a directed distance of the distribution $p(x)$ from the data, and allows a criterion of comparison of all reference distribution candidates. This suggests the following criterion:

The reference distribution should be selected such as to minimize the sum of the squares of the discontinuities in the minimum cross-entropy density function.

CONCLUSIONS

1. The type of distribution is usually unknown for any variable that occurs in technology or in nature and is modelled as random. Assumptions about distribution type in risk analysis are difficult to verify and justify. Unfortunately a reference distribution framework of some sort seems indispensable when dealing with continuous random variables. In the case of classical and Bayesian estimation, the solution space is thus restricted to a parametric family of tractable distributions. When the concern is with extreme and rare events, with disastrous consequences or with matters of grave public responsibility, it is best to make only weak and robust assumptions about distribution type.

2. An unknown element in a sequence of r+1 elements, each of which may or may not be an independent realization of a random variable, is a random variable with exactly known $i/(r+1)$-fractiles. These fractiles prescribe constraints for the process of estimation of the random variable when the only usable information is the sample.

3. Distribution estimation on the basis of moments only is a common approach that cannot be recommended. It will in general contradict the exact intrinsic property of random sampling mentioned above. Moreover, it discards an arbitrary and unknown amount of information contained in the sample.

4. The method of minimum cross-entropy is known to yield results that are invariant under monotonic variable transformations. This method is preferable over generating distributions of continuous random variables with prescribed fractiles. The solution is piecewise a constant multiple of the reference distribution. This solution can be determined algebraically.

5. The minimum value of the cross-entropy functional is a function of the reference distribution function at the quantiles. It is functionally independent of the values assumed by the reference at other points and it is not directly dependent on the reference density function.

6. To solve a distribution estimation problem in practice by the method of minimum cross-entropy, it is necessary to select a reference (or "prior") distribution that provides a function of interpolation between the fractiles and extrapolation outside the fractile range. The minimum cross-entropy can be interpreted as the directional distance from the reference distribution to the sample, which suggests that the reference should be chosen from a candidate set such as to minimize this minimum cross-entropy.

7. In general the minimum cross-entropy density function is discontinuous at the prescribed fractiles. The jumps in the density at a fractile adjacent to a tail can always be eliminated by choosing a reference distribution that contains all sample points.

8. Given a set of fractile constraints there exists a reference in any class of distributions that minimizes the discontinuities in the minimum cross-entropy density in the least squares sense. The reference distribution may be selected from a set of acceptable candidates such as to minimize the sum of the squares of the discontinuities in the minimum cross-entropy density function.

REFERENCES

1. B. W. Silverman, *Density Estimation for Statistics and Data Analysis*, Chapman and Hall, London (1986).
2. J. Shore and R. W. Johnson, Axiomatic Derivation of the Principle of Maximum Entropy and the Principle of Minimum Cross-Entropy, *IEEE Transactions on Information Theory* **IT-26(1)**:26-37 (1980).
3. J. Shore and R. W. Johnson, Properties of Cross-Entropy Minimization, *IEEE Transactions on Information Theory* **IT-27(4)**:472-482 (1981).
4. J. N. Kapur and H. K. Kesavan, *The Generalized Maximum Entropy Principle (with Applications)*, Sandford Educational Press, Waterloo, Ontario (1987).
5. S. N. Karbelkar, On the Axiomatic Approach to the Maximum Entropy Principle of Inference, *Pramana J. Phys.* **26(4)**:301-310 (1986).
6. D. M. Titterington, A. F. M. Smith, and U. E. Markov, *Statistical Analysis of Finite Mixture Distributions*, John Wiley and Sons, Chichester, UK (1985).
7. P. Ofverbeck, *Small Sample Control and Structural Safety*, Report TVBK-3009, Dept. Struct. Eng., Lund University, Lund, Sweden (1980).
8. E. T. Jaynes, Papers on Probability, Statistics, and Statistical Physics, D. Reidel, Dordrecht, Netherlands (1983).
9. H. Akaike, *Prediction and Entropy, A Celebration of Statistics*, A. C. Atkinson and S. E. Fienberg, eds., Springer-Verlag, New York, NY (1985).
10. W. Feller, *An Introduction to Probability Theory and its Applications*, 3rd ed., John Wiley and Sons, Inc., New York, NY (1968).
11. H. O. Madsen, S. Krenk and N. C. Lind, *Methods of Structural Safety*, Prentice-Hall Book Co., Inc., Englewood Cliffs, NJ (1986).
12. G. Matheron, *Estimating and Choosing*, Springer-Verlag, Berlin (1989).
13. N. C. Lind and V. Solana, *Estimation of Random Variables With Fractile Constraints*, IRR paper No. 11, Institute for Risk Research, University of Waterloo, Waterloo, Ontario, Canada (1988).

Human Error in the Transportation of Spent Nuclear Fuel

S. Tuler, R. E. Kasperson, and S. Ratick
Clark University
Worcester, MA

ABSTRACT

This paper summarizes work completed on human factors contributions to risks from spent nuclear fuel transportation. Human participation may have significant effects on the levels and types of risks from transportation of spent nuclear fuel by enabling or initiating incidents and exacerbating adverse consequences. Human errors are defined as the result of mismatches between perceived system state and actual system state. In complex transportation systems such mismatches may be distributed in time (e.g., during different stages of design, implementation, operation, maintenance) and location (e.g., human error, its identification, and its recovery may be geographically and institutionally separate). Risk management programs may decrease the probability of undesirable events or attenuate the consequences of mismatches. To be successful, they must be based in part on the analysis of human reliability data. This paper presents an overview of the availability and quality of human reliability data for spent fuel transportation risk assessments. In addition, we identify example prior occurrences of "human errors" during different stages and activities of spent nuclear fuel transportation. We have used such data, in conjunction with human error models, to develop a framework for the identification and management of potential mismatches.

KEYWORDS: Transportation, human reliability, nuclear, human error, risk management

INTRODUCTION

Despite the evident importance of reliable human performance in spent nuclear fuel transportation, no comprehensive analysis of human factors has to date been undertaken. In general, federal agency and industry activities reflect the belief that human actions are not significant contributors to risk in the transportation system. This attitude arises from the assumption that the probability associated with simultaneous human and technical failures leading to major accidents is negligible. However, the two prior risk assessments on which this conclusion is based[1,2] have been evaluated and shown to contain both methodological errors and faulty data.[3,4] We believe that careful consideration of human-task mismatches are likely to lead to much higher estimated transportation risks resulting from the shipment of spent fuel to a repository than those estimated in prior risk assessments.

The systematic evaluation of human reliability has become an important need as planning begins for a federal high level radioactive waste repository. The opening of such a

Risk Analysis, Edited by C. Zervos
Plenum Press, New York, 1991

site will greatly affect the magnitude of manufacturing, operational, and maintenance activities associated with spent fuel transportation. The potential for adverse events arising out of human actions will increase as the magnitude of the transportation system grows. We believe that careful consideration of human reliability is likely to lead to much higher estimated transportation risks than those estimated in prior risk assessments.

Adverse events arising out of human actions are frequently blamed on "human error;" the flip-side of "human reliability." The confluence of research resulting from both theoretical and applied work on human error suggests that they derive from interactions within a human-task system. "Human error" is defined as the result of a mismatch between perceived and actual system state and dynamics in human-machine or human-task systems.

Mismatches occur as a result of human variability, technical variability or failure, and required interactions that are incompatible with general human cognitive and motor control limitations or organizational constraints. They occur within a "socio-technical system" that includes system hardware (e.g., spent fuel casks, trucks, cranes), system personnel (e.g., drivers, crane operators, managers), organizational and institutional infrastructure (e.g., operations, maintenance, management, administration), and social-economic factors (e.g., regulations, legislation, economics, culture).[5] Mismatches may accumulate at these four different levels to cause system wide failures or disasters by (1) initiating risk events, (2) contributing to risk events, (3) altering the frequency of risk event sequences, (4) altering the structure of risk event trees by changing intervention strategies and reliability, and (5) altering couplings and interactions between subsystems and components.

In this paper, we summarize aspects of our on-going research related to the transportation of spent nuclear fuel to a national repository. Our concern is for the quality of data available to assess the likelihoods and consequences of human errors during all phases of the spent fuel transportation system. The intent of the paper is

1. to identify the characteristics of the spent fuel transportation system that suggest human reliability should be an important area of concern and research;

2. to discuss the adequacy of existing transportation accident and incident databases for providing human error data that can be used for both the identification of human error types before they occur and modes of control after they occur; and

3. to provide examples of human error in prior spent nuclear fuel transportation activities at all phases of system design, implementation, operation, maintenance, and accident recovery.

THE IMPORTANCE OF HUMAN RELIABILITY

To date there have been no severe incidents or accidents resulting in significant releases of radioactivity during spent fuel shipments. Indeed, several successful shipment campaigns for spent nuclear fuel have been completed.[6-8] On the other hand, the shipment campaigns were (1) small compared with the expected numbers after a repository opens, and (2) heavily regulated and closely observed to assure operational safety and system reliability.

A lack of concern over human error as a cause of accidents or incidents in the transportation system is apparent within the relevant regulatory agencies and national research laboratories. Many individuals are not convinced that human reliability in the transportation of spent fuel is an issue worth further study. The primary rationale for this limited attention is that the spent fuel transportation system is viewed as a simple system that does not require complex monitoring and problem solving tasks. This assumption, however, ignores the issue of emergency response-related decisions. In addition, it dismisses the ambiguities of inspection and monitoring activities and problems arising from inexperienced personnel.

Similarly, there are strong beliefs that technological features (e.g., cask integrity under severe accident conditions) and the reliability and thoroughness of regulatory requirements (e.g., route selection, equipment maintenance, quality assurance programs) will ensure system safety and reliability. However, responsibilities and control in the transportation system are distributed across many organizational and political boundaries, including several federal agencies, state agencies, private industry, and other public organizations (e.g., utilities, shippers, carriers).[4] Human reliability considerations are not usually specifically addressed by regulations. In addition, beliefs about technical reliability and safety in the transportation system are based on highly suspect data and assumptions.

However, four characteristics of spent fuel and other high-level radioactive waste transport suggest that human actions may indeed contribute significantly to both actual and perceived risk of the transportation system.[9] They are as follows:

1. The transportation of spent fuel involves a number of activities (Table 1), all of which depend on effective, safe, and reliable human performance. Those entities that must respond to events caused by "upstream" human actions are often separated temporally, spatially, and sectorally (i.e., institutionally) from the sources of the errors.

2. The magnitude of transportation activities for a national repository will be larger, more complex, and potentially more hazardous than any previous transportation program attempted. Historical evidence, however, suggest that the effectiveness of transportation risk management programs have previously not been completely effective in eliminating human errors during the transportation of spent nuclear fuel.

3. Even minor risk events in the transportation system for spent fuel have the potential for contributing to the social amplification of risk.[10] There has been little emphasis, however, on the avoidance of minor events and their effects on risk perceptions related to the assumption. The implications of small events are considered unimportant from a risk perspective.

4. Even under the best circumstances the transportation system for spent fuel will remain sensitive to the possibility of human error. Human factors research suggests that it is not possible to eliminate human errors in complex technological systems.[11-13] Human errors have also been estimated to account for at least 62% of hazardous material transportation accidents.[14]

HUMAN ERROR DATABASES

The effective and timely collection and evaluation of human error data are important inputs into effective risk management strategies. However, the collection of data adequate to support system design and modifications, as well as quantitative human reliability assessments, is fraught with difficulties.[11,15,16,17] For example, structured descriptions of events are needed, based on the sequence of cognitive functions and human behaviors prior to, during, and in response to events.[15] Similarly, current human error reporting systems typically are associated with the assignment of blame and responsibility that inhibit the reporting of required information.

Thus the adequacy of existing transportation databases are important considerations in the development of transportation risk management strategies. In our work we have

Table 1. Spent Fuel Transportation System Phases and Activities

Design

- regulations
- institutional structure
- planning criteria (e.g., routing, modes)
- hazard communication
- cask and equipment design

Implementation

- organizational
- technical
- personnel

Operation

- oversight
- pre-shipment activities
- packaging, loading, securing casks
- transportation and transshipment
- receipt and post-shipment activities

Maintenance

- technical
- personnel
- data collection and analysis

Accident response and recovery

- notification
- immediate response
- long-term activities

addressed questions relating to the accuracy, completeness, and usefulness of transportation related human error data in federal and state agencies and private institutions. Table 2 lists federal, state, and private databases that contain information related to human error.

The main sources of information about human errors during non-operations phases in the transportation system for spent fuel are inspection and maintenance reports. Sources for such information include the DOT, NRC, DOE, state inspection agencies, utilities, and carriers. For example, NRC data has been used to summarize prior inspection activities.[18] Other data sources are provided by incident investigations when some type of failure occurs during non-transit operational activities. Specific information available from these sources includes data on manufacture, use, and maintenance of casks and transportation equipment (e.g., vehicles, cranes) and personnel qualifications.

Previous reviews of federal, state, and private transportation accident and incident databases suggest that there are major generic inadequacies in the data they contain for supporting evaluation efforts.[14] For example, reporting compliance of transportation incidents is clearly not 100%, there is no centralized authority for transportation related data collection and analysis, and no uniformity exists in the types of data collected and definitions used.

Table 2. Transportation Databases Containing Human Error Accident and Incident Data

DATABASES	KEPT BY	YEARS	MODES
Hazardous Materials Information System	DOT, Office of Hazardous Materials Transportation, Research and Special Programs Administration	1971 to present	All
Radioactivie Materials Incident Report	Department of Energy, Oak Ridge National Laboratory	1971 to present	All
National Transportation Safety Board File	National Transportation Safety Board	---	All
Monthly Accident/Incident Reports	DOT, Federal Railroad Administration	1957 to present	Rail
Railroad Accident File	Association of American Railroads	1973 to present	Rail
SAFETYNET	DOT, Federal Highway Administrator, Motor Carrier Safety Assistance Program	Demonstration only	Highway
Truck and Rail Inspections	Illinois, Department of Nuclear Safety	1983 to present	Rail, Highway
Washington State Accident File	Washington State Utility and Transportation Commission	1978	Highway
Hazardous Material Spill Database	North Carolina, Department of Environmental Management	1978 to present	Highway
Inspection Reports	NRC, DOE, DOT	---	All

Although one might suspect that the problems would not be as severe for the more heavily regulated spent fuel transportation system, this is not necessarily the case because of the multiple agencies involved and the ineffectiveness of existing inspection programs.[4] For example, spent fuel transportation related incidents are not complete in the DOT or DOE databases and, when events do occur, they may not be entered immediately. Similarly, access to data is not always easy — for example, the NRC did not even start separating out data on transportation related issues from on-site inspection reports until 1981.

The state of Illinois is unique in that it maintains an extensive database of spent fuel rail and truck shipment inspections. Since 1983 the Illinois Department of Nuclear Safety has performed inspections on casks, vehicles, and drivers of all shipments passing through the state. In addition, the Illinois Commerce Commission has performed pre-departure inspections of all rail shipments. Specific problems that have been identified for both rail and truck shipments through Illinois are listed in Table 3.

Aside from the generic problems of data reporting and availability, specific problems arise in the data relating to human error. In fact, such data are less adequate for comprehensive analyses than other transportation related data (e.g., property damage, injury rates) because of the ambiguity of human error itself, difficulty in its evaluation, and the general disregard of causal information (i.e., only accident consequences need to be reported in many cases). This suggests in part why data in the Battelle and NRC reports on human error were substantially defective.

PRIOR EXPERIENCES OF HUMAN ERROR

Human reliability issues in spent fuel transport extend well beyond vehicle operation and cask loading. Consideration must be given to human activities at all phases of the transportation system, including technical designs, fabrication of equipment, management, maintenance, and emergency response (see Table 1). This section provides examples of human error events that have occurred during the different phases of spent nuclear fuel transportation.

The *design phase* includes the activities that develop the characteristics of the specific transportation system. These include the development of institutional structures through legislative action and regulatory promulgation, the design of equipment and manufacturing standards, and the design of accident prevention and response methods. Many of the human errors that have occurred in the transportation system can be traced back to situations where insufficient consideration has been given to human factors issues in this phase. Specific problems include:[3,4,19,20]

- errors in the analysis of spent fuel cask baskets,
- drop, puncture, and fire test standards for the most severe accident conditions are not based on historical data,
- cask trailer designs that are inadequate to hold heavy loads resulting in buckling during use,
- designs not tested for maintainability or ease of inspection,
- documentation errors related to cask designs and fabrication,
- methodological errors in risk assessments,
- incorrect value for railroad car miles used to estimate accident probabilities,
- errors in simulation data inputs, and
- mathematical errors in stress analysis.

Table 3. Example Records from the Illinois Spent Fuel Transportation Inspection Database

---

Rail Shipments

- Rather common paper work and labelling deficiencies.
- Security problems at an Illinois rail yard, involving a bomb threat.
- Security problems caused by media coverage, which included following a TMI spent fuel shipment with a helicopter.
- Potential security problems at another Illinois rail yard due to negligence.
- A rail/automobile collision (a 25 mph train-speed) in Missouri shortly after the train crossed the Illinois/Missouri border. No damage to the cask occurred.
- The buffer car between the casks in one shipment had a defective flange; the train had to be delayed for repair.

Truck Shipments

- Common paper work and labelling deficiencies.
- Vehicle problems, including a lost wheel in Indiana, misadjusted brakes, unoperable tail lights, several cases of air leaks in brakes, unoperative emergency flashers, and unsafe rear tires. In one case the trailer failed the safety inspection and the shipment was cancelled.
- Driver related problems, including a case where the driver was found sleeping in the cab, and expired training dates.
- Several cases of incorrect highway route plans.
- Security problems, including several failures to notify state authorities, security guards leaving the truck unattended, and several cases of inoperable mobile phones in trucks.

The *implementation phase* involves the development of the transportation system components, such as the fabrication of equipment, the training of personnel, and the implementation of inspection, enforcement, and emergency response programs. Errors have included the use of inadequate testing and licensing procedures for drivers. Other errors have occurred during cask fabrication that involved:[3,4,19]

- the installation of defective valves and rupture disks,
- the use of improper welding materials and defective bolts, and sealant,
- the use of improper cask welding
- the defective installation of shielding,
- the improper installation of valves,
- the use of a defective shell on an outer cask body, and
- the continued use of casks after the breakdown of quality assurance programs at the manufacturer.

The *operations phase* includes the entire sequence of activities from the selection of fuel for shipment to the unloading of the material at the final destination. A sequential view of the shipping procedure is a useful aid in the identification of potential hazards and includes the following stages (Fig. 1):

1. The packaging of spent fuel into casks, completed underwater in cooling pools, by personnel remotely controlling automated equipment with the use of video cameras and robotic equipment. A key aspect of this stage is the evaluation of spent fuel characteristics (e.g., age, cladding condition, burn-up rate) for shipment because they may influence the integrity of the fuel during transport activities, the selection of casks for shipment, and the handling, inspection, and emergency response needs at a repository. The inspection of casks prior to packaging are also important to determine if they are defective (e.g., leaking, warped).

2. The loading of casks onto a transport vehicle (e.g., truck-trailer or rail-car) and the completion of all required routing and labeling requirements (e.g., pre-notification, placards). This stage is completed after casks have been secured and inspected on the vehicle.

3. The actual material transport by truck or rail, including temporary stowage or transshipment as a result of modal mixing. Several road accidents have occurred during truck shipments, which fortunately did not result in releases.

4. The unloading and inspection of casks and the spent fuel upon arrival at its final destination.

There have been numerous examples of human errors during these activities; they are listed in Table 4.[3,4,8,19]

The *maintenance phase* occurs when equipment requires either scheduled or unscheduled repairs and is simultaneous with the operations phase. Specific activities include inspection, repair, calibration, testing, and verification tasks. Human errors in this phase have included:[3,4,19]

- improper repairs using improper materials,
- inspection failures (i.e., faulty equipment not identified),
- required repairs not performed on vehicles,
- failure to properly perform cask leak tests,
- failure to properly decontaminate casks and equipment,
- failure to routinely replace cask lid seals, and
- replacement of faulty cask valves with other faulty valves.

The *accident recovery phase* is initiated after either an incident or accident occurs in the transportation system. Specific activities range from the actions and decisions made at the very onset of an emergency (e.g., notification) and extend through long term monitoring and clean-up activities as needed. Errors involving the improper placarding and notification have previously resulted in inadequate emergency response measures being undertaken.[3,19] In one case emergency response personnel did not attempt to put out a fire resulting from an accident because they were erroneously led to believe that radioactive materials were involved. Additional problems have occurred because of inaccurate or false reports of accident consequences to emergency response personnel[21] and confusion resulting from unfamiliar personnel working together in novel situations.[22]

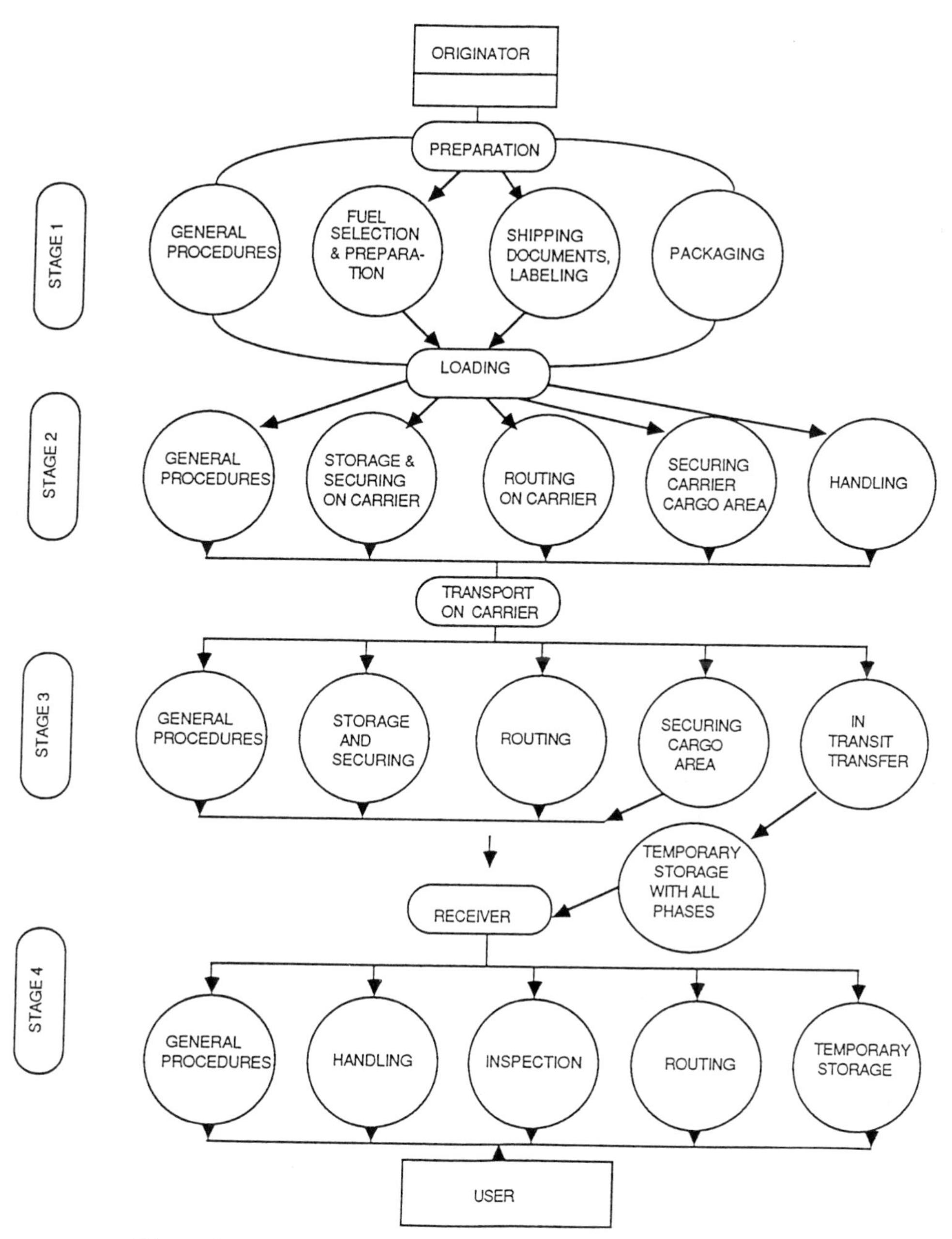

Fig. 1. Operational phase activities of spent fuel transportation.

CONCLUSIONS

Risks from human-task and human-machine mismatches during all phases of the spent fuel transportation system remain largely unexamined. Human error data collection and analysis have not usually been a priority of government regulators or industry groups and they are distributed among many different responsible agencies and organizations. This

Table 4. Human Errors During the Operational Phase of Spent Fuel Transportation

- incorrect fuel selection resulting from the use of outdated mathematical fuel-selection equations (the use of an improper equation led to the incorrect choice of fuel to transport in a particular cask)
- failure to properly drain pool water from casks (in one case this occurred when the incorrect valve was opened because of the absence of color-coded labeling on the valves)
- improper dry shipment of spent fuel
- incorrect placarding of shipments
- incorrect filling out of shipping papers
- improper securing of casks on truck beds
- surface contamination of cask and trailer
- improper pre-departure inspections of casks and vehicles
- improper loading of spent fuel into casks
- damage to fuel and casks during loading
- drivers' failure to adhere to preplanned routes
- rail shipments being "lost" and ending up in unprotected train yards
- co-drivers sleeping at unauthorized times
- inoperative driver communication equipment
- collapsing truck beds due to cask weight
- lack of proper escorts due to improper notification
- failure to notice radioactive contamination of equipment
- transport vehicle breakdowns and improper repairs
- a truck-trailer overturned during transit

problem is not unique to the spent fuel transportation system; it is also an important problem in hazardous material transportation generally.[14]

Although the historical experience from spent fuel and other high-level radioactive waste transportation is limited, some specific lessons related to human reliability are apparent. For example,

- significant problems in cask usage and transportation activities have resulted from insufficient attention to human factors issues in the design of equipment and procedures, and
- many problems occur during nondesign phase activities, including improper shipping paper completion, improper labeling and placarding, and hardware (e.g., vehicles, casks) maintenance, inspection, and mechanical failures.

The frequency of such failures in general transportation systems suggests that meticulous attention needs to be focused on inspection and enforcement programs, operator training, and quality control. Unfortunately, available data on particular hazardous material transportation incidents or accidents usually cannot support detailed error or accident investigations. A lack of systematic data collection and analysis limits the ability to perceive patterns of problems.

In our work we have developed a methodology for the systematic collection and identification of human error data that may be used in human reliability analyses.[4] It is a key component of our framework (1) for the identification of previous and potential future human errors in the transportation system, and (2) for the identification of risk management options that can be implemented to prevent, mitigate, or recover from human errors and their consequences.[9]

REFERENCES

1. Battelle Pacific Northwest Laboratories, An Assessment of the Risk of Transporting Sent Nuclear Fuel by Truck, PNL-2588, Battelle Pacific Northwest Laboratories, Richland, WA (1978).
2. Nuclear Regulatory Commission, Transportation of Radionuclides in Urban Environs: Draft Environmental Assessment, U. S. Nuclear Commission, NUREG/CR-0743, USGPO, Washington, DC (1980).
3. Nebraska Energy Office, A Review of the Effects of Human Error on the Risks Involved in Spent Fuel Transportation, Nebraska Energy Office, Lincoln, NE (1987).
4. S. Tuler, R. E. Kasperson, and S. Ratick, The Effects of Human Reliability on Risk in the Transportation of Spent Nuclear Fuel, unpublished manuscript, CENTED, Clark University, Worcester, MA (1988).
5. National Research Council, *Human Factors Research and Nuclear Safety*, Committee on Human Factors, National Research Council, National Academy Press, Washington, DC (1988).
6. R. W. Rasmussen, Duke Power Company Spent Fuel Storage and Transportation Experience, *Nuclear Safety* **27(4)**:512-518 (1986).
7. M. Ruska and D. Schoonen, Virginia Power and Department of Energy Spent Fuel Transportation Experience, Report EGG-2491, prepared for the Department of Energy by EG&G Idaho, Idaho Falls, Idaho (1986).
8. R. K. Kunita and A. R. Wallace, Interstation Transfer of Spent Nuclear Fuel, in *Fifth International Symposium on Packaging and Transportation of Radioactive Materials*, Las Vegas, NV, May 7-12, 1978.
9. S. Tuler, R. E. Kasperson, and S. Ratick, Human Reliability and Risk Management in the Transportation of Spent Nuclear Fuel, in *Reliability on the Move: Safety and Reliability in Transportation*, G. B. Guy, ed., Elsevier Applied Science, London (1989).
10. R. E. Kasperson, O. Renn, P. Slovic, H. S. Brown, J. Emel, R. Goble, J. X. Kasperson, and S. Ratick, The Social Amplification of Risk: A Conceptual Framework, *Risk Analysis* **8(2)**:177-188 (1988).
11. J. Rasmussen, What Can Be Learned from Human Error Reports? in *Changes in Working Life*, K. Duncan, M. Gruneberg, D. Wallis, eds., John Wiley and Sons, NY (1980).
12. L. Bellamy, Neglected Individual, Social, and Organizational Factors in Human Reliability Assessment, in *Proceedings of the Fourth National Reliability Conference*, Vol. 1, National Centre of Systems Reliability, Birmingham, England, July 6-8, 1983.
13. D. P. Miller and A. D. Swain, Human Error and Human Reliability, in *Handbook of Human Factors*, G. Salvendy, ed., John Wiley and Sons, NY (1987).
14. Office of Technology Assessment, The Transportation of Hazardous Materials, OTA-SET-304, USGPO, Washington, DC (1986).

15. L. Bainbridge, Diagnostic Skill in Process Operation, paper presented at the International Conference on Occupational Ergonomics, Toronto, Canada, May 7-9, 1984.
16. Nuclear Regulatory Commission, Nuclear Power Safety Reporting System, U. S. Nuclear Commission, NUREG/CR-4132, USGPO, Washington, DC (1985).
17. D. Lucas, Human Performance Data Collection in the Nuclear Industry, paper presented at the Conference on Human Reliability in Nuclear Power, London, England, October 22-23, 1987.
18. A. Grella, NRC Inspection Activities on Recent Shipments of Spent Fuel 1983-Present, Office of Inspection and Enforcement, U.S. Nuclear Regulatory Commission, unpublished speech at the Spent Nuclear Fuel Transportation Seminar, Chicago, IL, August 1, 1985.
19. M. Resnikoff, The Next Nuclear Gamble, Council on Economic Priorities, NY (1983).
20. J. R. Paschall, A Railroad Perspective on Transportation of Spent Fuel and High Level Waste and Recent ICC Decisions, paper presented at the Fifth International Symposium on Packaging and Transportation of Radioactive Materials, Las Vegas, NV, May 7-12, 1978.
21. J. C. Taylor, The Safe Transportation of Radioactive Material Shipping Containers Including Accident and Response Experience, paper presented at the Fifth International Symposium on Packaging and Transportation of Radioactive Materials, Las Vegas, NV, May 7-12, 1978.
22. M. Neuweg, Spent Fuel Transportation Accident — A State's Involvement, paper presented at the Fifth International Symposium on Packaging and Transportation of Radioactive Materials, Las Vegas, NV, May 7-12, 1978.

Estimation of Synergy in Risk Analysis Using Orthogonality Principles, Ancillary Variables and Multivariate Analysis

Turkan Kumbaraci Gardenier
TKG Consultants, Ltd.
Vienna, Virginia

ABSTRACT

This paper addresses an issue an issue in risk assessment which has often been acknowledged but for which reliable statistical analysis methods have not been synthesized: estimating synergy in the onset of risk event. Biological, environmental and habit-related factors all influence the detriment or detriments to health which we observe and research. Often, however, our data collection and data analysis strategy has had only the principles of "one-at-a-time" experiments — the possible risk factors have not been varied simultaneously in the planning of data collection. A "directed data collection and analysis" using multivariate statistical methods is advocated in this paper. The present author developed two systems, PRE-PRIM and POST-PRIM, which provide sampling and data collection specifications for research studies which explore synergistic effects. Design templates from PRE-PRIM use matrix orthogonality principles to assist in data collection for prospective or retrospective studies. POST-PRIM interfaces the data input matrix of hypothesized and ancillary variables with multiple output measures. A profile of multiple input-output links is thus generated.

KEYWORDS: Synergy, multivariate analysis, orthogonality, design matrix, retrospective sampling

INTRODUCTION

According to the Office of Technology Assessment[1] synergy occurs "when two or more substances enhance each other's effects producing more. . . than can be accounted for by adding the effects of each. The multiplicative effects of cigarette smoking and exposure to asbestos and of smoking and exposure to radiation are well-known examples of synergism."

The observed risk due to two or more compounds may be higher or lower than the sum of the risks of each compound observed alone. When the risk is higher, the interactive effect is denoted as "synergism"; if total risk is lower, the term used is "antagonism." For example, if chromium carbonyl is administered along with benzo(a)pyrene, the observed number of tumors in animal experiments was found to be higher than the sum of the number of tumors if each were administered to different groups of animals. Similar results are found in experiments that produce skin cancer when floranthene is administered along with benzo(a)pyrene. On the other hand, if copper and calcium are present along with cadmium, the onset of risk for anemia seems to be retarded. Similarly, protection against teratogenic effects is demonstrated if zinc is present along with cadmium, a suspected teratogen. For people with decreased vital capacity nitrogen oxides cause increased retention of harmful particulates. Bioavailability studies have also shown that a certain level of copper in the metabolism leads to a tolerance for high doses of zinc.[2]

Several laws have stressed the need to study the synergistic or antagonistic effects in determining the risk from substances to which we are exposed in the workplace or elsewhere in our daily life. The Toxic Substances Control Act [TSCA PL94-469, Oct. 11, 1976, Section 4(b)(2)(a) (90 STAT 2007)] has a testing requirement rule for chemical substances or mixtures. It requires standards and tests which will estimate "carcinogenesis, teratogenesis, behavioral disorders, cumulative and synergistic effects, and any other effect which may present an unreasonable risk of injury to health or the environment." Maximum allowable levels of contaminants such as lead, nitrogen oxides, nitrates and hydrocarbons have been documented in publications such as the *Handbook of Key Federal Regulations and Criteria for Multimedia Environmental Control*.[3] They are used in various criteria set by the National Institute for Occupational Safety and Health Administration (NIOSH) and in the National Ambient Air Quality Standards (NAAQS). Furthermore, compensating victims under workmen's compensation and personal injury action demands an ability to evaluate the composite effect of biological interactions in specific settings.

The recent calls for emergency response decisions at sites such as Love Canal and Three Mile Island also demand study protocols or data collection methods which will estimate interactive effects. When an emergency alarm appears, short-term studies are designed to gather data which will determine if the site is hazardous. Samples are usually taken from body fluids of residents, from soil, water and air. Multi-media data from such sources interact among themselves and with the biological characteristics of the individuals under attack. Maugh[4] stressed the importance and difficulty of analyzing data of this type.

ANALYTIC CONSIDERATIONS IN SYNERGY ESTIMATION

Statistical procedures for linking health and environmental effects have not adequately addressed the synergy and antagonism of multiple pollutants and biological predisposition. In most studies, health risk has been tested for the environmental concentration of a specific pollutant. Lave and Seskin[5] used multivariate regression procedures to associate death rates with (a) sulfur dioxide and particulate concentration in air, (b) socioeconomic data, and (c) home heating characteristics. Goldsmith and Hexter[6] and Azar[7] explored the relationship between blood and air concentrations of lead by plotting the logarithm of ambient air lead against blood lead levels of residents. In most correlational studies of this type, risk estimates have been obtained for only one pollutant, ignoring the effect of simultaneous exposure to others.

The PRE-PRIM approach to estimating synergy or antagonism is based upon a multivariate framework and stresses the significance of a "directed data collection" effort in prospective or retrospective studies. PRE-PRIM visualizes the concept of interaction as the cross-product of main effect terms in a design matrix. Templates are generated for input data retrieval or collection. Their design is dictated by (a) budget constraints, (b) the number of hypothesized influential or ancillary variables, and (c) the network of interactions to be tested for statistical significance. As will be demonstrated, this approach has proved cost effective in terms of sample size requirements.

THE MULTI-ATTRIBUTE APPROACH IN PRE-PRIM

PRE-PRIM approaches the risk decision as a composite of multiple inputs and multiple outputs. The multiple inputs consist of the sum total of the biological and environmental characteristics in a particular scenario. The multiple outputs are the "more than one" risk events elicited — data need to be collected for all hypothesized and ancillary endpoints, much like laboratory monitoring data in clinical trials.

Brainstorming as well as stringent statistical criteria dictates the contents of the multiple inputs.[8] First, let us conceptualize interaction graphically through Fig. 1.

If there is no synergy or antagonism between the two variables, X_i and X_j shown in Fig. 1, the numerical values on the dependent variable Y will increase or decrease in parallel. This is illustrated on the right-hand side. However, if a cross-over is noted in the plots of various partitions of X_j as X_i increases (or vice versa), an interaction is flagged. Researchers can demonstrate this graphically in most studies. The goal, however, is to be able to derive stable mathematical coefficients for a general model of risk estimation.

PRE-PRIM builds new parameters for such estimation into the data collection scheme. Let us first illustrate what is meant by a pre-processing matrix and template.

Multivariate regression analysis procedures have often been used merely for data analysis. The principles underlying the inherent design called for in the input data have often been overlooked. Figure 2 shows a data matrix consisting of (a) data collection criteria in columns 2-4 and (b) internally generated coefficients for parameter estimation in columns 5-12. Each of the 8 lines in the matrix corresponds to a specific observation: for example, mortality rate from lung cancer in a community as a function of (a) annual sulfur dioxide concentration (X_1), (b) cigarette smoking rate (X_2), and (c) proximity to a power plant (X_3). If we are interested in the synergy or antagonism among the three input variables, such interactions need to be built into the mathematical model. In Fig. 2 these are expressed as the last 4 terms in the regression model below the matrix and as columns 8 and 10-12 in the "effect matrix" portion of the diagram. Although data collection is based only on information in columns 2-4, columns 5-12 are essential to assuring reliability and stability in risk parameters estimated and documented.

Figure 2 tells us that with 8 observations it is possible to estimate the individual and joint effects of three input variables. This allows for no replication to estimate random error; not all estimable interactions may be clinically feasible. It is possible, through other features in PRE-PRIM, to design other templates for data collection which will evaluate fewer interactions but screen more input risk factors for statistical significance. Figure 3 shows a data collection design plan using 16 observations, 5 variables being screened for risk, and 4 interactions for investigation. We note in this design that the risk factors are taken two at a time, ignoring triple and higher order interactions which usually appear insignificant and are difficult to interpret.

Columns 2-4 in Fig. 2 and columns 2-6 in Fig. 3 constitute data collection specifications. Although at many risk sites input data may be more fine-tuned, PRE-PRIM calls for only for those values which can be specified as "+/-": that is, the experimenter's decision as to an appropriate choice of high and low levels. Further sensitivity can be attained by introducing non-linear terms into the model and using an intermediate value for each variable. This orientation to data collection is multi-faceted — it can be applied to prospective or retrospective studies given that the selection of the specific datapoints is unbiased. For example, "blinding" procedures need to be introduced similar to those used in randomizing among patients in clinical trials. These form a set of rules for the selection of targeted datapoints among those encountered in already collected databases.

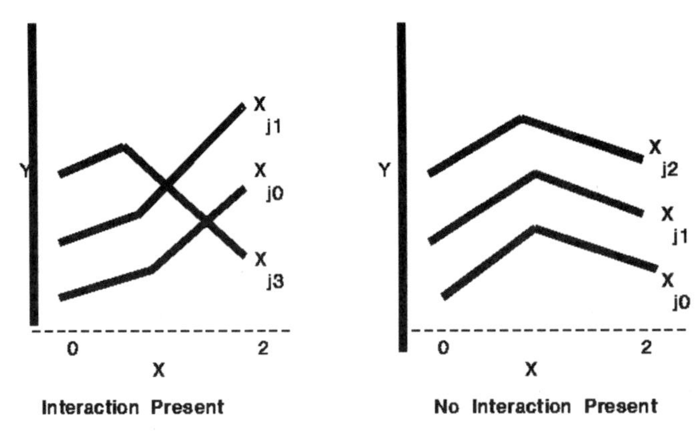

Fig. 1. Crossover patterns depicting interaction (Source: Gardenier[9]).

Observation	Representation By Signs			Effect Matrix							
	X_1	X_2	X_3	Mean	X_1	X_2	X_1X_2	X_3	X_1X_3	X_2X_3	$X_1X_2X_3$
1	-	-	-	+	-	-	+	-	+	+	-
X_1	+	-	-	+	+	-	-	-	-	+	+
X_2	-	+	-	+	-	+	-	-	+	-	+
X_1X_2	+	+	-	+	+	+	+	-	-	-	-
X_3	-	-	+	+	-	-	+	+	-	-	+
X_1X_3	+	-	+	+	+	-	-	+	+	-	-
X_2X_3	-	+	+	+	-	+	-	+	-	+	-
$X_1X_2X_3$	+	+	+	+	+	+	+	+	+	+	+

$$y = \beta_0 + \beta_1X_1 + \beta_2X_2 + \beta_3X_3 + \beta_4X_1X_2 + \beta_5X_1X_3 + \beta_6X_2X_3 + \beta_7X_1X_2X_3$$

Fig. 2. Data collection and pre-processing guidelines for synergy/antagonism estimation.

PRE-PROCESSING DEMANDS FOR ORTHOGONALITY AND BALANCE

A careful review of the columns in Figs. 2 and 3 will reveal two unique features:

1. the sum of each row of codes adds to zero, a criterion denoted as "balance;"
2. the sum of the cross-product of each pair of columns, taken in any combination, is also zero, a criterion denoted as "orthogonality."

We note specifically that the interaction columns, which will estimate the synergy or antagonism, are derived from multiplying the codes of the risk variables. Yet, in the two examples cited here and in all designs offered by PRE-PRIM, they maintain the features of balance and orthogonality. If data collection specifications are not formulated in this manner, the reliability of the coefficients obtained for a multivariate model is

RUN	X_1	X_2	X_3	X_4	X_5	X_1X_2	X_1X_3	X_1X_4	X_2X_4
1	-	-	-	-	-	+	+	+	+
2	+	-	-	-	+	-	-	-	+
3	-	+	-	-	+	-	+	+	-
4	+	+	-	-	-	+	-	-	-
5	-	-	+	-	+	+	-	+	+
6	+	-	+	-	-	-	+	-	+
7	-	+	+	-	-	-	-	+	-
8	+	+	+	-	+	+	+	-	-
9	-	-	-	+	-	+	+	-	-
10	+	-	-	+	+	-	-	+	-
11	-	+	-	+	+	-	+	-	+
12	+	+	-	+	-	+	-	+	+
13	-	-	+	+	+	+	-	-	-
14	+	-	+	+	-	-	+	+	-
15	-	+	+	+	-	-	-	-	+
16	+	+	+	+	+	+	+	+	+

Fig. 3. Target database of 16 observations to estimate 5 risk factors and 4 synergy/ antagonism effects.

questionable.[10] PRE-PRIM includes methods which give the risk analyzer the flexibility to select among interactions of interest for estimation, still maintaining minimal sample size as well as orthogonality and balance. Although the user does not handle the interaction component of the matrix, reliability is assured.

MULTIVARIATE REGRESSION INTERFACE

Data collected using the PRE-PRIM design templates are then interfaced (a) with synergy/antagonism sub-matrices and (b) multivariate regression analysis routines in POST-PRIM. A sample output is shown in Table 1. Six possible risk factors, denoted as X_1-X_6 are explored along with 4 interactions denoted as Z_1-Z_4. The coefficients to be used in the general linear model are displayed in the first column; the statistical confidence level associated with each such coefficient is given in the last column. The third and fourth columns refer to intermediate outputs. The reliability of the full multivariate regression equation is also shown in the last line.

In addition to providing a means to screen among relevant risk factors, this statistical capability also gives a handle on relevant interactions. These can be explored in greater detail in future studies designed specifically to examine synergy/antagonism.

The results in Table 2 refer to the association of multiple inputs and interactions with a single endpoint, Y_1. It was mentioned earlier that it is important to review the profile of multiple outputs consisting of possibly related primary and ancillary variables. POST-PRIM provides the capability to integrate such results. A sample matrix of multiple outputs, corresponding to the design shown in Fig. 2, is displayed in Table 2. Statistically significant results (showing the probability of error in claiming that they are significant) are shown on each of 9 output variables. A "non-significant" (N.S.) entry is made where this error exceeded 25%. The last line corresponds to the reliability of the full regression equation in terms of the coefficient of determination.

Interesting conclusions in Table 2 are that (a) endpoint variables differ in terms of their overall predictability, ranging from 22% to 90%, and (b) significant interactions cluster in certain endpoints.

Table 1. Sample Multivariate Regression Output of Coefficient Values and Confidence Levels for Risks and Interactions

	Coefficient	Term	Standard Error	T-Value	Confidence Coef <> 0	
		Regression Coefficients for Y_1				
	0.2513	1 (constant)	0.1853	1.356	75.8%	
	0.001971	X_1	0.0018	1.083	65.8%	
→	-0.002007	X_2	0.0012	1.611	82.7%	←
	0.000114	X_3	0.0001	0.8450	55.0%	
→	0.02444	X_4	0.0105	2.324	92.9%	←
→	0.2602	X_5	0.0966	2.693	95.3%	←
	-0.08333	X_6	0.1052	0.7922	52.3%	
→	0.08625	Z_1	0.0473	1.822	86.8%	←
→	0.08250	Z_2	0.0237	3.486	97.7%	←
→	0.1537	Z_3	0.0473	3.248	97.2%	←
	-0.02500	Z_4	0.0473	0.5281	38.8%	

Effect:

Standard deviation about the regression = 0.1894.

Explained variation about the mean (R-squared) = 89.81%.

Table 2. Multiple Output Profile Associating Risk Inputs and Their Interactions

Input/ Interaction	Output/Endpoints								
	Y_1	Y_2	Y_3	Y_4	Y_5	Y_6	Y_7	Y_8	Y_9
X_1	.99	.99	.99	.99	.92	.99	--	.99	.99
X_2	.99	--	.95	.99	.99	.99	--	--	.99
X_3	.96	--	--	.96	--	.95	--	.87	--
X_4	.83	--	--	--	--	--	--	--	.86
X_5	.99	.92	.86	.99	.02	--	.98	.99	--
				Interactions					
X_1 X_2	--	--	.92	.87	--	--	--	--	.91
X_1 X_4	--	--	--	--	.86	.97	--	--	--
X_1 X_5	--	--	--	--	--	.87	--	--	--
X_2 X_3	--	--	--	--	--	--	--	--	--
X_4 X_5	--	--	--	--	--	.97	--	--	--
R squared	.86	.79	.86	.89	.64	.80	.22	.87	.90

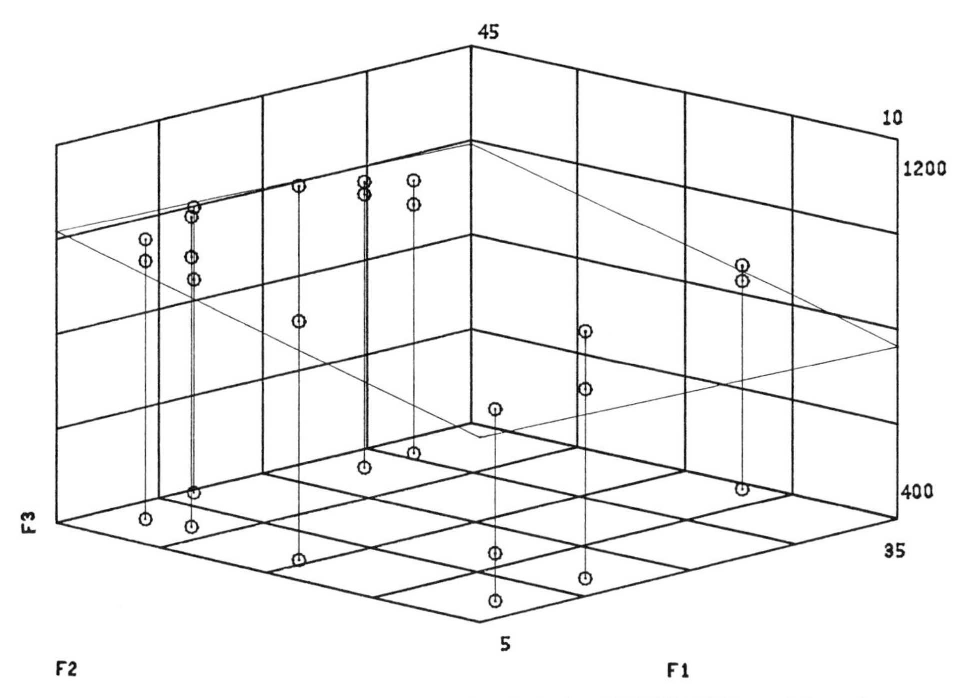

Fig. 4. Three-dimensional rotatable display featuring POST-PRIM model results.

RESPONSE SURFACE GRAPHICS FOR SCENARIO-RELATED DECISIONS

Tools in the form of multivariate profiles can be very useful in estimating the probability of risk.[11] Given that an equation with a certain degree of reliability is attained, researchers can substitute various intermediate levels of each risk factor and estimate the profile of expected results. PRE- and POST-PRIM applications to various simulated scenarios have demonstrated their robustness. The systems also have a "preventive" flavor in that they can estimate multiple risks in presence of synergy without the necessity of onset.

Users in these contexts are often interested in the interactive graphical display of results. POST-PRIM includes a graphical component: three variables can be simultaneously chosen; the expected output risk can be displayed. An example is displayed in Fig. 4. The best "response surface" is fitted to the mathematical model. Ranges of uncertainty are also indicated. POST-PRIM includes a rotational capability in the three-dimensional diagram.

SUMMARY

This paper has illustrated the integrated use of PRE- and POST-PRIM in designing appropriate inputs for a multiple input-output analysis of risks in the presence of synergistic/antagonistic effects. The necessity of a "directed data collection" is stressed, even in ex-post-facto data collection from already available databases. The importance of orthogonality and balance in the stability of results is stressed.

ACKNOWLEDGEMENTS

I am grateful to the staff of IIT Research Institute for encouraging my work in the application of experimental designs to multivariate studies and to projects at ANSER Corporation where the formulations were applied to large scale simulation models.

REFERENCES

1. Office of Technology Assessment, Assessment of Technologies for Determining Cancer Risks from the Environment, U.S. Congress, Washington, DC (1981).
2. Environmental Protection Agency, National Interim Primary Drinking Water Regulations, PB-267, 630, U.S. Environmental Protection Agency, Washington, DC (1976).
3. Environmental Protection Agency, *A Handbook of Key Federal Regulations and Criteria for Multimedia Environmental Control*, EPA-600/7-79-175, U.S. Environmental Protection Agency, Research Triangle Park, NC (1979).
4. T. H. Maugh, Just How Hazardous Are Dumps? *Science* **215**:490-493 (1982).
5. L. B. Lave and E. P. Seskin, *Air Pollution and Human Health*, Johns Hopkins University Press, Baltimore, MD (1977).
6. J. R. Goldsmith and A. Hexter, Respiratory Exposure to Lead: Epidemiological and Experimental Dose-Response Relationships, *Science* **158**:132-134 (1967).
7. A. Azar, R. E. Snee, and K. Habib, An Epidemiological Approach to Community Air Lead Exposure Using Personal Air Samples, *Environmental Quality and Safety*, Supplemental Vol. II-Lead:254-288 (1975).
8. T. K. Gardenier, PRE-PRIM As a Pre-Processor to Simulations, Internal Report #1, TKG Consultants, Ltd., Vienna, VA (1988).
9. T. K. Gardenier, Some Uses of Statistics in Simulation, in *Computer Modeling and Simulation: Principles of Good Practice*, pp. 129-139, J. McLeod, ed., Society for Computer Simulation, LaJolla, CA (1982).
10. G. E. P. Box, Use and Abuse of Regression, *Technometrics* **8**:625-629 (1966).
11. T. K. Gardenier, Principles of Simulation Metamodeling, *TIMS/ORSA Bulletin* **25**:249 (1988).

Risk Communication: Talking About Risk Reduction Instead of Acceptable Risk

Alfred Levinson
New Jersey Institute of Technology
Newark, NJ

ABSTRACT

The best way to communicate risk is NOT TO. Often the concern raised by people, ostensibly over the hazards associated with facilities in their community, tends to reflect a lack of trust of the firms that own those facilities and to a lesser extent the risks associated with their operation. To build trust companies must develop serious programs to reduce the risks facilities pose to the surrounding communities. They should include reduction of the use of toxic substances, reductions of emissions and reductions in the generation of hazardous waste. Risks faced by communities are classified into four types. Actions which can be take by companies wishing to build trust are identified for each type. Instances when it may be appropriate to communicate risk are illustrated but emphasis should be placed on risk reduction, not risk communication.

KEYWORDS: Risk communication, building trust, risk reduction, siting facilities

INTRODUCTION

Generally, the best way to communicate risk is NOT TO. Often peoples' concerns raised, ostensibly, over hazards associated with facilities in their community tend to reflect, primarily, lack of trust of the firms that own the facilities and secondarily the risks associated with the products they manufacture. Covello *et al.*[1] state that,

> "Often, actions are what people most want to know about. People want to know what you are doing to prevent an accident or how you are preparing for the possibility, not how likely you think one is. People want to know what you are doing to reduce emissions, not just how much is being emitted and how many deaths or illnesses may result. People often care about the competence and conscientiousness of the plant manager more than about the risk itself. Many people perceive mismanagement, incompetence and lack of conscientiousness as the central issues in risk assessment. Explaining what you have done, are doing and plan to do to reduce and manage the risk is at least as important as explaining how small you think it is."

Table 1. Risk Situation Types

Type	Actions To Reduce Community Concern
1. Continuing risk from an existing facility	Don't talk about risk other than to state that it is small (assuming it is) unless specifically asked. Instead talk about risk reduction activities of firm.
2. New risks from addition to or modification of existing facility	Talk about risk reduction activities of firm. Talk about the extent to which the addition (modification) will increase the risk.
3. New risks from proposed facility by firm new to region	You have the difficult task of convincing the community of the safety of the operation of the facility where there is no track record. Community may decide not to accept the facility under any conditions. Here, risk communication is irrelevant and may be counter-productive.
4. Incidental release	Primary concern of community: how to respond to release. Magnitude of risk is of secondary concern.

Peoples' concerns may also reflect fears that facility operation will result in lower property values and that the products made by other local firms may be tainted by their proximity to the hazardous substances generated by the facility of concern. Rather than devoting major efforts to playing down the environmental risks posed by a facility, it would be more productive to address these fears directly and the best way to do it is to build trust in the community.

Silbergeld[2] notes that trust is built through action and not through inaction and that companies must show what they are doing to reduce risks — to make their towns safer places to live. The chemical industry is responding by moving aggressively toward the reduction of risks from the operation of their plants.[3] This is the type of action that should be communicated, but additional trust building activities are required.

It is useful to classify the types of risky situations to which communities might be subjected. Consideration of risks will be limited to facilities that generate hazardous materials, release pollutants into the environment, or use toxic substances. Communities face risks of four types: (1) old risks from existing plants; (2) new risks from the modification or addition to existing facilities; (3) new risks from facilities proposed by firms new to the region; and (4) risks from incidental releases of toxic substances (Table 1).

CONTINUING RISK FROM AN EXISTING PLANT

In the past, concerns over risks from existing facilities have usually arisen as a result of incidental releases which heightened the community's awareness of neighboring facilities and the risks they pose. Often, tensions have been exacerbated by a company's lack of response to the community's need for information about an incidental release and by attempts by the firm to play down the seriousness of the release. Even where there have been no incidental releases, community concerns over continuing risks from existing facilities, will increase as a result of the Emergency Planning and Community Right-to-Know Act[4] and of the various State emergency planning and right-to-know laws.

As a result of the Community right-to-know laws, chemical companies will have to make greater efforts to build trust in their communities. A key component of such efforts will have to be greater emphasis on reductions in the generation of hazardous waste and in the use of toxic substances. Such emphasis will do more to mollify community concerns than any attempt to explain the precise magnitude and nature of risks (a rule of thumb is to give the actual magnitude of the risk only when it is specifically requested by members of the community).

Notification of local fire and police departments whenever there are above normal releases would be an important part of a trust building program, even if official emergency plans do not require it. In a community there may be people sensitive to unfamiliar odors or colored clouds of pollutants. They will probably want to know what they are and what action, if any, they should take.

There are other trust building activities companies might consider. For example, even though a firm may explain to the community that cancer risks from its pollutants are very low and continually reduced, trust will be built by offers of free cancer screening tests to concerned residents.

Thoughtless behavior on the part of one company can diminish the publics trust for the whole industry. Often companies under pressure to reduce their toxic emissions threaten to shut down their facilities. The case of the ASARCO copper smelting plant in Tacoma, WA, is an example.

ASARCO argued that if stringent EPA standards were imposed it would be forced to shut down its smelting operations because the facility was old and it did not pay to modernize it. As a result a less stringent standard was proposed as a compromise and ASARCO accepted it. The compromise solution was put to the vote of the residents of Tacoma, and after the community voted to accept it, ASARCO announced that it would have to close the facility, any way, due to poor copper market conditions.

Much time, effort, and ill feeling could have been saved if the proponents of the stringent standard had taken into account macroeconomic conditions. Anyone following the market should have known that there was a global overcapacity of copper smelters and copper prices were depressed. Copper producers, particularly in the United States, were scrapping their obsolete smelters as a means of reducing this overcapacity and reducing their costs of producing copper. Given these macroeconomic conditions, it would have been appropriate to ask ASARCO if they expected to be able to continue to operate the smelter, even under the existing standards. Although the company may not have been able to give an unqualified negative response, it is highly unlikely that their response would have been in the affirmative.

An alternative resolution of the ASARCO conflict would have been to inform the public that, given poor market conditions for copper, there was a good chance that the smelting operations would have to be terminated regardless of the emission standards. Imposition of the stringent standards could have been delayed for 3-5 years. Emission standards would thus have been removed as a political issue and Tacoma officials would have been told that the smelting jobs would be lost in any case giving them a good start to seek new industries.

NEW RISKS FROM AN ADDITION TO AN EXISTING FACILITY

Community concerns over proposed modifications and additions to existing facilities present a challenge to the industry. For a firm with a poor record in operating an existing plant it will be extremely difficult, if not impossible, to gain the neighboring community's support for a plant addition. One might cite cases such as that experienced by Ciba Geigy in Toms River, N.J. where the people in the community became so alienated the firm lost the support even of local business. Again, the risk to the community from the additional facility should only be given if it is specifically requested. When it announces the new facility, the company should emphasize its efforts at reducing its use of toxic substances, release of pollutants and generation of hazardous waste. It should follow the risk reduction strategy recommended by Levinson.[5]

A firm planning an addition to an existing facility should reduce the risk to the community from its current activities by an amount greater than the increase in the risk from the new facility. This reduction should be above and beyond whatever reductions would have been instituted if the firm had decided not to build the new facility. This risk reduction could come from a reduction in the emission of pollutants, a reduction in the use of toxic substances and a reduction in the generation of hazardous waste. However, it should be kept in mind that it will always be difficult to convince the public of such reductions.

Following is an example of how convincing might be accomplished. Consider the case where a company has decided to build a plant to replace an obsolete polluting plant. The new facility is likely to be less polluting because it is likely to be more efficient, use lesser amounts of toxic substances and generate less hazardous waste. If a different process were to be used, toxic substances might not be required at all.

In general, closing down obsolete facilities when planning to build new ones is a positive way to approach the problem of public trust. None of this will gain the community's acceptance of the new facility if the company does not already have a good rapport with the residents of the community.

The measures recommended above can only reduce the public anxiety to a level that will allow the firm's projects to go forth providing the anxiety level is not initially too high as a result of community antagonism to the firm. You can not build trust on distrust.

RISKS FROM A NEW FIRM'S FACILITY

A company wishing to locate a plant in a region where previously it has not operated one, may face a skeptical or even hostile public. It is likely that neither the company nor its track record will be known. It will therefore have the difficult task of convincing the community that it can safely operate the facility in the absence of a known track record to point to. In such cases, risk communication is irrelevant and possibly counterproductive. Essentially the company will be asking the community to accept an additional risk, no matter how small and in most instances, it will not matter how it communicates the additional risk. The people will not see any reason to accept increases. Emphasizing the "smallness" of the risk may actually increase their hostility toward the company. Offering compensation for acceptance of additional small risks will not usually placate the members of the community.

A good strategy to follow is not to locate the proposed plant in a greenfield area, with no extensive industry but to consider, instead, brownfield regions with similar industries. Fischhoff *et al.*[6] have shown that familiarity with the risks from such facilities will mean less fear and less resistance.

This strategy also provides opportunities for risk reduction tradeoffs with other firms in the area. For example, the new comer firm might offer to pay an existing company to modernize an old polluting plant in return for being allowed to locate in the region. The risk reduction to the community from the modernization of the existing plant must, of course, be greater than the increase in risk from the new facility. Only then would the approach be an effective way for a new firm to gain the trust of the community. It can also be appealing for siting hazardous waste facilities in brownfield areas. Baker[7] has shown that property values in a community can be affected by the siting of a hazardous waste facility. A firm can calm the community's fears about the potential loss of property values by offering to post a bond that could be used to cover any losses due to the facility experienced by property owners. Again, this should be seen as a trust building measure by the company.

INCIDENTAL RELEASES

The primary concern of residents of communities facing incidental toxics releases from neighboring facilities is how to respond. Interest in the magnitude of the risk is of secondary concern and is perceived by the residents as a determinant of the mode of response. First, they will want to know what immediate action they have to take. Later, they may want to know what long term effects the release might have on them to determine if any treatment or monitoring is needed. This is when they may wish to know the magnitude of the risk. If there have been releases of radiation from a nuclear power plant, for instance, informing them that it was comparable to a small number of X-rays could serve to calm fears. But again information should only be given when requested.

After an incidental release, the responsible company might find it in their interest to tell the potentially affected communities what measures have been taken to insure that this type of release does not occur again. If there is an outcry from the community over the release, even after these assurances have been given, this may indicate that public concerns go beyond the incidental release. In this eventuality, the firm should make an effort to identify them and institute remedial action.

CONCLUSION

Firms have been facing a growing neighboring community opposition to the continued operation of their facilities and to the siting of new facilities. Improving risk communication has been suggested as a means of mitigating this opposition. It has been shown that emphasizing the risks may be counterproductive. Companies can build trust with their communities emphasizing risk reduction efforts.

To insure that increased emphasis on risk reduction is not viewed as a public relations gimmick, the firms must make serious risk reduction efforts.

Other trust building measures might also be appropriate. Where the siting of new facilities is being sought and residents of the surrounding community are concerned over the adverse effects on property values, a firm could consider offering to post a bond to cover any losses in property values due to the facility. Risk communication is not the way companies can improve relationships with neighboring communities. The most productive approach is to build trust. Companies should establish serious risk reduction programs which must include efforts to reduce the use of toxic substances, reduce the emission of pollutants and reduce the generation of hazardous waste.

REFERENCES

1. Vincent Covello, Peter Sandman and Paul Slovic, Risk Communication, Risk Statistics, and Risk Comparisons: A Manual for Plant Managers, Chemical Manufacturers Association, Washington, DC (1988).
2. J. Clarence Davies, Vincent T. Covello and Frederick W. Allen, eds., Risk Communication, The Conservation Foundation, Washington, DC (1987).
3. Laurie Hays, Chemical Firms Press Campaigns to Dispel Their 'Bad Guy' Image, *The Wall Street Journal*, September 20, 1988.
4. Title III — Superfund Amendments and Reauthorization Act of 1986.
5. Alfred Levinson, Risk Reduction Strategies for Setting Redial Priorities: Hazardous Waste, in *Advances in Risk Analysis*, pp. 213-218, James J. Bonin and Donald E. Stevenson, eds., Plenum Press, New York (1989).
6. Baruch Fischhoff, Sarah Lichtenstein, Paul Slovic, Stephen L. Derby and Ralph L. Keeney, *Acceptable Risk*, Cambridge University Press, Cambridge (1981).
7. Brian Baker, Perception of Hazardous Waste disposal Facilities and Residential Real Property Values, *Impact Assessment Bulletin* **6(1)** (1988).

Development and Application of a Shower Risk Assessment Model

Jonathan Savrin
New Jersey Department of Health
Trenton, NJ

Richard Dime
New Jersey Department of Environmental Protection
Trenton, NJ

ABSTRACT

A risk assessment model was developed for calculating the inhalation risk posed by showering in contaminated water. The model was applied to three households near a hazardous waste site, where the groundwater had been contaminated by volatile organic chemicals (VOCs). Calculated exposures were less than the relevant verified reference doses, and calculated lifetime cancer risks from showering were in the range of 10^{-4} to 10^{-6}. The impact of assumptions that were used in the application of the model, along with uncertainties, are discussed.

Quantitative evaluations were performed on some of the activities that would lower exposure. Ventilating the bathroom at a reasonably fast rate reduces exposure by approximately 49%. As anticipated, taking shorter showers have a greater effect on the exposure than shortening the time in the bathroom after the shower. The lifetime cancer risks from showering were approximately the same as the lifetime cancer risks posed by ingesting 2 liters per day of the same water. These results indicate that inhalation exposures from activities like showering, washing clothes, and washing dishes need to be included in accurately assessing risks and in setting standards and guidelines for VOCs in drinking water.

KEYWORDS: Risk assessment, shower, drinking water, indoor air, inhalation

INTRODUCTION

Drinking water standards, guidelines, and criteria have been based on ingestion as the primary or only pathway for major exposure to contaminants present in drinking water. Similarly, most risk assessments involving potable water contamination have evaluated exposure via ingestion only. More recently, however, inhalation routes (i.e., the inhalation of contaminants that volatilize during activities such as showering, bathing, washing clothes, etc.) have been receiving greater attention,[1-6] and recent risk assessments have indicated that inhalation exposure pathways may be as significant or more significant than exposure via ingestion.[4,6,7]

The consideration of noningestion exposures from drinking water raises a number of important questions, including: Is there a need to include noningestion exposure pathways when setting drinking water standards? If people are advised to drink bottled water, should they also have alternative water sources for nonpotable uses to sufficiently reduce their risk? What actions other than alternative water sources can be taken to mitigate exposure? Have risk assessments been underestimating the risk that is posed by contaminants in drinking water?

A major source of inhalation exposure to contaminants in drinking water is the shower. Realizing the potential significance of showering as an exposure pathway and the need to better address the actual risk posed by showering in contaminated water, we conducted a review of risk assessment methodologies developed to assess inhalation exposure from showering in contaminated water.[4,7,8] Four assumptions were included in each of these methodologies that did not represent what intuitively occurs in a shower environment and could have significant impacts on the results and conclusions of the respective models. These assumptions were:

1. All of the volatilized contaminants were in the shower stall the instant that the shower started,
2. The air concentration of contaminants in the shower stall was constant from the time that the shower started until the shower ended,
3. Exposure to contaminants ceased as soon as the shower ended, and
4. No air exchange (room ventilation) occurred during the shower.

In reality, (1) contaminants cannot volatilize into the shower stall air until they have been introduced through the showerhead, (2) the air concentrations of volatiles increases as more water is introduced through the showerhead, (3) most people remain in the bathroom (and therefore are potentially exposed) after the shower ends, and (4) normal ventilation of the bathroom could play a significant role in reducing the concentration of volatiles in the shower stall and the bathroom.

This paper proposes a shower risk assessment model that corrects for these assumptions and applies it to a typical hazardous waste site with groundwater contamination. In addition, recommendations are presented to reduce exposures via inhalation.

EXPOSURE ASSESSMENT MODEL

Assumptions

There is a lack of information available on the volatilization of chemicals in the shower environment, so a number of assumptions must be made in any shower risk assessment model. In the proposed model, some of these assumptions are based upon site-specific conditions (variables). Others are standard risk assessment modelling assumptions, while others are areas of uncertainty, where additional research is needed.

The variable assumptions (i.e., assumptions that could be modified for specific shower situations) are:

1. 100 liters of water is used per shower.
2. An individual spends 15 minutes/day in the shower.
3. An individual remains in the bathroom for 15 minutes after the shower.
4. The volume of the shower stall is 3 cubic meters (3,000 liters).

5. The volume of the bathroom is 9 cubic meters (9,000 liters).
6. An individual weighs 70 kilograms.
7. A lifetime is 70 years.
8. Ventilation of the bathroom produces six air changes per hour in the bathroom.

Standard risk assessment assumptions that were used include:

1. Individual cancer risks are additive.
2. An individual breathes at a constant rate of 23 cubic meters/day while in the shower and bathroom.
3. Carcinogenic potencies and noncarcinogenic reference doses that were used are accurate.
4. Carcinogenic potencies via inhalation equal carcinogenic potencies via ingestion (when no inhalation potencies are available).

Assumptions that are typically made in risk assessment models include:

1. The concentrations of the contaminants in the water are constant.
2. The concentrations of the contaminants in the air are uniform.
3. Dermal absorption and accidental ingestion are not significant exposure pathways during a shower.
4. The estimated fraction of contaminants that volatilize and pulmonary absorption rates are accurate.
5. Contaminants in the air do not adsorb to surfaces in the bathroom and are available for intake.

In reality, (1) there is probably a higher concentration of contaminants in the water that has been setting in the pipes and is first used in the shower, (2) the concentration of contaminants in the breathing zone is likely to be greater than that in the rest of the bathroom as the water splashes off of the individual's upper body, (3) dermal absorption from water pooled in the bathtub and accidental ingestion could be significant, and (4) adsorption (condensation) of contaminants on towels and tiles in the bathroom could be significant.

Equations

The exposure model is based on a minute-by-minute calculation of the concentration of the contaminants in the air. The doses per minute of the contaminant are calculated from the air concentrations and summed to determine the total dose from the shower.

The calculation of the concentration of contaminants in the air during each proceeding minute is based on the continual input of contaminants as the shower progresses, the concentration of contaminants in the air from the previous minute, room ventilation, and contaminant removal due to intake into the body. The components of the equation developed to perform this calculation are described below.

The contribution of the concentration in air from the previous minute is based on the concentration during the previous minute and the room ventilation rate and is represented by:

$$(CA_n)(VE)(X),$$

where CA_n = concentration of the contaminant in air during the previous minute (μg/liter),
VE = ventilation rate of the bathroom (1/minute)
X = 1 minute (X = minutes)

The contribution of the additional contaminants that volatilized out of the water during the minute is based on the amount of water used during the minute, the concentration of the contaminant in the water, the fraction of the contaminant volatilized, and the size of the shower stall. It is represented by:

$$(CW)(WU)(VR)(X)/(SS)$$

where CW = concentration of the contaminant in the water (μg/liter),
WU = water introduced into the shower (liters/minute),
VR = fraction of the contaminant that volatilizes (dimensionless),
SS = size of the shower stall (liters).

The reduction in contaminant concentration in the air due to the contaminants being absorbed by the lungs is based on the dose during that minute and the shower stall size, and is represented by:

$$(DO)(X)/(SS)$$

where DO = dose per minute (μg/minute).

Therefore, the equation to calculate minute-by-minute concentrations of contaminants in the air during shower use is:

$$CA_{n+1}=\{[(CA_n)(VE)]+[(CW)(WU)(VR)/(SS)]-[(DO)/(SS)]\}(X), \qquad (1)$$

where CA_{n+1} = concentration of the contaminant in air during the current minute (μg/liter).

When the individual turns off the shower but remains in the bathroom, the dilution of the contaminants from the shower stall to the entire bathroom is represented by the following equation:

$$CA_{n+1}=(CA_n)(SS)/(BS) \qquad (2)$$

where BS = size of the bathroom (liters).

As there are no longer any contaminants being introduced into the bathroom, the equation for the concentration of contaminants in the air is:

$$CA_{n+1}=\{[(CA_n)(VE)]-[(DO)/(SS)]\}(X). \qquad (3)$$

The equations that were used to calculate the minute-by-minute dose (DO) were based on the minute-by-minute concentration of the contaminants in the air, the respiratory rate of the individual, and pulmonary absorption factor. The total dose per shower (TD) was the sum of the minute-by-minute doses. Minute-by-minute doses and total doses were calculated using the following equations:

$$DO=(CA_{n+1})(RR)(PA) \qquad (4)$$

and

$$TD=\Sigma(DO)(X), \qquad (5)$$

where RR = respiratory rate (liters/minute),
PA = pulmonary absorption factor (dimensionless),
TD = total dose (μg/day).

The carcinogenic risk of exposure to the contaminant(s) was calculated using the following equation:

$$CR=(TD)(CP)/(BW)/(CF), \quad (6)$$

where CR = lifetime cancer risk,
CP = carcinogenic potency (mg/kg/day),
BW = body weight (kg),
CF = conversion factor (1,000 μg/mg).

Cancer risks for time periods less than 70 years (assumed lifetime) are calculated by dividing the number of years exposed by 70 years.

Noncarcinogenic risks from showering were evaluated by comparing the total daily dose from showering (after dividing by the body weight) with reference doses for noncarcinogenic effects (e.g., verified reference doses or No Observed Effects Levels divided by appropriate safety factors).

Refinements can be made to the proposed shower risk assessment model to fit the specific situation. The model can be expanded to include both volatilization and aerosolization. The time periods (minute-by-minute) for which the concentrations of the contaminants in the air are calculated can be shortened, which would yield slightly more accurate doses and risk calculations.

Computer Program

A computer program, using Basic language, was developed and used to run the risk assessment model. Required inputs include the weight of the person, the room ventilation rate, the concentration of the contaminant in water, the inhalation carcinogenic potency of the contaminant, the liters of water per shower, the respiratory rate of the person, the pulmonary absorption factor, the fraction of the contaminant that volatilizes, the number of years showering with the contaminated water, the size of the shower stall, the size of the bathroom, the average number of minutes in the shower, and the average number of minutes in the bathroom after the shower. The computer program calculates and can print out the following information: the concentration of contaminants in the air on a minute-by-minute basis, the dose received on a minute-by-minute basis, the total cumulative dose on a minute-by-minute basis, the total dose from the shower, the lifetime cancer risk associated with the shower, and the cancer risk for the years showering with the contaminated water.

APPLICATION OF THE MODEL

A typical problem associated with hazardous waste sites is contamination of groundwater with volatile organic contaminants (VOCs). At some sites, groundwater contamination has extended beyond the boundaries of the site and reduced the quality of potable water supplies. Frequently, the response to such a situation has been to provide or recommend use of a temporary alternative water source (e.g., bottled water), while arrangements for a permanent alternative water source (e.g., extension of a water main) are being made. Residents could wait for many months to over a year to have a permanent solution. While the temporary alternative water supply can be used for ingestion, residents in the affected area may have no alternative to using the contaminated water for non-ingestion purposes (e.g., showering, bathing, dishwashing, toilets, and clothes washing).

The proposed shower risk assessment model was applied to a hazardous waste site where potable wells had been affected by contaminated groundwater and where it was expected that a permanent alternative water source would not be supplied for about one year. An alternative water source (bottled water) for drinking was recommended. Consideration was given to identifying actions that could be taken by residents to reduce exposure during showering.

The groundwater contaminants of concern at the site were chloroform, methylene chloride, tetrachloroethylene (PCE), and trichloroethylene (TCE). These four contaminants were used in this assessment. Three homes were used in the assessment. They were:

Household A — the household with the highest concentration of chloroform in the potable water supply,

Household B — the household with the highest concentration of methylene chloride in the potable water supply, and

Household C — the household where the residents expressed concern with showering in contaminated water.

The concentration of contaminants that were detected in the potable water supplies of the households are presented in Table 1. The fraction of each contaminant volatilized during showering was twice the calculated rate using a previously developed model.[4] These calculations yielded air concentrations that were comparable to, or slightly higher than, concentrations that have been measured in controlled shower environments.[1,9,10] Pulmonary absorption factors were assumed to be 75%, except for chloroform where a literature value (63%) was available. Carcinogenic potencies that were used were from the U.S. Environmental Protection Agency Carcinogen Assessment Group (EPA/CAG). The fraction of contaminant volatilized, the pulmonary absorption factors, and the carcinogenic potencies that were used for each chemical are presented in Table 2. Monitoring of the air in the shower stall was not conducted, due to difficulties in analyzing for trace chemicals in a shower environment (discussed below).

The exposure model was run on each chemical in each home to obtain both lifetime and one-year carcinogenic risks (since public water was likely to be supplied in a year). The carcinogenic risks for all the chemicals were then summed to yield a total lifetime and one-year carcinogenic risk. The model was run twice, once assuming that the air in the bathroom turned-over at a rate of six times per hour (see Table 3), and once assuming no ventilation of the bathroom (see Table 4).

Assuming that the bathroom is ventilated and that public water would be supplied in one year, there was only one household that had an incremental cancer risk greater than one in a million (Household A). Although this risk is a one-year risk and not a lifetime risk, the decision was made that the magnitude of the risk did not merit emergency actions. Instead, precautions were recommended to the residents. To reduce their exposure to contaminants in the shower for that year, the residents were advised to: (1) ventilate the bathroom during use, (2) take shorter showers, and (3) use colder water.

The total daily doses from showering were below the reference doses for the respective chemicals, and thus were not considered to pose an unacceptable chronic noncarcinogenic risk. There was some concern that the concentrations in the shower environment could cause skin or eye irritation, particularly if the skin is sensitized by the hot and humid environment.[5,11] However, no acceptable data base for assessing irritant effects of these chemicals could be found.

Table 1. Concentration of Contaminants in Water (in ppb)

	Household A	Household B	Household C
Chloroform	74.4	25	2
Methylene Chloride	14	415	190
Tetrachloroethylene	4.9	2	3
Trichloroethylene	ND	ND	1

ND = not detected.

Table 2. Contaminants' Volatilization, Potency, and Absorption Factor

	Percent of Contaminant that Volatilized	Carcinogenic Potency	Pulmonary Absorption Factor
Chloroform	80%	7.0E-2	63%
Methylene Chloride	88%	6.3E-4	75%
Tetrachloroethylene	74%	1.7E-3	75%
Trichloroethylene	80%	4.6E-3	75%

Table 3. Carcinogenic Risks from Showering With Ventilation

	Household A		Household B		Household C	
	Lifetime	1-year	Lifetime	1-year	Lifetime	1-year
Chloroform	1.4E-4	2.0E-4	4.8E-5	6.8E-7	3.8E-6	5.4E-8
Methylene Chloride	3.1E-7	4.5E-9	9.2E-6	1.3E-7	4.3E-6	6.1E-8
Tetrachloro-ethylene	2.5E-7	3.6E-9	1.0E-7	1.5E-9	1.5E-7	2.2E-9
Trichloro-ethylene	NA	NA	NA	NA	1.5E-7	2.1E-9
Total	1.4E-4	2.0E-6	5.7E-5	8.1E-7	8.4E-6	1.3E-7

NA = not applicable.

Table 4. Carcinogenic Risks from Showering Without Ventilation

	Household A		Household B		Household C	
	Lifetime	1-year	Lifetime	1-year	Lifetime	1-year
Chloroform	2.8E-4	4.0E-6	9.4E-5	1.3E-6	7.6E-6	1.1E-7
Methylene Chloride	6.2E-7	8.9E-9	1.8E-5	2.6E-7	8.4E-6	1.2E-7
Tetrachloro-ethylene	4.9E-7	7.0E-9	2.0E-7	2.8E-9	3.0E-7	4.3E-9
Trichloro-ethylene	NA	NA	NA	NA	2.9E-7	4.2E-9
Total	2.8E-4	4.0E-6	1.1E-4	1.6E-6	1.7E-5	2.4E-7

NA = not applicable.

DISCUSSION

The concentrations of chloroform in the air (assuming 50 ppb of chloroform in the water) versus the minutes in the shower were plotted (see Fig. 1). Curves were drawn for the model with ventilation, the model without ventilation, and a representative of the models that were used with the assumptions discussed above in the Introduction. The shape of the curve for both ventilation and no ventilation are similar to shower volatilization studies that have been reported in the literature. These curves also demonstrate that (1) the concentration of the contaminants in the air as the shower progresses, (2) the effect of room ventilation on the concentration of contaminants in the air, (3) the dilution effect when the contaminants are diluted into the entire bathroom, and (4) differences in this model versus models described in the Introduction.

Shortening the amount of time spent in the shower and/or the bathroom lowers the calculated cancer risk, as demonstrated by Table 5. As anticipated, shortening the time in the shower had a greater effect on the dose than shortening the time in the bathroom after the shower. Ventilating the bathroom while showering also reduced the calculated cancer risk. Ventilating the bathroom at a reasonably fast rate (six air changes per hour) reduced the total daily dose by approximately 49%.

The lifetime cancer risk from showering in a ventilated bathroom to drinking two liters of water per day was compared.[12] As demonstrated by Table 6, the risks from the two activities were remarkably similar. Other shower risk assessments have also demonstrated that the risks from showering and drinking two liters of water per day were similar in magnitude.

There are uncertainties that are associated with the assumptions that were used in this model. While most of the assumptions were conservative and may have led to an overestimation of the risk, some of the assumptions may have led to an underestimation of the risk. Among the assumptions that were made that would have a significant impact on the outcome of this assessment are: that the chemicals being evaluated are carcinogens (none of the four chemicals evaluated are proven human carcinogens), that carcinogenic potencies via inhalation are the same as carcinogenic potencies via ingestion, that the concentration of

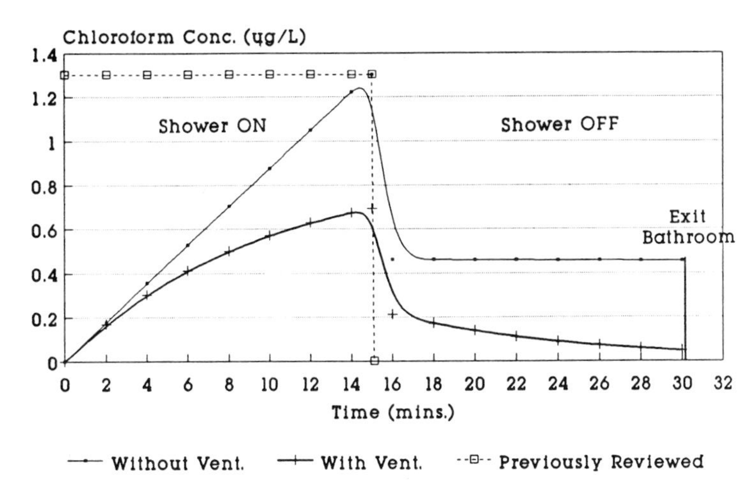

Fig. 1. Contaminant concentration in air during and after showering (50 ppb Chloroform in water).

Table 5. Lifetime Cancer Risks Based on Time in Shower/Bathroom[a]

Time in Shower/Bathroom (minutes)[b]	Cancer Risk	Percent Reduction of Cancer Risk[c]
15 in Shower and 15 in Bathroom	1.0E-4	0%
15 in Shower and 7 in Bathroom	9.4E-5	7%
7 in Shower and 15 in Bathroom	4.1E-5	59%
7 in Shower and 7 in Bathroom	3.6E-5	64%

[a]Assuming water contains 50 ppb of chloroform.

[b]Assuming ventilation.

[c]Assuming ventilation, 15 minutes in shower, 15 minutes in bathroom.

contaminants in the bathroom is uniform, that the fractions of contaminants volatilized are accurate, and that the concentration of contaminants in the water is uniform.

CONCLUSIONS

The results of the application of the shower risk assessment raise the question of how drinking water standards are set. While drinking water standards are primarily set on drinking two liters of water per day, the shower risk assessments indicate that showering and other indoor volatilization exposure pathways need to get as much or more attention.

Table 6. Lifetime Cancer Risks—Showering Versus Ingestion

	Showering[a]	Ingestion[b]
Household A	1.4E-4	1.5E-4
Household B	5.7E-5	5.7E-5
Household C	8.4E-6	7.7E-6
Chloroform (50 ppb)	1.0E-4	1.0E-4

[a]Assuming ventilation.

[b]Assuming ingestion of 2 liters per day.

The house that had the highest cancer risk was the house with the highest concentration of chloroform in the potable water (74.4 ppb). Even when the concentration of methylene chloride was much higher than chloroform (Household B), the cancer risk from chloroform was greater. The current Maximum Contaminant Level (MCL) for trihalomethanes (including chloroform) in chlorinated potable water is 100 ppb. Although this MCL is not health-based, this shower risk assessment supports the argument that the MCL for trihalomethanes is too high.

The model demonstrated that ventilating the bathroom while showering and taking shorter showers reduces exposure to the contaminants. Using colder water would further lower the fraction volatilized of the contaminant and thus reduce exposure.

There have been studies conducted to evaluate the total exposure to contaminants from drinking water in the household. Other potentially significant sources of exposure include washing dishes, washing clothes, and flushing toilets.[2,3,10] Future research can address assumptions and uncertainties of indoor air risk assessment models (discussed above), and can be aimed at making adjustments in these models. Analyzing air samples in a shower environment is difficult and sometimes inaccurate due to the humidity and low concentration of contaminants.[13] However, developing a methodology of accurately sampling and analyzing the air in a shower environment is necessary to verify shower exposure models. Refinements to the shower risk assessment models, along with other indoor risk assessment models, would increase our understanding of the total exposure to indoor air contamination from drinking water. A better understanding of how people are exposed to volatile chemicals in their home would increase our ability to recommend actions that would best and most efficiently reduce exposure. In addition, it is apparent that there is a need to change the basis by which we currently set drinking water standards, criteria, and guidelines.

ACKNOWLEDGMENTS

Special thanks to Drs. Terry Shehata, Dhun Patel, Robert Hazen, and Ron Harkov for their review of the model, to Dr. Kate Joyce for her assistance in the computer program, and to Shirley Markman for her assistance.

REFERENCES

1. J. B. Andelman, Human Exposures to Volatile Halogenated Organic Chemicals in Indoor and Outdoor Air, *Environmental Health Perspectives* **62**:313-318 (1985).
2. J. M. Clark and C. Fuller, A Total Exposure and Risk Analysis for Carcinogens Found in Drinking Water, Presentation at 1988 Annual Conference of the Society for Risk Analysis.
3. C. R. Cothern, W. A. Coniglio, and W. L. Marcus, Estimating Risk to Human Health, *Environmental Science and Technology* **20**:111-116 (1986).
4. A. Foster and P. C. Chrostowski, Integrated Household Exposure Model for Use of Tap Water Contaminated with Volatile Organic Chemicals, 79th Annual Meeting of the Air Pollution Control Association, June 1986.
5. T. Shehata, A Multi-Route Exposure Assessment of Chemically Contaminated Drinking Water, *Toxicology and Industrial Health* **1**:277-298 (1984).
6. United States Environmental Protection Agency, Office of Drinking Water, Exposure to Volatilized Drinking Water Contaminants Via Inhalation—Importance Relative to Ingestion (draft), June, 1987.
7. R. A. Dime, Shower Risk Assessment, unpublished, 1985.
8. United States Environmental Protection Agency, Office of Toxic Substances, Methods for Assessing Exposure to Chemical Substances, Vol. 5, pp. 142-144, August 1985.
9. J. B. Andelman, Personal Communication, 1986.
10. J. B. Andelman, Inhalation Exposure in the Home to Volatile Organic Contaminants of Drinking Water, *The Science of the Total Environment* **47**:443-460 (1985).
11. T. Shehata, Personal Communication, 1986.
12. United States Environmental Protection Agency, National Primary Drinking Water Regulations: Synthetic Organic Chemicals, Inorganic Chemicals and Micro-organisms, *Federal Register* **50(219)**:46944, November 13, 1985..
13. R. Harkov, Personal Communication, 1986.

The Transboundary Movement of Hazardous Products, Processes and Wastes from the U.S. to Third World Nations: A Prognosis

Allen L. White
Tellus Institute
Boston, MA
and
Clark University
Worcester, MA

ABSTRACT

Hazards exports from the U.S. to developing nations occur in three principal forms: (1) the siting of industrial facilities by multinational corporations (MNCs); (2) exports of intermediate and final consumer products; and (3) shipments of hazardous wastes for treatment and/or disposal. I examine the underlying forces and current scale of each using North-South economic-political relations as an organizing theme. Facility siting and product exports are linked to the emergence of the MNC as the dominant post-War economic entity. In contrast, waste exports are viewed as unrelated to the MNC phenomenon. The 1990s will witness an acceleration of recent trends in hazards exports as the international marketplace in capital and technology becomes even more fluid than in previous decades. Whether such exports will translate into a commensurate increase in risk to host countries will depend on both corporate conduct and the rate at which regulatory capabilities are expanded.

KEYWORDS: Hazards, exports, Third World, technology transfer, wastes

INTRODUCTION

This paper examines three dimensions of a phenomenon which has attracted increasing attention among risk analysts and managers: international movements of hazardous products processes and wastes between industrial and developing nations. The phenomenon is not new, but its complexity and implications for human health and the environment have accelerated during the last decade and captured the attention of multilateral bodies ranging from the World Bank[1] and United Nations[2] to the Brundtland Commission on environment and development.[3] These developments reflect a recognition that transboundary flows of hazards have evolved as part of a globalization of markets for materials, labor, capital and technology, all of which are mobilized and channeled through new organizational structures which facilitate the search of investors and firms for efficient

Risk Analysis, Edited by C. Zervos
Plenum Press, New York, 1991

locations and maximum market opportunities. The very nature of post-war industrial organization, coupled with demographic trends worldwide, has thus reshaped the map of technological hazards, leading observers to ask how extant risk management institutions should be restructured to meet these new patterns of technological risks.

While focus on these long-term, macro level trends intensifies after major acute events such as the Bhopal chemical disaster[4] and the Goiania (Brazil) radiation poisoning episode,[5] systematic analyses within a broader causal and policy context are few, particularly those concerned with ethical and value aspects in contrast to measurement and economic consequences of such actions.[6]

In this paper, I examine some of the issues of the problem of transboundary transfers of hazards by looking at its three principal dimensions. First, global industrial location patterns, perhaps the most obvious agent of risk redistribution, are considered. The focus is on how new forms of corporate organization have freed firms from historical locational constraints while enhancing the movement of capital resources to regions of maximum economic returns. In the course of this internationalization, hazardous technologies and manufacturing processes have moved abroad as a result of corporate locational choices.

Second, I examine the movement of hazardous products between the U.S. and developing nations, with emphasis on the well documented case of agricultural pesticides and other chemicals. Again, these products are used to illustrate larger market and regulatory conditions which have reshaped the global distribution of hazards.

Finally, the movement of hazardous wastes, the most recently documented of the three dimensions of transboundary hazards, offers further substance to formulation of my central thesis. Here I draw on the burgeoning number of actual and attempted shipments of chemical and radioactive wastes to the Third World, and the nature and rapidity of government and multilateral responses to such shipments. I then draw together these three dimensions—industrial location, agricultural chemical exports and waste exports—into a prognosis of hazards exports during the next decade and beyond.

INDUSTRIAL PLANT LOCATION

The fugitive firm hypothesis is based on the interplay of post-war industrial reorganization and neoclassical economic concepts of comparative advantage and factor mobility in the face of variable prices. The significance of the organizational characteristics may be viewed within the context of how multinational corporations (MNCs) manage resources differently from smaller scale national enterprises. Pearson[7] identifies three such characteristics. First, because MNC operations are by definition transboundary, managers are inclined to appropriate the firm's surplus—broadly construed as profits, rent, productivity improvements—across all its operations and investors worldwide. Thus, in the absence of host country restraints in the form of taxes, profit restrictions and royalty repatriation, profits will flow according to some corporate-wide, transboundary optimization pattern.

Second, MNCs as a group are among the world's largest corporations and, at the same time, disproportionately concentrated in pollution-intensive industries. Pearson reports worldwide sales in 1984 for the 15 largest average $38 billion and net assets average $14 billion. Such strength translates into superior financial, marketing, technological and managerial resources, all of which give an advantage to such MNCs in bargaining with host Third World nations. The same strengths, of course, also offer sizable potential benefits in terms of risk management. Pollution control technologies, the capacity to respond to acute events and the know-how to husband natural resources in the long run are, in concept, more available to MNCs than small, less sophisticated domestic corporations.

Third, and in transition to neoclassical economic arguments, is the idea that MNCs enjoy unrivaled capacity to move production facilities to other sites when local environmental regulations become too onerous. In these circumstances, the argument goes, MNCs may forgo or reduce new investments in favor of less stringent conditions found elsewhere in their production network. This scenario is most applicable to manufacturing firms not engaged in natural resource extraction or otherwise tied to country-specific labor and consumer markets.

Placing these MNC characteristics within the context of neoclassical economic analysis allows us to flesh out the fugitive firm argument. The assimilative capacity of air, water and land is itself a factor of production, and a particularly important one to pollution-intensive industries. Under conventional theories of comparative advantage, firms will seek locations in which key production factor costs are lowest. From a national perspective, countries will be inclined to import products which use large amounts of scarce resources and export products which consume abundant resources. Insofar as the environment's assimilative capacity is "cheaper" in Third World nations owing to their biophysical characteristics or more lenient regulatory regimes, pollution-intensive industries will be drawn to such locations. These tendencies may be reinforced when one accounts for the particular strengths of MNCs in diffusing their intangible, fixed managerial and organizational assets abroad; capitalizing operations abroad to more easily penetrate foreign markets and retain domestic market share through utilization of low cost labor; and vertically integrating with foreign supplies of raw materials.[8] Of course, these features apply to MNCs in general; they are not peculiar to MNCs which are pollution-intensive or technologically risky. However, because such firms as a group are disproportionately represented among MNCs, we may infer a propensity to establish Third World operations. The causal factor here is not environmental escapism but the nature of modern MNC organization, which allows superior access to capital to respond to global production and market opportunities. That risky industries are frequently the beneficiaries of such internationalization of capital does nothing to fortify either the economic or regulatory arguments which purport to explain selective industrial flight, or hazards transfer, to Third World nations.

To what extent does empirical evidence support this line of reasoning? Beginning in the early 1970's, the mass media triggered a number of investigations into the phenomenon of "environment-induced locational shifts." Gladwin,[9] one of the first to examine the behavior of MNCs with respect to environmental regulations, argued that the significance of such regulations was greatly exaggerated. He pointed to a host of other variables falling into several broad categories which are at least as influential as environmental control costs in shaping MNC locational behavior, namely the industrial organization of the sector in which the MNC competes (for example, degree of oligopoly among producers and technology transfer practices); business investment conditions; relative political stability and risks of overseas versus domestic locations; organization behavior of the MNC in regards to growth, profit and market share expectations; international economic conditions, such as exchange rate conditions and comparative resource endowments; and other "economics" besides environmental control costs, for example, labor and energy availability and costs.

The concern with fugitive firms, however, has persisted, in large part owing to the expansion of MNCs as the preeminent form of industrial organization in the most pollution-intensive industries. Overall, by the early 1980's it was estimated that 500 MNCs were responsible for 80 percent of direct foreign investment,[10] and that internationalization of capital markets would continue as a permanent feature of the U.S. economy.[11] In the chemical, petroleum, metals, and other industry sectors accounting for a disproportionate share of environmental residuals, MNCs continue to control a substantial portion of all direct foreign investment in Third World nations. Since their 10 percent growth in output in the 1970s was double that of the gross world product,[12] it is clear that decision making within MNCs would continue to be critical to forecasting the spatial distribution of technological hazards over time.

The persistence of the fugitive firm/pollution haven argument was sustained by continuing media coverage of hazards transfers to the Third World as well as by industry specific studies of industry relocation. Castleman's 1979 study,[13] which was used as part of a 1978 Congressional investigation of U.S. regulatory policy on hazards exports, identified several pollution intensive industries which may be inclined to seek relief abroad from U.S. occupational and environmental health regulations. Among these are asbestos fiber, arsenic trioxide, mercury and lead, representatives of classes of mining and manufacturing for which pollution control costs as a percent of capital spending are above nationwide averages. These, by inference, are likely to lead industry shifts toward overseas production operations in the face of increasingly stringent and costly domestic controls. Castleman later reaffirmed his case in the context of the double standard in occupational health regulations, arguing that different standards of occupational and environmental health and pollution control present not only inducements to industrial flight but also fundamental issues of corporate values and ethics vis-a-vis Third World populations.[14]

Arguments depicting an impending large-scale relocation of hazardous manufacturing have been critiqued by several researchers. Levenstein and Eller,[15] for example, reject this thesis, pointing to unconvincing reliance on the asbestos and arsenic industries as indicators of larger industrial trends, although they do not preclude the possibility that future Third World industrialization may be accompanied by inadequate environmental and occupational health protection. Leonard[16] essentially concurs with this prognosis, concluding that only a few specific mineral-processing and specialty chemical industries—asbestos, benzidine dyes and selected pesticides—have demonstrated tendencies to escape U.S. regulations. By and large, however, spatial investment patterns in pollution intensive manufacturing, including most mineral processing, chemicals (including petrochemicals) and pulp and paper, have not been substantially altered by U.S. regulations. This is not to say environmental compliance is absent from the corporate decision calculus, only that it rarely is decisive and is more commonly one ingredient among many economic forces which shape locational choices, e.g. prices, interest rates, product demand and overall domestic economic conditions.

In sum, the fugitive firm, or pollution haven, arguments appear to rest on weak foundations. While few selected, pollution-intensive processes have sought Third World locations in search of regulatory relief, this can hardly be characterized as endemic among firms which utilize hazardous technologies. Insofar as hazardous firms have shifted investments abroad, it appears that such transfers reflect broader trends in the globalization of capital markets which position MNCs to rapidly identify and exploit production and marketing opportunities. That hazardous industries are identified with these trends speaks more to the capital-intensiveness of their operations than to the costs of avoiding relatively rigid environmental controls. This is not to deny the possibility of future shifts in hazardous industries due to either regulatory costs or a more complex mix of factor costs, markets and investment climates which are favorable to expansion abroad. Indeed, for pollution-intensive industries like basic chemicals, fertilizers, pesticides and resins, the long-term prospects are for demand growth in developing countries to be double that of developed nations.[17] MNCs will respond to these through a variety of subsidiary, licensing and joint marketing arrangements, most of which will require majority or equal ownership by host country interests. Regardless of such arrangements, however, or the motives driving MNCs to overseas locations, technological hazards are likely to appear in greater volume in the environmental landscape of Third World nations.

HAZARDOUS PRODUCTS

Years before the emergence of the fugitive firm controversy, large volumes of hazardous products manufactured in the U.S. and other developed nations were regularly exported to Third World nations. Led by the post-WWII expansion of the chemical industry, the volume of agricultural chemicals, pharmaceuticals and consumer products exports to Third World nations has steadily expanded, giving rise to regulatory, corporate organizational and ethical questions similar to those which define the fugitive firm debate. Debate over the appropriate role of U.S. regulators, and legal questions of marketing domestically banned products abroad, has been fueled by such exports as garments treated with Tris (a mutagen in bacteria and carcinogen in animals); Phosvel insecticide for cotton crops; and Depo-Provera contraceptive injection.[18] Recent controversies surrounding application of malathion and ethylene dibromide insecticides in Central America,[19] MNC tobacco marketing efforts in the Third World and Japan,[20] and field testing in Argentina of genetically engineered vaccines for animals[21] developed by a Philadelphia laboratory underscore the scope and political volatility of regulating the export of hazardous products to developing nations.

Among all such exports, agricultural chemicals probably have drawn the most attention owing to the duration, volume and economic significance to Third World economies. Beginning with the development and export of DDT in the late 1930s, U.S. manufacturers found receptive markets for agricultural chemicals throughout Latin America, Africa and Asia. Accelerated post-war transformation of mixed-use, small scale farming to monocultural, large scale farms to supply international markets with cotton, bananas and other farm products primed the export market for insecticide, pesticide and herbicides. U.S. MNCs, often in collaboration with smaller national firms, spearheaded these changes, which required managerial, marketing and financial strength to bring to fruition. By the late 1950s, the Green Revolution in rice and wheat production spurred additional demand for agricultural chemicals to achieve maximum output from hybrid seeds which lay at the heart of the new high-yield technologies.

Cotton production in Central America exemplifies the forces and consequences of this agricultural conversion. In the late 1940's, ideal soil and climatic conditions on the western coastal plain of the Central American isthmus attracted large amounts of foreign capital in response to a rapid increase in world demand for cotton fiber.[22] Although cotton production had been attempted in the area as early as the 1870's, only the introduction of synthetic chemicals permitted control of the various pests which historically plagued production. By the mid-1950's, with the consolidation of small food crop farms into large scale, export-oriented cotton monoculture, intensive dusting with DDT, toxaphene, ethyl parathion and methyl parathion became commonplace. Supply of prepackaged insecticides, and later in-country mixing and packaging under the protection of tariff-free imports and intermediate products, was largely controlled by U.S. MNCs. With heavy government and multi-lateral involvement in credit provision and infrastructural development (especially road building), the domination of cotton throughout the western coastal region was assured. Pesticide usage grew faster than cotton acreage itself, reflecting the typical practice of intensifying applications to cope with pests. By the mid-1960s in Nicaragua, for example, economically significant pests had increased from five (in the mid-1950s) to nine, applications had increased from about 5-10 to 28 per year and the tonnage per acre of cotton steadily grew.[23]

Reliance on pesticides for cotton production illustrates the interaction of economic and political forces which create dual standards of health and safety in many hazardous products. Many compounds, perhaps as many as one-third of all U.S. exports to developing nations in 1976, were banned or restricted for use in the U.S. Many of these, such as endrin, dieldrin, kepone, leptophos, lindane, and DDT, played instrumental roles in Central America's cotton economy. Health risks associated with such compounds, the basis for their prohibition or restriction in the U.S., are elevated by careless use in Third World nations where farm and factory occupational health regulations are poorly enforced or simply non-existent.[24] These conditions, coupled with the heavy concentration of the workforce in agricultural activities, make pesticide poisoning one of the region's principal public health problems.[25]

Relative to their historical role in transferring hazardous products to the Third World, the mechanisms and boundaries of MNCs involvement have become less clear-cut overtime. MNCs now do business using a wide variety of arrangements which have blurred the distinction between the MNCs home and host country. Various forms of marketing/distributorship agreements, product/equipment supply agreements, technology licenses, joint equity ventures and joint development agreements cloud the distinction between the source and responsibility for the transfer of hazardous products.[26]

In India, for example, where pesticide use increased by a factor of 20 between 1960 and 1980 and domestic production increased approximately 13-fold between 1970 and 1980, imports increased in dollar terms seven-fold between 1978 and 1980 alone.[27] Chemical industry growth overall since Indian independence has been among the nation's most robust, now accounting for 20 percent of the nation's fixed industrial assets. Thus, hazards transfers materialize through a combination of foreign MNC exporters, finished products and domestic manufacturers in the form of state, quasi-state and private enterprises. Together these two will share an estimated market of 99,000 tons in 1984-85 to 119,000 tons (forecasted) in 1989-90.[28] As in the Central American case, an estimated 70 percent of such products are prohibited or severely restricted in Western nations. The outcomes, too, are consistent with such intensive pesticide use. About one third of all pesticide poisonings in the Third World occur in India, concentrated in the relatively large scale wheat, rice and cotton producing regions of the country. On the production side, a recent study estimated that 73 percent of pesticide plant workers show signs of toxic poisoning and 35 percent have cardiovascular and gastrointestinal problems.[29]

HAZARDOUS WASTES

The third dimension of hazards transfers is the export of hazardous wastes from the U.S. to Third World nations. We refer here only to those hazardous byproducts of industrial activities located within the boundaries of the U.S., not to wastes generated within Third World nations by MNCs operations. The exporting of hazardous waste differs from process and product exports in at least two respects. First, it is a relatively recent phenomenon, identified (though not actually occurring) only during the last few years during which time it has surfaced as a potentially significant vehicle of hazards exports. Second, all indications point to little or no involvement of MNCs, a situation likely to continue in the foreseeable future. These features may be explained by reference to the changing U.S. regulatory and liability climate, currency-starved Third World nations and, in contrast to process and product exports, the minimal barriers to entry in the form of capital and marketing resources.

Prior to the major environmental legislation of the early 1970s, waste generators had few incentives to seek alternatives to land burial of chemical wastes either on-site or at commercial facilities. The enactment of the Resource Conservation and Recovery Act (RCRA) in 1976 and the Superfund Act of 1980 signaled the end of the era of cheap and abundant waste disposal. Since then, gradual implementation of cradle-to-grave tracking of wastes, expansive liability and explicit performance standards have reduced the supply and increased the demand for licensed treatment and disposal facilities. At the same time, price escalation has pushed disposal costs to levels 5-20 times their mid-1970's levels. Amendments to RCRA in 1984 and Superfund in 1986 reinforced these market trends by shifting waste management practices to source reduction, imposing strict limitations of land disposal options, increasing the number of generators regulated and defining higher standards for storage, treatment and disposal facilities.[30] In addition, a number of state level regulations have, or likely will, impose additional economic costs on waste generators which go beyond current federal regulations. Most prominent among these are pending reclassification of municipal waste incinerator ash residue, the exemption of which from RCRA as a "household waste" is likely to end in at least several Northeastern states.

As other Western nations have joined the U.S. in implementing waste controls, the market for waste disposal services has moved from national and regional markets to a more global configuration. The lure of highly lucrative opportunities for sending industrial waste to low cost disposal sites in Third World nations has attracted middlemen, brokers, phantom corporations, legitimate shipping firms, property owners and, in some instances, government officials. Even a small fraction of the $20 billion per year waste disposal business represents a sizable inducement for firms to enter the business, especially with the limited capital requirements.[31] In the absence of uniform international standards for waste disposal and handling and definitions of what constitutes a hazardous waste, a climate of uncertainty fosters the rapid turnover of shipments among various middlemen, each of whom extracts a mark-up for handling what amounts to a commodity liability.

Because waste exporting often operates on the margins of legitimacy, the figures of actual tonnage and composition shipped are subject to enormous uncertainty. Officials of the International Register of Potentially Toxic Chemicals believe that waste exports to Africa from industrial nations are at least a decade old.[32] EPA reports that in 1987, 230,000 tons of waste were proposed for shipment to Mexico, though only 30,000 tons of recyclables were actually accepted.[33] Proposals to ship U.S. wastes to Africa in the first part of 1988 exceeded the figure for the previous four years.[34] An inventory of active waste importing schemes by Greenpeace International reports active plans in the African nations of Benin, Equatorial Guinea, Gabon, Guinea, Guinea-Bissau, Morocco, Senegal and South Africa; historical shipments in Nigeria, South Africa and Zimbabwe; and rejected shipments to the Congo, Djibouti, Guinea and Guinea-Bissau.[35] In Latin America, active plans are reported in Argentina, Brazil, the Dominican Republic, Guyana, Haiti, Mexico, Netherland Antilles, Paraguay, Peru, Surinam and Uruguay; historical shipments to only two countries, the Dominican Republic and Mexico; and rejected shipments to more than a dozen nations, four of which fall into the active category.

The diversity of actual and potential destinations indicates the breadth, scope and regulatory complexities of controlling waste exports to the Third World. Typically, the number of nationalities represented in a single scheme may easily reach a half dozen when a full accounting is made of the generators, brokers, shippers and government agencies in both sending and recipient nations. These kinds of complex linkages, for example, have occurred in cases involving actual or attempted shipments of U.S. wastes to India, South Korea, Nigeria, Zimbabwe, Honduras and Panama[36] as well as the Bahamas and Haiti;[37] Italian wastes to Nigeria,[38] Djibouti and Venezuela;[39] and British and Swiss-based firms' waste to Guinea-Bisseau.[40] The multiplicity of actors in part reflects the complexity of international marine shipping in which the registry, owner and operator of cargo vessels are often different parties and nationalities. It also reflects the ease with which corporate entities are formed in response to short-term business opportunities and just as quickly disappear to escape responsibility for illicit actions attendant upon such opportunities. Finally, as a number of the African and Latin American incidents have demonstrated, both host countries agencies and individuals are susceptible to accepting waste imports because of hard currency and personal gains linked to such deals.

Current U.S. control of waste exports is authorized under regulations promulgated pursuant to RCRA (issued in 1980) and HSWA (issued in 1986).[41] The first set forth only two requirements: (1) notification to EPA four weeks in advance of the first shipment in a calendar year and (2) submission of an annual report of shipments. Subsequent amendments to RCRA expanded controls by requiring a more detailed notification procedure, consent of the recipient country, and provisions for bilateral agreements, which subsequently have been enacted for Canada and Mexico. Despite these expanded controls, EPA recognizes the proliferation of "sham recyclers" and the "criminal intent" among waste exporters, as well as the stimulus to such actors caused by increasingly restrictive and costly land disposal requirements contained in HSWA.[42] Activities in Congress reflect concern with what some view as inadequate controls. Current proposals for new legislation range from outright ban of all hazardous waste exports (except to Canada and Mexico) to requirements that facilities in recipient nations meet U.S. standards before exports are allowed. In addition, EPA is exploring the advantages of relying more on bilateral agreements such as those that currently in force with Canada and Mexico instead of the case-by-case prior notification/acceptance process currently in place.[43]

Outside the U.S., a number of multilateral efforts by the United Nations as well as groups of exporting and importing nations are aimed at establishing international standards for waste trading between Western and Third World nations. The European Community (EC) in June, 1988, came close to approving an outright ban on waste shipments to Third World nations.[44] The British delegate responsible for the defeat described the proposed unilateral prohibition as "commercial colonialism," underscoring the tension between policies of self-determination and external economic control imposed by Western nations. While discussions continue, the only concerted EC policy relies on earlier agreements to notify receiving governments of the nature of wastes and to insure that sufficient technical capacity is available for proper disposal. At this juncture, however, only three of twelve EC members have implemented these regulations.

Among receiving nations, the Organization of African Unity (OAU) in May 1988, approved a resolution for member nations to refrain from entering agreements which allow disposal of nuclear or hazardous wastes within their territories.[45] The Organization of Eastern Caribbean States also announced plans to subscribe to international conventions as they become available. Such resolutions and intentions, of course, do not insure enforcement. As long as the economic returns are so powerful, both to private persons and national governments enticed by major infusions of foreign currency, these types of regional agreements are unlikely to regulate effectively the flow of wastes to subscribing nations.

As the multilateral efforts proceed, the United Nations has moved toward replacing its weak guidelines and principles for hazardous waste management with a more detailed and comprehensive convention.[46] With the objective of a signed agreement by March 1989, negotiations during 1988 have uncovered several areas of North-South disagreement, including prior informed consent of third party nations through which wastes in transit travel, penalties on exporting nations in the event of violations, and definition of wastes to be included in the convention. A January 1989 meeting organized by United Nations Environmental Program (UNEP) highlighted further unresolved matters: treatment offshore or dependent territories which do not maintain the same environmental laws as the motherland, control of ships flying flags of convenience, e.g., Panama and Liberia, liability and compensation rules for environmental and human injury, and specific criteria for certifying shipments and disposal sites.[47] Should agreement be reached, current efforts by the Organization for Economic Cooperation and Development (OECD) may be set aside in favor of a global agreement.[48]

CONCLUSIONS

In the preceding discussion, I have attempted to place the transfer of hazards in the form of process, product and waste exports to the Third World in the context of larger economic forces which have restructured international capital markets and industrial organizations. When viewed in this framework, the transboundary movement of hazards to the Third World becomes one among many manifestations of increasingly fluid global markets for technology, products and wastes. This perspective in effect regards the fugitive firm as an exception while not rejecting the idea that hazardous technologies in the post-war period have diffused, and will continue to diffuse to Third World nations with increasing intensity. The underlying cause of these trends, however, is not the individual firm or industry seeking a pollution haven but the globalization of corporate enterprise which allows MNCs to respond to production and marketing opportunities with unprecedented adeptness and agility.

The same perspective appears equally applicable to process and production hazards as to product hazards. The same financial strength and organizational versatility that facilitate global production decisions allow MNCs to identify, cultivate and penetrate new product markets. Such penetration is achieved increasingly through a variety of bilateral agreements in which host countries often act as partners through the formation of state or quasi-state enterprises. Thus, the transfer of hazardous products, historically in the form of finished products, increasingly is in the form of raw material or intermediate inputs. Neither host country nor international regulations have kept pace with the complexity of hazardous product manufacture and marketing arrangements. Indeed, the reorientation of agriculture in the post-war years has deepened dependence on agricultural chemicals, many of which remain banned or severely restricted in Western nations. The ethical issues surrounding such dual standards of health and safety remain as key policy and political issues in hazards transfers.

Finally, in the arena of hazardous wastes, our conceptual framework offers fewer, though still some worthwhile, insights. MNCs are clearly not directly involved in the growing global traffic in waste exports, although certain waste management firms certainly qualify as MNCs. Because of modest capital requirements, waste exports to date are dominated by relatively small firms whose principal attributes are aggressivenss and daring rather than technological and marketing prowess. Relatively few barriers to entry, short-term profitability and the virtually infinite supply of potential Third World disposal sites make waste exports especially difficult to regulate. Current controversies over how such regulations should be structured reflect these features of international waste markets.

REFERENCES

1. Environmental Requirements of the World Bank, *The Environmental Professional* **7**:205-212 (1985); R. Batstone, World Bank to Prevent Chemical Disasters, *Technology Review*, pp. 66-67, April 1986.
2. United Nations Environment Programme, Environmental Law Guidelines and Principles No. 8, *Environmentally Sound Management of Hazardous Wastes*, June 17, 1987.
3. The World Commission on Environment and Development, *Our Common Future*, Oxford University Press, Oxford (1987).
4. B. Bowonder, J. X. Kasperson, and R. E. Kasperson, Avoiding Future Bhopals, *Environment* **27**:6 (1985).
5. M. Simons, Radiation Accident in Brazil Stirs Misgivings Over Nuclear Program, *New York Times*, p. A14, October 13, 1987; M. Simon, Deaths Raise Brazil's Fear of Radiation, *New York Times*, p. A3, October 29, 1987; J. S. Petterson, Goiania Incident Case Study: Report on Followup Study of Goiania Incident, prepared by Impact Assessment Inc. for the Yucca Mountain Socioeconomic Project, June 8, 1988.
6. R. A. Shaikh, The Dilemmas of Advanced Technology for the Third World, *Technology Review*, pp. 58-64, April 1986; N. A. Ashford and C. A. Ayers, Policy Issues for Consideration in Transferring Technology to Developing Countries,

Ecology Law Quarterly **12**:871-905 (1985); J. Ives, *The Export of Hazard*, Routledge; and Kegan Paul, Boston (1985). See also H. Brown *et al.*, Value Issues in the Transfer of Hazardous Technology to Developing Countries, proposal submitted to the National Science Foundation by the Center for Technology, Environment and Development, Clark University (1988).

7. C. S. Pearson, *Down to Business: Multinational Corporations, the Environment and Development*, World Resources Institute, Washington, DC (1985).
8. C. S. Pearson, *op. cit.*, pp. 49-50.
9. T. N. Gladwin and J. G. Welles, Environmental Policy and Multinational Corporate Strategy, in *Studies in International Environmental Economics*, I. Walter, ed., John Wiley & Sons, New York (1976).
10. R. Jenkins, *Transnational Corporations and Uneven Development*, Methuen, New York (1987).
11. J. Graham *et al.*, Restructuring in U.S. Manufacturing: The Decline of Monopoly Capitalism, *Annals of the Association of American Geographers* **78**:473 (1988).
12. T. N. Gladwin and J. G. Welles, *op. cit.*, p. 177.
13. B. I. Castleman, The Export of Hazardous Factories to Developing Nations, *Int. J. of Health Services* **9**:569 (1979).
14. B. I. Castleman, The Double Standard in Industrial Hazards, in *The Export of Hazard*, J. Ives, ed., *op. cit.*
15. C. Levenstein and S. W. Eller, Exporting Hazardous Industries: 'For Example' Is Not Proof, *The Export of Hazard*, J. Ives, ed., *op. cit.*
16. H. J. Leonard, *Are Environmental Regulations Driving U.S. Industry Overseas?* The Conservation Foundation, Washington, DC (1984).
17. United Nations Industrial Development Organization, *Industry and Development: Global Report 1986*, Vienna (1986).
18. R. A. Shaikh, *op. cit.*
19. D. Dumanoski, U.S. Medfly Plan in Guatemala Draws Fire, *Boston Globe*, p. 19, July 12, 1987.
20. ALPHA Testimony: U.S. Pushes Tobacco Exports on Other Nations, *The Nation's Health*, p. 1, March 1988.
21. K. Schneider, Argentina Protests Use of Live Vaccine by Scientists of U.S., *New York Times*, p. 1, November 11, 1986.
22. R. G. Williams, *Export Agriculture and the Crisis in Central America,* University of North Carolina Press, Chapel Hill, NC (1986).
23. S. L. Swezey, D. L. Murray, and R. G. Daxi, Nicaragua's Revolution in Pesticide Policy, *Environment* **6**, January/February 1986.
24. D. Michaels, C. Barrera, and M. G. Gacharna, Occupational Health and Economic Development of Latin America, in J. Ives, ed., *op. cit.*, pp. 94-114.
25. Report Urges Better Chemical Controls Abroad, *Conservation Foundation Letter*, No. 2, The Conservation Foundation, Washington, DC (1988).
26. The Bhopal accident was recently settled after years of protracted debate over such issues. See S. Hazarika, Bhopal Payments Set at $470 Million for Union Carbide, *New York Times*, p. 1, February 15, 1989.
27. Center for Science and Environment, *The State of India's Environment 1984-1985: The Second Citizen's Report*, p. 195, Ravi Chopra, New Delhi (1985). Part of this increase is undoubtedly due to oil price escalation during that period.
28. Y. P. Gupta, Pesticide Misuse in India, *The Ecologist* **16**:36 (1986).
29. Study reported by Y. P. Gupta, *op. cit.*, conducted by S. K. Kashyap, Indian Institute of Occupational Health, Ahmedabad (Gujarat).
30. Formally known as the Hazardous and Solid Waste Amendments of 1984 (HSWA) and the Superfund Amendments and Reauthorization Act (SARA) of 1986.
31. J. Dufour and C. Denis, The North's Garbage Goes South, *World Press Review*, pp. 30-32, November 1988; Only the Ruthless Need Apply, excerpted from *L'Express* and *Financial Times London.*
32. The Dumping Grounds, *South*, pp. 37-41, August 1988.

33. Philip Shabecoff, Irate and Afraid, Poor Nations Fight Efforts to Use Them as Toxic Dumps, *New York Times*, p. C4, July 5, 1988.
34. Greenpeace USA, *International Trade in Toxic Wastes: Policy and Data Analysis*, p. 7, Washington, DC, June 1988.
35. Greenpeace International, *op. cit.*. See also *Greenpeace Waste Trade Update* **1**, August 1, 1988.
36. A. Porterfield and D. Weir, The Export of U.S. Toxic Wastes, *The Nation*, p. 325, October 3, 1987.
37. Greenpeace USA, *op. cit.*
38. L. Jenkins, After Dumping on Nigeria, Italy Takes It All Back, *The Washington Post*, p. A38, September 4, 1988.
39. Greenpeace USA, *op. cit.*
40. Africa: The Industrial World's Dumping Ground? *African Business*, p. 10, July 1988.
41. EPA Enforcement; Strategy on Hazardous Waste Exports (March 1988), *Environment Reporter*, pp. 9-19, Bureau of National Affairs, May 5, 1988.
42. EPA Enforcement Strategy. . ., *op. cit.*
43. "U.S. Would Tie Waste Exports to Bilateral Agreements," Thomas says, Bureau of National Affairs, *International Environmental Reporter* [hereafter BNA/*IER*], p. 472, September 14, 1988.
44. Dirty Games in Brussels, *South*, p. 41, August 1988.
45. *Greenpeace Waste Trade Update*, *op. cit.*
46. Waste Shipment Incidents Spur Interest in UNEP Agreement to Deal with Problem, BNA/*IER*, September 14, 1988; D. A. O'Sullivan, *C&EN*, p. 24, September 26, 1988.
47. Delegates of 50 Countries Fail to Agree on Draft Covering Movement of Toxic Wastes, and Western, African Nations Fail to Agree on Transboundary Movement of Toxic Wastes, BNA/*IER*, p. 49, February 8, 1989.
48. For a discussion OECD initiatives, see B. Piasecki and W. Grieder, Waste Havens and Waste Transfers: International Transboundary Issues, in *America's Future in Toxic Waste Management: Lessons from Europe*, B. Piasecki and G. Davis, eds., Quorum Books, New York (1987)

Development of a Generic Knowledge-Based Risk Assessment System

Jane Silber, Serdar Uckun, Kazuhiko Kawamura, and Shigeru Ozaki
Vanderbilt University
Nashville, TN

ABSTRACT

In recent years, artificial intelligence (AI) programs have appeared which contribute significantly to the field in which they are applied. Risk assessment and risk management (RA/RM) is an ideal candidate for such a program, and researchers at the Center for Intelligent Systems of Vanderbilt University are investigating the application of AI techniques to RA/RM, specifically within the context of a knowledge-based system, or expert system. Knowledge-based systems are one of the better known fruits of AI research and offer many benefits. Chief among these are the ability to make expert knowledge available to non-experts, the ability to explore "what it" scenarios safely, improved communication channels, and methods of handling uncertainty. This paper describes the development of a generic knowledge-based risk assessment system. By identifying an underlying representation common to many risk assessment fields (a network), the same architecture and construction techniques embodied in this generic system may be used in numerous individual applications. The system architecture and design principles, as well as the benefits they will provide, are described.

KEYWORDS: Artificial intelligence (AI), expert system, knowledge-based system, risk assessment/risk management (RA/RM)

INTRODUCTION

The effective assessment and management of risks has become an increasingly significant concern of policy makers and the public.[1,2] The conception and maturation of risk assessment in the last decade can be attributed to various political, economic, and technical changes. As the political, economic and technical environments continue to change, risk assessment and risk management practices will reflect those changes. One of the most important recent developments in the technical world is the emergence of artificial intelligence (AI) and its increasing acceptance in both the academic and business communities.

AI is the study of ideas which allow computers to behave intelligently. Definitions of "intelligent behavior" vary greatly, and the AI field encompasses an equally wide range of research areas. Planning, problem-solving, learning, vision, and natural language processing are examples of what has been considered intelligent behavior. Perhaps the most widely researched area within AI, however, has been the development of "knowledge-based" systems, also known as "expert systems."

A knowledge-based system is an AI-based computer program which uses expert knowledge to attain high levels of performance in a specific problem area. Knowledge-based systems have been successfully deployed in such diverse fields as medical diagnosis,[3,4] mineral exploration,[5] computer system configuration,[6] and intelligent tutoring.[7,8] The power of expert system technology comes from a large body of knowledge, acquired from human experts and stored in a declarative, modular format as heuristic rules and facts. Further, powerful explanation capabilities, essential for any intelligent system which must have a great deal of interaction with the user, can be implemented. This way the user can easily explore different scenarios using "what-if" hypotheses on-line. Finally, expert systems offer the possibility of dealing with uncertainty in an understandable manner, a critical feature in the domain of risk assessment.

Expert system technology offers possible solutions to many of the problems facing traditional risk assessment programs. Risk assessment consumes valuable resources, such as time and money, and therefore often does not receive sufficient attention. Also, a reliable risk analysis must be conducted by one or more experts, and it is often difficult to determine the underlying reasoning and explanations in a risk analysis. A generic knowledge-based system for risk assessment can alleviate many of these problems.

SYSTEM DESIGN

The Center for Intelligent Systems at Vanderbilt University has undertaken a long-term research project to develop a generic risk assessment expert system. The risk assessment system has been designed to take full advantage of AI methods to improve uncertainty management, system modeling, and risk communication.

To design a generic system for use in many risk assessment applications, a common ground among applications must be identified. The commonality identified in this system is a network structure. Most risk assessment applications may be represented in some form of network, such as a causal model[9] or a fault or event tree.[10] A causal model is a more general form of a fault or event tree and provides a functional representation of the application model. In addition to representing the input and output events, a causal network shows the functional events that connect the input to the output. These connections facilitate the reasoning process, as well as helping provide explanations of the reasoning.

One of the fundamental design principles for this risk assessment system has been the wide applicability of network structures. In fact, network functions provide one of the basic building blocks on which specific risk assessment applications will be constructed. The system architecture contains four conceptual layers which correspond to four distinct layers in the system design. The multi-layer architecture is shown in Fig. 1, and each layer is described in detail below.

Kernel

The kernel layer provides the foundation for the system. It contains the software tools and techniques with which the higher layers are constructed. Growing interest in the AI community in object-oriented programming (OOP) systems led to the investigation of Smalltalk as the kernel language for this system.

OOP languages are fundamentally different from traditional procedural languages. The basic unit of data abstraction in an object-oriented environment is the "object," which combines properties of procedures and data; all action in an OOP system is derived from

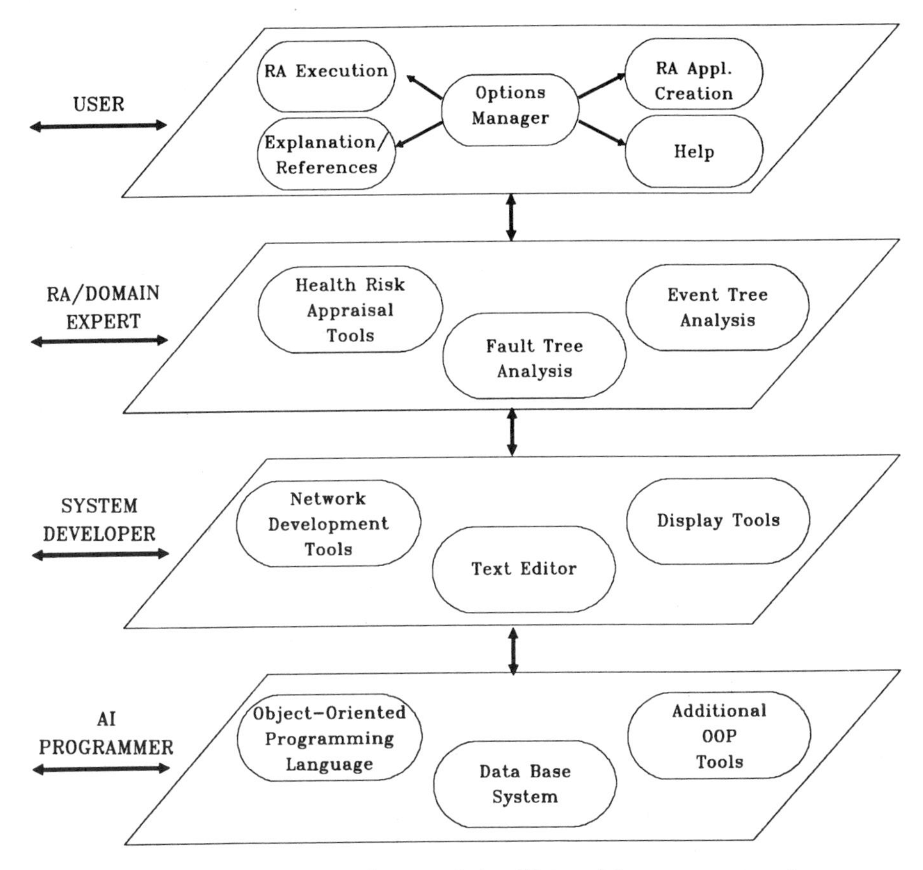

Fig. 1. Design concept of a generic intelligent risk assessment system.

passing messages between objects. In addition, OOP environments provide inheritance properties which allow objects and methods to be organized hierarchically. The hierarchical organization leads to very modular and portable code, which, in turn, allows development of functional modules for the higher layers in the system architecture.

The current system is being developed in the Smalltalk-80 environment from ParcPlace Systems. Many third party software tools have been developed for the Smalltalk environment, including NodeGraph-80 from Knowledge Systems Corporation. NodeGraph-80 is a toolkit for developing directed node graph representations and structures. NodeGraph-80 provides much of the support required for the second conceptual layer, the network development layer, as well as graphics functions used in the user interface layer. Other software tools used in the system include a data base management system to handle the various data bases and historical information.

Network Development Layer

The network development layer includes a set of generic tools which may be used for a variety of applications including, but not limited to, risk assessment. Three major groups of tools are included in this layer. The first group is the network development tools (NDT). Generic networking tools are critical in many risk assessment applications, such as modeling event and fault trees and describing qualitative or causal models of the system under study.

The main functions of the network development tools are summarized in Table 1. The first family of functions is related to the creation of a network and its graphical display. Another set of functions helps the user to modify the network and change data about specific nodes, and a third group of support functions deals with saving and loading networks to/from disk files.

A second set of tools in this layer contains a module which aids in the design of user interfaces. An effective user interface is crucial not only for risk communication but also to allow accurate risk assessment by a non-expert. The capabilities of possible users must be considered in developing the user interface, and no standard user interface will be adequate for all levels of user expertise. An alternate approach is to customize user interfaces for different users.

A third set of tools is derived from conventional Smalltalk-80 file editors. These editors are available to be plugged into risk assessment applications. These file/text editors can be used to create text files that can be attached to certain network nodes to provide explanation, advice or reference information.

Risk Assessment/Domain Expert Layer

The third layer contains the risk assessment expertise and domain specific knowledge. Creating a generic risk assessment system is difficult due to the large number of assessment procedures. Our strategy is to prepare many components of a complete risk assessment package, including all necessary inference procedures, risk calculation algorithms, interfaces to causal networks created by the network development tools, and interfaces to user interfaces created by the display customizing tools. Therefore, complete risk assessment systems will be constructed easily by putting three modules together: a causal network, a user interface, and a risk assessment procedure to connect them.

The set of risk assessment tools will include, among others, fault tree analysis, event tree analysis, dose-response analysis, and probabilistic risk assessment. Additional modules may be added at any time.

User Interface Layer

There are many issues involved in user interface design. The complexity of the task is increased due to the desire to accommodate users with varying degrees of expertise. The first user of the system will be a risk assessment expert. The expert will use the network development tools to create a risk assessment network. The second user, a "naive user," will use the system simply to run a risk assessment. This user will not necessarily know the fundamentals of risk assessment.

To accommodate both types of users, the interface must be flexible yet well structured. The expert user will need a flexible environment in which he can easily and quickly define the network or networks. Instructions and on-line help should be available to guide the use of the network development tools. The naive user, on the other hand, requires a very structured system which will lead him through the risk assessment process. This "structured" aspect of the interface should anticipate the naive user's moves and always have help or explanations available. These explanations will generally focus on the domain information provided by the expert.

A sample screen from a health risk assessment application is shown in Fig. 2. The interface consists of several windows, each with a designated purpose. The menu selections across the top of the screen allow the user to move through the risk assessment system. The middle window, or pane, supports graphics functions for network display and creation. The

Table 1. List of Risk Assessment Tools

- **Network Development Tools**: A set of tools to develop structural backbones and graphical representations of causal networks of the risk assessment domain.

- **Display Customizing Tools**: A set of tools for creation of user interfaces customized for different levels of users, incorporating various graph, text and gauge representations.

- **Risk Assessment Modules**: Several modules for different risk assessment procedures.

- **Supervisory Module**: A controlling module that will integrate the risk assessment module, the causal network and the user interface as a complete risk assessment system.

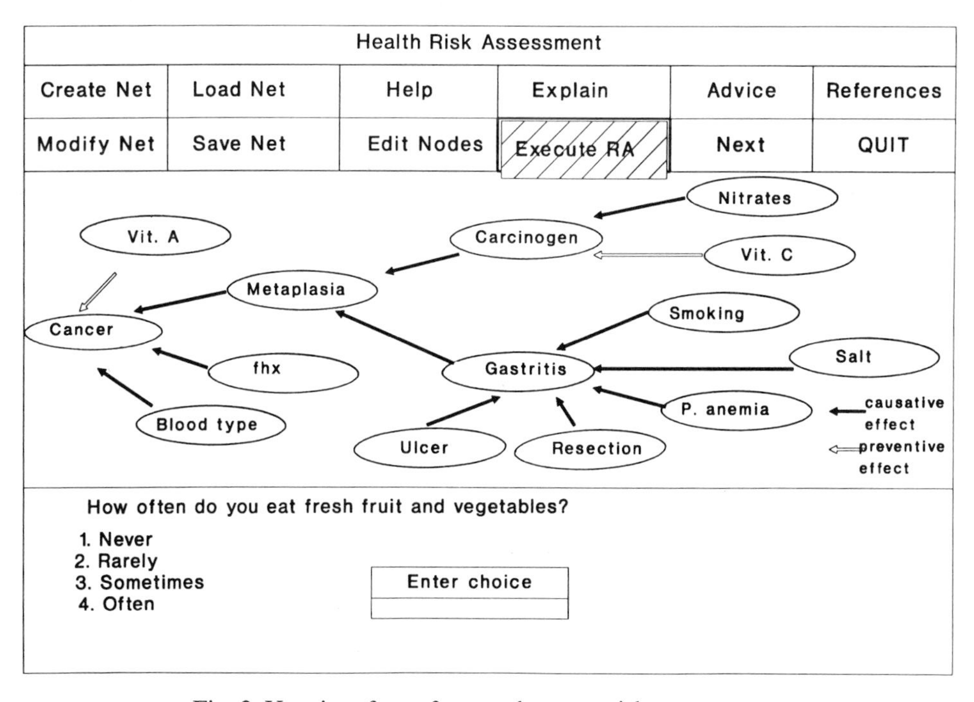

Fig. 2. User interface of stomach cancer risk assessment.

bottom window serves as a system transcript for user queries and system guidance. The interface is mainly mouse driven, with new menus and windows appearing as needed.

PROTOTYPE IMPLEMENTATION

The first step in the development of the risk assessment expert system described above was the implementation of a prototype system. The prototype was developed on an

IBM-AT compatible personal computer with EGA color graphics. The Smalltalk/V programming environment was used.

The prototype development concentrated on two major areas: (1) a generic tool set for creating causal networks or any other network structure and (2) a health risk assessment application which was developed using the network development tools. Figure 2 depicts a causal model developed for the assessment of stomach cancer mortality risk.

Starting with a small prototype system, it was possible to conceptualize and validate many approaches in system development. Work is on-going to create a more complete and robust system on a larger machine. As discussed above, the complete system will be based on a Hewlett Packard workstation in Smalltalk-80. This version will differ from the prototype in that it will be more generic. The Smalltalk-80 version will also offer a larger set of tools at the network development layer and the risk assessment application layer.

CONCLUSION

There is much evidence to validate the knowledge-based approach to risk assessment. A generic risk assessment expert system will allow rapid development of risk assessment applications and facilitate repeated analysis under different conditions (a "what-if" analysis). In addition, because the knowledge of a risk assessment expert is stored in the computer system, the knowledge will be made available to a wider range of people and applications.

In addition to the development of the proposed system, the idea of knowledge-based risk assessment has afforded a number of interesting areas of basic research. For example, this project has spawned other projects in hypertext research, uncertainty management, and machine learning, all of which will be incorporated into the final risk assessment system. Also, a related project is being undertaken at Vanderbilt to study applications of qualitative modeling to knowledge-based risk assessment studies.[11] In this project, models of technological processes are used to generate fault and event networks for hypothesized fault situations in various engineering domains.

ACKNOWLEDGEMENTS

The authors acknowledge the System Research & Development Institute of Teijin Limited, Tokyo, Japan, for partial support of the research described in this paper.

REFERENCES

1. Conservation Foundation, State of the Environment: An Assessment at Mid-Decade, Washington, DC (1984).
2. National Research Council, *Risk Assessment in the Federal Government: Managing the Process*, National Academy Press, Washington, DC (1983).
3. B. G. Buchanan and E. H. Shortliffe, eds., *Rule-Based Expert Systems: The MYCIN Experiments of the Stanford Heuristic Programming Project*, Addison-Wesley, Reading, MA (1984).
4. R. A. Miller, H. E. Pople, Jr., and J. D. Myers, Internist-1, An Experimental Computer-Based Diagnostic Consultant for General Internal Medicine, *The New England Journal of Medicine* **307(8)**:468-476 (1982).
5. R. Duda, P. E. Hart, N. J. Nilsson *et al.*, Development of the PROSPECTOR Consultation System for Mineral Exploration, SRI Report, SRI International, Menlo Park, CA (1978).

6. J. McDermott, J., R1, A Rule-Based Configurer of Computer Systems, *Artificial Intelligence* **19**:33-88 (1982).
7. W. J. Clancey, *Knowledge Based Tutoring: The GUIDON Program*, The MIT Press, Cambridge, MA (1987).
8. D. Sleeman and J. S. Brown, eds., *Intelligent Tutoring Systems*, pp. 227-282, Academic Press, New York (1982).
9. M. Bunge, *Causality and Modern Science*, Dover Publications, Inc., New York (1974).
10. N. Rasmussen, Reactor Safety Study: An Assessment of Accident Risks in U.S. Commercial Nuclear Power Plants, U.S. Nuclear Regulatory Commission Report No. NUREG 75/014 (WASH1400), October, 1975.
11. G. Biswas, K. Debelak, and K. Kawamura, Applications of Qualitative Modeling to Knowledge-Based Risk Assessment Studies, Technical Report CS-88-11, Vanderbilt University (1988).

The Role of Salient Fates and Anxiety in Hazard Perception

Linda-Jo Schierow
Massachusetts Institute of Technology
Cambridge, MA

ABSTRACT

Social psychologists investigating perceptions of technological and natural hazards have identified critical characteristics of hazards that account for much of the variance in assessments of risk acceptability by non-experts. Additional explanations of variance are being sought through studies of cognitive generalizations (e.g., stigmatization) which simplify, and social interactions which amplify or attenuate, risk judgments.[1] This paper examines the possible role of fear in modulating risk perceptions. It is hypothesized that hazards may be judged more or less acceptable depending on the quality of negative consequences which are salient and on evaluative responses to salient consequences. A basic assumption underlying this hypothesis is that there are fates associated with hazards which are perceived to be "worse than death." It is expected that the degree of anxiety aroused on contemplation of the potential fates of those exposed to hazards will be related directly to the amount of deviation of perceptions from objective risk estimates, although other variables are expected to obscure the relationship.

KEYWORDS: Risk perception, fear, hazard evaluation, affective dimensions, environmental attitude

INTRODUCTION

Pioneering research on risk perceptions has demonstrated that both reason and sentiment influence hazard evaluations.[2-6] This result is consistent with the more general conclusion by psychologists that both cognitive and motivational components affect judgment.[7,8] It appears, for example, that attitudes toward technologies, activities, and storms are influenced by the estimated probability of personal fatality, given hazard exposure,[9] and by dread of globally-catastrophic and uncontrollable events and consequences.[10] These and other critical beliefs about hazards explain much of the variance in assessments of overall riskiness by research subjects. Additional cognitive explanations of variance are being sought through studies of hazard generalizations (e.g., stigmatization) which simplify, and social interactions which amplify or attenuate, risk judgments.[1]

In the United States, the emotional (affective) dimension of hazard perceptions is less studied and less understood than the cognitive dimension. Sjoberg's *Risk and Society*,[11] however, includes several articles by Europeans on the subject, and there is a large body of relevant literature on the psychology of motivation, fear, stress, and coping, in general. This paper is based on that literature and focuses on the possible role of fear in modulating risk perceptions.

FEAR OF HAZARDS

The potential importance of fear often is acknowledged, and generally is assumed, in the risk perception literature. Fear has been evoked to explain risk-averse behaviors, for example, and has been discussed as an irrational response to misperceived risks. Nevertheless, the role of fear in the process of hazard appraisal and the factors eliciting fear have received little serious attention, with a few notable exceptions.

Research by Slovic and others[10] has demonstrated that hazards which survey respondents judge least acceptable are those for which they believe people have a great dread. More recently, Green *et al.*[12] have shown that "worry" can be measured relatively easily, and that in some cases it is a rational response to real threat. Stallen and Tomas[13] found that manifest anxiety was a function of the assessment of a threat, of the opportunities for specific personal control, and of optimism regarding one's power to improve the environment. Moreover, they observed that anxiety increased along with knowledge of the hazard and its safety mechanisms. The most comprehensive discussion of fear and its relevance to hazard perceptions research is found in articles by Blomkvist.[14,15] Menkes[16] and Lyttgens[17] also have discussed anxiety as a social force affecting hazard appraisal.

There are several reasons why fear is an important topic for research related to hazard perceptions. First, fear focuses attention on the perceivers and their individual differences and similarities, which may allow identification of clusters of subjects with similar perspectives. Secondly, because fear is associated with salient experiences or objects—that is, with experiences or objects which come to mind readily—it may reveal the attributes of hazards or situational characteristics which lead to stigmatization, attenuation (through habituation), or amplification of perceived risks.[17] In addition, the various manifestations of fear facilitate measurement and allow assessment of the validity and reliability of fear indicators. Finally, fear is of interest because of the generally stable association of fears with their sources. Fear, therefore, may be a reliable predictor of evaluative response to hazards, a welcome contrast to the more labile values attached to positive goals.[14]

INVESTIGATING THE ROLE OF FEAR IN HAZARD EVALUATION

Psychologists have demonstrated that fear is a potent influence on cognitive processes and behavior[18,19] and have suggested it functions as a negative goal, focusing attention, motivating information processing, and increasing the tendency to respond with escape or avoidance behaviors (see Ref. 20, p. 217; and Ref. 21). It competes with other positive and negative goals for cognitive dominance, however, so that avoidance responses may be suppressed (or not elicited) if fear is weak.[22] In addition, social influences can obscure expressions of fear, and habituation can weaken the relative importance of avoidance over time (see Ref. 19, pp. 11 and 41). A little fear may even be satisfying, providing a thrill of sensation (see Ref. 19, p. 11; and Ref. 22). In general though, the stronger the fear, the more potent its influence on thought and behavior, and the more certain the direction of its influence. Greater fear dislodges other considerations and focuses attention on the source of fear and how best to avoid it (see Ref. 18; and Ref. 20, pp. 225-227).

My general thesis is that hazards may be judged as more or less acceptable depending on the quality of negative consequences which are salient and on the direction and strength of evaluative responses to salient consequences. It is expected that the degree of fear aroused on contemplation of consequences associated with a hazard will be directly related to the size of deviation of overall hazard evaluations from hazard assessments based on subjective probability estimates of mortality, given exposure. The relationship between fear and hazard evaluation is expected to be obscured, however, by the influence of other critical parameters—e.g., level of knowledge, decision-making procedure, and degree of uncertainty—associated with various hazards and their potential consequences. But, if sufficient fear is elicited during hazard evaluation, the result should be an increased tendency to avoid the hazard, and subjects' evaluations should be more risk averse than they would be in the absence of fear. Furthermore, it is possible that the utility of avoiding fairly small amounts of fear would have a relatively large negative impact on an evaluation, whereas beyond a certain level of fear, further increments would have relatively smaller impacts. In other words, the disutility of fear might be described by a concave function because it represents a desire to avoid loss rather than a desire to achieve safety. Several studies have demonstrated that utility functions tend to be sharper for relative losses than for relative gains.[23,24] This point is theoretically significant because small differences in the perceived severity of a threat might have stronger and more measurable effects on hazard evaluations than would small increments in perceived safety gains.

The relative importance of fear, compared to other independent variables, as a predictor of a hazard's acceptability depends on the degree of independence of fear from subjective estimates of the probability of personal mortality: if fear were only evoked by thoughts of death, then at least a portion of its effect on hazard appraisal is incorporated into current conceptual models. It is reasonable to hypothesize, however, that fear could be aroused by contemplation of fates other than death (for example, see the articles in Refs. 11, 14, 15, and 17). Students in a study reported by Green[25] identified two injuries to which death was preferred—brain damage and permanent paralysis from the neck down. Alternatively, the level of fear aroused in response to risks of death perceived to be equal might vary depending on the imagined conditions surrounding different modes of dying. For example, Hinton[26] has noted that an important aspect of the fear of death is the expectation of pain and suffering.

Fear and probability of mortality only can be completely independent, however, if there are "fates worse than death" that are salient consequences associated with hazards. If there are such fates, then the reliance of risk assessment experts on annual fatality rates is based on a simple normative judgment—that death is the fate of greatest importance. Other norms would be equally valid foundations for rational (or quasi-rational) risk assessments. This is the issue which originally steered my thinking toward motivational factors in risk perception research. As a scientist myself, I wondered how people I regarded as reasonably intelligent and logical sometimes decided to ignore the relatively high probability of fatal consequences.

For example, consider the people who refuse to buckle their safety belts. Different people express different explanations for this obviously irrational behavior if the worst consequence is death. Traditional explanations for this behavior concern the relative importance of comfort, convenience, or other benefits which must outweigh the perceived cost of a very small probability of a fatal accident on a single occasion of automobile use. Alternatively, one might argue that people fail to use seatbelts simply because they forget; perhaps they are locked into a pattern of behavior that begins with opening the car door.

An equally convincing explanation, offered by the drivers themselves, is that they fear the consequences of seatbelt use in the event of a serious accident. Two feared consequences dominate among my acquaintances: fire and entrapment. Usually the fear is of being trapped in a fire. How common are these fears and how powerful in the "average" person? Which is more salient in decisions about seatbelt use—the perceived probability of an accident or the quality of the consequences? Is the most salient consequence for an individual always most salient, across hazards and contexts, given that it is an attribute of the hazard?

These are the kinds of questions I am addressing in a series of studies. This research is in a formative stage and still is wide open to suggestions and constructive criticisms. It is hoped that this brief outline and presentation of preliminary results will encourage feedback that may lower my risk of stumbling into blind alleys and pitfalls.

The first step has been to test the underlying assumption that there are "fates worse than death" which are salient. In a preliminary survey of graduate students in Public Health, I asked students to list up to seven outcomes or events which would be "fates worse than death," or almost as bad as death. I told them that these should be fates they personally would die to prevent if necessary. Students had no trouble thinking of responses in the five minutes they were given. There were 114 different fates among the 118 fates listed by the 30 students who responded to this question. Most students listed three to four fates.

Classification of responses is difficult, but, in addition to four sets of duplicate responses, many of the fates listed by different students were similar. Some fates were described in ambiguous terms. (For example, the response "loss of child" could be interpreted as death or separation from a child who is one's own or whose parents are strangers.) Other responses were very specific, e.g., "losing a limb on my body therefore restraining me from taking care of myself." To date I have resisted over-generalization and kept a large number of categories so as to retain all the relevant detail of the responses. The physical fates mentioned in at least 5 percent of responses included: death; chronic, terminal disease, usually AIDS; more or less complete physical or mental incapacitation; some other condition causing dependence; other disabilities; and temporary, probably painful situations such as torture. In addition to the physical conditions, 3 to 4 percent of responses identified each of the following internal states: situations endangering others for which the respondent is responsible; apathy; and failure. Horrifying situations mentioned in at least 5 percent of responses included poverty or debt and isolation or confinement. Other popular responses related to interpersonal relationships and to political or broad social conditions such as racism or war.

Clearly these students believe that there are fates worse than death. The results also point to areas needing further investigation. It is interesting, for example, that 17 different students, more than half of the respondents, linked at least one fate with a specific victim, usually a family member. This result is consistent with work reported by Rachman (see Ref. 19, pp. 8-9, 35-36, 146), which found fear of one's own death to be uncorrelated with fear of death of others and that fear for loved ones, especially one's children, often is more salient than fear for oneself. The possible importance of situational variables such as time also is indicated by survey responses: one-third of the students specifically noted that the fates were long-term.

Additional studies should clarify these preliminary results, and identify fates which are most feared. The results also may generate hypotheses about the qualities of consequences feared by individuals across hazards and consequences. For example, what is it about war that terrifies different individuals who have never seen combat? For some it may be chaos, for others perhaps the possibility of injury to their children. If particular qualities of consequences are salient, and if the same qualities are associated with each consequence feared by an individual, it might be possible to predict the individual's response to other hazards with similar attributes. The existence of underlying dimensions of fear is suggested in the results of recent research by a psychologist at the University of Illinois at Chicago, Steven Reiss, who has found a surprisingly small number of fear categories which can predict a wide range of individual differences in fearfulness. Given that a subject fears one or more objects or situations in the same category, other fears can be predicted. For example, certain subjects fear injuries and, therefore, tend to fear snakes, heights, and other objects or situations likely to cause injury. Exploratory research, then, should seek the underlying dimensions of feared situations, objects, and events associated with natural and technological hazards. In some cases, the consequence identified by respondents may be specific and irreducible—e.g., pain—but, in other cases, an underlying dimension may be more meaningful—e.g., if the consequence is AIDS, the underlying dimension may be long-term dependence, pain, shame, or some other factor. If dimensions emerge, factor analysis could be used to evaluate associations between dimensions and consequences across people. Further analysis by individual across hazards, rather than in the more usual way by hazard across individuals, might allow clustering of respondents with similar patterns of responses.

The preliminary study on fates worse than death demonstrated the difficulties that will be involved in designing better survey instruments. Eliciting the underlying dimensions of feared fates may be particularly difficult: on the one hand, elicitation of salient attributes requires an open-response format, while on the other hand, classification is facilitated by more structured responses. Personal, structured interviews probably will be necessary, at least initially, to guide survey development.

Identification of common fears and their underlying dimensions cannot help to predict responses to emerging technologies until it is known whether these fearful situations are cognitively linked to existing technologies that are perceived to be hazardous, and whether these are the most salient elements during hazard appraisal. In a separate study, therefore, identification should be attempted of the consequences that are salient when subjects think about hazards. At the same time, subjects should identify the consequences they most fear. Results should reveal whether the salient fates and fears for hazards are the same as the fates and fears that come to mind when hazards have not been mentioned. If the same fates and fears are salient, regardless of the context, their impacts might be expected to generalize to new or newly significant hazards.

A rough measure of the potential explanatory power of fear for predicting attitudes toward hazards can be obtained by analyzing the co-occurrence among respondents of feared, salient fates with high levels of perceived overall riskiness for a variety of hazards. For this study, the order in which subjects are asked about overall risk and associated fates of hazards should be varied to avoid focusing effects. As shown by Von Winterfeldt *et al.*,[9] when thoughts are focused first on a particular set of characteristics—e.g., probabilities or feared fates—the influence of those characteristics on hazard rankings can be exaggerated.

CONCLUSION

My research agenda is long, and investigations have just begun. The studies I have planned are exploratory, so analysis will be gross and results may be negative. But if results indicate that further research is warranted in this direction, detailed measures of fear will be developed that permit more sensitive analysis. Existing measures, such as the fear survey schedule of Wolpe and Lang[27] or the worry index of Green *et al.*[12] might be useful starting points.

There are many interesting research questions about the role of fear and other motivational influences in hazard evaluation that have not been raised in this brief report and which are beyond the scope of my present research interests. These are fertile areas for interested investigators.

REFERENCES

1. R. E. Kasperson, O. Renn, P. Slovic, H. S. Brown, J. Emel, R. Goble, J. X. Kasperson, and S. Ratick, The Social Amplification of Risk: A Conceptual Framework, *Risk Analysis* **8(2)**:177-187 (1988).
2. B. Fischhoff, P. Slovic, S. Lichtenstein, S. Read, and B. Combs, How Safe Is Safe Enough? A Psychometric Study of Attitudes Towards Technological Risks and Benefits, *Policy Sciences* **9(2)**:127-152 (1978).
3. G. Grosser, W. Wechsler, and M. Greenblatt, eds., *The Threat of Impending Disaster*, Massachusetts Institute of Technology Press, Cambridge, MA (1964).
4. C. Hohenemser, R. W. Kates, and P. Slovic, The Nature of Technological Hazard, *Science* **220(4595)**:378-384 (1983).
5. C. Vlek and P.-J. Stallen, Rational and Personal Aspects of Risk, *Acta Psychologica* **45(1-3)**:273-300 (1980).
6. G. White, ed., *Natural Hazards: Local, National, Global*, Oxford University Press, NY (1974).
7. H. J. Einhorn and R. M. Hogarth, Behavioral Decision Theory: Processes of Judgment and Choice, *Annual Review of Psychology* **32**:53-88 (1981).
8. E. J. Johnson and A. Tversky, Affect, Generalization, and the Perception of Risk, *Journal of Personality and Social Psychology* **45(1)**:20-31 (1983).
9. D. Von Winterfeldt, R. S. John, and K. Borcherding, Cognitive Components of Risk Ratings, *Risk Analysis* **1(4)**:277-288 (1981).
10. P. Slovic, B. Fischhoff, and S. Lichtenstein, Facts and Fears: Understanding Perceived Risk, in *How Safe Is Safe Enough?* pp. 181-216, R. C. Schwing and W. A. Albers, Jr., eds., Plenum Press, NY (1980).
11. L. Sjoberg, *Risk and Society* Allen & Unwin, Boston, MA (1987).
12. C. H. Green, E. C. Penning-Rowsell, and D. J. Parker, Estimating the Risk from Flooding and Evaluating Worry, in *Advances in Risk Analysis: Uncertainty in Risk Assessment, Risk Management, and Decision Making,* Vol. 4, pp. 159-176, V. T. Covello, L. B. Lave, A. Moghissi, and V. R. R. Upppuluri, eds., Plenum Press, NY (1987).
13. P. J. M. Stallen, and A. Tomas, Public Concern About Industrial Hazards, *Risk Analysis* **8(2)**:237-245 (1988).
14. A.-C. Blomkvist, Psychological Aspects of Values and Risks, in *Risk and Society*, pp. 89-112, L. Sjoberg, ed., Allen & Unwin, Boston, MA (1987).
15. A.-C. Blomkvist, Public Transportation Fears and Risks, in *Risk and Society*, pp. 159-173, L. Sjoberg, ed., Allen & Unwin, Boston, MA (1987).
16. J. Menkes, Risk or Angst? *Risk Analysis* **4**:237-240 (1981).
17. H. Lyttgens, Human Anxiety, in *Risk and Society*, pp. 115-129, L. Sjoberg, ed., Allen & Unwin, Boston, MA (1987).
18. I. L. Janis and L. Mann, *Decision Making—A Psychological Analysis of Conflict, Choice, and Commitment*, The Free Press, NY (1977).
19. S. J. Rachman, *Fear and Courage*, W. H. Freeman and Company, San Francisco, CA (1978).
20. H. Gleitman, *Basic Psychology*, 2nd ed., W. W. Norton & Co., NY (1987).
21. H. A. Simon, Alternative Visions of Rationality, in *Judgment and Decision Making: An Interdisciplinary Reader*, pp. 97-113, H. R. Arkes and K. R. Hammond, eds., Cambridge University Press, NY (1986).
22. H. F. Harlow, The Nature of Love, *American Psychologist*, **13(12)**:673-685 (1958).
23. D. Kahneman and A. Tversky, Prospect Theory: An Analysis of Decision Under Risk, *Econometrica* **47(2)**:263-291 (1979).
24. D. Kahneman and A. Tversky, Choices, Values, and Frames, in *Judgment and Decision Making: An Interdisciplinary Reader*, pp. 194-210, H. R. Arkes and K. R. Hammond, eds., Cambridge University Press, NY (1984).
25. C. H. Green, Risk: Beliefs and Attitudes, in *Fires and Human Behaviour*, p. 277-291, D. Canter, ed., John Wiley & Sons, NY (1980).

26. J. Hinton, *Dying*, 2nd ed., Penguin Books, London (1972).
27. J. Wolpe and P. J. Lang, A Fear Survey Schedule for Use in Behavior Therapy, *Behaviour Research and Therapy* **2(1)**:27-30 (1964).

Development of Robust Measures of Attitude Towards Risk

Beverly Fleisher
Office of Science and Technology Policy
Washington, DC

ABSTRACT

The concept of an attitude towards risk that is unique to the individual is used in predicting and prescribing preferred responses to risk. Because it is expensive and time consuming to measure attitude towards risk, one measurement or estimate of an individual's risk attitude is often used to predict or prescribe actions in different decision contexts. However, empirical evidence shows that one of the most commonly used measures of risk attitude, the Arrow-Pratt coefficient of absolute risk aversion, varies over time, income levels and decision contexts. It can be shown that for the Arrow-Pratt coefficient to be a reliable indicator of risk attitude, individuals must exhibit (1) constant marginal utility for money, (2) homogeneous preferences, and (3) coherence of preference orderings over certainty and uncertainty. Experimental data indicate consistent violation of these conditions. As a result, the Arrow-Pratt coefficient confounds risk attitude and strength of preference for particular goods. A new measure of intrinsic risk attitude that removes the confounding influence of strength of preference for particular goods is developed and its use demonstrated.

KEYWORDS: Attitude towards risk, strength of preference, Arrow-Pratt coefficient, expected utility hypothesis (EUH)

INTRODUCTION

The concept of an attitude towards risk that is unique to the individual is used both formally and informally in decision theory and risk management. The most commonly used measure of attitude towards risk is the Arrow-Pratt coefficient of absolute risk aversion.[1,2] Because determination of risk attitudes is costly and time consuming, one measurement or estimate of an individual or group's risk attitude is often used to predict or prescribe actions in different decision contexts. In the few instances when risk attitudes have been determined in more than one decision context or over time, individuals' attitudes towards risk appear to be unstable.

Most reviews of the axioms of the expected utility hypothesis (EUH), from which the Arrow-Pratt coefficient is derived, focus on their mathematical content. The EUH and the Arrow-Pratt coefficient are elegantly derived and are internally consistent. The critical question is whether the underlying behavioral assumptions actually correspond to individuals' preferences.

Risk Analysis, Edited by C. Zervos
Plenum Press, New York, 1991

Closer examination shows that the seemingly unstable risk attitudes obtained using the Arrow-Pratt coefficient stem from violations of the behavioral assumptions associated with the use of the EUH. More specifically, violation of the assumptions of constant marginal value for money, homogeneity of preferences, and additivity of preferences over attributes leads to a confounding of attitudes towards risk and strength of preference for the goods involved in a specific decision. Thus, development of a robust measure of risk attitude requires isolating pure or intrinsic risk attitude from the confounding influence of strength of preference for goods under certainty.

The results presented here extend previous work on measurement of intrinsic attitude towards risk by allowing for non-additivity of preferences. To understand why this extension is necessary for a robust measure of risk attitude, we first examine the implications of violation of the assumptions underlying the EUH and Arrow-Pratt coefficient of absolute risk aversion.

WHAT DOES THE ARROW-PRATT COEFFICIENT ACTUALLY MEASURE?

The utility function used in the expected utility hypothesis takes as its domain preferences over probability distributions over outcomes. If the representation theorem provides a mapping which preserves all relations and orderings in the domain (a homomorphic mapping), the resulting utility function incorporates both preferences over probability distributions and preference orderings over outcomes. The former, referred to here as a value function, may be viewed as containing information about preferences for riskless outcomes, while the latter, referred to here as a utility function, contains information about both preferences for riskless outcomes and attitude towards risk.

The obvious question, then, is if the utility function whose range is the real line incorporates information about both preferences for riskless outcomes and attitudes towards risk, can we use the rate of bending of the utility function as a measure of attitude towards risk? The answer, as we will soon see is yes, but only under very restrictive conditions. These conditions are that:

1. individuals have constant marginal value for money;
2. preferences are homogeneous; and
3. preferences are independent and additive.

Where have these assumptions come from?

For money to serve as a measuring rod of utility, each individual must have constant marginal value for money.[1] The assumption of constant marginal value for money stems from the early cardinalists' argument that money could be used as a measuring rod for utility and, as such, must have constant units of value just as each inch on a standard ruler must represent the same unit of measure. Acceptance of this assumption infers rejection of the economic tenet of diminishing marginal utility.

The assumption of homogeneity of preferences stems from Marshallian demand theory which argues that the last unit of a good purchased by any individual gives him equal value or satisfaction as the monetary equivalent of that unit of good. Since in a perfectly competitive market at equilibrium, each individual faces identical prices, it is argued that individuals' marginal utility is equal. Thus, all individuals would obtain the same degree of satisfaction of needs from the last unit purchased which is, in turn, the same degree of satisfaction they would obtain from having an amount of money equivalent to the price of that good.

This precept of economics cannot be derived from the hypothesis of diminishing marginal utility unless it is also assumed that individuals are making decisions in a world where there is only one commodity, such as money. Without the assumption of a one commodity world, Marshallian demand theory contradicts the economic assumption that individuals' marginal utility for money will remain constant even in the face of changes in prices and income. If this difficulty is avoided by giving up the assumption of constant marginal utility of money, then money can no longer provide the measuring rod for utility, and we can no longer express the marginal utility of a commodity in units of money.

The assumptions of constant marginal value of money and homogeneity of preferences are not only mathematically required by the EUH, but explicitly recognized by von Neumann and Morgenstern[3, p.8]:

> "We shall therefore assume that the aim of all participants in the economic system, consumers as well as entrepreneurs, is money, or equivalently, a single monetary commodity. This is supposed to be unrestrictedly dividable (sic) and substitutable, freely transferable and identical, even in the quantitative sense, with whatever 'satisfaction' or 'utility' is desired by each participant."

If individuals' preferences meet the conditions implied by these two assumptions, their indifference curves for any two goods, or any one good and money, are straight lines with slope of negative one and each individual must value goods at their market price. Indifference curves of this type can be obtained when an individual's value and utility functions over multiattributed outcomes are additive. If both the utility and value functions meet these conditions, the utility function must be a positive linear transformation of the value function. This positive linear transformation mathematically ensures that preferences are invariant under certainty and uncertainty.

Empirical evidence does not lend credence to the use of these assumptions. What happens when the assumptions of constant marginal value for money and homogeneous preferences are violated can be demonstrated graphically. Specifically, it can be shown that, even if an individual actually has stable attitudes towards risk, if his preferences for riskless outcomes do not conform to the three assumptions, his risk attitude, measured using the Arrow-Pratt coefficient, will appear unstable.

Consider a risk neutral individual who exists in a world that consists of one monetary commodity. Risk neutrality implies that this individual's risk premium will be zero and his certainty equivalent will be equal to the mean of the lottery. If the individual has constant marginal value for money, as is shown in panel a of Fig. 1, and is presented with a choice of an equal probability gamble between \$2 and \$6, or \$4 with certainty (which is also the mean of the lottery), he will be indifferent between the two because his certainty equivalent is equal to the mean value of the lottery:

$$0.5 \times v(\$2) + 0.5 \times v(\$6) = 0.5 \times (2) + 0.5 \times (6) = 4 . \quad (1)$$

If the individual does not have constant marginal value for money, as is shown in panel b of Fig. 1, he would not be indifferent between the gamble and the sure thing. In this case, he would prefer the sure thing over the gamble. Using our current notions of attitude towards risk, we would say that this indicated that the individual was risk averse with regard to lotteries with monetary outcomes. But in this case, that conclusion is not justified. The value of the lottery for the individual is:

$$0.5 \times v(\$2) + 0.5 \times v(\$6) = 0.5 \times (4) + 0.5 \times (6.25) = 5.125 , \quad (2)$$

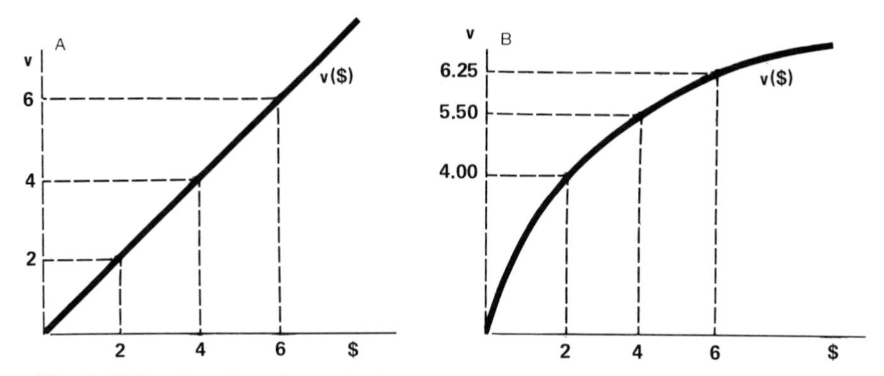

Fig. 1. Value functions for an individual with (panel a) and without (panel b) constant marginal value for money.

which is less than the value of the sure consequence since for him v($4) = 5.5. In this case, the apparent risk averseness of our subject is due to his non-constant marginal value for money, not the requirement for a risk premium.

Figure 2 shows the case where one individual is faced with two different decisions in a multi-commodity world. In the first case the decision involves receiving tractor services; in the second case the decisions involves receiving services from a car. Note that the individual has constant marginal value for money but does not have homogeneous preferences; the transformation between car services and money is non-linear while the transformation between tractor services and money is linear. When presenting the individual with the standard choice between $4 for sure and an equal chance gamble between $2 and $6 when he is concerned with car services, we find that he prefers the gamble to the sure thing since:

$$
\begin{aligned}
&0.5 \times v(\$2) + 0.5 \times v(\$6) \\
&0.5 \times v(2 \text{ units of car services}) + 0.5 \times v(6 \text{ units of car services}) \\
&0.5 \times (3) + 0.5 \times (8) = 5.5
\end{aligned}
\tag{3}
$$

while the value of $4 of car services is 5. When presenting him with the standard choice between $4 for sure and an equal chance gamble between $2 and $6 when he is concerned with tractor services we find that he is indifferent because both the conditions of constant marginal value of money and homogeneity preferences between money and tractor services hold. Does this mean that the individual's risk attitudes have changed? No, the "instability" in risk attitude only reflects heterogeneity of preferences for riskless outcomes.

Obviously, more complex examples could be developed for combinations of cases where marginal value for money is not constant and individuals do not have heterogeneous preferences. However, these would serve only to make the same point: to accept the Arrow-Pratt coefficient as a measure of attitude towards risk, we would have to be able to justify use of the assumptions that the value functions were linear and of identical slope for each individual across commodities and that they are, in addition, of identical slope for all individuals.

THE CONCEPT OF INTRINSIC RISK ATTITUDE

The axioms of the EUH comprise a representation theorem which provides a homomorphic mapping from the domain of preferences over probability distributions over outcomes to a utility function whose range is outcome space on the real line. This mapping

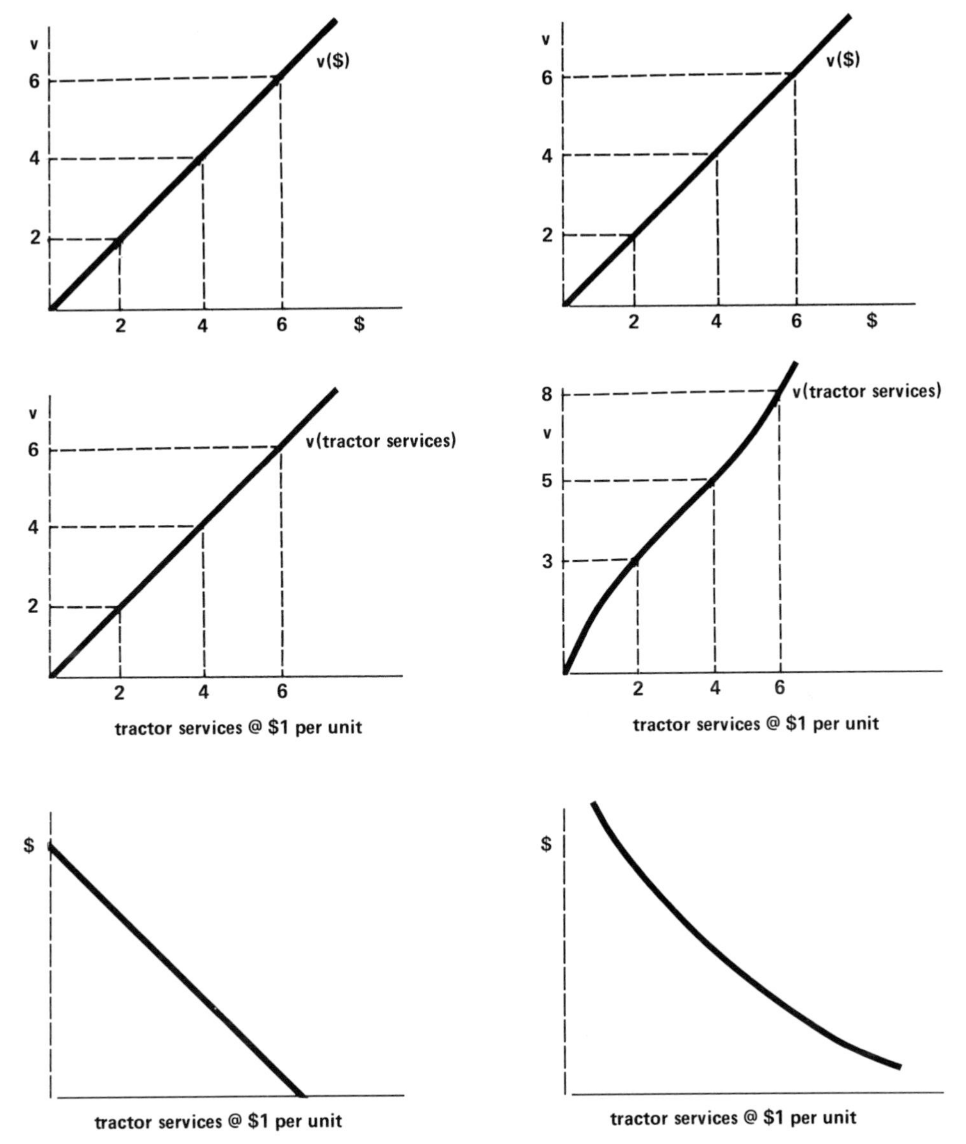

Fig. 2. Value functions and indifference curves of one individual in two situations with constant marginal value of money and heterogeneous preferences.

can be decomposed to isolate preferences for probability density functions (or attitudes towards risk) from preferences for the goods themselves under certainty.

In theory, separating the mapping of risk attitude from that for preferences for goods is simple. In practice, however, it is not yet possible to measure directly individuals' pure attitude towards risk. But such a measure can be derived from a two-step process. First, both value and utility functions are elicited. Then the transformation between the two is calculated. This transformation encapsulates pure attitude towards risk as is shown in Fig. 3.

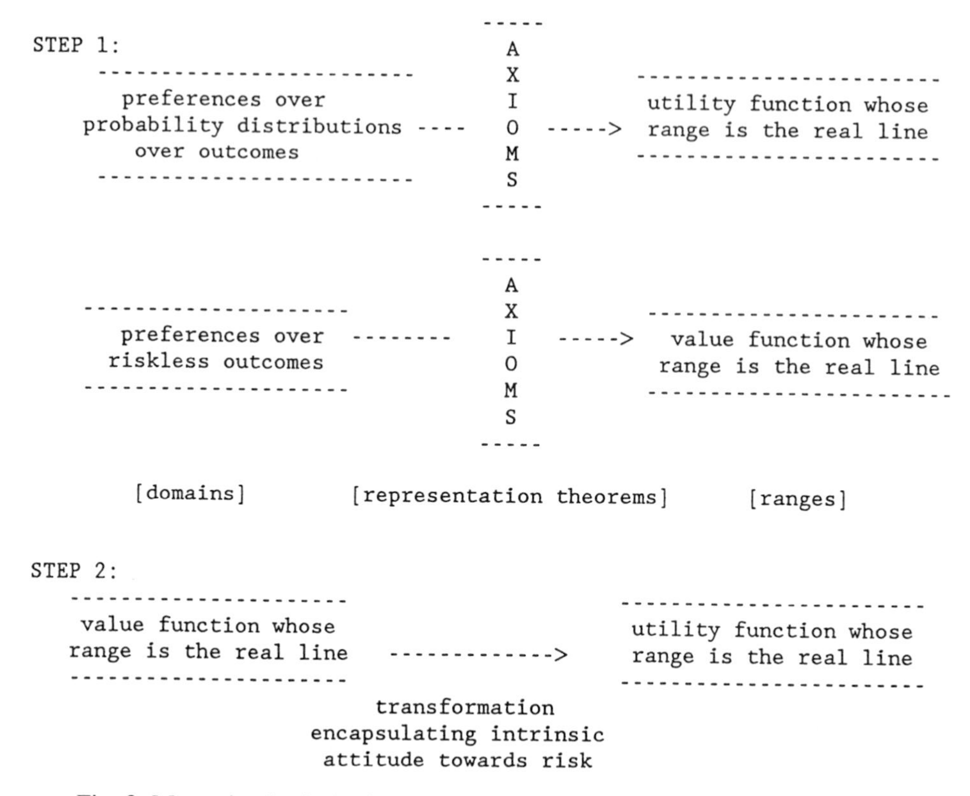

Fig. 3. Measuring intrinsic risk attitude as a function transforming value functions to utility functions on the real line.

The idea of using the transformation between value and utility functions to isolate individuals' intrinsic attitude towards risk was first introduced by Bell and Raiffa.[4] Dyer and Sarin[5] refined Bell and Raiffa's work. They argue that to discover an individual's intrinsic risk attitude, we need to look at the rate of bending of the utility function relative to the rate of bending of the individual's value function.

It is assumed that both the measurable value function $\mathrm{v}(x)$ and the von Neumann-Morgenstern utility function $u(x)$ are monotonically increasing in X and are continuous and twice differentiable. Using the Arrow-Pratt coefficient of absolute risk aversion, defined as

$$r(x) = -\frac{\ddot{u}(x)}{\dot{u}(x)} ,$$

as a model, a local measure of the strength of preference for an asset under certainty at level x can be defined as

$$m(x) = -\frac{\ddot{\mathrm{v}}(x)}{\dot{\mathrm{v}}(x)} .$$

Just as $r(x)$ >,=,< 0 respectively indicate "risk aversion," risk neutrality," or "risk proneness," $m(x)$ >,=,< 0, respectively indicate decreasing, constant, or increasing marginal value at x. Value functions have another parallel with utility functions. A measure of satiation sacrifice is derived in the same manner as the risk premium for a utility function.

When v(x) is not equal to $u(x)$, the relationship between $m(x)$ and $r(x)$ can be used to define a local measure of intrinsic risk aversion. An individual is said to be intrinsically risk averse, intrinsically risk neutral, or intrinsically risk prone as $m(x)$ is respectively less than, equal to, or greater than $r(x)$. If $m(x) = r(x) > 0$, the individual would be risk averse in the Arrow-Pratt sense, because $r(x) > 0$, but intrinsically risk neutral because $m(x) - r(x) = 0$. In other words, risk attitude can only be attributed to that degree of bending of the utility function that is not a direct result of the curvature of the value function as is shown in Fig. 4.

When a von Neumann-Morgenstern utility function is elicited, it incorporates both the individual's preferences for riskless outcomes and his attitude towards risk. A value function incorporates only preference for riskless outcomes. We can define a utility function which maps only the individual's preference for the riskiness of outcomes independent of his preferences for the outcomes themselves. This is equivalent to eliciting u(v). The measure of the rate of bending of the function u(v), denoted $b(x)$, is

$$b(x) = \frac{r(x) - m(x)}{\dot{\mathrm{v}}(x)} \quad . \tag{4}$$

Like the Arrow-Pratt coefficient of absolute risk aversion, Dyer and Sarin's measure of intrinsic risk aversion is a local measure. If individuals exhibit constant intrinsic risk attitude in risky situations, then the hypothetical utility function for riskiness of outcomes should take one of the following forms:

$$u(x) \text{ is a linear transform of } -e^{-b\mathrm{v}(x)} \text{ iff } b(x) = b > 0; \tag{5}$$

$$u(x) \text{ is a linear transform of } \mathrm{v}(x) \text{ iff } b(x) = 0; \tag{6}$$

$$u(x) \text{ is a linear transform of } e^{b\mathrm{v}(x)} \text{ iff } b(x) = b < 0. \tag{7}$$

These three functional forms are nearly identical to the forms of the utility function $u(x)$ that Pratt proves are required in the cases of constant absolute risk aversion, constant absolute risk neutrality, and constant absolute risk proneness. However, in the case of intrinsic risk attitude, the transformations are from v(x) to $u(x)$ rather than from x to $u(x)$.

At first glance, it looks like Dyer and Sarin have solved the problem at hand. They have shown a way to separate attitude towards risk from preference for riskless outcomes. However, their development of the concept of intrinsic risk attitude contains a troublesome assumption. By using holistic preference judgments, Dyer and Sarin implicitly assume either that (1) all decision problems are simple value problems, i.e., that outcomes have only one attribute, or (2) preferences for attributes in a multiattributed world are independent and additive.

We know that decision makers are often concerned with more than one dimension or attribute of an outcome. For example, agricultural producers are concerned not only with profit maximization in this period; they may also be concerned about their asset/debt ratio, quality of life, maintaining soil productivity, or implications of current decisions for future flexibility in the organization of the farm firm. Therefore, to develop a measure of attitude towards risk which can be used to predict preferred action choices for realistic decisions, we cannot assume one-dimensionality.

Abandoning the simplifying assumption of a one-dimensional world means we must examine the second possible condition: preferences for attributes are independent and additive. Empirical work by Fleisher[6] confirms earlier findings by Tversky,[7] Fischer,[8] Keeney,[9] and Krzysztofowicz[10] that individuals' preferences do not necessarily conform to the independence conditions required for additivity of value or utility functions.

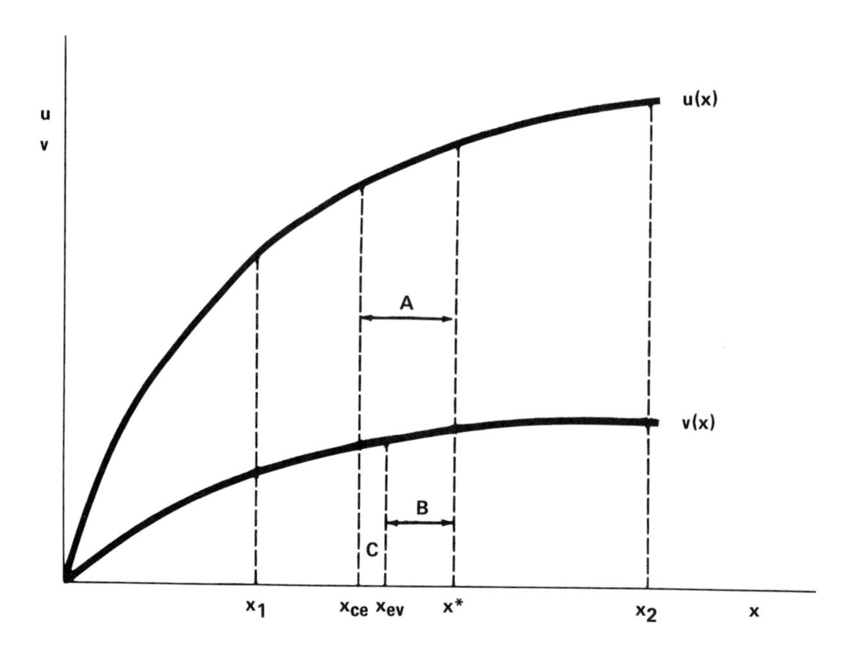

A = risk premium $x^* - x_{ce}$
B = satiation sacrifice $x^* - x_{ev}$
C = risk premium due to only attitude towards risk $x_{ev} - x_{ce} > 0$

Fig. 4. Value and utility functions for the case of intrinsic risk aversion.

A NEW MEASURE OF ATTITUDE TOWARDS RISK

A robust measure of intrinsic attitude towards risk must reflect findings that individuals' preferences do not conform to the assumptions made in formulating earlier measures: individuals do not treat marginal value of money as constant, preferences are not homogeneous, and conditions required for additivity of preferences for multiple attributes are not met. Dyer and Sarin's work presents a possible solution for the first two problems. Multiattribute utility theory is used to adapt the measure of intrinsic risk attitude so that it does not require that preferences meet strong independence conditions required for additivity over attributes or holistic preference judgments over multiattributed outcomes.

Independence Conditions

Using one of several representations theorems, value and utility functions can be constructed that preserve orderings among multiattributed riskless or risky outcomes. The form of the value or utility function (additive or multiplicative) depends upon the independence conditions met by the decision maker's preferences. The standard independence conditions used in multiattribute utility theory must be modified to allow for the preference reversals that are an important consideration in agricultural settings. For example, one could expect that preferences for rain would increase or decrease with existing soil moisture levels or the amount of sunshine. It is not possible to have preference reversals with additive value and utility functions. However, weakened forms of standard independence conditions allow for preference reversals for multiplicative multiattribute value and utility functions. Figure 5 shows the relationships between preference independence conditions.

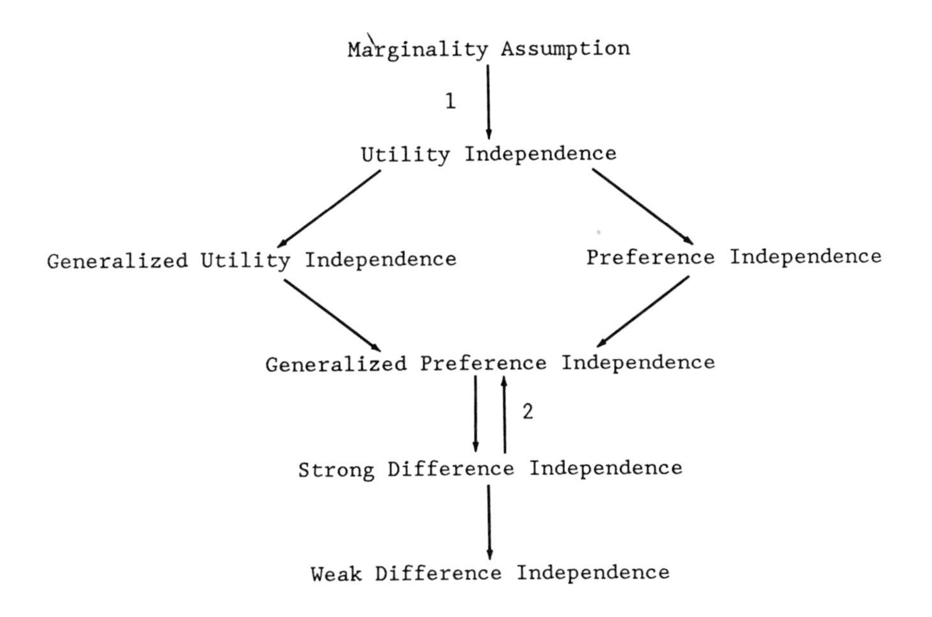

1. Given y, y',x,x'∈X, x preferred to y and x' preferred to y'
2. Given $X = X_1 \times X_2 \times \ldots \times X_n$ for some positive integer n, each X_i is a convex subset of a finite dimensional Euclidean space and: $\Sigma a(x)u(x) > \Sigma b(x)u(x)$ iff a is preferred to b for all a, b∈A holds for some u: X -> Re which is continuous in the relative usual product topology for X.

Fig. 5. Relationships among independence concepts. (Adapted from Ref. 11, p. 300 and Ref. 12.)

Additive value functions require that preferences meet the conditions of mutual preference independence and strong difference independence. An attribute, *Y* is said to be preferentially independent of its complement, *Y*′, if the preference order of consequences involving only changes in the levels of *Y* does not depend on the levels at which attributes in *Y*′ are held fixed. Mutual preference independence simply requires that this also holds for attributes in *Y*′ with respect to *Y*.

An attribute, *Y*, is said to be strong difference independent of the remaining attributes if the preference difference between two levels of *Y* is not affected by fixed levels of the other attributes.

For a value function to be multiplicative, preferences must meet the weaker conditions of generalized preference independence and weak difference independence. Generalized preference independence is also known as sign dependence[13] or the sign axiom.[14] Y_1 is generalized preferentially independent of Y_2 if, given any two levels of Y_2, the two orderings of Y_1 are either identical, reversals of each other, or indifference exists among the Y_1. *Y* is weak difference independent of the remaining attributes if the ordering of preferences on *Y* does not depend on the fixed level of the other attributes.

Similarly, additive and multiplicative utility functions can be distinguished on the basis of the restrictiveness of the independence conditions that preferences meet. Additive utility functions require that the condition of utility independence and the marginality assumption are met. An attribute *Y*, where $Y \in X$, is said to be utility independent of its complement Y' if the conditional preference order for lotteries involving only changes in the levels of attributes in Y does not depend on the levels at which the attributes Y' are fixed.

The marginality assumption states that attributes Y where $Y \in X$, are additive independent if preferences over lotteries on Y depend only on their marginal probability distributions and not on their joint probability distributions. The marginality assumption is sometimes difficult to intuit, but can be made clearer using the following example. The marginality assumption requires that for any $a \in Y_1$ and $b \in Y_2$, the decision maker is indifferent between lotteries

$$l_1 = p(a,b) + (1-p) \cdot (a^*,b^*)$$

and

$$l_2 = p(a,b^*) + (1-p) \cdot (a^*,b).$$

For a utility function to be multiplicative, weaker conditions of generalized utility independence and generalized preference independence must hold. Y_1 is generalized utility independent of Y_2 if the conditional preference order for lotteries involving only changes in the levels of attributes in Y_1, given any two levels of Y_2, are either identical, reversals of each other, or indifference exists among the Y_1. Generalized preference independence for multiplicative multiattribute utility functions is the same as that for multiplicative multiattribute value functions.

Multiattribute Value and Utility Functions

If preferences meet the independence conditions required for additivity, an additive multiattribute value function is written as:

$$\mathrm{v}(x) = \Sigma\, w_i \cdot \mathrm{v}_i(x_i)\,, \tag{8}$$

where v_i is a single attribute value function and w_i is a scaling constant between zero and one.[a]

If preferences meet the independence conditions required for multiplicativity, a multiplicative multiattribute value function is written as:

$$(\mathrm{sgn}\ w)(1 + w\mathrm{v}(x)) = (\mathrm{sgn}\ w)\Pi[1 + ww_i\mathrm{v}_i(x_i)]\,, \tag{9}$$

where w is a constant reflecting the type and degree of non-additivity present.[b]

Similarly, if preferences meet the independence conditions required for additivity, an additive multiattribute utility function is written as:

$$u(x) = \Sigma\, k_i u_i(x_i)\,, \tag{10}$$

where u_i is a single attribute utility function and k_i is a scaling constant between zero and one.

---

a. Scaling factors serve to compress or stretch the scales of the value or utility functions over individual attributes so that they are consistent. Scaling factors are not a measure of an attribute's relative importance to the decision maker.

b. w must be either $-1 \leq w \leq 0$ or $w > 0$ and solve the conditions $1+w = \Pi \cdot (1+ww_i)$. The constants w and k have received various economic interpretations including that they indicate the complementarity or substitutability of attributes.

If preferences meet the independence conditions required for multiplicativity, a multiplicative multiattribute utility function is written as:

$$(\text{sgn } k)(1 + ku(x)) = (\text{sgn } k)\prod[1 + k_i u_i(x_i)] \tag{11}$$

where k is a constant reflecting the type and degree of non-additivity present and must meet the conditions specified for w in footnote b.

Economic Interpretation of Parameters *k* and *w*[c]

Consider the two equal probability lotteries <A,C> and <B,D> shown in Fig. 6 and assume that preferences are increasing in both Y and Z. It will be assumed that individuals' value functions are homogeneous. It can be shown that if <A,C> is preferred to <B,D>, $k > 0$ and Y and Z can be viewed as complements. If <A,C> is indifferent to <B,D>, k=0, indicating an additive utility function and preferences for Y and Z are independent, while if <B,D> is preferred to <A,C>, $k < 0$ and Y and Z can be viewed as substitutes.

The lotteries are structured so that for <A,C> the individual will either receive a high level of both Y and Z or a low level of both. For lottery <B,D>, the individual will receive either a high level of Y or Z, but not a high level of both. If <A,C> is preferred, it is as if the individual needs an increase in Y to complement an increase in Z in going from A to C. Otherwise, the full worth of the increase in Z could not be exploited. On the other hand, to prefer <B,D> implies that it is important to receive a high level of at least one attribute and, given a high level of, say, Y, the increased preference due to an increase in Z is not as much. Thus, Y and Z can be thought of as substitutes for each other.

To illustrate a complementary case, consider a farm manager who is thinking of investing in the use of a new, pest sensitive, high yielding variety of grain and a new, more expensive pest management system. Attribute Y can be viewed as the productivity of the new variety on his field, given existing soil types, drainage, etc. Attribute Z can be viewed as the successfulness of the new pest management system. If both the high yielding variety and the new pest management system are successful, the farm manager is very happy. However, if either fails, the financial consequences may be as bad as if both had failed.

To illustrate a case of substitution, consider a farm manager who is thinking of using a new variety of corn on two separate fields which have very different soil and drainage characteristics. Attribute Y, in this case, is the yield from one field while attribute Z is the yield from the other. Although the farm manager would like it if both fields flourished, achievement of attributes Y and Z would, most likely, be substitutes.

Fischer[8] sets forth another interpretation for k. He argues that a $k > 0$ could be indicative of complementary attributes or the simple fact that the individual is willing to give up a sure thing in either attribute for the chance of receiving something which is better with regard to both attributes, i.e. risk prone behavior. Similarly, a $k < 0$ could indicate attributes which are substitutes or simply an aversion to high variance outcomes.

These two interpretations of k are not necessarily contradictory; both can add insight into the formation of attitudes towards risk. If Keeney and Raiffa's interpretation of k is applied to the interpretation of w, then if $w > 0$, the attributes can be said to be complements, and if $w < 0$, the attributes can be said to be substitutes. Because a multiattribute utility function, like a von Neumann-Morgenstern utility function, incorporates information about both attitudes towards risk and the individual's value function, examination of k without information about w does not allow us to determine what portion of k is due to the

---

c. Parts of this discussion are adapted from Ref. 15, pp. 240-241.

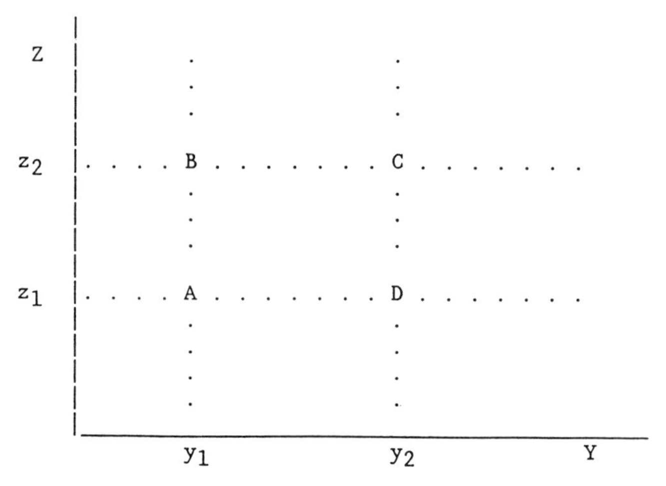

Fig. 6. Using lotteries to interpret k in a multiplicative multiattribute utility function.

complementarity or substitutability of the attributes and what portion is due to attitude towards risk.

Allowable Transformations Between Value and Utility Functions

A common way to relate $\mathrm{v}(x)$ and $u(x)$ is through the uniqueness theorems of their respective measurement theoretic representations. Here, however, we will rely on the use of Cauchy's four fundamental functional equations. This greatly simplifies proofs and allows departure from the standard assumptions about the additivity of value functions.

Cauchy's four fundamental functional equations can be used to determine that:

- If the value and utility functions are additive:

$$u = \mathrm{v} \tag{12}$$

- If the value function is additive and the utility function is multiplicative:

$$1 + ku = (1 + k)^{\mathrm{v}} \tag{13}$$

- If the value function is multiplicative and the utility function is additive:[d]

$$u = \frac{\ln(1 + w\mathrm{v})}{\ln(1 + w)} . \tag{14}$$

- If the value and utility functions are multiplicative:

$$1 + ku = (1 + w\mathrm{v})^{\frac{\ln(1+k)}{\ln(1+w)}} . \tag{15}$$

---

d. Actual cases where the utility function is additive and the value function is multiplicative are rare. From a strictly measurement theoretic point of view, this condition is impossible since the independence conditions for additive utility imply the conditions for additive value. However, in some cases, economic theory or *a priori* knowledge about the attributes of outcomes involved may dictate that a multiplicative value function be used in conjunction with an additive utility function.

APPLYING THE RESULTS

To envision how these results can be applied in determining an individual's intrinsic attitude towards risk, consider the individual whose value and utility functions are shown in Fig. 7. Assume that the individual's value function is additive and that:

$$v_i(x_i) = \ln x_i \,, \tag{16}$$

and that the individual's utility function is multiplicative and that:

$$u_i(x_i) = (x_i - 1) \cdot \frac{1}{e-1} \;. \tag{17}$$

Note from panel a of Fig. 7 that the utility function is linear. The Arrow-Pratt coefficient of absolute risk aversion, taken at any $x \in X$ will be zero, indicating risk neutrality.

But our concern is not with the utility function alone; we are interested in separating pure attitude towards risk from the effects of non-constant marginal value. We may proceed in several directions, depending on what information is available about the individual's value and utility functions.

If we had actually elicited the individual's multiattribute utility function and determined k, which in this example is assumed to be $e-1$, we could test for the validity of the hypothesized transformation between additive value functions and multiplicative utility functions. Taking the transformation of Eq. (13) and substituting Eqs. (16) and (17) and the value for k we obtain:

$$1 + (e-1)\left[(x-1) \cdot \frac{1}{(e-1)}\right] = (1 + e - 1)^{\ln x} \;, \tag{18}$$

which has the solution:

$$x = x \,, \tag{19}$$

and thus, the transformation is valid.

Similarly, the value of k could be predicted from Eqs. (13), (16), and (17) and tested against the estimated k. In this case:

$$1 + k\left[(x-1) \cdot \frac{1}{(e-1)}\right] = (1 + k)^{\ln x} \;, \tag{20}$$

which has the solution:

$$k = e - 1 \tag{21}$$

How do we interpret the k value? In this case, $k > 0$, which indicates risk prone behavior. This can be seen more intuitively by examining the function $u(v)$ in panel b of Fig. 7 which is of the form:

$$u(v) = \frac{e^v - 1}{e - 1} \;. \tag{22}$$

The function is convex to the origin. A measure of the rate of bending of this function, analogous to the Arrow-Pratt coefficient, is:

$$-\frac{\frac{\delta^2 u}{\delta v^2}}{\frac{\delta u}{\delta v}} = -1 \quad \text{at all } v \;, \tag{23}$$

which indicates constant risk proneness.

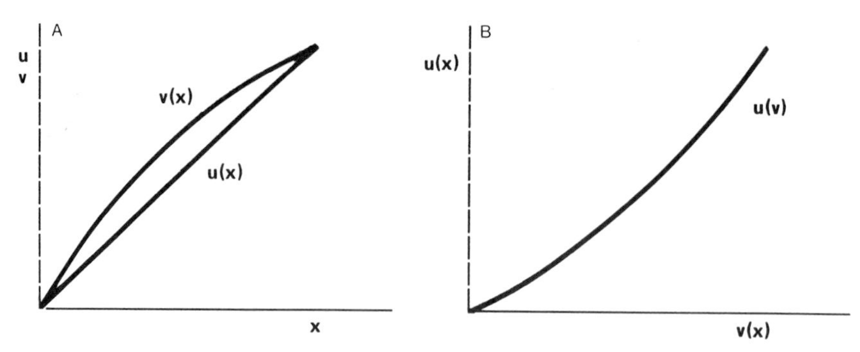

Fig. 7. v(x) and $u(x)$ for an intrinsically risk prone individual when v(x) = Σ ln x.

This information about the individual's pure attitude towards risk can be used in predicting preferred action choices in other situations. Assume that in a different decision situation, the decision maker's value function is again additive with

$$\mathrm{v}_i(x_i) = x_i^2 \ . \tag{24}$$

Using our knowledge of the transformation between additive value functions and multiplicative utility functions, and the value of k, the individual's von Neumann-Morgenstern utility function is easily obtained:

$$u(x) = \frac{e^{x^2} - 1}{e - 1} \ . \tag{25}$$

The Arrow-Pratt coefficient at a point x on this function is:

$$r(x) = \left[2e^{x^2} \cdot \frac{(2x^2 - 1)}{(e - 1)}\right] \left[\left(\frac{e^{(1-x^2)}}{2x}\right) - \left(\frac{1}{2xe^{x^2}}\right)\right] , \tag{26}$$

which, when evaluated at x = 1.5, is −3.67, indicating risk proneness as would be expected from the convex curvature of $u(x)$ shown in panel a of Fig. 8.

But again, if we are concerned with separating the pure risk attitude from the effects of non-linearity in the value function, we want to know the rate of bending of u(v), not $u(x)$. Because u(v) is:

$$u(\mathrm{v}) = \frac{e^{v} - 1}{e - 1} , \tag{27}$$

the function, shown in panel b of Fig. 8, is convex to the origin. Measuring the rate of bending of this function yields:

$$-\frac{\frac{\delta^2 u}{\delta \mathrm{v}^2}}{\frac{\delta u}{\delta \mathrm{v}}} = -1 \quad \text{at all v} \ , \tag{28}$$

which indicates constant risk proneness.

If only the Arrow-Pratt coefficient were to be examined, we would surmise that the individual's attitude towards risk had changed from risk neutrality to risk proneness between the two situations. But we can see from this example that the individual's pure attitude towards risk has not changed; the change in the rate of bending of $u(x)$ was due to a change in the value function, not a change in pure attitude towards risk.

Preliminary empirical results suggest that the rate of bending of an individual's utility function over v, u(v), is constant over all levels of v(x) in one decision context and across decision contexts when the value function is additive. However, it is not constant over all

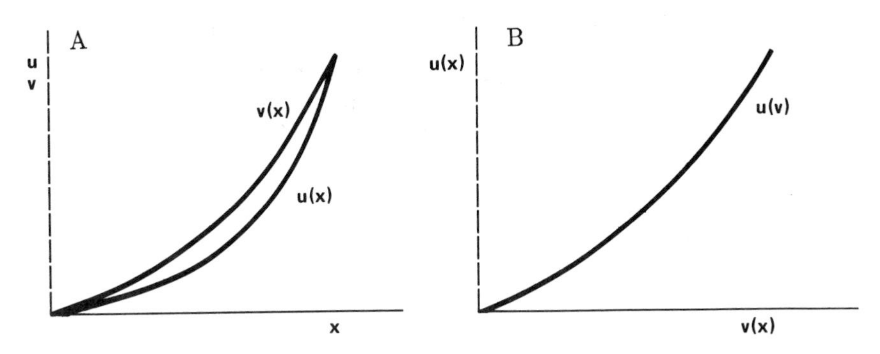

Fig. 8. v(x), u(x) and u(v) for an intrinsically risk prone individual when v(x) = Σx^2.

levels of v(x) in one context in cases where the value function is multiplicative. Even in this context, however, the intrinsic attitude towards risk will be constant at a given level of v(x) across decision contexts.

USES OF THE NEW MEASURE

Neither the new measure of intrinsic risk attitude nor the measure of strength of preferences for riskless outcomes can, by itself, replace the expected utility hypothesis as a means of predicting preferred action choices under uncertainty. However, intrinsic attitude towards risk can provide a justifiable means of generalizing across situations for one individual or comparing risk attitudes among individuals.

Empirical application of the new measure will require the collection of more information to elicit any one individual's attitude towards risk. Both a von Neumann-Morgenstern utility function and a value function must be elicited. Once the individual's intrinsic risk attitude is known, however, its use in new decision contexts will only require knowledge of the decision maker's preferences under certainty for the goods of concern. This information can be either directly elicited from the individual or obtained indirectly using one of a wide variety of tools developed through studies in consumption economics and marketing.

Perhaps more important than the empirical application is the enhancement that this measure brings to our conceptual understanding of decision making. In models used to predict decision maker behavior in response to policy changes or other exogenous factors, we can explicitly recognize what has been known on a practical level all along: individual decision makers are motivated by many factors, including profit, attitude towards risk, and simple preferences for goods or activities themselves. Attributing all behavior to any one of these factors is misleading.

REFERENCES

1. K. Arrow, *Aspects of the Theory of Risk Bearing*, Helsinki, Yrjo Jahhssonin Saatio (1965).
2. J. Pratt, Risk Aversion in the Small and in the Large, *Econometrica* **32**:122-136 (1964).
3. J. von Neumann and O. Morgenstern, *The Theory of Games*, Princeton University Press, Princeton (1944).
4. D. Bell and H. Raiffa, Marginal Value and Intrinsic Risk Aversion, Harvard Business School Working Paper No. 79-65 (1979).

5. J. Dyer and R. Sarin, Relative Risk Aversion, *Management Science* **28**:875-886 (1982).
6. B. Fleisher, A New Measure of Attitude Towards Risk, unpublished Ph.D. thesis, Michigan State University Department of Agricultural Economics (1985).
7. A. Tversky, Additive Utility and Subjective Probability, *Journal of Mathematical Psychology* **4**:175-201 (1967).
8. G. Fischer, Multidimensional Utility Models for Risky and Riskless Choice, *Organizational Behavior and Human Performance* **17**:127-146 (1976).
9. R. Keeney, Multiplicative Utility Functions, *Operations Research* **22**:22-34 (1974).
10. R. Krzysztofowicz, Strength of Preference and Risk Attitude in Utility Measurement, *Organizational Behavior and Human Performance* **31**:88-113 (1983).
11. P. Fishburn and R. Keeney, Seven Independence Concepts and Continuous Multiattribute Utility Functions, *Journal of Mathematical Psychology* **11**:294-327 (1974).
12. P. Fishburn and R. Keeney, Generalized Utility Independence and Some Implications, *Operations Research* **23**:928-940 (1975).
13. D. Krantz, H. Luce, P. Suppes, and A. Tversky, *Foundations of Measurement*, Vol. 1, Academic Press, New York (1971).
14. R. Roskies, A Measurement Axiomatization for an Essentially Multiplicative Representation of Two Factors, *Journal of Mathematical Psychology* **2**:266-267 (1965).
15. R. Keeney and H. Raiffa, *Decisions with Multiple Objectives: Preferences and Value Tradeoffs*, John Wiley and Sons, New York (1976).

Platitudes and Comparisons: A Critique of Current (Wrong) Directions in Risk Communication

Timothy C. Earle and George Cvetkovich
Western Washington University
Bellingham, WA

ABSTRACT

The current directions in risk communication research and practice have been staked out by Covello and Allen's "seven cardinal rules"[1] and by Covello, Sandman and Slovic's guide to the use of risk comparisons.[2] We argue that these directions lead to increased conflict over risk management rather than to effective risk communication. The "seven cardinal rules" are wrong because they are platitudes that assume an idealized state in which the public is as involved and concerned about the hazard as its managers are. The guide to the use of risk comparisons is wrong because it assumes that risk comparisons are as useful to the public as they are to hazard managers. These errors in plotting the path of risk communication result from the adoption of the hazard manager's frame or way of defining the risk problem rather than the appropriate public frame. These two frames differ on three basic dimensions: (1) level of involvement, (2) degree of personal relevance, and (3) level of information processing ability. Hazard managers tend to be high on these dimensions, most members of the public low. Risk comparisons, therefore, are appropriate for communicating with hazard managers but not with the public. A map of alternative directions toward effective public risk communication is provided.

KEYWORDS: Communication, risk, management

INTRODUCTION

Risk communication researchers are frequently confronted by questions regarding the practical usefulness of their work. This is good, an indication that risk communication is a socially significant activity. It is also dangerous, however, because the identification of a need also creates a strong desire to fill it. This motive to do good, to contribute to the solution of important social problems, can sometimes overwhelm the countervailing motive to be correct.

In this paper we present a critique of several recent efforts to translate risk communication research into practical risk communication advice. Most prominent among these compilations of wisdom have been guidebooks aimed at managers of hazardous materials plants[2] and representatives of government agencies.[3] It is not our purpose to review such efforts comprehensively. We wish to use selected examples to illustrate what we conclude are wrong current directions in advice regarding risk communications. While these manuals warn readers that "there are no easy prescriptions for effective risk

Risk Analysis, Edited by C. Zervos
Plenum Press, New York, 1991

communication" (see Ref. 2, p. 2), they nonetheless boldly announce that a good deal of useful information is known about the risk communication process. Covello and Allen,[1] for example, have established the "Seven Cardinal Rules of Risk Communication." It is our contention that these rules, and much of the remaining advice in current risk communication manuals, consist more of hollow platitudes than solid guides to successful hazard management.

Using the first of Covello and Allen's Seven Cardinal Rules as an example, we argue that students of risk communication know a lot less than the guidebooks would lead us to believe.[4] Second, we contend that these guidebooks are products of a general approach to risk communication, the *technocentric*, that, due to inherent limitations, is unlikely to be successful. Finally, this constrained technocentric approach is contrasted to a general social teamwork alternative; several reasons for the superiority of the latter are offered.

PLATITUDES DISGUISED AS RULES

The first Cardinal Rule of Risk Communication is this: "Accept and Involve the Public as a Legitimate Partner."[1] The goal of risk communication should be "to produce an informed public that is involved, interested, reasonable, thoughtful, solution-oriented and collaborative." The following guidelines are given: "Demonstrate your respect for the public and your sincerity by involving the community early, before important decisions are made. Make it clear that you understand the appropriateness of basing decisions about risk on factors other than the magnitude of the risk. Involve all parties that have an interest or a stake in the particular risk in question." Are these guidelines useful?

First, can the community "be involved" before important decisions are made? In many cases, no. Hazards have histories.[5] The decisions to produce nuclear wastes were made long before the decisions on how to dispose of them. Plants producing hazardous materials were located in heavily populated areas when people were unaware of and unconcerned about the hazards (e.g., Superfund sites; ASARCO Copper Smelter in Tacoma, WA; Ref. 6). For these and for many major hazards, it is simply impossible to "involve the public as a legitimate partner" in making the crucial early decisions. The deeds have been done. The hazards exist, creating economic and other factors that may limit a plant manager's willingness to share his/her decision-making powers with the public. In these cases, efforts to "involve the public" may appear disingenuous. The public may come to view them as a manipulating strategy to produce acceptance of a foregone conclusion.

Second, is it likely that a plant manager will espouse "the appropriateness of basing decisions about risks on factors other than the magnitude of the risk?" Our research comparing the risk judgment policies of hazard managers and risk analysts, on the one hand, with the policies of laypersons, on the other, has demonstrated dramatic differences between the two.[7,8] The basic difference, of course, is that technically-trained managers and analysts focus on the "magnitude of the risk," while the public uses other factors.[9] Acknowledgment by plant managers that risk decisions should be based on qualitative as well as quantitative factors would seem to contradict their basic beliefs. Why would they allow their decisions to be affected by factors that they believe to be wrong? It is more likely that a plant manager will attempt to convince the public of the correctness of his/her professional (technical) judgment policy.

Third, can a plant manager "involve all parties that have an interest or stake in the particular risk in question?" What is meant by involvement? We have argued elsewhere[10,11] that psychological involvement with an issue is a key factor affecting the success of risk communication. Involvement in this sense refers to the personal importance of an issue for an individual. This can best be understood by the use of concepts from the psychology of information processing: when a person is involved with an issue, he/she has thought about it previously and has stored models in memory that link specific features of the hazard with the self. Presented information about a hazard, an individual will search his/her memory for a model that is similar to that produced by the message.[12,13,14] If a match is found, the issue is identified as personally important to the individual, and he/she is said to be involved. A person who is highly involved in an issue will seek out and systematically process information about it. A person who is not involved will process information in a rapid, intuitive way, if at all.

This brief presentation of the psychology of involvement illustrates two points. First, the involvement of a person in a risk issue is the product of a subjective judgment by the individual. This cognitive and affective involvement normally precedes and is necessary for the type of behavioral involvement referred to in the first Cardinal Rule. An involved person is a concerned person, concerned about risks or costs or other features of a plant's operations. Persons who are not concerned, who do not feel threatened, are unlikely to spend their limited resources of thought, emotion, energy and time on an issue that does not directly affect them. People who do become involved as the result of information about the hazard, on the other hand, are not likely to be considered "interested, reasonable, thoughtful, solution-oriented and collaborative" by plant management.

Our analysis of involvement also illustrates the deep complexity of risk communication processes. Involvement is only one of dozens of key concepts invoked in the Seven Cardinal Rules. Each of these concepts — trust, credibility, fairness, audience segmentation, cooperation with the news media, etc. — carries its own burden of complexity and difficulty. Yet they are blithely linked together in a few simple steps to success.

When confronted with the complex difficulties of risk communication, we clearly must apply the best tools at hand. In criticizing the Seven Cardinal Rules and the other similar risk communication manuals, we are not advocating surrender. We believe there is a better set of tools. The usefulness of the Rules and the manuals is severely limited for two general reasons. First, the Rules are not guides for action, informing hazard managers about what to do to communicate successfully with the public about risk. Instead, they are platitudes disguised as rules. The rules are platitudes because they convey the appearance and feeling of confident guidance although their substance consists only on non-specific, banal truisms: involve the public; plan carefully; listen to your audience; be honest; collaborate with credible sources; meet the needs of the media; speak clearly. All one can say is, "Yes, of course! But how? How can I do these things, in my situation, now?" The Seven Cardinal Rules unfortunately do not address the needs of the individual hazard manager. And it is our contention that they cannot.

The second general limitation on the usefulness of current risk communication rules and manuals is what we call their "technocentrism." That is, guidance on how to communicate with the public is presented from the points of view of hazard managers and risk analysts. These persons are, of course, the audience for the guidance. They, therefore, might find the guidance reasonable and potentially useful. The public, however, the intended risk communication audience, is likely to remain unconvinced. The negative effects of technocentrism on risk communication are discussed next.

TECHNOCENTRISM DISGUISED AS NEUTRALITY

The technocentric approach to risk communication defines the problem as: "How can we get the public to understand and accept our technical analysis of this hazard?" Attempts may be made to address some public concerns, but the general thrust remains the same: from the technical analyst to the public. As Burger[15] has so succinctly illustrated, risk communication from the technocentric point of view boils down to a matter of scientific literacy: The public should be persuaded to understand and accept "true risk" and relinquish any reliance on invalid indicators.

Recent risk communication manuals reveal their technocentric bias through their reliance on "risk comparisons." As the term indicates, a risk comparison consists of a statement comparing the risks of two or more hazards. These comparisons can be made in many different ways using a wide variety of measures. The job of the risk communicator is to assess the relative effectiveness or acceptability of various types of comparisons.[2] Within its limited scope, this is a worthy endeavor; some risk comparisons clearly convey more useful information than others. Nonetheless, the risks being compared are the "true," quantitatively-measured risks. Improved comparisons of this type will no doubt benefit communication within the community of hazard managers and risk analysts. But what about the less scientifically literate public? There is no evidence that technocentric risk comparisons can facilitate public understanding of complex hazard management issues. Baird[6] demonstrated to the contrary that public risk judgments tend to ignore available technical risk estimates.

There is of course nothing inherently wrong with the risk analyst's technical approach to risk management. The safety of our society depends to a great extent on the risk analyst's knowledge. The analyst's error, and that of many managers and risk communicators, lies in the assumption that the technical point of view is the one true understanding of risk: technocentrism. From a wider societal perspective, risk can be seen to wear a variety of guises, appearance varying with point of view. Within any community there are several general points of view on risk. Risk communication can be profitably thought of as an effort to bring these points of view together into a community hazard management team. Together these team members form the social teamwork alternative to the technocentric approach to risk communication.[7]

THE SOCIAL TEAMWORK ALTERNATIVE

There are three fundamental distinguishing features of the social teamwork approach to risk communication. First, the social teamwork approach recognizes multiple legitimate perspectives to risk management decisions. The technocentric perspective is one of several. Second, risk communication is assumed to be a team-level problem rather than a problem of one group selling its point of view to another. The goal is teamwork: team-wide understanding; team-wide cooperation and collaboration in risk management. Third, effective risk communication is facilitated by professional risk communicators who are independent from any of the other team members. The goal of the independent risk communicator is not to sell any particular point of view. The goal of the independent risk communicator is to use effective risk communication as a tool to help the community hazard management team to meet its safety goals.

Membership in our community hazard management team is of course a bit arbitrary. But for purposes of simple illustration, we offer the following.

> **The professional hazard managers.** These are the persons hired by communities and businesses to solve their hazard management problems. Professional hazard managers tend to use systematic decision making techniques in the application of a variety of tools: technological fixes, regulation, education. In using these tools, the hazard manager employs two different kinds of information: technical knowledge (from risk analysts) and social knowledge (from the public). The hazard manager's basic problem is the integration of these two different kinds of knowledge into an effective hazard management strategy.

The risk analysts. They are the scientific and technical experts on hazards. It is their technical approach to hazards that sets risk analysts apart from the other members of the community hazard management team. Technology is the risk analyst's greatest strength in understanding hazards. But it is also his/her greatest weakness in communication to other team members about risk.

The public and stakeholder groups. The public consists of non-technically trained citizens, affected by hazards but with no special training in understanding them. Stakeholder groups are organized members of the public who are concerned about a hazard or set of hazards and who want to bring about change in hazard management. Stakeholders are deeply involved; they serve to activate larger segments of the general public.

The news media. By helping the community to communicate about hazards, the news media help build teamwork within the hazard management team. The news media raise early warnings about new and dangerous threats, and they give us information on how to deal with the chronic hazards in our lives.

The risk communicator. The risk communicator is an advocate of none of the individual points of view within the hazard management team. The risk communicator is independent. By allowing team members to see the problem from the points of view of others, the risk communicator presents diversity of opinion in a positive way. Diversity becomes an aspect of group strength rather than weakness.

At first glance, the technocentric and social teamwork approaches to risk communication may appear similar. Both approaches recognize the existence of multiple perspectives on risk. The whole thrust of the technocentric approach, however, is to gather all other points of view unto itself. Most significantly for risk communication, it is the job of the risk communicator within the technocentric perspective to convince dissenters of the errors of their ways. We reject the technocentric approach to risk communication because it rejects the strength of democratic decision-making: diversity of opinion. We are all, in our different ways, groping toward adaptation to an ever-changing hazardous environment. If we all follow a single, narrow path, disaster will result if we are wrong.

The social teamwork approach to risk communication seeks to benefit from diversity. The job of the risk communicator is to enable the hazard management team to serve the community as a whole, a team. The risk communicator works to facilitate optimal use of the community's diverse resources to make it a safer place to live for everybody. The risk communicator is also a research scientist, working to develop an integrated theory of risk communication based, not on empty platitudes, but on fundamental information processing principles. As a consultant and as a researcher, the risk communicator recognizes that no one individual or group controls access to the truth. We are all wrong in our own ways. And the stakes are too high to risk going it alone.

REFERENCES

1. V. Covello and F. Allen, Seven Cardinal Rules of Risk Communication, U.S. Environmental Protection Agency, Washington, DC (1988).
2. V. Covello, P. Sandman, and P. Slovic, Risk Communication, Risk Statistics, and Risk Comparisons: A Manual for Plant Managers, Chemical Manufacturers Association, Washington, DC (1988).

3. B. J. Hance, C. Chess, and P. M. Sandman, Improving Dialogue with Communities: A Risk Communication Manual of Government, New Jersey State Department of Environmental Protection, Trenton, NJ (1987).
4. P. Stallen and R. Coppock, About Risk Communication and Risky Communication, *Journal of Risk Analysis* **7**:4 (1987).
5. B. B. Johnson, Accounting for the Social Context of Risk Communication, *Science and Technological Studies* **5**:103-111 (1987).
6. B. Baird, Tolerance for Environmental Health Risks: The Influence of Knowledge, Benefits, Voluntariness and Environmental Attitudes, *Risk Analysis* **6**:425-436 (1986).
7. T. C. Earle and G. Cvetkovich, Being Safe: The Importance of Risk Communication to Modern Society, WISOR Series OM/RS 88-12, Western Washington University (1988).
8. M. K. Lindell and T. C. Earle, How Close Is Close Enough?: Public Perceptions of the Risks of Industrial Facilities, *Risk Analysis* **3**:245-254 (1983).
9. P. Slovic, Perception of Risk, *Science* **236**:280-285 (1987).
10. T. C. Earle and G. Cvetkovich, Risk Communication: A Marketing Approach, Battelle Human Affairs Research Centers, Seattle (1984).
11. T. C. Earle and G. Cvetkovich, Risk Judgment, Risk Communication and Conflict Management, in *Human Judgment: The Social Judgment Theory Approach*, B. Brehmer and C. R. B. Joyce, eds., North-Holland, Amsterdam (1988).
12. R. S. Wyer and T. K. Srull, Human Cognition Is Its Social Context, *Psychological Review* **93**:322-359 (1986).
13. G. Cvetkovich and T. C. Earle, Hazard Images, Evaluation, and Political Actions — The Case of Toxic Wastes Incineration with Implications for Hazard Communication, in *Communication Health and Safety Risks: International Perspectives*, R. Kasperson and P. Stallen, eds. (1990).
14. G. Cvetkovich and G. Keren, Mental Models and Communicating Fundamental Hazard Information: Prospects, Practice and Problems, WISOR Series DM/RC 88-10, Western Washington University (1988).
15. E. Burger, How Citizens Think About Risks to Health, *Risk Analysis* **8**:309-314 (1988)

Cancer Risk Prediction for Carbon Tetrachloride Using Pharmacokinetic and Cell-Kinetic Models

Kenneth T. Bogen
Lawrence Livermore National Laboratory
Livermore, CA

ABSTRACT

Multistage cancer risk models that account for clonal growth of intermediate, premalignant cell populations have been successfully used to describe age-specific incidence trends for human and experimentally induced animal tumors. Currently there is keen and growing interest in applying "cell-kinetic multistage" (CKM) models, which distinguish between mutations and cell population kinetics as separate processes influencing the rate of tumor formation, to the problem of predicting human cancer risk that may be posed by environmental agents. This paper illustrates the application of such models to cancer risk prediction for carbon tetrachloride (CCl_4), taking into account rodent cancer-bioassay data and CCl_4 pharmacokinetics in rodents and humans. The increased importance of knowledge concerning exposure scenarios when using CKM models for risk extrapolation, as opposed to more traditional approaches, is illustrated. The presumption, made in most CKM models considered to date, that preneoplastic cell growth is exponential over time, is critically evaluated along with the impact on predicted CCl_4-induced cancer risk of using a more biologically realistic cell-growth model. Because the potential application of CKM models to cancer risk prediction could have important consequences on public health measures directed at controlling environmental exposure to chemicals, the biological plausibility of specific CKM models considered for application deserves renewed scrutiny.

KEYWORDS: Carbon tetrachloride (CCl_4), cell-kinetic multistage (CKM) models, pharmacokinetic (PBPK) models, cancer-risk extrapolation

INTRODUCTION

Multistage cancer-risk models that account for clonal growth of intermediate (initiated, premalignant) cell populations, or "cell-kinetic multistage" (CKM) models, have long been successfully used to describe age-specific incidence trends for human cancer and experimentally induced tumors in animals.[1-3] More recently, a 2-stage stochastic model allowing for birth and death of initial and intermediate cells has been used to model human-cancer incidence in particular and has been proposed to be capable of describing spontaneous and induced carcinogenesis in general.[4-6] Currently there is keen and growing interest in the possibility of applying this 2-stage model to the problem of predicting the human cancer risk posed by environmental agents.[7-11] Because CKM models distinguish between mutations and cell-population kinetics as separate processes that influence the rate of tumor formation, such models can predict widely different cancer risks for agents affecting only one process (e.g., promotion via induced cell proliferation, assuming a dose-response threshold) but not the other (e.g., mutagenesis, assuming a no-threshold dose-response relationship). Such an approach allows for distinct treatment of genotoxic carcinogens and nongenotoxic tumor promoters, provided the latter can be operationally defined. This approach has been advocated[11-13] but has not yet been incorporated into widely used cancer-risk-assessment procedures.[14,15]

This paper illustrates issues involved in the application of CKM models, in conjunction with physiologically based pharmacokinetic (PBPK) models, to the problem of cancer-risk extrapolation for the case of CCl_4 using the following approach. Appropriate PBPK models for predicting effective dose in rodents and humans as a function of CCl_4 exposure are first identified. It is presumed here that CCl_4 is not effective in producing mutations assumed (by the CKM approach) to be necessary to the carcinogenic process, but that CCl_4 is an effective "promoter" by virtue of an ability, at cytotoxic doses, to selectively increase the rate of net cell growth within premalignant cell clones. Hence, an appropriate model is fit to rodent data on the dose-response relationship for CCl_4-induced cell proliferation. This dose-response relationship is assumed to be the same for humans. An increase in cell proliferation is then presumed to correspond to a proportional increase in the value of the growth parameter of a 2-stage CKM model fit to a rodent-bioassay data set on increased cancer risk above background associated with different effective CCl_4 doses, which in turn correspond (using the rodent PBPK model) to the exposure scenario used in the bioassay selected as the basis for risk extrapolation.

Increased risk to humans associated with a given effective CCl_4 dose is then either presumed to be identical to predicted increased risk to rodents or calculated by fitting a corresponding 2-stage CKM model to human incidence data for cancer of the same type observed to be significantly increased in the selected rodent bioassay. These predicted relationships between effective dose and cancer risk are then transformed into corresponding relationships between human exposure and cancer risk using an appropriate human PBPK model and a scenario for human exposure to CCl_4 in drinking water. Because almost all CKM models considered to date have assumed that premalignant cells may proliferate exponentially over time *in vivo*, this paper also examines the implications of using an alternative, perhaps more biologically reasonable, assumption[16] that such cells grow geometrically over time. Finally, a comparison is made between the "virtually safe dose" (corresponding to a lifetime cancer risk of 10^{-6}) predicted using the CKM/PBPK approach illustrated here and that predicted using the more conservative approach typical in regulatory cancer-risk assessment.

DATA ON CCl_4-INDUCED CARCINOGENICITY IN RODENTS

Experimentally induced carcinogenic effects of CCl_4 observed in mice, rats and hamsters have led scientific and regulatory bodies to consider this compound a probable human carcinogen.[17-19] Dose-response data on induced cell proliferation (see below) are only available for mice. Therefore, cancer-risk extrapolation for the present analysis will be based on cancer-bioassay data derived from studies on mice by the National Cancer Institute (NCI). In particular, data will be used from the NCI studies[20-22] of female B6C3F1 mice weighing about 28 g that received 0, 1250, and 2500 mg/kg-d of CCl_4, 5 days/wk for 78 wk, by oral gavage using a corn-oil vehicle. Dosing began at 7 wk of age and surviving mice were observed up to 14 wk after dosing was stopped. Hepatocellular carcinomas were observed in one of the 80 pooled control female mice, 40 of the 40 low-dose mice, and 43 of the 45 high-dose mice.

Because 100% incidence was observed in the low-dose mice, these data cannot be used directly to derive a traditional estimate of hepatocarcinogenic potency for CCl_4 in mice. Nevertheless, the data indicate that a dose of 35 mg CCl_4 per animal on the NCI dosing regimen yielded a cumulative risk of liver cancer greater than (40-1)/40 or 97.5% by 97 wk of age in these mice. The value of >97.5% is used as a lower bound on incidence rate in the analysis below.

PBPK MODELS

The PBPK model of Paustenbach *et al.*[23] was adapted to estimate uptake and metabolism of CCl_4 in mice and humans in the present study. Here, CCl_4 metabolism in rats was assumed to be described by a single saturable pathway with V_{max} equal to 0.40 mg/hr-kg or, equivalently (by the body-weight scaling approach used here and described by Paustenbach *et al.*[23]) 0.14 mg/hr for a 225-g rat (the value empirically determined[24,25] for rats cited, but then not used for simulation purposes[23]). Corresponding scaled V_{max} values used here for modeling 30-g mice and 70-kg humans are 0.034 mg/hr and 7.78 mg/hr, respectively. The present analysis makes use of the partition coefficients for rats and humans used by Paustenbach *et al.*[23] and assumes that mice have the same partition coefficients as the rats of the latter model. All other physiological parameter values for 25-g mice and 70-kg humans were taken to be the reference values reported by the U.S. Environmental Protection Agency (U.S. EPA),[26] except that the latter reported human alveolar ventilation rate was increased from 5.0 to a more realistic 5.6 liters/hr. Numerical implementation of the model was done as previously described.[27,28] Other details and the results of PBPK analyses undertaken are described in the following sections.

A study[29] of the absorption kinetics of four chlorinated organic compounds administered by a single gavage dose to rats in aqueous and corn oil vehicles demonstrated that, over a 5-hr observation period, a corn oil vehicle decreases the rate and extent of uptake of these compounds relative to that observed using an aqueous vehicle; the greatest decrease in uptake observed was for trichloroethylene, the least water-soluble compound tested. For the present analysis, oral absorption kinetics for CCl_4 were presumed to be similar to those observed[29] for trichloroethylene administered in 10 mL/kg of corn oil to 400-g Wistar rats, which yielded a roughly constant, 90-min absorptive pulse of equivalent to a clearance of compound from the vehicle at a rate of about 0.11 mL vehicle/kg-min. The resulting total dose was about one 170th of that obtained using an aqueous vehicle (which, in turn, was assumed to be 100% of the administered dose). The vehicle-clearance rate of 0.11 mL/kg-min used here was assumed to scale to the –0.26 power of body weight[27] and to apply only to single-dose exposure scenarios. The effect of using a corn oil vehicle on absorption efficiency of chronically administered oral doses of similar compounds is currently unknown.

DOSE-RESPONSE FOR INDUCED CELL PROLIFERATION

Dose-response data on CCl_4-induced hepatocellular proliferation in 30-g male CD-1 mice were obtained from a recent study by Doolittle *et al.*[30] The mice in this study were given single (or daily) oral doses of from 0 to 100 mg/kg CCl_4 in 10 mL/kg corn oil, and measurements were made of the percent of hepatocytes in S-phase (%S) 48 hr after dosing and the concentration of selected enzymes in blood serum at various times after dosing. To estimate metabolized doses corresponding to the applied doses used in this study, one 170th of the ingested CCl_4 was assumed to be cleared from the corn oil vehicle at the constant rate of 0.22 mL/kg-min, yielding a 45-min pulse injected into the liver compartment (see discussion above). The results of the PBPK analysis scaled to apply to the mice used by Doolittle *et al.* are shown in Fig.1a.

Studies of rats exposed to CCl_4 by gavage have demonstrated that metabolism of this compound is the cause of its hepatotoxicity in rats.[31-34] One recent study further

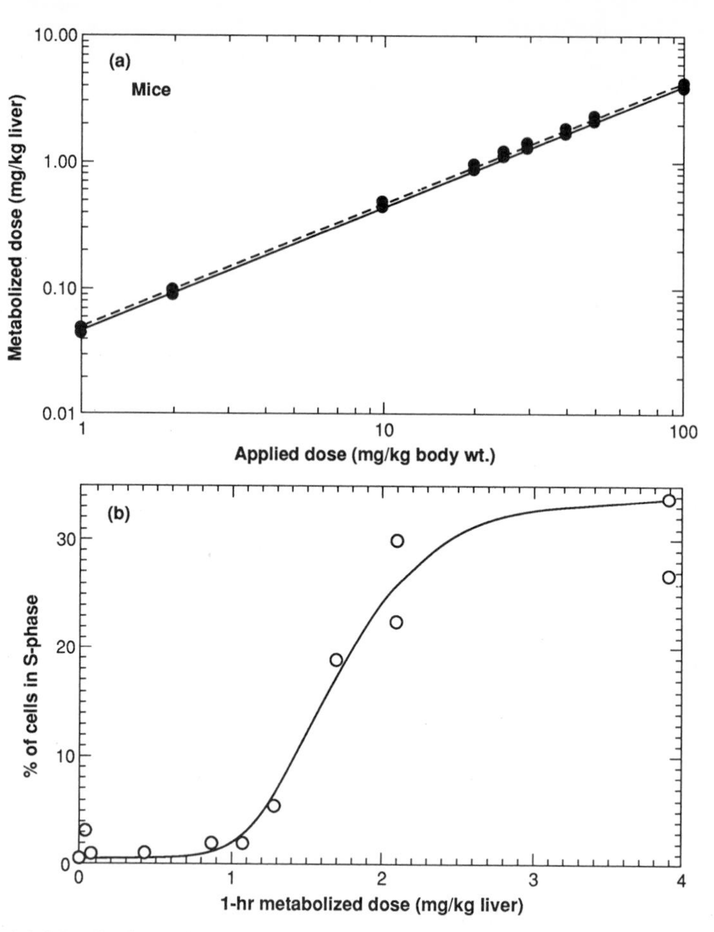

Fig. 1. **(a)** Metabolized dose as a function of orally administered dose of CCl_4 in corn oil to 30-g mice, based on the physiologically based pharmacokinetic model of Paustenbach *et al.*[23] modified and parameterized as explained in the text. Solid and dashed curves represent 1-hr and 24-hr total metabolized doses, respectively. Solid points indicate the administered doses used in the study by Doolittle *et al.*[30] referred to in the text. **(b)** Data (open circles) of Doolittle *et al.*[30] on the percent of hepatocytes in S-phase 48 hr after a single gavage dose (or in some cases the first of daily doses) of CCl_4 in corn oil to rats, as a function of the corresponding presumed effective (1-hr total metabolized) dose derived from (a) above. Solid curve is the function given by Eq. (1) in the text, fit to the data by least-squares optimization.

demonstrated that rats primarily metabolize CCl_4 to CO_2 and found that the rate of CO_2 production within 1 hr of dosing was the measure of CCl_4 metabolism most highly correlated (R^2=0.88) with the observed degree of liver injury as measured by elevation in serum glutamate-pyruvate transaminase (SGPT) concentration.[35] It was therefore assumed, for the present analysis, that the total amount of CCl_4 metabolized in 1 hr is the most appropriate metric of effective dose, *d*, for the cytotoxic effects observed by Doolittle *et al.*

The relationship between estimated values of *d* (from Fig. 1a) and the corresponding values of %S observed by Doolittle *et al.* is shown in Fig. 1b. Also shown is the log-normal dose-response model

$$\%S_d \;=\; \frac{100\%}{3}\,\Phi\left(\frac{\log_{10}(d)-a}{b}\right) \;+\; \%S_0 \;, \tag{1}$$

in which Φ is the cumulative normal distribution function, $\%S_0$ is the background level of %S (0.5% in the mice studied), and d is 1-hr metabolized dose. The model was fit to the data shown using least-squares optimization of the location and shape parameters a and b (yielding best-fit values of 0.23 and 0.13 mg/kg-hr, respectively). This dose-response function for CCl_4-induced cell proliferation is a quasi-threshold model, based on the assumption that such proliferation represents regenerative cell growth following necrosis caused by acute toxicity of a sufficiently high dose of CCl_4. The factor of 100%/3 in the model accounts for the fact that %S was measured by Doolittle *et al.* as a fraction of total hepatocytes undergoing replicative DNA synthesis at 48 hr post exposure, whereas not all hepatocytes induced into S-phase are involved in synthesis precisely at that time. Clearly, a synchronous induction of 100% of hepatocytes into S-phase would be lethal. Detailed experiments have shown that CCl_4 intoxication or partial hepatectomy induces in rats and mice a wave of regenerative hepatocellular proliferation corresponding to an S-phase pulse commencing between 24 and 48 hr after administration and persisting between approximately 24 and 36 hr.[36-39] In fact, such proliferative response kinetics have been shown to be quite heterogeneous within rat liver, with hepatocytes in most liver zones reaching maximum %S values of between 20 and 35% at various times post injury.[37-38] This is consistent with the estimated upper bound of 33.3% for %S used in Eq. (1), based on an average S-phase duration of about 8 hr (in rats)[38] and an average duration of sustained induced peak S-phase activity of approximately 24 hr.[36-39]

The Doolittle *et al.* study included some investigation of how chronic (daily) dosing affects %S and serum enzyme levels in mice as compared to single dosing. Their results indicate that %S is lower with daily as opposed to single CCl_4 dosing by a factor of 2 to 3.[30] For the present analysis, it was therefore assumed that the factor 100%/3 in Eq. (1) must be replaced by 100%/9 when this model is applied to chronic dosing situations. The latter assumption implies that no chronic effective dose, regardless of its magnitude, would produce a value of %S greater than 11.6%.

An analysis of the Doolittle *et al.* data on CCl_4-induced increases in %S and 24-hr SGPT concentration (Fig. 2) shows that the correlation between these two indices of hepatotoxicity may be sufficient to enable increased SGPT to be used as a quantitative predictor of increased %S according to the relation

$$\%S_d \ = \ c\left[\log_{10}\left(\frac{\mathrm{SGPT}_d}{\mathrm{SGPT}_0}\right)\right] \ + \ \%S_0 \ , \qquad (2)$$

in which the slope constant c is equal to 10.9%. Figs. 3a-3c summarize an investigation of this hypothesis using data on induced changes in SGPT levels in male 225-g rats given single oral doses of CCl_4 in 2.5 mL/kg corn oil from a study by Reynolds *et al.*[35] The PBPK analysis for this study (Fig. 3a) assumed that one 170th of the ingested CCl_4 was cleared from the corn oil vehicle at a rate of 0.13 mL/kg-min, yielding a 19-min pulse injected into the liver compartment (see discussion above). The relation shown in Fig. 2 was then used to derive predicted %S values corresponding to observed elevations in SGPT at the estimated effective doses of CCl_4 to rats for the Reynolds *et al.* study. Eq. (1) was then fit to these predicted %S values as a function of effective dose as described above, yielding the parameter estimates a=0.93 and b=0.12 mg/kg-hr corresponding to the dashed curve shown in Fig. 3b, where this fit is compared to the one pertaining to mice from Fig. 1b. Fig. 3c shows that the dose-response models fit to the mouse data and the estimated rat data on elevated %S are approximately identical only if a from Eq. (1) for mice is assumed to increase by a factor of 5 and if c from Eq. (2) is assumed for rats to be 5.45 (i.e., half the value referred to above pertaining to mice). The first assumption suggests that the value of V_{max} for mice used in the PBPK analysis discussed above may be too low by a factor of 5, which is plausible in light of the fact that V_{max} for mice in this analysis was simply assumed to be identical to an estimate obtained for rats (i.e., mice may have a higher

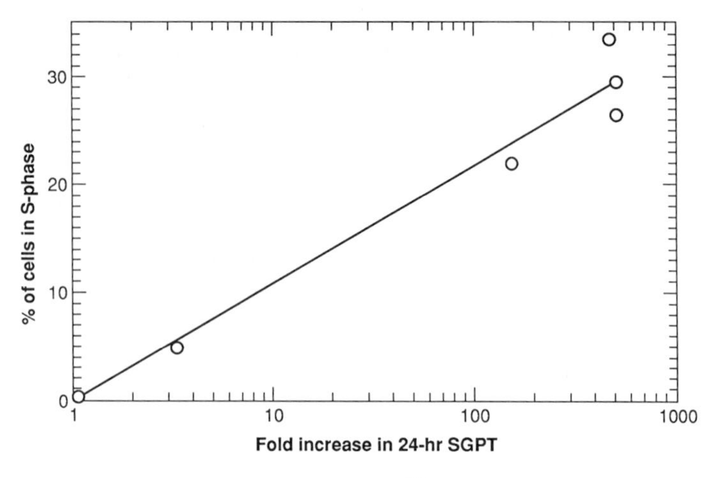

Fig. 2. Data (open circles) of Doolittle *et al.*[30] on percent of hepatocytes in S-phase (%S) 48 hr after gavage administration of various doses of CCl_4 in corn oil to 30-g mice, as a function of the fold increase (F) in SGPT concentration observed in these mice 24 hr after dosing. Solid line is the function given by Eq. (2) in the text, fit to the data by log-linear least-squares optimization.

capacity to metabolize CCl_4 than would be expected based simply on allometric scaling from an experimentally based estimate for rats). The second assumption suggests that the relation indicated by Eq. (2) and Fig. (2) may be species-specific.

CKM MODELS APPLIED TO CANCER LIVER DATA FOR MICE

The simple 2-stage CKM models used in the present analysis are described elsewhere[16] and are reviewed in the Appendix. Specifically, the exponential and geometric CKM models used here to predict cumulative cancer risk, R, as a function of age (minus a latency period here assumed to be 0) for a constant, lifetime exposure scenario, incorporate Eqs. (E-3) and (G-3) in the Appendix, where these are replaced by Eqs. (E-8) and (G-8), respectively, for scenarios involving n distinct exposure periods (i.e., in cases involving a sequence of n sets of parameter values governing mutation and cell proliferation rates). Because the NCI bioassays for CCl_4[20-22] involved preexposure, exposure, and postexposure periods (see discussion above), Eqs. (E-8) and (G-8) were used with n set equal to 3 to model hepatocellular cancer risk to the mice used. The cell-growth parameters of these models, g and a respectively (see Appendix), were fit to each of the single data points R_0=0.0125 and R_d=0.975 for the exposure scenario described above under the assumption that CCl_4 is a "pure promoter," i.e., acts only to increase the proliferation rate of initiated cells. Here, d is the effective (1-hr total metabolized) dose to liver tissue for NCI bioassay mice, estimated to be 21.1 mg/kg liver using the PBPK model described above, scaled to 28-g mice under the assumption that 100% of the chronically applied doses were absorbed. (Note that since 100% of these mice got liver cancer, R_d>0.975 so the corresponding models actually describe a plausible lower bound on true risk. Fig. 1b suggests that a similar response would have occurred had the effective dose been up to about 10 times less than it was.) To fit these models, it was also assumed that the NCI mice had 1.5×10^8 hepatocytes/g liver tissue[40] at risk throughout their lives of which roughly 25% were diploid cells at risk for malignant transformation,[41] yielding a total of 6×10^7 cells for 28-g mice with 5.5% liver tissue by weight, and that the two interstage mutation rates were each equal to 10^{-7}. The growth parameter values predicting the risks R_0 and R_d, $\{g_0,g_d\}$ and $\{a_0,a_d\}$ for the geometric and exponential CKM models respectively, produce the CKM functions shown in Fig. 4a.

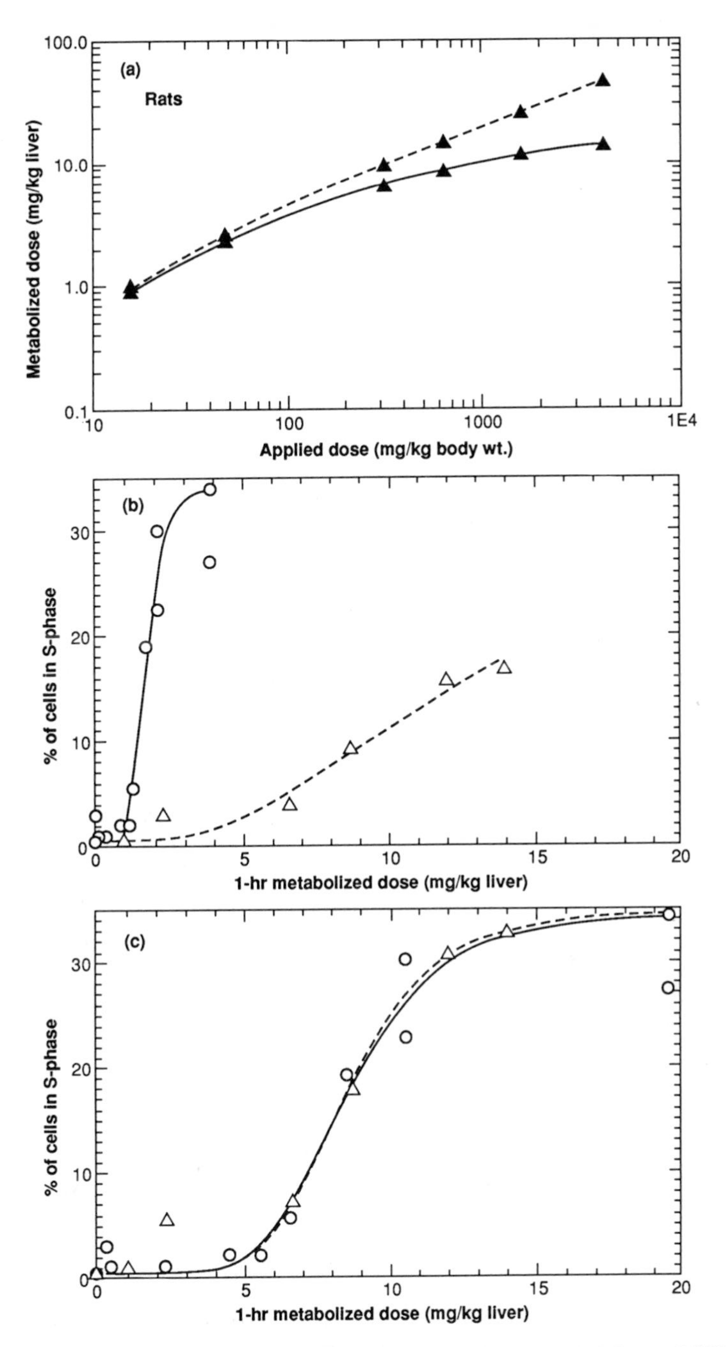

Fig. 3. **(a)** Metabolized dose as a function of orally administered dose of CCl_4 in corn oil to 225-g rats, based on the PBPK model of Paustenbach *et al.*[23] as explained in text. Solid and dashed curves represent 1-hr and 24-hr total metabolized doses, respectively; solid triangles indicate administered doses used in the Reynolds *et al.*[35] study. **(b)** Open triangles represent the predicted % in S-phase 48 hr after single gavage doses of CCl_4 in corn oil to rats extrapolated from Fig. 2 and from (a), using Eq. (1) from text; solid curve and associated data points redrawn from Fig. 1(b) for comparison. **(c)** The two curves in (b) converge if parameters are changed as explained in text.

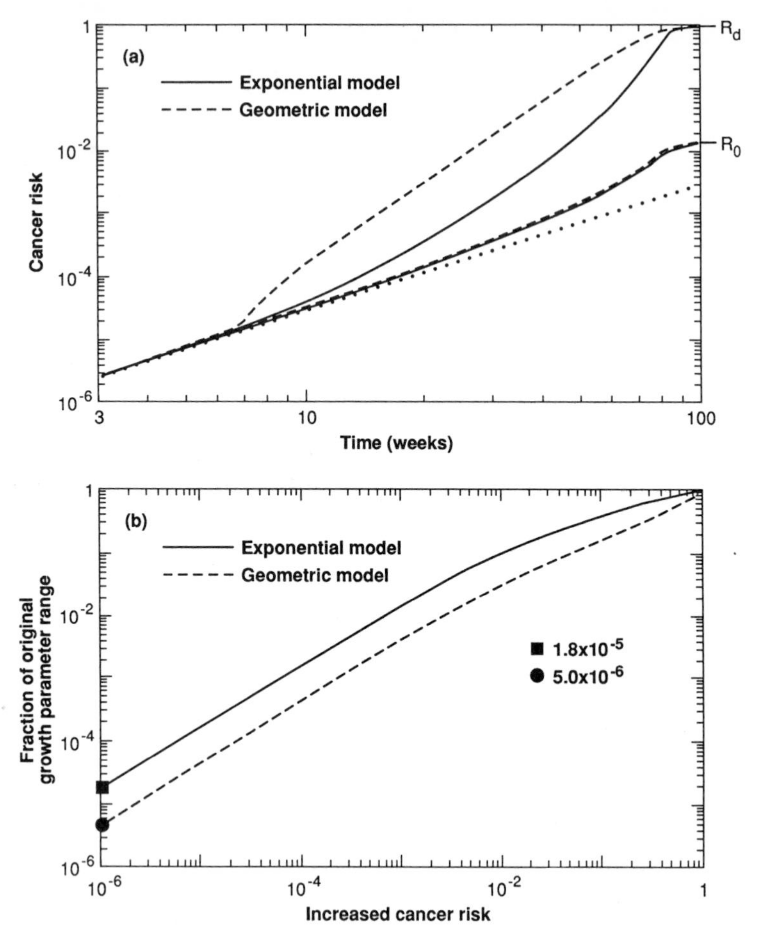

Fig. 4. Exponential and geometric cell-kinetic multistage models fit to tumor response data[20-22] for female mice exposed to CCl_4. **(a)** Solid and dashed curves are the functions 1-exp(E) and 1-exp(G), respectively, where E and G are given by Eqs. (E-3) and (G-3) in the Appendix, respectively, for which the constant $X_0 m_1 M_1$ is set to 6×10^{-7}. The functions are fit to the points R_0=0.0125 and R_d=0.975 at 97 wk, yielding the fitted exponential and geometric growth parameter values of $\{g_0=1.91, g_d=6.54\}$ and $\{a_0=0.939$ and $a_d=12.7\}$, respectively. The dotted line represents both models if the growth parameter is taken to be 0. **(b)** The fraction f corresponding to the growth parameter $z = z_0+f(z_d-z_0)$ (where z is either g or a) used in the models from (a) to predict a given risk R, as a function of increased risk $(R-R_0)/(1-R_d)$ for $R_0 \leq R \leq R_d$.

To proceed in the analysis, the background risk R_0 was assumed to be independent such that increased risk is defined as $A = (R-R_0)/(1-R_0)$, where $R_0 \leq R \leq R_d$, and that premalignant (stage-1) clones are resistant to the cytotoxicity of necrogenic doses of CCl_4, but are stimulated to proliferate to the same extent that surrounding normal hepatocytes are during regenerative growth following dosing.[42] It was further assumed that a change in %S by a given fraction f of its observed range corresponds to the same fractional change in net growth of premalignant cells, i.e., that

$$f = \frac{\%S - \%S_0}{\%S_d - \%S_0} = \frac{z - z_0}{z_d - z_0} , \tag{3}$$

where $0 \leq f \leq 1$ and where $z_0 \leq z \leq z_d$ for z equal to g or a. Thus, by decreasing f from 1 to 0, the curves leading to R_d in Fig. 4a are decreased until they converge to those leading to R_0. These assumptions and the information from Fig. 4a were then used to calculate f as a function of A for the exponential and geometric CKM models (Fig. 4b). Figure 4b shows that, based on the NCI mouse bioassay data, a reduction in f from 1 to between 5 and 20×10^{-6} is needed to ensure that $A=10^{-6}$.

CKM MODELS APPLIED TO LIVER CANCER DATA FOR HUMANS

The same approach taken above for using CKM models to describe liver cancer risk to the female NCI mice was applied to data on liver cancer incidence for human females. In this case, R_0 was taken to be 0.0005, the cumulative risk of getting liver cancer by age 75 for U.S. females during the period 1969-1971.[43] For humans receiving the same effective dose of CCl_4 that the NCI mice received, the corresponding lower bound on increased risk R_d was assumed to be approximately that applicable to the NCI mice. CKM models fit to each of these risk values are shown in Fig. 5a, and the corresponding relation of f to A shown in Fig. 5b demonstrates that, based on female liver cancer incidence data, a reduction in f from 1 to between 5 and 40×10^{-5} is needed to ensure that $A=10^{-6}$.

EXTRAPOLATION OF LIVER CANCER RISK TO HUMANS

Figure 6a shows effective dose as a function of f based on the data of Doolittle *et al.*[30] This relation was derived from Eq. (3) and the inverse of the relation specified in Eq. (1), appropriately modified to reflect a chronic dosing assumption. The analyses in the previous two sections indicate that, at minimum, a reduction in f from 1 to between 5 and 400×10^{-6} is needed to ensure that $A=10^{-6}$, which, in light of Fig. 6a, corresponds to an effective chronic CCl_4 dose rate of between 0.46 and 0.63 mg/kg liver per day. It was next assumed that this predicted range of "virtually safe" effective dose applies to humans as well as mice. To complete the analysis, a PBPK model for CCl_4-exposed 60-kg human females (with parameter values obtained as discussed above) was implemented using a chronic, daily scenario of ingestive exposure to CCl_4, e.g., in drinking water. Exposures were presumed to occur once per day, each modeled to result in a constant 6-min infusion of 100% of ingested CCl_4 into the liver compartment, and simulated exposures were repeated (for 7 simulated days) until dynamic equilibrium in effective (1-hr total metabolized) dose was approximated. The resulting relation of chronic applied to effective dose is shown in Fig. 6b. This information, combined with the previous analyses, leads to the prediction that an upper bound for the "virtually safe" dose rate of ingested CCl_4 for 60-kg humans is 3 to 5 mg/d, or 0.05 to 0.08 mg/kg-d, or 2 liters of water per day containing roughly 2 mg CCl_4 per liter. Recall that these represent upper bound figures because 100% of the low-dose NCI bioassay mice developed liver cancer.

DISCUSSION

The CKM-based approach to cancer risk assessment illustrated here for the case of CCl_4 differs fundamentally from more traditional risk assessment methods. Because the CKM model allows for a threshold-type dose response for agents considered to be "pure promoters," CKM-based risk estimates associated with exposure to such agents will typically be much lower than those based on "linear no-threshold" risk extrapolation methods. Using the latter methods, for example, the U.S. EPA[44] and the State of California[19,45] have, on the basis of animal cancer bioassay data such as the NCI study considered above, predicted a 10^{-6} (upper bound) increased cancer risk to be associated with ingestion of 4 sym(180) 10^{-6} and 5×10^{-5} mg/kg-d of CCl_4, respectively, which are from 3 to greater than 4 orders of magnitude lower than the corresponding upper bound

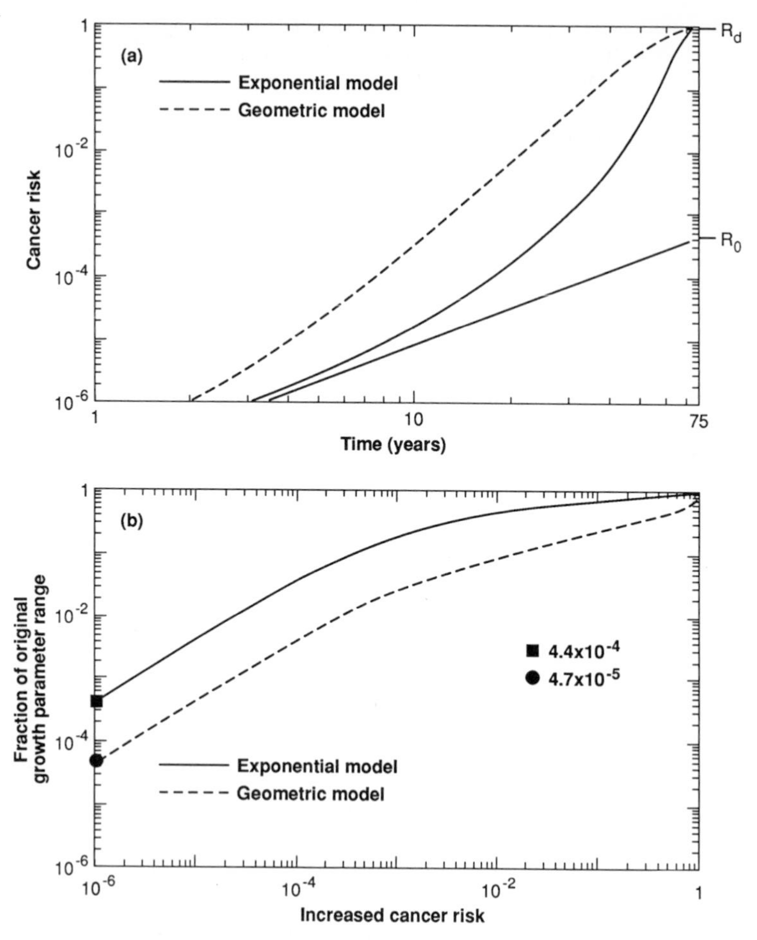

Fig. 5. Exponential and geometric cell-kinetic multistage models fit to the liver cancer incidence rate[43] (R_0=0.0005) for 75 yr-old U.S. females during 1969-1971 and to a much larger risk (R_d=0.987) presumed to be associated with a high-level, lifetime exposure to CCl_4. **(a)** Solid and dashed curves are the functions 1-exp(E) and 1-exp(G), respectively, where E and G are given by Eqs. (E-3) and (G-3) in the Appendix, respectively, for which the constant $X_0 m_1 M_1$ is set to 1.8×10^{-7} (the highest value possible to allow a fit to the risk values mentioned. The fitted exponential and geometric growth parameter values obtained are $\{g_0$=0.0,g_d=0.181$\}$ and $\{a_0$=0.0 and a_d=0.568$\}$, respectively. **(b)** The fraction f corresponding to the growth parameter $z = z_0+f(z_d-z_0)$ (where z is either g or a) used in the models from (a) to predict a given risk R, as a function of increased risk $(R-R_0)/(1-R_d)$ for $R_0 \leq R \leq R_d$.

"virtually safe" dose rates estimated above using the CKM-based approach. Even if a reduction in the latter values by 1 to 2 orders of magnitude is made to account for the 100% response in the NCI bioassay mice and for interindividual variability in humans, the CKM approach used here still predicts a much higher "safe" dose of CCl_4 than do the more traditional approaches.

It must be emphasized, however, that large uncertainties remain in defining the most appropriate way to implement CKM-based cancer risk extrapolation, even assuming the CKM approach is correct. The most fundamental source of uncertainty lies in the assumption made regarding the extent to which the observed carcinogenicity of a given

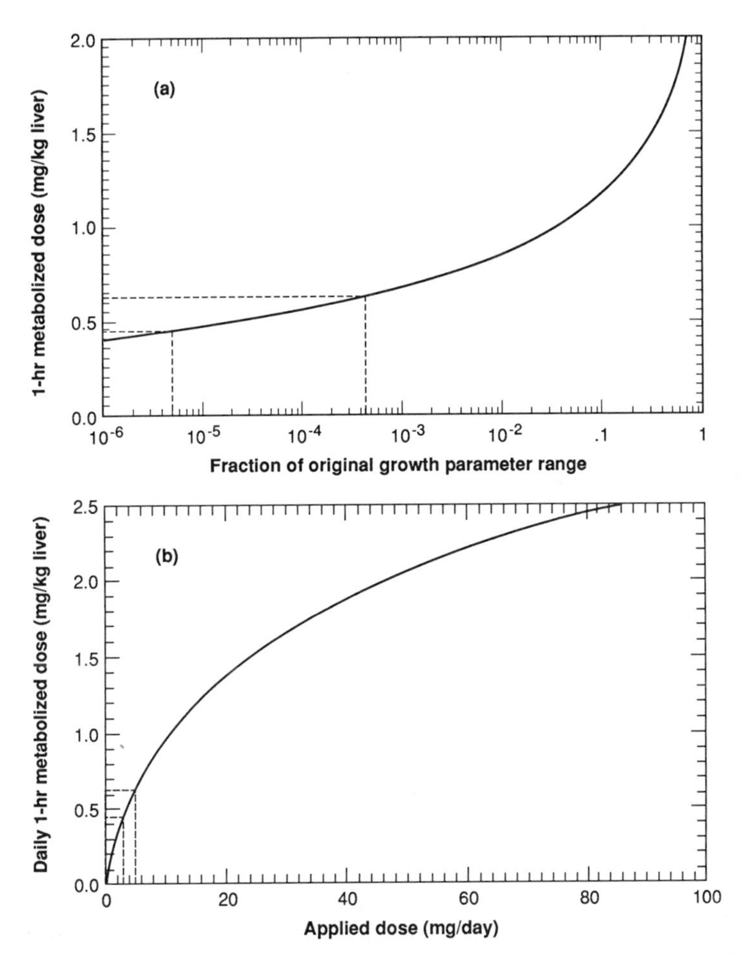

Fig. 6. **(a)** Predicted cytotoxically effective dose to mice as the function of f defined by Eq. (3) in the text, based on the inverse of the function specified by Eq. (1) in the text (in which the constant, 3, is replaced by 9 to account for the effect of chronic dosing). Dashed lines represent the range in values of f corresponding to a 10^{-6} risk from Figs. 4(b) and 5(b). **(b)** 1-hr total metabolized dose at dynamic equilibrium as a function of daily oral dose of CCl_4 to 60-kg humans, based on the physiologically based pharmacokinetic model of Paustenbach *et al.*[23] modified and parameterized as explained in the text. Dashed lines correspond to those in (a).

compound (say, in bioassay animals) is due to "promotion" (enhanced cell proliferation rates) alone, which reasonably can be presumed to have a threshold-type dose-response relationship, and how much is due to increased interstage transition rates (enhanced mutation rates), which is presumed by 2-stage CKM models to have a linear-quadratic dose-response relationship. Clearly, if a compound is assumed to have any degree of mutagenicity at all, this effect will ensure that the CKM dose-response relationship will be linear at sufficiently low doses.[46] The analysis above assumed that CCl_4 is a "pure promoter," which, despite the very limited evidence for CCl_4-induced genotoxicity *in vivo*,[44] may not strictly be the case. Other sources of uncertainty in this analysis include the effects of corn oil vehicle and chronic dosing on ingestive uptake of CCl_4 (sources not specific to CKM modeling), the selection of the most appropriate form of CKM model to use, and the quantitative relationship between changes in %S (or in SGPT levels) and changes in proliferation (birth minus death) rates in premalignant cells.

Despite these uncertainties, the CKM approach incorporates the emerging facts regarding carcinogenesis to a far greater extent than do the more traditional risk extrapolation models. Thus, even when data available to implement a CKM-based risk extrapolation for a given compound are limited, consideration of this approach may provide heuristic advantages. For example, the present application to CCl_4 suggests that levels of serum enzymes (such as SGPT) associated with cytotoxicity and/or induced cell proliferation be routinely collected from animals during cancer bioassays, and that application of linear or quasi-linear risk extrapolation methods to data obtained from such bioassays be ruled out for those dose groups exhibiting significantly elevated levels of such enzymes.

ACKNOWLEDGMENTS

This work was performed under the auspices of the U.S. Department of Energy at the Lawrence Livermore National Laboratory with funds provided by the State of California, Department of Health Services, and the U.S. Air Force, H.G. Armstrong Aerospace Medical Research Laboratory, Toxic Hazards Division.

REFERENCES

1. P. Armitage and R. Doll, A Two-Stage Theory of Carcinogenesis in Relation to the Age Distribution of Human Cancer, *Br. J. Cancer* **11**:161-169 (1957).
2. P. Armitage and R. Doll, Stochastic Models for Carcinogenesis, Fourth Berkeley Symposium on Mathematics, Statistics, and Probability, pp. 19-38, University of California Press, Berkeley, CA (1961).
3. A. Whittemore and J. B. Keller, Quantitative Theories of Carcinogenesis, *SIAM Rev.* **20**:1-30 (1978).
4. S. H. Moolgavkar and D. J. Venzon, Two-Event Models for Carcinogenesis: Incidence Curves for Childhood and Adult Tumors, *Math. Biosci.* **47**:55-77 (1979).
5. S. H. Moolgavkar, N. E. Day, and R. G. Stevens, Two-Stage Model for Carcinogenesis: Epidemiology of Breast Cancer in Females, *J. Natl. Cancer Inst.* **65**:559-569 (1980).
6. S. H. Moolgavkar and A. G. Knudson, Mutation and Cancer: A Model for Human Carcinogenesis, *J. Natl. Cancer Inst.* **66**:1037-1052 (1981).
7. S. H. Moolgavkar, Model for Human Carcinogenesis: Action of Environmental Agents, *Environ. Health Perspect.* **50**:285-291 (1983).
8. T. W. Thorslund, C. C. Brown, and G. Charnley, Biologically Motivated Cancer Risk Models, *Risk Analysis* **7**:109-119 (1987).
9. J. A. Swenberg, F. C. Richardson, J. A. Boucheron *et al.*, High- to Low-dose Extrapolation: Critical Determinants Involved in the Dose Response of Carcinogenic Substances, *Environ. Health Perspect.* **76**:57-63 (1987).
10. S. H. Moolgavkar, A. Dewanji, and D. J. Venzon, A Stochastic Two-Stage Model for Cancer Risk Assessment. I. The Hazard Function and the Probability of Tumor, *Risk Analysis* **8**:383-392 (1988).
11. J. D. Wilson, Risk Assessment Reappraisals, [Letter] *Science* **240**:1126 (1988).
12. J. H. Weisburger and G. M. Williams, The Distinct Health Risk Analyses Required for Genotoxic Carcinogens and Promoting Agents, *Environ. Health Perspect.* **50**:233-245 (1983).
13. G. M. Williams, Definition of a Human Cancer Hazard, in *Nongenotoxic Mechanisms in Carcinogenesis (Banbury Report 25)*, pp. 367-380, B. E. Butterworth and T. J. Slaga, eds., Cold Spring Harbor Laboratory, Cold Spring Harbor, NY (1967).

14. E. L. Anderson and the Carcinogen Assessment Group of the U.S. Environmental Protection Agency, Quantitative Approaches in Use to Assess Cancer Risk, *Risk Analysis* **5**:277-295 (1985).
15. U.S. Environmental Protection Agency (EPA), Guidelines for Carcinogen Risk Assessment, *Federal Register* **51**:33992-34003 (1986).
16. K. T. Bogen, Cell Proliferation Kinetics and Multistage Cancer Risk Models, *J. Natl. Cancer Inst.* **81**:267-277 (1989).
17. U.S. Environmental Protection Agency (EPA), Health Assessment Document for Carbon Tetrachloride, EPA-600/8-82-001F, U.S. EPA Environmental Criteria and Assessment Office, Cincinnati, OH (1984).
18. IARC, International Agency for Research on Cancer, Some Halogenated Hydrocarbons, *IARC Monographs on the Evaluation of Carcinogenic Risk of Chemicals to Man* **20**:371-399 (1979).
19. N. R. Reed, R. Babapour, W. Reed, L. Beltran, and D. P. H. Hsieh, Health Risk Assessment of Carbon Tetrachloride in California Drinking Water, Report prepared for the California Public Health Foundation on behalf of the California Department of Health Services, Department of Environmental Toxicology, University of California, Davis, CA (1988).
20. National Cancer Institute (NCI), Report on the Carcinogenesis Bioassay of Chloroform, Carcinogenesis Program, Division of Cancer Cause and Prevention (1976).
21. National Cancer Institute (NCI), Report on the Carcinogenesis Bioassay of Trichloroethylene, National Cancer Institute Technical Report Series, No. 2, NCI-CG-TR-2 (1976).
22. National Cancer Institute (NCI), Bioassay of 1,1,1-Trichloroethane for Possible Carcinogenicity, National Cancer Institute Technical Report Series, No. 3, NCI-CG-TR-3 (1976).
23. D. J. Paustenbach, H. J. Clewll, III, M. L. Gargas, and M. E. Andersen, A Physiologically-Based Pharmacokinetic Model for Inhaled Carbon Tetrachloride, *Toxicol. Applied Pharmacol.* **96**:191-211 (1988).
24. M. L. Gargas, P. G. Seybold, and M. E. Andersen, Modeling the Tissue Solubilities and Metabolic Rate Constant (V_{max}) of Halogenated Methanes, Ethanes, and Ethylenes, *Toxicol. Letters* **43**:235-256 (1988).
25. M. L. Gargas, M. E. Andersen, and H. J. Clewell, III, A Physiologically Based Simulation Approach for Determining Metabolic Constants from Gas Uptake Data, *Toxicol. Appl. Pharmacol.* **86**:341-352 (1988).
26. U.S. Environmental Protection Agency (EPA), Reference Physiological Parameters in Pharmacokinetic Modeling, EPA-600/6-88/004, NTIS PB88-196019, U.S. EPA Office Research and Development, Office of Health and Environmental Assessment, Washington, DC (1988).
27. K. T. Bogen, Pharmacokinetics for Regulatory Risk Analysis: The Case of Trichloroethylene, *Regulatory Toxicol. Pharmacol.* **8**:447-466 (1988).
28. K. T. Bogen and L. H. Hall, Pharmacokinetics for Regulatory Risk Analysis: The Case of 1,1,1-Trichloroethane (Methyl Chloroform), *Regulatory Toxicol. Pharmacol.* **10**:26-50 (1989).
29. J. R. Withey, B. T. Collins, and P. G. Collins, Effect of Vehicle on the Pharmacokinetics and Uptake of Four Halogenated Hydrocarbons from the Gastrointestinal Tract of the Rat, *J. Appl. Toxicol.* **3**:249-253 (1983).
30. D. J. Doolittle, G. Muller, and H. E. Scribner, Relationship Between Hepatotoxicity and Induction of Replicative DNA Synthesis Following Single or Multiple Doses of Carbon Tetrachloride, *J. Toxicol. Environ. Health* **22**:63-78 (1987).
31. J. V. Bruckner, W. F. MacKenzie, S. Muralidhara, R. Luthra, G. M. Kyle, and D. Acosta, Oral Toxicity of Carbon Tetrachloride: Acute, Subacute, and Subchronic Studies in Rats, *Fundam. Appl. Toxicol.* **6**:16-34 (1986).
32. H. G. Shertzer, M. P. Niemi, F. A. Reitman, M. L. Berger, B. L. Myers, and M. W. Tabor, Protection Against Carbon Tetrachloride Hepatotoxicity by Pretreatment with Indole-3-carbinol, *Exp. Mol. Pathol.* **46**:180-189 (1987).

33. G. Labbe, V. Descatoire, P. Letteron, C. Degott, M. Tinel, D. Larrey, Y. Carrion-Pavlov, J. G. G. Amouyal, and D. Pessayre, The Drug Methoxsalen a Suicide Substrate for Cytochrome P-450, *Biochem. Pharmacol.* **36**:907-914 (1987).
34. H. G. Shertzer, M. L. Berger, and M. W. Tabor, Intervention in Free Radical Mediated Hepatotoxicity and Lipid, *Biochem. Pharmacol.* **37**:333-338 (1988).
35. E. S. Reynolds, R. J. Treinen, H. H. Farrish, and M. T. Moslen, Metabolism of [14C] Carbon Tetrachloride to Exhaled, Excreted and Bound Metabolites: Dose-Response, Time-Course and Pharmacokinetics, *Biochem. Pharmacol.* **33**:3363-3374 (1984).
36. C. M. Leevy, R. M. Hollister, R. Schmid, R. A. MacDonald, and C. S. Davidson, Liver Regeneration in Experimental Carbon Tetrachloride Intoxication, *Proc. Soc. Exp. Biol. Med.* **102**:672-675 (1959).
37. H. Gerhard, A Quantitative Model of Cellular Regeneration in Rat Liver After Partial Hepatectomy, in *Liver Regeneration after Experimental Injury: III Workshop on Experimental Liver Injury*, pp. 340-346, R. Lesch and W. Reutter, eds. Stratton Intercontinental Medical Book Corporation, NY (1973).
38. H. M. Rabes, H. V. Tuczek, and R. Wirsching, Kinetics of Hepatocellular Proliferation After Partial Hepatectomy as a Function of Structural and Biochemical Heterogeneity of the Rat Liver, in *Liver Regeneration after Experimental Injury: III Workshop on Experimental Liver Injury*, pp. 35-55, R. Lesch and W. Reutter, eds., Stratton Intercontinental Medical Book Corporation, NY (1973).
39. B. Schultze, H. Gerhard, and W. Maurer, A Quantitative Model of Liver Regeneration in the Mouse After CC14 Intoxication, in *Liver Regeneration after Experimental Injury: III Workshop on Experimental Liver Injury*, pp. 330-339, R. Lesch and W. Reutter, eds., Stratton Intercontinental Medical Book Corporation, NY (1973).
40. S. Petersen, Flow Cytometry of Human Colorectal Tumors: Nuclear Isolation by Detergent Technique, *Cytometry* **6**:452-460 (1985).
41. H. Danielsen, H. B. Steen, T. Lindmo, and A. Reith, Ploidy Distribution in Experimental Liver Carcinogenesis in Mice, *Carcinogenesis* **9**:59-63 (1988).
42. T. A. Dragani, G. Manenti, and G. D. Porta, Enhancing Effects of Carbon Tetrachloride in Mouse Hepatocarcinogenesis, *Cancer Lett.* **31**:171-179 (1986).
43. National Cancer Institute (NCI), Third National Cancer Survey: Incidence Data, National Cancer Institute Monograph 41, DHEW Publication No. NIH 75-787, p. 100, U.S. Department of Health, Education and Welfare, Bethesda, MD (1975).
44. U.S. Environmental Protection Agency (EPA), Health Assessment Document for Carbon Tetrachloride, EPA-600/8-82-001F, Environmental Criteria and Assessment Office, U.S. EPA, Cincinnati, OH (1984).
45. California Department of Health Services, Proposition 65 Risk-Specific Intake Levels: Carbon Tetrachloride, Draft report, Reproductive and Cancer Hazard Assessment Section, Office of Environmental Health Hazard Assessment (1988).
46. C. J. Portier, Statistical Properties of a Two-Stage Model of Carcinogenesis, *Environ. Health Perspect.* **76**:125-131 (1987).

APPENDIX

For cell-kinetic multistage (CKM) models in general,[16] the stage-j cell populations of a k-stage process of carcinogenesis are represented by the stochastic processes $X_j(T)$, j=1,...,k, over the period $0 \leq t \leq T$, where $X_j(0)=0$; $X_0(T)$ is a deterministic nonnegative (DN) ("driving") function; and $m_j(T)$, for j=0,...,$k-1$ and $m_j(T)T<<1$, are DN functions (stage-specific mutation rates) such that the probability of a unit gain by $X_{j+1}(T)$ caused by a simultaneous unit loss from $X_j(T)$ during the interval $[T,T+dT)$ is approximately $m_i(T)dT$, and the probability of more than one such event occurring in this interval is negligible. In semi-stochastic CKM models, $w_j(T)$, j=1,...,$k-1$, are DN impulse-response (or weighting) functions used to represent (premalignant) cell proliferation subsequent to the occurrence of each new stage-j clone arising by mutation of a stage-$(j-1)$ cell, where $w_k(T) = 1$. Finally, let $R(t) = \text{Prob}\{X_k(t) \geq 1\}$, i.e., $R(t)$ is the cumulative distribution of the waiting time for the occurrence by time t of the first increment in $X_k(t)$, representing the first cancer cell. It has been shown for semistochastic CKM models in general that $R(t) \approx EX_k(t)$ for $R(t) << 1$ and that $R(t) \approx 1-\exp(EX_k(t))$ is a first-order approximation for all $R(t)$, where E denotes the expectation operator.[16]

Derived below are the approximate solutions for 2-stage (i.e, k=2), semistochastic, exponential and geometric CKM models of carcinogenesis in the case that parameter values governing mutation rates and cell proliferation in intermediate-stage (here, in stage-1) cells change at times t_i for i=1,...,n, where t_0=0, $t_{i-1} \leq t_i$, and t_n=t. Here it is assumed that $X_0(T)$ is equal to the constant X_0 and that $m_j(t_{i-1} \leq T \leq t_i)$ for j=0 and j=1 are equal to the constants m_i and M_i, respectively. From these assumptions, it follows[16] that for both exponential and geometric CKM models,

$$EX_1(t_n) \approx \sum_{i=1}^{n} \int_{t_{i-1}}^{t_i} X_0 m_i w_1(t_i - T)dT \quad , \text{ and} \tag{A-1}$$

$$EX_2(t_n) \approx EX_2(t_{n-1}) + \int_{t_{n-1}}^{t_n} M_n EX_1(T)dT \quad . \tag{A-2}$$

In the following evaluations of Eqs. (A-1) and (A-2), the growth response function, $w_1(T)$, for all proliferating premalignant (i.e., stage-1) cells is taken to be a function of the growth parameter z, where z is designated g and a in exponential and geometric CKM models, respectively, and where z at time T equals the constant z_i for $t_{i-1} \leq T \leq t_i$, i=1,...,n. Also, p_i will be used to denote the vector $\{m_i, M_i, z_i\}$ of mutation- and growth-related parameter-values in operation over the period from t_{i-1} to t_i, i=1,...,n.

I. Exponential 2-Stage CKM Models

For 2-stage exponential CKM models, $w_1(T) = e^{gT}$ when n=1, so that Eqs. (A-1) and (A-2) yield

$$EX_1(t_1) \approx X_0 \frac{m_1}{g_1}(e^{g_1 t_1} - 1) \tag{E-1}$$

$$= EX_1(p_1, t_1) \quad , \text{ and} \tag{E-2}$$

$$EX_2(t_1) \approx X_0 \frac{m_1 M_1}{g_1^2}(e^{g_1 t_1} - g_1 t_1 - 1) \tag{E-3}$$

$$= EX_2(p_1, t_1) \quad . \tag{E-4}$$

To consider cases in which n>1, we first define

$$\in_{r,s} = \begin{cases} \sum_{i=r}^{s} g_i(t_i - t_{i-1}) & \text{for } r \leq s \\ 0 & \text{for } r > s \end{cases} \tag{E-5}$$

and note that $w_1(T) = \exp(g_i T + \in_{i+1,n})$ during the period t_{n-1} to t_n for stage-1 clones arising at time T where $t_{i-1} \leq T \leq t_i$. Upon substitution, Eqs. (A-1) and (A-2) yield

$$EX_1(t_n) \approx \sum_{i=1}^{n} \int_{t_{i-1}}^{t_i} X_0 m_i \exp(g_i(t_i - T) + \in_{i+1,n})dT \quad , \tag{E-6}$$

$$\approx \sum_{i=1}^{n} X_0 \frac{m_i}{g_i} \Big[\exp(\epsilon_{i,n}) - \exp(\epsilon_{i+1,n}) \Big] \quad , \text{ and} \tag{E-7}$$

$$EX_2(t_n) \approx \sum_{i=1}^{n} EX_2(p_i, t_i - t_{i-1}) + \sum_{i<j\leq n} \Big[X_0 \frac{m_i M_j}{g_i g_j} (\exp(\epsilon_{i,i} - 1))$$

$$\cdot \; (\exp(\epsilon_{j,j} - 1)) \; \exp(\epsilon_{i+1,j-1}) \Big] \quad . \tag{E-8}$$

II. Geometric 2-Stage CKM Models

For 2-stage geometric CKM models in the case that n=1, it has been shown[16] that $w_1(T) = (aT+1)^x$ (where in the text x=3 to model premalignant clones assumed to grow spherically with radial growth proportional to time). For these geometric CKM models, Eqs. (A-1) and (A-2) yield

$$EX_1(t_1) \approx X_0 \frac{m_1}{(x+1)a_1} \left[\Big(a_1 t_1 + 1 \Big)^{x+1} - 1 \right] \tag{G-1}$$

$$= EX_1(p_1, t_1) \quad , \text{ and} \tag{G-2}$$

$$EX_2(t_1) \approx X_0 \frac{m_1 M_1}{(x+1)(x+2)a_1^2} \left[\Big(a_1 t_1 + 1 \Big)^{x+2} - \Big((x+2) a_1 t_1 \Big) + 1 \right] \tag{G-3}$$

$$= EX_2(p_1, t_1) \quad . \tag{G-4}$$

To consider cases in which n>1, we first define

$$\gamma_{r,s} = \begin{cases} 1 + \sum_{i=r}^{s} a_i (t_i - t_{i-1}) & \text{for } r \leq s \\ 1 & \text{for } r > s \end{cases} \tag{G-5}$$

and note that $w_1(T) = (a_i T + \gamma_{i+1,n})^x$ during the period t_{n-1} to t_n for stage-1 clones arising at time T where $t_{i-1} \leq T \leq t_i$. Upon substitution, Eqs. (A-1) and (A-2) now yield

$$EX_1(t_n) \approx \sum_{i=1}^{n} \int_{t_{i-1}}^{t_i} X_0 m_i \left[\Big(a_i (t_i - T) + \gamma_{i+1,n} \Big) \right]^x dT \quad , \tag{G-6}$$

$$\approx \sum_{i=1}^{n} X_0 \frac{m_i}{(x+1)a_i} \Big(\gamma_{i,n}^{x+1} - \gamma_{i+1,n}^{x+1} \Big) \quad , \text{ and} \tag{G-7}$$

$$EX_2(t_n) \approx \sum_{i=1}^{n} EX_2(p_i, t_i - t_{i-1}) + \sum_{i<j\leq n} \left[X_0 \frac{m_i M_j}{(x+1)(x+2) a_i a_j} \right.$$

$$\left. \cdot \; \Big(\gamma_{i,j}^{x+2} - \gamma_{i,j-1}^{x+2} - \gamma_{i+1,j}^{x+2} + \gamma_{i+1,j-1}^{x+2} \Big) \right] \quad . \tag{G-8}$$

A General Model for Quantitative Risk Comparisons

Hector A. Munera
Cisatec Ltd.
Bogota, Colombia, South America

ABSTRACT

One important aspect of risk analysis is the individual and societal comparison of probability distributions over a set of undesirable outcomes. To compare all possible distributions it is mandatory to assign one single value (called an index) to each distribution. Typical indices are the expected value and the expected utility model; the paper notes some theoretical and practical limitations of these indices. The paper briefly describes the author's linearized moments model (LMM) that gives consideration to individual risk perceptions and that takes into account the shape of the probability distribution including the low-probability high-consequence tail. The LMM solves the main theoretical and practical inconsistencies of the expected utility model. It is noted that current indices like the expected value, the expected utility model and the prospect theory are special cases of the LMM.

KEYWORDS: Linearized moments model, decision analysis under uncertainty, quantitative risk comparisons, risk perception, utility theory

INTRODUCTION

One important aspect of risk analysis is the individual and societal comparison of probability distributions over a set of undesirable outcomes. An intrinsic weakness of stochastic dominance approaches (and for that matter of any risk theory based on partial orderings) is that in many instances a definite answer can not be obtained from the risk comparison. An example of practical interest that can not be resolved by stochastic dominance of first-order is the comparison of two designs of a technological device with the same mean (say a nuclear power plant), when lower probabilities in the high-consequence region are traded for higher probabilities in the low-consequence region.

A general methodology for quantitative risk comparisons should yield complete orderings among all non-deterministic alternatives. One way to attain this is use of indices of dispreference as discussed in this paper. Typical indices are the expected value and the expected utility, whose theoretical and practical limitations are well known. I will not elaborate on the now abundant literature pointing out the inadequacies of the expected utility model (EUM), see, e.g., McCord and de Neufville.[1] The situation is summarized by Cohen *et al.*[2]: "These facts have created a fairly widespread belief in the field that new descriptive and normative models must be sought."

Risk Analysis, Edited by C. Zervos
Plenum Press, New York, 1991

Over the last ten years I have developed and tested a linearized moments model (LMM) that gives consideration to individual risk perceptions and that takes into account the shape of the probability distribution including the low-probability high-consequence tail. The LMM eliminates the main theoretical and practical inconsistencies of the EUM.

This paper briefly discusses some currently used risk indices, summarizes the LMM, and concludes with notes that expected value, utility models, and prospect theory are special cases of the LMM.

CURRENTLY USED RISK INDICES

For risk analysis the objects undergoing comparison are unfavorable non-deterministic alternatives $A = (Z; P)$. These are continuous (discrete) probability density (mass) functions PDFs. Here we limit consideration to the discrete case of the form

$$A = (Z; P) = (z_j; p_j) \tag{1}$$

where

$j = 0,1,..n,$

$Z = \{z_j\}$ is the set of (potential) unfavorable consequences, and

$P = \{p_j\}$ is the corresponding probability measure.

The state z_0 is neutral and may represent a (dynamic) status-quo or the "normal" conditions when there are no accidents. Extension to more complicated situations (like continuous outcomes and/or infinite number of consequences) can be made with due care. Examples of unfavorable outcomes are "monetary loss" and "loss of life" — or more detailed descriptions like "early fatalities," "delayed deaths," "occupational deaths," and so on.

An index of dispreference is a real number $I(A)$ attached to a non-deterministic alternative A. The index represents the scale of individual or societal preferences. More formally, we say that $I(.)$ is an index of dispreference if, and only if, $I(A) < I(B)$ implies that alternative B is strictly not preferred to alternative A or, equivalently, that A is strictly preferred to B.

The Expected Value

The simplest index of dispreference is the average or expected value $I_a(.)$ given by

$$I_a(A) = E(Z) = \sum_j p_j z_j \tag{2}$$

Even today, specially in engineering applications, there exists the naive concept that $I_a(.)$ is a "natural" index to represent individual scales of preferences for non-deterministic alternatives. However, it is a well known fact that any probability distribution, in particular the non-deterministic alternatives of interest herein, may be characterized by $2n+1$ moments, all taken together (for there are $n+1$ outcomes and $n+1$ probabilities that must add to unity). Then, it is fairly obvious that selecting only one of them (say, the expected value, the variance, etc.) to represent a whole PDF is a very strong value judgment that may not be always acceptable.

The inapplicability of an average index for decision making was already noticed in the eighteenth century in the context of the famous St. Petersburg Paradox described in many textbooks on probability and decision theory. It is noted in passing that the PDF in the St. Petersburg gamble shares with the PDFs of some modern technological accidents a common feature: a long tail of potential high-consequences with low-probabilities. This suggests that concepts of risk based on I_a are far from being universally acceptable. For further discussion see Ref. 3.

The Expected Utility Model

Ever since the 18th century Daniel Bernouilli[4] interpreted the St. Petersburg Paradox as meaning that the expected value was not an appropriate index. He introduced the concept of "moral utility" $B(.)$ over monetary consequences z, and proposed for it a logarithmic function: $B_z = \ln(z)$. Furthermore, he suggested that a suitable index I_b for ranking alternatives would be the expected moral utility, i.e.,

$$I_b(A) = E[B(Z)] = \sum_j p_j B(z_j) = \sum_j p_j \ln(z_j) \ . \tag{3}$$

A small finite value for I_b solves the St. Petersburg's paradox. However, the fundamental weakness of Bernouilli's model, shared by other recent methodologies for non-deterministic decision making (e.g., portfolio theory) is their ad-hoc nature. Indeed, there are no logically compelling reasons for selecting one model while excluding others. In order to find indices that may eventually attain some form of universal acceptability, it may be reasonable to adopt an axiomatic approach, i.e., to define *a priori* a set of logically appealing principles and properties. A dispreference index compatible with such principles and properties should have some logically binding power to those individuals accepting the axioms. In an axiomatic framework an index itself can not be challenged, but the acceptability of the underlying axioms may be, and certainly is, challenged in many occasions.

Nearly half a century ago John von Neumann and Oskar Morgenstern[5] (vN-M) first succeeded in defining a set of rules from which they derived an index, similar to Bernouilli's proposal, that was also labelled "expected utility." When applied to unfavorable alternatives, it becomes an index of dispreference $I_u(A)$ given by

$$I_u(A) = E[u(Z)] = \sum_j p_j u(z_j) \ , \tag{4}$$

where the individual disutilities $u(z_j)$ are such that $u(z_1) < u(z_2)$ implies that z_2 is strictly dispreferred to z_1, and conversely.

It is trivial to note that the expected value index $I_a(A)$ defined by Eq. (2) is a special case of Eq. (4) when $u(z_j) = z_j$. This is a typical example of normal scientific progress, whereby newer and more comprehensive theories contain the previous theory as a particular case.

After vN-M's pioneering breakthrough, all succeeding EUMs also adopted an axiomatic approach. It is noted in passing that not all EUMs are alike. In fact, some are based on "objective" probability, see, e.g. Ref. 5 and 6, but other EUMs make use of "subjective" interpretations of probability, sometimes completely detached from any physical reality.[7]

It is our contention that the input to risk comparisons, i.e. to the decision making model represented by a risk index, should be as "objective" as possible. By this it is meant that both probability and consequences should be linked to physical realities only, without reflecting individual attitudes towards risk or uncertainty. In the words of Hagen[8]: a probability is "rational" if its "estimate is the same whether the event is desirable or not." In our view, subjective risk feelings should be an explicit component of the risk index, thus facilitating controversy and compromise among different opinions.

The previous remarks indicate preference for objective over subjective EUMs. The Luce and Raiffa (L-R) model applies exactly to the class of finite discrete alternatives of interest here. The axioms that have immediate intuitive appeal, are as follows:

1. *Complete ordering of consequences.* All elements of the deterministic set Z can be ordered in a transitive fashion.
2. *Reduction of compound alternatives.* If A is a compound alternative of the form $A=(B_k;s_k)$ having as potential outcomes non-deterministic alternatives $B=(Z;Q)=(z_j;q_j)$, it is possible to express A directly in terms of the deterministic consequences z_j, that is, $A=(z_j;p_j)$ by calculating p_j in terms of s_k and q_j according to the ordinary probability calculus (where s, q and p are probabilities).
3. *Continuity.* For every deterministic consequence z_j there is always an equivalent non-deterministic alternative A_j of the form $A_j=(b,w;\ u_j,1-u_j)$, where b and w (elements of Z) are the best and worst potential consequences, and u_j is a probability.
4. *Substitutability.* In any non-deterministic alternative $A=(Z;P)$, it is possible to exchange any deterministic consequence z_j for its equivalent non-deterministic A_j as defined by axiom 3.
5. *Transitivity.* Preference and indifference between non-deterministic alternatives are transitive relations.
6. *Monotonicity.* The non-deterministic alternative $A=(b,w;\ p,1-p)$ is preferred or indifferent to $A'=(b,w;\ p',1-p')$ if and only if $p \geq p'$.

Since the EUM is proposed as a normative theory for decision making, the obvious question is whether there are real individuals that accept all the six axioms underlying the model; otherwise, the theory is irrelevant for decision making in the real world.

All axiomatic systems include transitivity and some form of stochastic dominance which, for idealized—"normative" if you wish—decision making seem to be logically acceptable principles. In the L-R these assumptions are contained in axioms 1, 5 and 6 (i.e, deterministic transitivity, non-deterministic transitivity and monotonicity, respectively).

A principle of continuity is also present in all EUM derivations (axiom 3 in the L-R model). It has been already amply documented that some individuals may show discontinuities when probability tends to one. This is the "certainty effect" identified by Kahneman and Tversky.[9] Such phenomenon may be explained in simple words as: an infinite gap between something possible and something impossible. The opinion here is that for societal decision making some weak form of continuity may be desirable. The L-R model also includes an explicit assumption for the reduction of compound alternatives (axiom 2). Provided that there are no intermediate choice nodes in the decision tree, this assumption is an innocuous rule of arithmetic probability.

The really controversial assumption is axiom 4, the substitution principle (SP). Criticisms to the SP take two forms:

1. Theoretical or philosophical weaknesses.[10,11,12] The argument is that axiom 4 implies the elimination of some possibilities for choice (these take the form of choice nodes in a decision-tree representation) which decreases the flexibility available to the decision maker.
2. Empirical violations to the pattern of choice prescribed by the SP. The most famous is the Paradox posed by Allais.[13] In the context of Allais' problem many individuals, including Savage and Samuelson, who were some of the best EUM

theoreticians and champions, have made choices opposite to the prescriptions of the EUM. Identical violations of predictions of the EUM have been recently observed by Kahneman and Tversky (see Ref. 9, pp. 265-66) when the prizes are small and the probabilities intermediate. All in all, it is widely acknowledged, even by the most convinced defenders of the EUM, that when confronted with decisions like those in the Allais' Paradox at least some individuals will make choices in violation of the prescriptions of the EUM.

Some defenders of the EUM solve the paradox by saying that the individual made a "non-rational" choice, or in the milder opinions that he made a mistake. Opponents of the EUM resolve the paradox by arguing that the EUM is not always applicable. Here an alternative choice model is presented: the LMM summarized in the next section. The LMM predicts that in Allais' problem there may exist up to four choice patterns, those actually observed. Thus, the existence of the paradox is preempted. For further details see Munera.[11,12,14]

There are other two groups of empirical observations contradicting the EUM:

1. The so-called "preference reversals,"[15-17] which are also predicted by our LMM[18]; and,

2. The dependence of the utility function upon the probabilities used for its assessment.[1,19] (According to EUM, utility is unique up to a positive linear transformation.) Such behavioral patterns can also be explained by the LMM.[11]

THE LINEARIZED MOMENTS MODEL (LMM)

The Descriptive Model

As a result of the growing awareness that the EUM is not founded on a universally valid theory, there are already several proposals for alternative choice models. An example is prospect theory advanced by Kahneman and Tversky[9] to explain the behavior of the majority of their subjects. A more general proposal is Allais' suggestion[13] to include all moments of the probability distribution over "psychological values." Specific models belonging to this class are the works of Hagen,[8] Munera,[11,14,19] and Munera and de Neufville.[12] In the following I will concentrate on the LMM which has two basic strengths: (a) compatibility with all non-controversial axioms of the EUM, and (b) compatibility with empirical observations contradicting the EUM, like the Allais Paradox,[11,12,14] dependence of "utility" on probability,[11] preference reversals,[18] certainty effects and other violations.[20]

From a different vantage point, the LMM radically departs from most theories of choice with respect to the most fundamental and implicit assumption: the description of the problem. Indeed, current models invariably use an analytic representation for the PDF, either by listing the mass probabilities or the complementary cumulative distribution function (CCPDF). Axioms of those theories refer, therefore, to preferences over probabilities; for instance, axioms 3 and 6 (continuity and monotonicity) in L-R.[6] The same approach is present even in theories opposing the EUM, like the axiom of absolute preference proposed by Allais (see Ref. 13, p. 457) and discussed by Munera.[21]

Contrarywise, the LMM describes PDFs synthetically by using linearized moments M_k, monotonically related to the moments around some reference point m_k by

$$M_k = m_k^{1/k} \tag{5}$$

Both representations for PDFs, analytic and synthetic, are completely equivalent; choosing one representation or another is a matter of convenience. Therefore, some of the axioms and definitions in the LMM must refer to preferences over moments rather than to preferences over probabilities.[19] For example, in the LMM two alternatives A and B are equivalent if $M_k(A) = M_k(B)$ for all $k = 1, 2, ..., 2n+1$.

Assuming a complete ordering over deterministic consequences is standard practice in all theories of choice leading to preference indices. For instance, in L-R it is axiom 1. In the LMM it is also assumed that there exists a deterministic index of dispreference $h(.)$ mapping sure outcomes $z \in Z$ onto the real line such that if outcome a is preferred to outcome b, then $h(a) < h(b)$, and conversely. Index $h(.)$ is a "riskless" construct similar to the value functions discussed by Keeney and Raiffa (see Ref. 22, Chapter 3) and Krzysztofowicz[23]; $h(.)$ encodes the strength of dispreference and does not have any risk content whatsoever. Hence, in general, $h(.)$ is not equivalent to the utility function $u(.)$ of the EUM.

It is further assumed that individual decision makers (DMs) are capable of assigning certainty equivalents $c \in Z$ behaviorally equivalent to the non-deterministic alternatives $A(Z;P)$. This assumption effectively maps the space (Z,P) onto the real line; in symbols: $h(c) = H(A)$, where $H(.)$ is a functional.

The functional $H(A)$ proposed by Munera[11,14,19,20] and Munera and deNeufville[12] is a LMM. For prospects leading to monetary losses most individuals are consistent with the following version of the LMM[20]:

$$H(A) = h(z_0) + \sum_k r_k M_k , \tag{6}$$

where $k = 1,2,...,2n+1$ and

$$m_k = \sum_j p_j \, [h(z_i) - h(z_0)]^k = \sum_j p_j \, [h_j - h_0]^k . \tag{7}$$

For descriptive purposes a three-moments model (TMM)[20] suffices:

$$H(A) - h_0 = r_1 M_1 + r_2 M_2 + r_3 M_3 . \tag{8}$$

Note that the moments are over preference indices $h(.)$, relative to some reference state z_0. The coefficients r_k are the attitude-towards-randomness (ATR) parameters, different for each individual, obtained by fitting Eq. (6) to observation. This means that each individual is represented by a point in a $(2n+1)$-dimensional ATR-space, which for the TMM is 3-dimensional. Without further restrictions the LMM of Eq. (6) — or the TMM of Eq. (8) — is a descriptive model only with a very high descriptive capability, but without axiomatic foundations. In the following section it will be shown that there are regions of the ATR-space that are forbidden by the introduction of axioms which the author prefers to call prescriptive conditions.

The Prescriptive Conditions

Let us define homogeneous and heterogeneous alternatives. For each individual, let the consequence set Z be partitioned into three subsets relative to his current status: favorable (Z_f), neutral (Z_n), and unfavorable (Z_u) consequences. The corresponding probability subsets are P_f, P_n, and P_u, respectively. Three groups belong in the class of homogeneous alternatives: (a) if P_u is empty, the alternative is favorable; (b) if P_f is empty, the alternative is unfavorable; and (c) if both conditions apply, the alternative is neutral which is the trivial case of an alternative behaviorally equivalent to current conditions. The class of heterogeneous alternatives is defined by both P_u and P_f being non-empty.

The simplest non-degenerate homogeneous alternatives are gains $G = (g,0; p,1-p)$ and losses $L = (l,0; p,1-p)$, and the simplest heterogeneous prospect is a lottery ticket $T = (g,l; p,1-p)$, where g and l respectively are favorable and unfavorable outcomes, and $p>0$.

Let us now restrict attention to particular individuals, defined by being consistent with some prescriptive conditions, which may be imposed one at a time or several simultaneously.

Monotonicity. Consider lottery tickets $T = (g,l; p,1-p)$ and $T' = (g,l; p',1-p')$. Monotonicity requires that T be preferred to T' if $p>p'$, and conversely. This condition is similar to the L-R model's axiom 6 and is a restricted form of first-degree stochastic dominance (FDSD).

Continuity. Consider lottery ticket T as above. For any consequence z in $[l,g]$, it is possible to find a p in $[0,1]$ such that z is the certainty equivalent of T.

Attitude-Towards-Security. Even for simple alternatives like G, L, and T, there is empirical evidence[9] suggesting the existence of a "certainty effect," i.e., a discontinuity at $p = 1$. To avoid misunderstandings in the interpretation of this expression (sometimes linked to mid-probability effects), the following expressions are used interchangeably in this paper: "certainty effect," "security effect," and "attitude towards security." For a given individual, let g^* and l^* be the certainty equivalents of G and L, respectively when $p \to 1$. Three cases are possible for each alternative: g^* (>=<) g and l^* (>=<) 1, for a total of nine different behavioral patterns. *A priori*, one would expect that some patterns would be observed more often than others. In the following we list several behavioral descriptions and the corresponding interpretation as a security effect:

- "Preference for security in the neighborhood of sure gains" is discussed by Allais (Ref. 13, pp. 88-92). Attitude towards security: $g^* < g$ with no restrictions on L.

- "Preference for randomness in the neighborhood of sure losses" is the opposite twin of the previous case. Attitude towards security: $l^* > l$ with no restrictions on G. These two descriptions together correspond to the "reflection effect" discussed long ago by Friedman and Savage[24] and more recently by Kahneman and Tversky.[9]

- "An almost sure loss is a sure loss, but an almost sure gain is not a sure gain" is the pessimistic condition discussed by this author elsewhere.[11,12] Attitude towards security: $l^* = l$ and $g^* \neq g$. In relation to Kahneman and Tversky's certainty effect,[9] pessimism is equivalent to a certainty effect for favorable prospects only.

- "An almost sure gain is a sure gain, but an almost sure loss is not a sure loss" is the author's optimistic condition.[11,12] Attitude towards security: $g^* = g$ and $l^* \neq l$. Optimism is equivalent to certainty effect for unfavorable prospects only. Optimism and pessimism may be grouped under the single heading of "partial consistency with certainty."

- "Full consistency with certainty" is the same continuity condition present in the EUM. Attitude towards security: $g^* = g$ and $l^* = l$. Out of the nine patterns, this is the only case that does not depict any certainty effect.

There are two extreme subcases that I expect to be exhibited by a very small fraction of DMs, namely:

- Randomness abhorrence: a DM would pay for not receiving G. Attitude towards security: $g^* < 0$.

- Randomness propensity: a DM would pay for receiving L. Attitude towards security: $l^* > 0$.

First-Degree Stochastic Dominance (FDSD). The LMM is compatible with partial FDSD over homogeneous alternatives. In fact, the model contained in Eq. (6) exhibits FDSD over favorable prospects provided that all ATR-parameters be non-negative.[14] Note that the FDSD condition is valid in one direction only, i.e., the LMM is compatible with FDSD for homogeneous prospects, but the LMM does not imply FDSD.[21]

It is worth stressing that in the EUM, FDSD is imposed for all alternatives (both homogeneous and heterogeneous). The LMM is also compatible with such strong requirement by simply letting all even ATR-parameters be zero: $r_2 = r_4 = ... = 0$. This leads to a large class of LMMs containing odd-order linearized moments only; clearly, the EUM is the simplest case.

Let us now present two examples of ATR-spaces for the TMM. Figure 1 shows the space compatible with monotonicity, continuity and optimism[11,12,14] while Fig. 2 is the ATR-space compatible with partial FDSD, consistent with certainty for gains and excluding randomness propensity.[20]

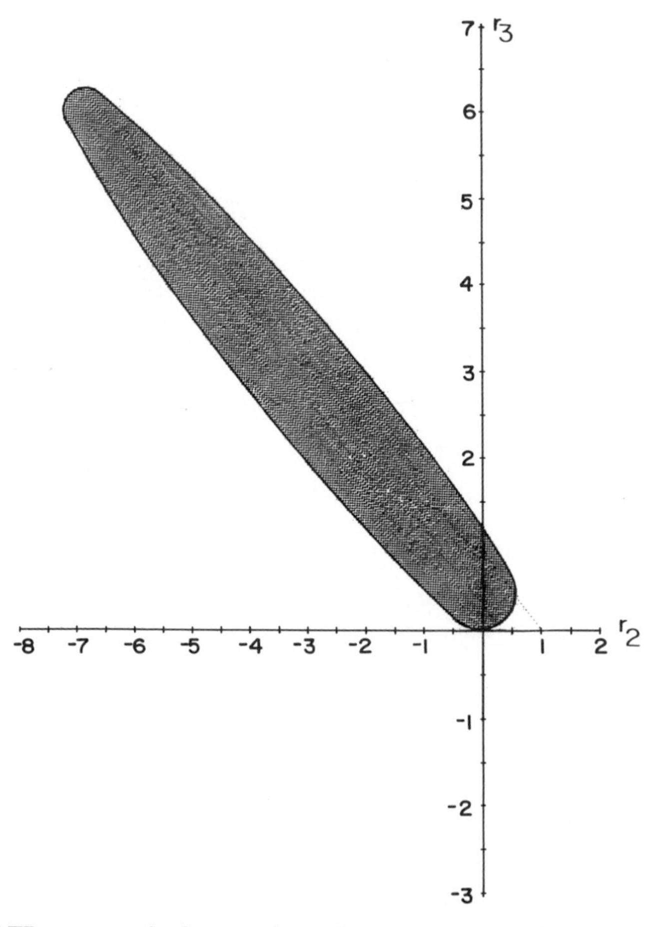

Fig. 1. ATR-space: attitude-towards-randomness space. Individuals consistent with monotonicity, continuity, and optimism.

From previous discussion, it should be obvious that the size and shape of the feasible region changes with the number and strength of the prescriptive requirements. For instance, if full consistency with FDSD is imposed then the ATR-space reduces to the vertical axis, which is further reduced by imposing the substitution principle, thus obtaining the EUM, whose feasible region is just the point (1,0,0). (This is the origin in Figs. 1 and 2.)

To assess the individual ATR-parameters, the very same methods used for the assessment of utility in the EUM may be used. Typically p-prospects and 50-50 prospects are used. For details see Munera.[11,20]

CONCLUSION

In this paper I briefly described the LMM which is consistent with a set of prescriptive conditions similar to the axioms of EUM. On the descriptive side the LMM explains the main criticisms addressed to the EUM and predicts many of the empirical observations violating the predictions of the EUM.

A model similar to the EUM is obtained by taking $r_1 = 1$ and all other ATR-parameters equal to 0. The expected value model is a further subcase when $h(z) = z$. Prospect theory is based on simple prospects (G and L in our notation). For these the LMM reduces to a product $s(p)f(z)$ which is the same prospect theory, except that $s(p)$ is a function of objective probability and not a subjective and/or defective probability as interpreted by Kahneman and Tversky.[9]

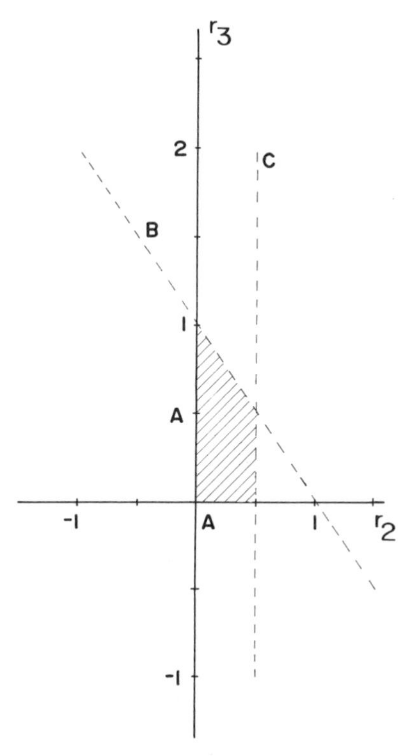

Fig. 2. ATR-space: attitude-towards-randomness space. Individuals compatible with (a) FDSD for favorable prospects, (b) consistency with certainty for gains, and (c) exclusion of randomness propensity.

To conclude, I mention several advantages that the TMM has, in my view, over other competing decision models:

- The probability is given exogenously and may be related to physical realities only.[25]
- Empirical parameters are few (only two). This may be contrasted with subjective probability approaches where the whole probability distribution becomes a set of parameters to be fitted.
- It has the capability of explaining both favorable and unfavorable prospects with a single general model.[20]
- It has the capability of incorporating directly as part of the prescriptive conditions the individual attitude-towards-security, which simply is the experimentally observed violation of continuity at certainty.

REFERENCES

1. M. McCord and R. de Neufville, Fundamental Deficiency of Expected Utility Decision Analysis, in *Multi-Objective Decision Making*, S. French, L. C. Thomas, R. Hartley, and D. J. White, eds., Academic Press, London (1983).
2. M. Cohen, J. Y. Jaffray, and T. Said, Individual Behavior Under Risk and Under Uncertainty: An Experimental Study, *Theory and Decision* **18**:203-228 (1985).
3. H. A. Munera, Expected Value Optimization Decreases Deaths But May Shorten Survival, *Risk Analysis* **9**:17-19 (1989).
4. D. Bernouilli, Exposition of a New Theory on the Measurement of Risk, translated from Latin in 1738 by L. Sommer, *Econometrica* **22**:22-36 (1954).
5. J. von Neumann and O. Morgenstern, *Theory of Games and Economic Behavior*, Princeton University Press, 3rd. ed., Science Editions, John Wiley & Sons, New York (1964).
6. R. D. Luce and H. Raiffa, *Games and Decisions*, John Wiley and Sons, Inc., 2nd printing, New York (1958).
7. L. J. Savage, *The Foundations of Statistics*, 2nd revised ed., Dover Publications, New York (1972).
8. O. Hagen, A New Axiomatization of Utility Under Risk, *Teorie a Metoda* **IV(2)**:55-80 (1972).
9. D. Kahneman and A. Tversky, Prospect Theory: An Analysis of Decision Under Risk, *Econometrica* **47**:263-291 (March, 1979).
10. E. F. McClennen, Sure-Thing Doubts, in *Foundations of Utility and Risk Theory with Applications*, B. P. Stigum and F. Wenstop, eds., D. Reidel Publishing Co., Dordrecht, Holland (1983).
11. H. A. Munera, Modeling of Individual Risk Attitudes in Decision Making under Uncertainty: An Application to Nuclear Power, Ph.D. dissertation, Department of Engineering, University of California, Berkeley, California (September 1978).
12. H. A. Munera and R. de Neufville, A Decision Analysis Model When the Substitution Principle Is Not Acceptable, in *Foundations of Utility and Risk Theory with Applications*, B. P. Stigum and F. Wenstop, eds., D. Reidel Publishing Co., Dordrecht, Holland (1983).
13. M. Allais, The Foundations of a Positive Theory of Choice Involving Risk and a Criticism of the Postulates and Axioms of the American School, in *Expected Utility Hypotheses and the Allais Paradox*, M. Allais and O. Hagen, eds., D. Reidel Publishing Co, Dordrecht, Holland (1979).
14. H. A. Munera, The Generalized Means Model (GMM) for Non-Deterministic Decision Making: Its Normative and Descriptive Power, Including Sketch of the Representation Theorem, *Theory and Decision* **18**:173-202 (1985).

15. S. Lichtenstein and P. Slovic, Reversals of Preference Between Bids and Choices in Gambling Decisions, *Journal of Experimental Psychology* **89**:46-55 (1971).
16. H. R. Lindman, Inconsistent Preferences Among Gambles, *Journal of Experimental Psychology* **89**:390-97 (1971).
17. P. Slovic and S. Lichtenstein, Preference Reversals: A Broader Perspective, *The American Economic Review* **73**:596-605 (September 1983).
18. H. A. Munera, Prediction of 'Preference Reversals' by the Linearized Moments Model, in *Understanding Economic Behavior*, K. G. Grunert and F. Olander, eds., D. Reidel Publishing Co., Dordrecht, Holland (in press).
19. H. A. Munera, A Theory for Technological Risk Comparisons, in *Risk Analysis as a Decision Tool*, G. Yadigaroglu and S. Chakraborthy, eds., Verlag TUeV Rheinland, Cologne (1985).
20. H. A. Munera, A Large Scale Empirical Test for the Linearized Moments Model (LMM): Compatibility Between Theory and Observation, in *Risk, Decision and Rationality*, B. R. Munier, ed., D. Reidel Publishing Co., Dordrecht, Holland (1988).
21. H. A. Munera, On Absolute Preference and Stochastic Dominance, *Theory and Decision* **21**:85-88 (1986).
22. R. L. Keeney and H. Raiffa, *Decisions with Multiple Objectives: Preferences and Value Tradeoffs*, John Wiley, New York (1976).
23. R. Krzysztofowicz, Risk Attitude Hypotheses of Utility Theory, in *Foundations of Utility and Risk Theory with Applications*, B. P. Stigum and F. Wenstop, eds., D. Reidel Publishers, Dordrecht, Holland (1983).
24. M. Friedman and L. J. Savage, The Utility Analysis of Choice Involving Risk, *J. Pol. Econ.* **56**:279-304 (1948).
25. H. A. Munera, A Deterministic Event Tree Approach to Uncertainty, Randomness and Probability in Individual Chance Processes, *Theory and Decision* (in press).

Strength of Preference and Risky Utility: An Empirical Study of Hazardous Waste Facility Siting

Thomas H. Hatfield
California State University
Northridge, CA

ABSTRACT

This paper presents evidence that a strength of preference function is not equivalent to a risky utility function. The differences between these functions, referred to as "relative" risk premiums, may provide a more accurate measure of attitudes toward uncertainty. A questionnaire distributed in Oklahoma used direct ratings and lotteries to evaluate the potential siting of a hazardous waste incinerator. Three attributes were evaluated: transportation distance, population, and cost of development. For the population attribute, statistically significant differences were found between direct ratings and lotteries, and between risk premiums and relative risk premiums. The distinctions between strength of preference and risky utility are shown to be both plausible and useful for hazardous waste management. An important remaining task is to determine when these differences should be measured for other attributes and for other policy issues.

KEYWORDS: Risk premium, relative risk premium, strength of preference, hazardous waste incinerator, risky utility

INTRODUCTION

This paper examines the relationship between a strength of preference function and a risky utility function. Broadly speaking, the former function measures preferences among known consequences (e.g., direct ratings) while the latter considers uncertain consequences (e.g., lotteries). In a long standing debate, numerous authors have argued that risky utility may not measure the strength of preference among consequences.[1-6] Others have argued that the two functions are equivalent.[7-10] Formal conditions have been derived for establishing equivalence between these two functions;[11] however, surprisingly little data have been presented that address this issue.

This debate can be critical to the assessment of attitudes toward risk. For example, if these two functions are equivalent, then analysts may use a variety of assessment techniques, and differences in assessments may be attributed to method variance or assessment error. However, if these two functions are not equivalent, then their differences may provide an important measure of attitudes toward uncertainty.[11] This measure, referred to as a "relative" risk premium, is formally defined in the next section. Given the

Risk Analysis, Edited by C. Zervos
Plenum Press, New York, 1991

uncertainties of risk analysis, an improved measure of attitudes toward uncertainty is worth careful consideration, and different sides of the debate have called for empirical studies on this question.[10,11]

This paper presents evidence that a strength of preference function may not be equivalent to a risky utility function. The evidence was gathered from a questionnaire on siting a hazardous waste incinerator in Oklahoma. A crucial finding of this study is that the data are robust to potential errors of assessment. Moreover, by drawing on existing rhetoric of hazardous waste issues, the case is presented that these differences are not only statistically significant, but also represent plausible distinctions that are important to hazardous waste management.

This paper proceeds with four major sections. The next section provides a more formal set of definitions for strength of preference, risky utility, and theoretical distinctions between the two. The subsequent section describes the evaluation attributes, assessment methods, statistical tests, and participants in the study. The ensuing section presents answers to two statistical questions:

1. Are there differences between risky utility and strength of preference? and
2. Are there differences between risk premiums and "relative" risk premiums?

Finally, the last section relates these results to the rhetoric of hazardous waste issues, and objections to relative risk premiums are addressed in this context. I conclude with suggestions for further research.

STRENGTH OF PREFERENCE AND RISKY UTILITY

Strength of preference [denoted $v(x)$] refers to the relative value of consequences rather than the absolute value for a single consequence. This approach focuses on the "closeness" or "similarity" of preferences for consequences, rather than statements that one consequence is "twice as good" as another.[11] Strength of preference can be assessed by various techniques, including direct ratings.[12]

A utility function under risk [denoted $u(x)$] introduces lotteries as a basis for assessing attitudes. Utility functions are assessed by various techniques, including a 50-50 lottery between most preferred consequence x'' and least preferred consequence x', denoted (x'', x'). For example, suppose that a decision maker believes x is equally desirable to lottery (x'', x'). We refer to x as the "certainty equivalent" of (x'', x'). Furthermore, if we set $u(x'') = 1$ and $u(x') = 0$, then $u(x) = 0.5$.

Using this notation, risk aversion can be measured by the risk premium (RP), which is the difference between the certainty equivalent x and the expected value of the 50-50 lottery Eq. (1). In contrast, the relative risk premium (RRP) is the difference between risky utility $u(x)$ and strength of preference $v(x)$ Eq. (2). For the sake of comparison, RP can be normalized to the same scale as RRP Eq. (3).

$$\mathrm{RP} = x - [(x'' + x') / 2] \tag{1}$$

$$\mathrm{RRP} = u(x) - v(x) \tag{2}$$

$$\mathrm{RP} = [(x-x') / (x''-x')] - 1/2 \tag{3}$$

Relying on these definitions, we can rephrase the two statistical questions raised in the introduction:

1. Does $u(x) = v(x)$? and
2. Does RP = RRP?

This notation will help clarify the subsequent study design. For example, it is crucial to recognize that the above two questions are not equivalent. If each question can be answered yes or no, this creates four possible cases (yes/yes, yes/no, no/yes, and no/no). The first case (yes/yes) can be met only by linear functions of $u(x)$ and $v(x)$. An informal proof for this theorem relies on the definition of RRP Eq. (2) and the two conditions that define the first case Eqs. (4) and (5):

$$\text{RRP} = u(x) - v(x) \tag{2}$$

$$u(x) = v(x) \tag{4}$$

$$\text{RP} = \text{RRP} \tag{5}$$

Replacing Eq. (2) with Eqs. (4) and (5):

$$\text{RP} = 0 \tag{6}$$

If RP = 0, then $u(x)$ is defined as a linear, risk neutral function. Because of Eq. (4), $v(x)$ is also a linear function.

In the second case (yes/no), $u(x) = v(x)$ but RP does not equal RRP. Thus, RRP = 0 [$u(x) = v(x)$], but RP does not equal 0 (RP does not equal RRP). However, an important question for empirical testing is whether $u(x) = v(x)$ for all applications. This constitutes our first statistical question.

In the third case (no/yes), RP = RRP but $u(x)$ does not equal $v(x)$. Thus, both RRP and RP do not equal 0. In this case, RRP is redundant of RP. The critical question here is whether RRP always equals RP. This constitutes our second statistical question.

The least restrictions apply to the fourth case (no/no). The next section elaborates on how each of these conditions was verified in actual assessments.

DESIGN OF THE STUDY

Three attributes were selected for evaluation: transportation distance, population, and cost of development (see Table 1). "Transportation distance" was defined as the average distance from industrial centers to a proposed incinerator site. In Oklahoma, this was determined to be 0 to 300 miles. "Population" was defined as the number of residents within 5 miles of an incinerator site. A range of 0 to 500,000 was derived from demographic records. "Cost of development" represented a composite of cost categories, which included costs for preparing the site, installing the incinerator, and complying with regulations. A cost of 20 to 70 million dollars was estimated for a rotary kiln incinerator handling 70,000 tons per year.[13] The strength of preferences within each criterion was assessed by direct ratings. The technique used in the questionnaire is illustrated below in Fig. 1.

A major objection to the relative risk premium is that method variance and measurement error will overshadow any distinctions between these two measures.[10] This argument is especially formidable because it may be impossible to account for all possible assessment errors. However, close attention to potential sources of error may test the robustness of any assessed differences. Consequently, this concern was addressed by

Table 1. Attributes

Transportation Distance	Population	Cost of Development
0 miles	0	$20 million
50 miles	100	$30 million
100 miles	1,000	$40 million
150 miles	10,000	$45 million
200 miles	100,000	$50 million
250 miles	250,000	$60 million
300 miles	500,000	$70 million

Assume that an incinerator is proposed at a site with one of the "residential populations" shown below. Using the following scale, indicate your "direct ratings" for each of these populations. PLEASE BE SURE TO USE BOTH A "0" AND A "10" IN YOUR EVALUATION.

Direct Rating Scale

least preferred — most preferred

0 1 2 3 4 5 6 7 8 9 10

Residential Population	Direct Ratings
0 residents	______
100 residents	______
1,000 residents	______
10,000 residents	______
100,000 residents	______
250,000 residents	______
500,000 residents	______

Fig. 1. Direct ratings.

assessing the certainty equivalent for lottery (x'', x') as a range between L (low value of the certainty equivalent) and H (high value of the certainty equivalent), where:

$$H \text{ is preferred to } (x'', x'), \text{ and} \tag{7}$$

$$(x'', x') \text{ is preferred to } L\,.$$

The technique used in the questionnaire is illustrated below in Fig. 2. This approach can account for substantial measurement error, because the certainty equivalent x is treated as any point between L and H. In comparing $u(x)$ with $v(x)$, we set both $u(L) = 0.5$ and $u(H) = 0.5$.

```
In the appropriate boxes below, indicate your preference
for Site 1 or Site 2. If both sites are equally appealing
to you, mark both boxes. Your answers will not imply that
any of these sites are acceptable. We are interested only
in how you evaluate uncertain conditions.

|__| Site 1                                  |__| Site 2

50% chance of 500,000 residents          250,000 residents
50% chance of       0 residents
----------------------------------------------------------
|__| Site 1                                  |__| Site 2

50% chance of 500,000 residents          100,000 residents
50% chance of       0 residents
----------------------------------------------------------
|__| Site 1                                  |__| Site 2

50% chance of 500,000 residents          10,000 residents
50% chance of       0 residents
----------------------------------------------------------
|__| Site 1                                  |__| Site 2

50% chance of 500,000 residents          1,000 residents
50% chance of       0 residents
----------------------------------------------------------
|__| Site 1                                  |__| Site 2

50% chance of 500,000 residents          100 residents
50% chance of       0 residents
```

Fig. 2. Lotteries.

The corresponding $v(L)$ and $v(H)$ were determined by direct ratings on a scale of 0 to 10 that were normalized to a scale of 0 to 1. Assessment errors in $v(x)$ were addressed by changing the direct ratings of 4 or 6 to 5. Consequently, $v(x)$ differed from $u(x)$ [at both $u(L) = 0.5$ and $u(H) = 0.5$] only if $u(x) - v(x) > 0.1$ on a scale of 0 to 1. In other words, at the low certainty equivalent (L):

$$\begin{aligned} \text{define:} \quad & u(L) = 0.5 \\ \text{if:} \quad & v(L) = 0.5 \ \ (\text{or } 0.4 \text{ to } 0.6) \\ \text{then:} \quad & v(x) = u(x) \ \ (\text{at } L) \end{aligned}$$

The above conditions were repeated for the high certainty equivalent (H).

Sign tests addressed the statistical questions raised in the introduction. For the first question, if $v(x)$ is not equivalent to $u(x)$, then paired comparisons between $v(x)$ and $u(x)$ should be significantly different. For the second question, if RRP is different from RP, then paired comparisons between RRP and RP should be significantly different.

Participants were distinguished by membership in environmental organizations (e.g., Sierra Club, Audubon Society). However, this sample was not intended to survey a region. The statistical differences in this analysis are useful for the questions in this paper, but they cannot lead to appropriate conclusions about the distribution of attitudes in Oklahoma.

RESULTS

Eighty-seven questionnaires were received. Of the mailed samples, the overall response rate was 71%, and the differences in response rates among identified groups were not statistically significant. Respondents identified themselves as members of environmental groups or as non-members.

Paired comparisons of $u(x)$ with $v(x)$ are shown in Table 2. For the majority of respondents, $u(x) = v(x)$ for transportation distance and cost of development. Furthermore, the remaining respondents did not suggest any trend of $v(x)$ being less than or greater than $u(x)$. However, for the "population" attribute, $v(x)$ was less than $u(x)$ for a majority of respondents, and the differences were statistically significant.

An additional distinction, however, became apparent in assessing $v(x)$ and $u(x)$ — direct ratings were not always monotonically increasing or decreasing. Under such conditions, $u(x)$ cannot be assessed as a monotonic function. Without the direct ratings, this limitation could not have been ascertained from the $u(x)$ assessments. Therefore, both functions may be useful for a more accurate interpretation of responses.

Using only monotonic functions, paired comparisons of RP and RRP showed no statistically significant differences for transportation distance or cost of development (Table 3). However, a significant difference was found in paired comparisons within the criterion "population." Also, the range of RP was risk prone while the range of RRP was relative risk averse (Table 4).

DISCUSSION

The evidence from this study supports the argument that a strength of preference function may differ from a risky utility function. For the attribute "population," this difference is statistically significant even when we account for substantial assessment error. Furthermore, statistically significant differences were found between risk premiums and relative risk premiums (for "population," the average RP was risk prone, whereas the average RRP was risk averse).

Given the risk averse rhetoric on population exposure near hazardous waste facilities, RRP appears to measure risk aversion more accurately. However, this does not explain why the risk premiums indicated risk proneness. A likely explanation for this outcome is that the lottery in the questionnaire offered a 50% chance for 0 population and a 50% chance for 500,000. Most participants were so opposed to any population near a facility that they preferred a 50% chance of 0 population to even an extremely small population. Consequently, their preferences for the lottery made them appear risk prone. Situations like this may not be interpreted correctly if analysts rely exclusively on the risk premium measure.

Von Winterfeldt and Edwards[10] have offered four major reasons for dismissing any distinction between strength of preference and risky utility. In light of the evidence presented, it may be useful to re-evaluate their reasoning. First, they argue that there are no "sure things" in life, and therefore all evaluations imply risk. For example, a respondent may offer direct ratings for "known" consequences with the knowledge that these consequences are not "sure things." However, it may be more appropriate to say there are different levels of uncertainty — for example, some hazardous waste facilities may be more thoroughly investigated than others. These levels of uncertainty should be distinguished and apparently have been distinguished by the evidence in this paper.

Second, they argue that risk aversion can be explained by diminishing marginal utility. For example, a risk averse utility function may simply represent a strength of preference function with diminishing marginal utility. However, this argument supports the need for both assessments, because the relative risk premium may be a more accurate

Table 2. Paired Comparisons of $v(x)$ and $u(x)$

Attributes	% of participants $v(x)<u(x)$	$v(x)=u(x)$	$v(x)>u(x)$	p*
Transportation Distance	19%	57%	24%	.81
Population	57%	38%	5%	.00
Cost of Development	12%	64%	24%	.30

*Sign test.

Table 3. Risk Premium (RP) versus Relative Risk Premium (RRP)

Attributes	% of participants RP<RRP	RP=RRP	RP>RRP	p*
Transportation Distance	12%	74%	14%	1.00
Population	60%	38%	2%	.00
Cost of Development	7%	79%	14%	.50

*Sign test.

Table 4. Risk Premium (RP) versus Relative Risk Premium (RRP)

Attributes		Mean Values* low	high
Transportation Distance	RP	–.23	.18
	RRP	–.09	.12
Population	RP	–.61	–.01
	RRP	.19	.34
Cost of Development	RP	–.18	.17
	RRP	–.06	.14

*Positive values denote risk aversion.

reflection of risk aversion (in their particular example, RRP would equal 0). Indeed, numerous evaluations from the Oklahoma questionnaire replicated their example.

Third, they argue that most decisions are repetitive in nature, and risk aversion disappears with repetitive choices. However, not all decisions are equally repetitive. The siting of a major facility may affect an area for decades and therefore may not be a highly repetitive choice. Moreover, some individuals make more risk decisions than others. This may result in different attitudes toward uncertainty, and these differences should be evaluated more accurately.

Perhaps their most challenging argument is that assessment errors overshadow the distinctions between value and utility (e.g., direct ratings and lotteries). Of course, there may be circumstances where distinctions between value and utility are indeed spurious, and analysts must be cautious in their interpretation of relative risk premiums. However, assessment error may not adequately explain the differences observed in this study. Some of these distinctions are quite strong, even if we account for substantial assessment error. Moreover, these differences appear plausible and even useful to hazardous waste management.

Clearly, further empirical studies are needed. However, this paper demonstrates that a distinction between strength of preference and risky utility can be measured, and it can reflect important policy issues. The essential question, then, is not whether to distinguish these measures in general but to understand when it is important to attempt a distinction in the first place.

An important clue for answering this question may lie in the nature of the population attribute. As Dyer and Sarin[12] have suggested, attributes that exhibit extreme convexity of assessed attitudes may be the very attributes where relative risk premium is different from risk premium. In fact, Dyer and Sarin predicted that the population attribute would exhibit these characteristics.

In searching for other attributes where relative risk premium is a distinctive measure, the outcome undoubtedly will depend on the particular decision problem, the definition of a particular attribute, and the population being sampled. Empirical studies are needed in other areas that will refine our answers to this important question.

REFERENCES

1. D. Ellsberg, Classic and Current Notions of Measurable Utility, *Econ. J.* **64**:528-556 (1954).
2. R. D. Luce and H. Raiffa, *Games and Decisions*, Wiley, New York (1956). W. H. Baumol, The Cardinal Utility Which Is Ordinal, *Econ. J.* **68**:665-672 (1958).
3. K. J. Arrow, *Social Choice and Individual Values*, 2nd ed., Wiley, New York (1963).
4. P. C. Fishburn, Utility Theory with Inexact Preferences and Degrees of Preference, *Synthese* **21**:204-221 (1970).
5. P. C. Fishburn, *Utility Theory for Decision Making*, Wiley, New York (1970).
6. J. S. Dyer, W. Farrel, and P. Bradley, Utility Functions for Test Performance, *Mgmt. Sci.* **20**:507-519 (1973).
7. W. Edwards, Public Values: Multi-Attribute Utility Measurement for Social Decision Making, in *Conflicting Objectives*, D. Bell, R. Keeney, and H. Raiffa, eds., Wiley, New York (1977).
8. J. C. Harsanyi, Bayesian Decision Theory and Utilitarian Ethics, *Am. Econ. Rev. Papers and Proc.* p. 68 (1978).

9. D. von Winterfeldt and W. Edwards, *Decision Analysis and Behavioral Research*, Cambridge University Press, New York (1986).
10. R. K. Sarin, Strength of Preference and Risky Choice, *Operations Research* **30(5)**:982-996 (1982).
11. J. S. Dyer and R. K. Sarin, Measuring Risk Attitudes in Risk Analysis, in *Risk Evaluation and Management*, V. Covello, J. Menkes, and J. Mumpower, eds., Plenum, New York (1986).
12. California Air Resources Board, Southern California Hazardous Waste Incineration: A Feasibility Study (1984).

Risk Aversion and Utility Function of Health: Experimental Determinations

Thomas Tam
City University of New York
New York, NY

ABSTRACT

This paper examines the utility values assigned by individuals to different states of health involving risk-taking behaviors in seeking medical treatment. Findings are based on surveys of various socio-economic-cultural groups in New York City: Chinatown residents, college students, and graduate public health students. Two scales of value measurement, category scaling, and standard gamble were used to compare respondents' values. Scores from the two scales were found to have a monotonic relationship. The difference in values between the two scales was used as a measure of risk aversion.

It was found that higher education and income were related to higher risk aversion. The hypothesis that respondents who worked longer hours would be less risk averse was confirmed among Chinese respondents, implying a tradeoff between health and financial security. Between respondents who worked and those who did not work, differences were significant at the 0.05 level in category scaling, and not significant in standard gamble. The notion of risk aversion and utility function of health was further examined in other groups in relation to their health status and behaviors.

KEYWORDS: Risk aversion, category scaling, standard gamble, utility function of health, value measurement

INTRODUCTION

The construction of health status index as a rational approach to the allocation of scarce resources, has its intellectual genesis in Jeremy Bantham, the 18th century founder of the Utilitarian school of economics. The belief that an individual derives happiness, or utility from the possession of money has led to the development of a theoretical system whereby resources may be allocated in such a way so that the happiness, or welfare of a society is maximized.

The construction of a social welfare function based only on money income and the associated happiness may sound somewhat simple minded. A firmer foundation is possible if an individual's health can be viewed as the manifestation of happiness. Not only does health affect an individual's consumption and production activities which have important economic consequences, but it lends itself to a more objective measurement than the elusive notion of happiness. While interpersonal comparison of happiness may be questionable,[1]

Risk Analysis, Edited by C. Zervos
Plenum Press, New York, 1991

interpersonal comparison of health should leave less room for argument. To define a society's health status as an aggregation of all the individuals' health states may provide a more acceptable basis for the construction of a social welfare function.

TWO APPROACHES TO THE CONSTRUCTION OF HEALTH STATUS INDEX

Since the sixties, health researchers have set out to gather quantitative data and to construct health indicators to describe society's health status. Two basic approaches can be distinguished. The one headed by Chiang,[2] Chen,[3] and Linder,[4] focused on the amount of time lost due to mortality and morbidity. The approach pioneered by Sullivan[5] on the other hand, did not dwell on morbidity and mortality per se, but on their effects on a person's ability to function physically, mentally and socially.

Sullivan's approach has been further elaborated by other researchers.[6] It is also the approach adopted in the present study because it appeared to be more comprehensive and promising. In essence, health is assumed to be a continuum stretching from death to total well-being. Certain points on this continuum, or health states, can be defined. If an individual's preference ratings for this series of health states are known, and if at the same time, the distribution of a population among these health states is also known, then the individual will be able to assign a value indicating the health status of the population. Let m be the finite number of states selected from the health continuum, h_i be the quantity of health contained in the ith state, $U(h_i)$ be the value of the ith state, n_i be the number of persons who are in the ith state. Then, an individual's health status index for the population at time t, may be defined by the following summation:

$$H(t) = \sum_{i=1}^{m} U(h_i)\, n_i(t) \ .$$

It should be clear that for individuals with different sets of values, the health status index will be different accordingly.

HEALTH VIGNETTE CONSTRUCTION

The health vignettes used in this study were originally constructed by Patrick,[7] and later adopted by the Health Policy Project of the University of California, San Diego. They were translated into Chinese language for the non-English speaking residents of Chinatown.

The thirty vignettes which are the major concerns of the survey, describe specific days in the lives of people who were in various states of health (see Tables 1 and 2). Each vignette refers to a different person and is made up of five components: age, mobility, physical activity, social activity and symptoms or problem complexes. Each vignette contains information about the age group in which the person falls, what activities he performed, what symptoms or problems he had, and whether or not he could travel freely or was confined to the house, hospital, or special care unit on that day. The thirty vignettes are combinations of different levels of these five components, representing various levels of health or well-being. They can be viewed as "snap shots" of particular points in the health continuum.

CARDINAL UTILITY AND ITS MEASUREMENT

A major point of research interest focused on the value of these health vignettes. Past surveys by researchers[8,9] have indicated that such values were highly stable over time. Controversy remained, however. On the one hand, the validity of measurement has been reinforced by a convergence of values obtained through different methods such as category

Table 1. Vignette Descriptions

No.	Age	Mobility	Physical Activity	Social Activity	Symptom and Problem Complexes
1	School Age 6-17	Needed more help than usual for age to use car, bus or train.	Walked with physical limitations	Did school work but limited in other activities	Pain in chest, stomach, side, back or hips
2	Adult 18-64	Confined in house	Moved own wheelchair without help	Needed help with self-care activities	Burn over large areas of face, body, arms or legs
3	Older Adult 65+	Unable to drive or needed help to use bus or train	Walked without physical problems	Limited in amount or kind of work or housework	Pain or discomfort in one or both eyes, such as burning or itching
4	School Age 6-17	Confined in hospital	Walked with physical limitations	Performed self-care as usual for age, but not schoolwork	General tiredness, weakness, or weight loss
5	School Age 6-17	Confined in special care unit	Walked with physical limitations	Performed self-care as usual for age, but not schoolwork	One foot or leg missing, deformed, paralyzed, or broken, include wearing artificial limbs or braces
6	School Age 6-17	Confined in special care unit	Walked without physical problems	Performed self-care as usual for age, but not schoolwork	One hand or arm missing, deformed, paralyzed, or broken, include wearing artificial limbs or braces
7	Small Child < 6	Used car, bus or train as usual for age	Walked or moved body as usual for age	Limited in amount or kind of play	Overweight for age and height
8	Older Adult 65+	Drove car and used bus or train without help	Walked without physical problems	Worked or did housework, but limited in other activities	Painful, burning, or frequent urination (passing water)
9	Small Child < 6	Used car, bus or train as usual for age	Walked or moved body as usual for age	Played and did other activities	Taking medication or staying on strict diet for health reasons
10	School Age 6-17	Used car, bus or train as usual for age	Walked with physical limitations	Did school work and other activities	Pain, stiffness, or discomfort of neck, arms, hands, feet, legs, or several joints
11	Small Child < 6	Confined in special care unit	Confined in bed or chair	Needed more help with self-care than usual for age	Pain, bleeding, itching, or discharge (drainage) from sexual organs
12	Adult 18-64	Confined in house	Confined in bed or chair	Performed self-care, but not work, school or housework	Sore throat, lips, tongue, gums or stuffy, runny nose
13	School Age 6-17	Needed more help than usual for age to use car, bus or train.	Walked without physical problems	Did school work but limited in other activities	Sick or upset stomach, vomiting, or diarrhea (watery bowel movements)
14	Adult 18-64	Confined in house	Confined in bed or chair	Needed help with self-care activities	Itching, bleeding, or pain in rectum
15	Older Adult 65+	Drove car and used bus or train without help	Walked without physical problems	Worked or did housework and other activities	No symptom or problem

Source: Patrick et al., "Toward an Operational Definition of Health", Journal of Health and Social Behavior, 14(1): 6-23, March 1973

Table 2. Vignette Descriptions

No.	Age	Mobility	Physical Activity	Social Activity	Symptom and Problem Complexes
16	Older Adult 65+	Confined in hospital	Confined in bed or chair	Needed help with self-care activities	Trouble learning, remembering, or thinking clearly
17	Small Child < 6	Confined in house	More limited in walking than usual for age	Played but limited in other activities	Two legs missing--includes wearing artificial limbs or braces
18	Older Adult 65+	Unable to drive or needed help to use bus or train	Walked with physical limitations	Limited in amount or kind of work or housework	Trouble seeing--includes wearing glasses or contact lenses
19	Older Adult 65+	Confined in hospital	Confined in bed or chair	Performed self-care, but not work, school or housework	missing or crooked
20	Small Child < 6	Confined in hospital	Walked or moved body as usual for age	Performed self-care as usual but did not play	Earache, toothache, or pain in jaw
21	Adult 18-64	Drove car and used bus or train without help	Walked with physical limitations	Limited in amount or kind of work, school or housework	Cough, wheezing, or shortness of breath
22	Adult 18-64	Confined in house	Moved own wheelchair without help	Performed self-care, but not work, school or housework	Weak or deformed (crooked) back
23	Adult 18-64	Drove car and used bus or train without help	Walked with physical limitations	Did work, school or housework but other activities limited	Fever or chills with aching all over and vomiting or diarrhea (watery bowel movement)
24	Adult 18-64	Confined in special care unit	Walked with physical limitations	Needed help with self-care activities	Cough and fever or chills
25	Small Child < 6	Used car, bus or train as usual for age	Walked or moved body as usual for age	Played and did other activities	Hernia or rupture of abdomen (stomach)
26	Older Adult 65+	Confined in hospital	Moved own wheelchair without help	Performed self-care, but not work, school or housework	One arm or one leg deformed, paralyzed, or broken, include wearing artificial limbs or braces
27	School Age 6-17	Needed more help than usual for age to use car, bus or train	Moved own wheelchair without help	Limited in amount or kind of work, school or housework	Two legs deformed, paralyzed, or broken, include wearing artificial limbs or braces
28	Adult 18-64	Drove car and used bus or train without help	Walked without physical limitations	Did work , shool or housework and other activities	Breathing smog or unpleasant air
29	Older Adult 65+	Confined in hospital	Moved own wheelchair without help	Performed self-care, but not work, school or housework	One arm and one leg deformed, paralyzed, or broken, include wearing artificial limbs or braces
30	Small Child < 6	Confined in special care unit	Confined in bed or chair	Needed more help with self-care than usual for age	Loss of consciousness such as seizures (fits) fainting, or coma (out cold or knocked out)

Source: Patrick et. al., "Toward an Operational Definition of Health", Journal of Health and Social Behavior, 14(1): 6-23, March 1973

scaling (Fig. 1), direct magnitude estimation, and equivalence tradeoff.[10,11] On the other hand, the presence of systematic difference in ratings by some other methods has brought doubts about their interpretation.[12,13] This paper presents the comparison of two methods in particular, category scaling (Fig. 1) and standard gamble (Fig. 2).

VALUE MEASUREMENT IN CERTAINTY AND UNCERTAINTY

In this study, the values assigned for each health vignette was obtained in two ways: (1) under certainty conditions and (2) under uncertainty conditions. By certainty conditions, it is meant that individuals are asked to state the values representing their preference ordering of the health state. It is assumed that, through a process of introspection, an individual is able to differentiate the health states, and to assign appropriate values to each. Alternatively, the value of a health vignette may be measured by an individual's willingness to give up the health state as described in the vignette for a risky medical process which has a probability of either leading to total well-being or leading to death. This was the method first proposed by Von Neumann and Morgenstern which became the theoretical basis for the famous experiment to determine the utility of money.[14] More recently, it has been employed to elicit utility values of health states by various health researchers.[15,16]

For respondents who were assigned the standard gamble method, their preference rating of each vignette is determined by a method suggested by the expected utility theorem.[17] The value of a health state is assumed to be bounded by the two extremes of the continuum, death and total well-being, with the corresponding values of zero and one hundred. It is determined by the respondent's choice of whether or not to accept a risky medical process with a probability ($P\%$) leading to death, and a probability ($1-P\%$) leading to total well-being.

The value of the ith vignette may be expressed mathematically as follows:

$$U(h_i) = P_i \, U(h_d) \; + \; (1 - P)U(h_{twb}) \quad ,$$

where P_i is the maximum allowable probability value for the ith vignette that the medical process will lead to death, and ($1-P$) is the minimum probability that it will bring total well-being. $U(h_d)$ is the value of death, which is arbitrarily chosen to be zero. $U(h_{twb})$ is the value of total well-being, which is arbitrarily set to be one hundred.

Each respondent, when presented with the vignette descriptions, will decide the value of P, above which he would not accept the medical process. A horizontal box of 20 slots, printed beneath the vignette descriptions, will represent equally spaced increasing probabilities (P) that the medical process will bring death, or equivalently, the slots will also represent equally spaced decreasing probabilities ($1-P$) that the medical process will bring total well-being. When P is very small, the respondent is assumed to accept the gamble because the expected value of the gamble is greater than the value of the sure outcome. He will reject it when the expected value of the gamble is less than the value of the given health states. Starting from zero probability of death for the medical process, P=0, the respondent is asked to increase this probability until a point where he will not accept the risky medical process. This is the point when the expected value of accepting the medical process equals that of not accepting it. In other words, this is where the respondent is indifferent between a sure outcome of a health vignette, and a gamble which may lead to either total well-being or death. In essence, the respondent is offered a series of gambles, each with a different probability of death and a different expected value of the gamble. By subjectively varying the value of this probability, the respondent is able to decide the point where the utility value of the health state and the expected value of utility of the gamble are indifferent. Since the value of death has been chosen to be zero, value of the ith vignette therefore equals $U(h_i)$=100–P.

VIGNETTE # 2

Adult (18-64 years)
Confined in house
Moved own wheelchair without help
Needed help with self-care activities
Burn over large areas of face, body, arms or legs

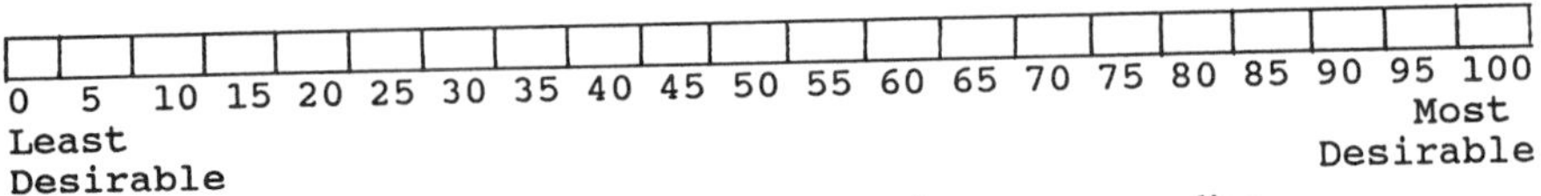

Fig. 1. Sample of vignette measurements by category scaling.

VIGNETTE # 6

School age (6-17 years)
Confined in special care unit
Walked without physical problems
Performed self-care as usual for age, but not school work.
One hand or arm missing, deformed, paralyzed, or broken --- includes wearing artificial limbs or braces

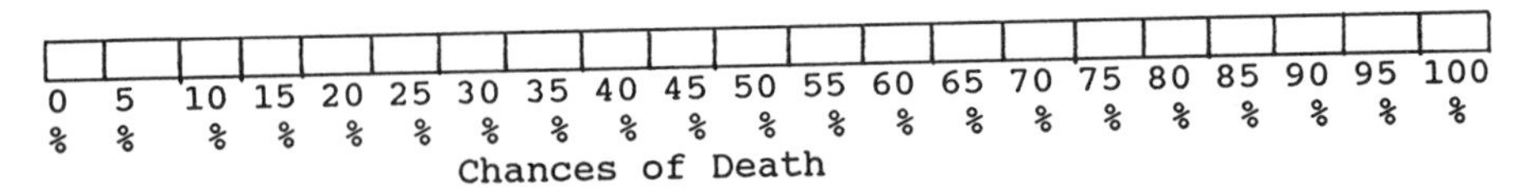

Indicate the chance of death above which you would not accept the medical treatment

Fig. 2. Sample of vignette measurement by standard gamble.

Respondents, who were randomly assigned the category scaling method, were asked to evaluate how desirable they think each vignette is. Respondents were specifically instructed to base their evaluation on how desirable such vignette appears to him, and not to the persons described. After the respondent has understood the vignette description, he is instructed to indicate his preference for the vignette by checking one of the slots in a horizontal box, printed underneath the descriptions. The box, with 20 slots, represents a scale from zero for the least desirable health state, to one hundred for the most desirable health state.

HOMOGENEITY OF RESPONDENTS

Respondents of this survey were residents in New York City's Chinatown, randomly selected from telephone directory listings. Out of the 307 respondents, 171 or 56% were assigned category scaling and 134 or 44% were assigned standard gamble. Due to the nature of random selection, it may be reasonable to assume that the two groups of respondents are similar enough so that the scores given by those using standard gamble are equally likely to be given by those who had used category scaling. This assumption, which should be justified, is necessary in comparing the two different measures of health preference.

In a comparison of characteristics between respondents who used category scaling and those who used standard gamble (see Fig. 3), the mean age of respondents who used category scaling was 45.78, compared to those who used standard gamble, 47.85. The average hours worked per week for the former was 30.56 hours, compared to the latter, 28.26 hours. The two groups were also found to have similar distribution along several important variables: income, education and health status. The two groups of respondents were therefore treated as equivalent.

CORRESPONDENCE BETWEEN CATEGORY SCALING AND STANDARD GAMBLE

The respondents' preference ratings were measured by category scaling and standard gamble. The ratings can be considered a manifestation of interaction between respondent characteristics and vignette components. Values assigned to each vignette may be determined by respondent characteristics such as health status and education. They may also be determined by the different components described in the vignette. Despite large dispersion of values for each health vignette, the mean preference ratings as determined by the two methods have remarkable correspondence. In general, the rank order of the vignettes is preserved in both methods. Preference rating by standard gamble is higher than that by category scaling. The difference is larger at the lower end of the health spectrum, and becomes progressively smaller towards higher levels of health functioning. Both methods show a monotonically increasing relationship, demonstrating the ordinal property of the values of health. Social preference for health may therefore by measured consistently by either method since the direction of increase or decrease will be similar in both cases. Category scaling, being an easier method to apply to the general public, perhaps should be the preferred choice. For the elicitation of utility values, however, standard gamble must be employed.

EFFECTS OF VIGNETTE DIFFERENCE

Ratings from the two methods indicated that the rank order of vignettes is maintained in both scales. A minor anomaly, however, is worth mentioning. Vignette 21 (see Fig. 4), which scored two ranks higher than vignette 23 (see Fig. 4) by category scaling, is found to be six ranks lower by standard gamble. The two vignettes are almost identical except the ability to work and the symptoms/problem complexes. Thus, it is not surprising to find that the scores of the two vignettes have approximately the same ranks by category scaling. The limited ability to work for an adult, however, may bring so much disutility to an individual that he is willing to take much larger risks, that is, to accept a medical process with a much higher probability of death, to restore full ability to work. This is evidenced by the drastic rank change of the two vignettes.

EFFECT OF RESPONDENT CHARACTERISTICS

Socioeconomic characteristics of the respondent may also determine his reaction to the vignette descriptions. For example, a respondent who has physical or social limitations may value the vignettes differently than someone who does not have first hand knowledge of such limitations. From a different perspective, a respondent who worked or who worked longer hours may be more willing to tradeoff some of his health for some financial security. It is possible that such a person has a lower utility value for health. Finally, as an individual's level of income and education rises, he is able to find more alternatives and

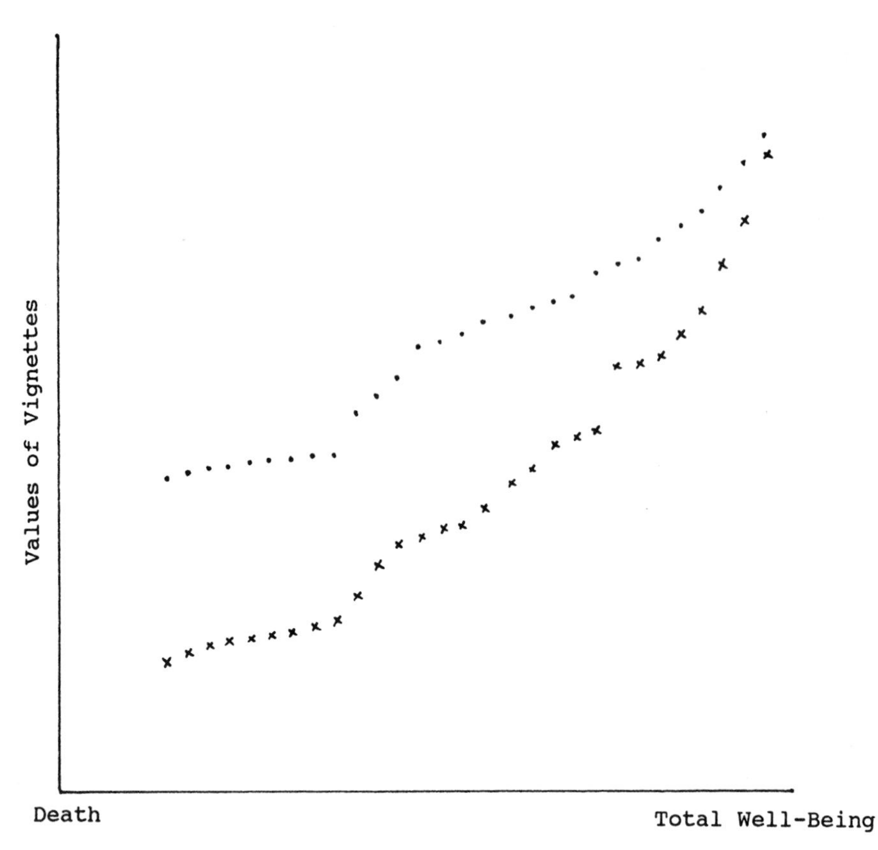

Fig. 3. Plot of vignette values by category scaling (.) and standard gamble (x) for entire group.

VIGNETTE 21	VIGNETTE 23
Adult (18-64 years) Drove car and used bus or train without help Walked with physical limitations Limited in amount or kind of work, school or housework. Cough, wheezing, or shortness of breath	Adult (18-64 years) Drove car and used bus or train without help Walked with physical limitations Did work, school or housework, but other activities limited Fever or chills with aching all over and vomiting or diarrhea

VIGNETTE NUMBER	CATEGORY SCALING MEAN	RANK ORDER	STANDARD GAMBLE MEAN	RANK ORDER
21	49.99	9	62.46	17
23	48.47	11	67.39	12

Fig. 4. Comparison of values for two vignettes.

support available for each of the health states, making them more tolerable. Thus, the value of each health state may be higher for such an individual than someone with a lower level of income and education.

A comparison of utility values by standard gamble indicated that respondents who worked are willing to accept riskier medical processes for all the vignettes except nine. Similarly, respondents who are less educated are also willing to accept riskier medical processes for all the vignettes except eight.

In a general linear regression model, the scores of vignettes are assumed to depend on several characteristics of the respondents: age, education level, income, hours worked and existence of long term illness. The coefficient estimates and significance levels of each variable were averaged across thirty vignette scores to determine the overall effect of each variable, in terms of magnitude and direction. In category scaling, with the exception of the income variable, all the others produced negative effects, particularly the variable of long term illness. In standard gamble, where the scores represent probability values assigned by respondents, all variables produced negative effects except the variable workhour.

VALUE MEASUREMENT AND RISK AVERSION

In the comparison of scores between the two methods of value measurement, it can be seen that sometimes conflicting results may occur. Respondents who worked are found to assign higher values to the vignettes by category scaling, but they seemed to assign lower values to the vignettes by standard gamble. This apparent contradiction leads one to believe that although both methods reveal respondents' values for the health states, under different conditions, the two methods may be measuring different substances. Respondents' values in certainty, scored by category scaling, may indeed measure the "quantity" of health perceived to be contained within the vignette, whereas values in uncertainty, scored by standard gamble, may measure the "utility" of the health state to the respondent.

In comparison to respondents who worked, it is thus conceivable that those who did not work could assign lower values to the vignettes because they thought the vignettes contain less health. At the same time, they could assign higher values to these vignettes because they were less willing to give up these health states for some risky medical process. Despite the lower level of health contained in the vignettes, respondents who did not work perhaps were able to derive more utility from these health states than those who worked.

Of course, it should be noted that the difference in means of neighboring health states do not truly represent marginal utility change of health, since the health states may not be equally spaced along the horizontal axis. There is no reason why the vignettes so picked should be arranged in ascending equal intervals. A better assumption is to let the category scaling score indicate the quantity of health (h) contained within the vignette. If we further let the standard gamble score represent the utility assigned to the vignette, then it is possible to construct a utility function of health (Fig. 5). Following Friedman and Savage,[18] the notion of risk aversion can be measured by the difference of utility value and the mathematical expectation of each standard gamble.

In the particular situation where utility of each health vignette equals the amount of health contained in it, $U(h)=h$, the mean scores by category scaling will provide us with a straight line 45 degrees to the axis. The values of each vignette on this line are identical to the mathematical expectation of utility of the standard gamble. The amount of health (h_i) contained in the vignette is equal to the probability ($1-p_i$) that should be assigned by a rational individual with neutral tendency towards risk taking.

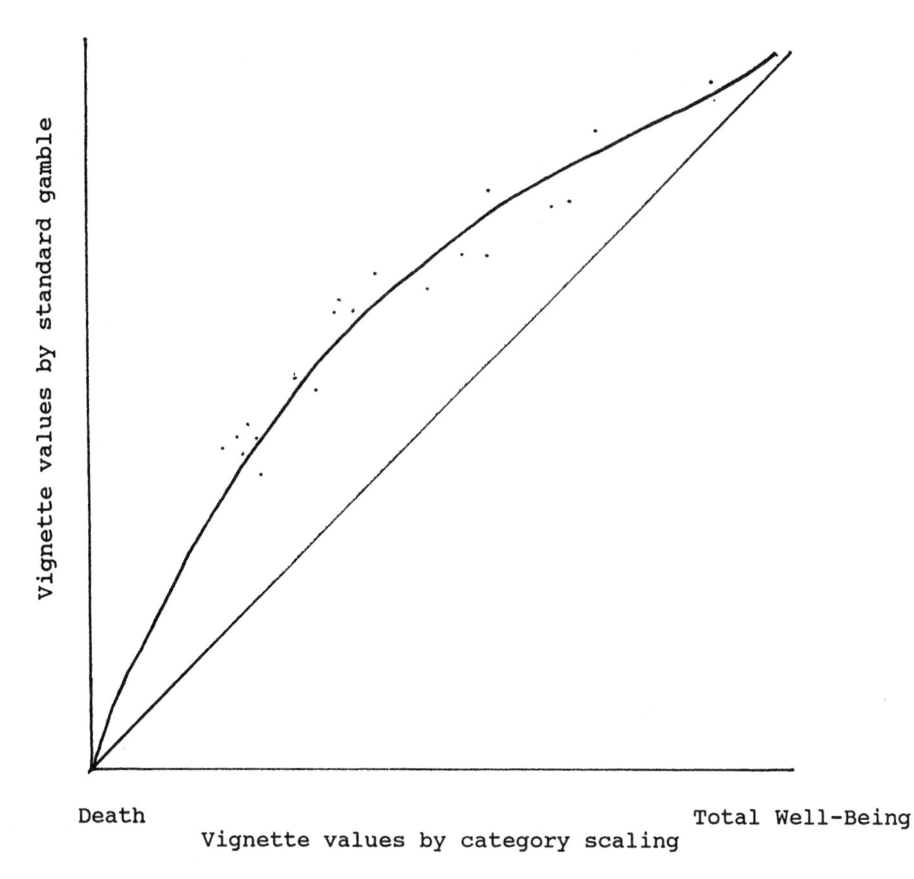

Fig. 5. Utility function of health standard gamble vs. category scaling.

Results from the survey, however, show that the utility values assigned by the respondents are uniformly larger than that suggested by the mathematical expectation of utility. In other words, the respondents are risk averse. They would allow their health to deteriorate before they would accept a risky medical process.

COMPARING RISK AVERSION AMONG DIFFERENT GROUPS

In a comparison of risk aversion between two groups of respondents, those who reported that they have long term illness were found to be more risk averse than those who did not have long term illness. Their degrees of risk aversion are higher in 24 out of 30 vignettes. The six remaining vignettes for which risk aversion was less are located in the region near death.

Obviously, health is not the only commodity that an individual may desire. There are other competing commodities such as financial security that also offer utility to an individual. If the consumption of these two commodities is constrained by the time available, then an individual may be willing to trade off some of his health to achieve some sort of financial security. If we make the assumption that those respondents who worked longer hours may be considered to want more financial security, it is possible that their utility of health may be lower than those who work less. This hypothesis may be tested by a comparison of the means of the two groups (Tables 3 and 4).

Table 3. Mean Vignette Scores by Group

	DID WORK PAST WEEK				DID NOT WORK PAST WEEK			
RANK ORDER	VIG #	C.S. MEAN	S.G. MEAN	RISK AVERSION	VIG #	C.S. MEAN	S.G. MEAN	RISK AVERSION
1	15	92.09	94.95	2.86	15	91.22	96.93	5.71
2	9	80.28	86.83	6.55	9	78.35	88.2	9.85
3	28	73.22	82.92	9.7	28	73.25	86.93	13.68
4	8	67.61	75.89	8.28	8	66.31	77.9	11.59
5	7	64.77	81.63	16.86	7	62.11	79.93	17.82
6	18	62.32	77.3	14.98	18	59	80.09	21.09
7	3	59.64	71.76	12.12	3	58.68	73.8	15.12
8	25	59.51	72.51	13	25	58.06	75.2	17.14
9	23	51.8	66.62	14.82	19	49.5	76.14	26.64
10	21	51.35	61.28	9.93	21	47.81	63.5	15.69
11	19	49.43	69.49	20.06	23	44.37	68.09	23.72
12	10	46.34	69.6	23.26	10	42.43	65.81	23.38
13	13	46.29	67.43	21.14	16	39.12	71.23	32.11
14	16	38.97	65.01	26.04	13	38.62	64.04	25.42
15	29	38.46	62.31	23.85	1	35.43	57.91	22.48
16	20	38.35	64.53	26.18	26	33.68	68.26	34.58
17	1	36.3	56.91	20.61	20	33.67	59.82	26.15
18	26	35.39	59.74	24.35	29	32	68.86	36.86
19	12	33.06	54.6	21.54	12	29.31	55.53	26.22
20	4	28.12	51.52	23.4	4	25.93	54.16	28.23
21	22	25.95	46.96	21.01	2	21.56	46.35	24.79
22	16	23.86	47.38	23.52	24	21.18	47.54	26.36
23	11	23.62	45.42	21.8	22	21	43.53	22.53
24	2	23.44	45.12	21.68	14	19.75	44.74	24.99
25	6	22.5	48.19	25.69	11	18.12	47.37	29.25
26	14	22.48	44.26	21.78	6	17.93	43.72	25.79
27	24	22.24	45.14	22.9	27	17.91	45.12	27.21
28	27	20.73	44.59	23.86	17	16.62	41.96	25.34
29	5	20.05	45.23	25.18	5	15.93	41.68	25.75
30	30	12.31	25	12.69	30	8.18	24.18	16

In comparing to those who worked in the past week, it can be seen that those who did not work show greater risk aversion for every vignette except one. Similarly, among the respondents who worked in the past week, it is found that those who worked less also have a higher risk aversion than those who worked more. Risk aversion of the former is higher for every vignette except three.

RISK AVERSION AND PHYSICIANS

The implication that the more one works, the more one is willing to accept a risky medical process, appears to be contradicted in a subsequent survey of Chinese physicians. The physicians, who worked much longer hours than the average community respondents, were found to be much more risk averse than the rest of the population. Not only did they assign higher values for the health conditions described in each vignette, but they accepted much lower chances of death for each risky medical process. Difference in risk aversion was found to be greatest for vignettes concerning children and teenagers who are confined in bed or chair, within a hospital or special care unit and whose social activities are severely restricted. Physicians were most reluctant to accept risky medical processes for this group of young dependent individuals. (See Table 5.)

Table 4. Mean Vignette Scores by Group

	WORKED MORE THAN 40 HOURS				WORKED LESS THAN 40 HOURS			
RANK ORDER	VIG #	C.S. MEAN	S.G. MEAN	RISK AVERSION	VIG #	C.S. MEAN	S.G. MEAN	RISK AVERSION
1	15	92.07	92.53	0.46	15	91.41	96.98	5.57
2	9	85.65	91.62	5.97	9	77.79	86.1	8.31
3	28	73.73	81.62	7.89	28	73.09	85.61	12.52
4	8	69.34	77.65	8.31	8	66.35	76.6	10.25
5	7	67.76	85.88	18.12	7	62.64	79.3	16.66
6	18	66.97	78.82	11.85	18	59.02	78.58	19.56
7	3	65.5	72.53	7.03	25	58.86	73.08	14.22
8	25	60.47	75.88	15.41	3	57.31	72.9	15.59
9	21	54.47	60.74	6.27	21	48.71	63.06	14.35
10	19	53.94	70.3	16.36	19	47.89	73.06	25.17
11	23	51.05	65.3	14.25	23	47.73	68.12	20.39
12	10	49.02	71.32	22.3	10	43.72	66.9	23.18
13	13	45.52	66.32	20.8	13	42.17	66.07	23.9
14	20	43.55	62.21	18.66	16	39.28	60.64	21.36
15	16	38.81	62.24	23.43	1	36.86	58.16	21.3
16	29	38.28	66.91	28.63	20	34.65	62.65	28
17	26	38.15	61.5	23.35	29	34.43	64.6	30.17
18	1	35.78	55.91	20.13	26	33.42	64.3	30.88
19	12	31.84	49.71	17.87	12	31.42	56.99	25.57
20	4	30.26	46.97	16.71	4	26.69	54.87	28.18
21	17	30.26	41.5	11.24	22	22.84	46.55	23.71
22	22	26.71	42.8	16.09	24	22.72	48.42	25.7
23	2	25.73	42.24	16.51	2	22.31	47.07	24.76
24	6	24.07	42.53	18.46	14	21.8	46.89	25.09
25	11	23	39.85	16.85	11	20.78	48.73	27.95
26	5	22.36	39.44	17.08	6	20.18	47.78	27.6
27	14	22.07	37.94	15.87	27	19.58	46.14	26.56
28	27	20.26	41.67	21.41	17	17.85	46.4	28.55
29	24	19.6	40.44	20.84	5	17.33	45.43	28.1
30	30	12.23	23.12	10.89	30	10.63	25.68	15.05

Table 5. Comparison of Risk Aversion Between Physicians and Entire Group of Respondents (Vignette Values Are by Age Group and Degree of Dependency)

	RISK AVERSION	DEPENDENT VIGNETTES					INDEPENDENT VIGNETTES			
AGE	VARIABLE	#11	#20	#30			#7	#9	#17	#25
-6	PHYSICIANS	56.5	39.5	44.5			15.5	21	55.5	16.5
	ENTIRE GRP	25.17	25.9	14.05			17.23	7.98	24.53	14.59
	RISK AVER	31.33	13.6	30.45			-1.73	13.02	30.97	1.91
		#4	#5	#6			#1	#10	#13	#27
6-17	PHYSICIANS	53.44	49.5	52.5			39.5	31.5	33	38
	ENTIRE GRP	25.36	25.44	25.39			20.97	23.14	23.23	25.29
	RISK AVER	28.08	24.06	27.11			18.53	8.36	9.77	12.71
		#2	#12	#14	#22	#24	#21	#23	#28	
18-64	PHYSICIANS	34.44	36.5	38.5	40	40.5	31	34.5	7	
	ENTIRE GRP	22.78	23.6	22.73	21.88	24.35	12.48	18.93	11.4	
	RISK AVER	11.66	12.9	15.77			18.52	15.57	-4.4	
		#3	#16	#19	#26	#29	#8	#15	#18	
+65	PHYSICIANS	27	449	33.5	33.5	38.56	16.5	6	29.5	
	ENTIRE GRP	13.69	28.56	23.12	29.11	29.91	9.86	4.29	17.86	
	RISK AVER	13.31	420.44	10.38			6.64	1.71	11.64	

The notion of risk aversion is derived from the shape of the utility function of health which is constructed from two measurements: utility and quantity of health. Any shift in either of these measurements will affect the curvature of the utility curve. Thus, risk aversion is not measured simply by a change in utility values from standard gambles. It is also affected by the quantity values from category scaling. Higher values in both scales therefore imply opposing forces. Higher values from standard gamble shift the utility curve upward from the diagonal signifying higher risk aversion. Higher values from category scaling, however, shift the utility curve towards the diagonal in the right, signifying less risk aversion. The resultant risk aversion is therefore dependent on the magnitude and direction of the shifts. In the case of physicians, although their high values in category scaling pull this utility curve closer towards the diagonal than the entire group, their higher values in standard gamble push it up so much further that the resultant risk aversion of physicians is higher than the entire group.

EFFECT OF EDUCATION

The somewhat conflicting result of the physician survey may be explained by a confounding variable: education. As an individual's level of education rises, he is able to find more alternatives and support available for each of the health state, making them more tolerable. Thus, the value of each health state increases for the individual. In terms of employment, there are more work opportunities open to an individual with higher education. A more educated individual is less dependent on his physical health state in order to earn a living. For example, a college professor whose legs are paralyzed can nonetheless carry on his responsibilities with very little loss of effectiveness. Even for those higher educated individuals whose work must depend on their physical ability, their higher level of education will enable them to seek successfully other types of work that do not require their physical ability but still generate equivalent income or satisfaction. The same cannot be said of individuals with very little education who must sell their physical labor to earn a living. They are less able to substitute other types of work that do not require their physical well-being. For them, the loss of physical ability would mean an immediate threat to their survival. Therefore, the less educated individuals have lower values for the health states. They would take much bigger risks in order to restore total physical well-being.

In a comparison of two groups of respondents in the survey, those who are more educated are found to be more risk averse than their counterpart. Their degree of risk aversion is higher in 23 out of 30 vignettes. The difference came from two sources: the more educated respondents assigned higher values to 22 out of 30 vignettes by standard gamble, and lower values by category scaling in 19 out of 30 vignettes. Thus, they pull the utility curve up, and push it away from the diagonal line. The more educated are more reluctant to give up the health states for a risky medical process.

EFFECTS OF WORK HOURS

Following the same line of analysis, we can see that the respondents who worked are less risk averse, because they are more willing to accept a risky medical process to bring them to total well-being even though it may have a high chance of leading to immediate death. Their risk aversion is diminished because they might thing that the vignettes contain more health. The standard gamble values of those who worked are lower in 21 out of 30 vignettes. The category scaling values are higher in 27 out of 30 vignettes. Exactly the same ratio is observed among the respondents who worked longer hours.

Looking from a different perspective, the higher values of health assigned by those who worked longer hours reflect their willingness to accept the risky medical process because they value total physical health as being more important to their being able to work.

DISCUSSION

Risk aversion has been observed to depend on scores on two scales which measure the quantity and the utility of health contained in the vignettes. The large variance in the scores probably arose from two sources: (1) insufficient training of interviewers and (2) inadequate preparation of respondents. It is believed that precision can be increased in the future with more rigorous training of interviewers and improved preparation of respondents.

In addition to the factors mentioned above, other variables have also been examined. Respondents who were older, or who had been living in the United States over ten years, both exhibited higher degrees of risk aversion. There was no marked difference between the sexes. Males, however, appeared to be more risk averse for the vignettes located in the better health region while the females seemed to be more risk averse for vignettes that are located in the lower health regions near death.

Risk aversion so far has been measured by the difference of values in category scaling and standard gamble. These measures, however, focused only on the individual health states, and not on the entire health spectrum. A more comprehensive measure of risk aversion may be defined as the area enclosed between the utility curve and the diagonal line. Larger area would signify greater total risk aversion. If the functional dependence of utility on health is known, the area enclosed may be determined by the difference between the area beneath the utility curve and the triangular area beneath the diagonal line. Risk aversion may be expressed as the following integral:

$$\text{RISK AVERSION}= \int_{h_d}^{h_{twb}} U(h)dh \;-\; \frac{1}{2}[(h_{twb} - h_d) \times (U_{twb} - U_d)] \;.$$

In the case where the exact functional dependence remains unknown, and the health spectrum is represented by a distribution of discrete vignette points, total risk aversion may be approximately determined by the following summation:

$$\text{RISK AVERSION}= \frac{1}{2} \sum_{i=1}^{30} U(h_i) \times [(h_i - h_{i-1}) \;+\; (h_{i+1} - h_i)] \;-\; \frac{1}{2}[(h_{twb} - h_b) \times (U_{twb} - U_d)]$$

In the case of the entire group of Chinese respondents, average area under the utility "curve" was found to be 988.06 units of risk aversion. For those respondents who did work, it can be seen that their total risk aversion of 874.19 units is indeed smaller than that (1254.08 units) of respondents who did not work.

REFERENCES

1. A. A. Alchian, The Meaning of Utility Measurement, *American Economic Review*, pp. 26-50 (1953).
2. C. L. Chiang, An Index of Health: Mathematical Models, *Public Health Science Publication 1000* 2:5, Washington, D. C. (1965).

3. M. K. Chen, The G Index for Program Priority, in *Health Status Indexes*, R. L. Berg, ed., pp. 28-39 (1972)
4. F. E. Linder, National Health Interview Surveys, *World Health Organization Public Health Papers* **27**:78-112 (1965).
5. D. Sullivan, Conceptual Problems in Developing an Index of Health, *Public Services Publication 1000* **2**:17 (1965).
6. D. Patrick, J. Bush, and M. Chen, Methods for Measuring Levels of Well-Being for a Health Status Index, *Health Services Research* **8(3)**:228-245 (1973).
7. D. Patrick, J. Bush, and M. Chen, Toward an Operational Definition of Health, *Journal of Health and Social Behavior* **14(1)**:6-23 (1973).
8. R. M. Kaplan, J. M. Bush, and C. C. Berry, The Reliability, Stability, and Generalizability of a Health Status Index, American Statistical Association Proceedings of the Social Statistics Section, pp. 704-709 (1978).
9. R. M. Kaplan, J. W. Bush, and C. C. Berry, Health Status: Types of Validity and the Index of Well-Being, *Health Services Research* **11(4)**:478-507 (1976).
10. R. M. Kaplan, J. M. Bush, and C. C. Berry, Health Status Index, Category Rating versus Magnitude Estimation for Measuring Levels of Well-Being, *Medical Care* (1979).
11. G. W. Torrance, Social Preferences for Health States: An Empirical Evaluation of Three Measurement Techniques, *Social Economic Planning Sciences* **10**:129-136 (1976).
12. J. L. Read, R. J. Quinn, D. M. Berwick, H. V. Fineberg, and M. C. Weinstein, Preferences for Health Outcomes: Comparison of Assessment Methods, *Medical Decision Making* **4(3)**:315-329 (1984).
13. H. Llewellyn-Thomas, H. J. Sutherland, R. Tibshirani, A. Ciampi, J. E. Till, and N. F. Boyd, The Measurement of Patients' Values in Medicine, *Medical Decision Making* **2(4)**:449-462 (1982).
14. F. Mosteller, and P. Nogee, An Experimental Measurement of Utility, *Journal of Political Economy*, pp. 371-404 (1951).
15. G. W. Torrance, Toward a Utility Theory Foundation for Health Status Index Models, *Health Services Research*, pp. 349-369 (1976).
16. G. W. Torrance, Measurement of Health State Utilities for Economic Appraisal: A Review, *Journal of Health Economics* **5**:1-30 (1986).
17. M. Friedman and L. J. Savage, The Expected Utility Hypothesis and the Measurability of Utility, *Journal of Political Economy*, pp. 463-474 (1952).
18. M. Friedman and L. J. Savage, The Utility Analysis of Choices Involving Risk, *Journal of Political Economy*, pp. 279-304 (1948).

New Technologies, New Hazards? A Systematic Approach

S. S. Raymond, D. Golding, S. K. Hammond,
J. Himmelstein, R. E. Kasperson, M. H. Melville,
F. Noonan, S. Ratick, and F. R. Tuler
New Technologies Safety and Health Institute
Worcester, MA

ABSTRACT

Hazards generated by new technologies may differ from those associated with established technologies, not only owing to differences in the processes employed and the products produced, but also stemming from the lack of data, monitoring capability, regulation, and management protocol for those technologies. The power to anticipate the sources and consequences of hazards in these rapidly developing technologies is the first step toward more effective hazard management. This paper describes the preliminary results of a systemtatic analysis of the hazards of new technologies undertaken by the New Technologies Safety and Health Institute. The methodology calls on innovation theory for the identification of new technologies, and on the CENTED Hazards Taxonomy for the classification and rating of their associated hazards. The resulting comparison of new with established technologies along twelve descriptor categories suggests a different configuration of hazards for each of the two groups.

KEYWORDS: Technologies, hazards, innovation, taxonomy, analysis

INTRODUCTION

If hazards generated by new technologies differ in type, configuration, or frequency from hazards associated with established technologies, then specialized strategies may need to be developed and marshalled to manage those hazards. A means toward identifying any new patterns in technological hazards is, therefore, the first step toward more effective hazard management.

This paper presents a proposed methodology for the systematic analysis of the hazards of new technologies, calling on innovation theory for identifying new technologies, and on the CENTED hazards taxonomy for classifying and rating their associated hazards. This method of analysis has been applied to a very limited set of new technological hazards as part of a larger study in process at the New Technologies Safety and Health Institute (NTSHI). Preliminary results of that study are presented, including some possible characteristics of the hazards of new technologies, a few probable limitations to the methodology, and several suggestions for further research.

Risk Analysis, Edited by C. Zervos
Plenum Press, New York, 1991

THE METHODOLOGY

Identifying New Technologies — Innovation Theory

New technologies are variously labelled in the literature as high technologies, emerging technologies, or as leading or strategic technologies. High technologies tend to be capital-intensive rather than labor intensive.[1] Emerging technologies characteristically record large research and development commitments relative to total annual expenditures,[2,3] have products that may not yet be commercial, and evidence a high potential for overlap and synergism between technologies.[4] New technologies also may be regarded as leading or strategic technologies, as they tend to fuel and shape the economic development of nations in a competitive world market.[2]

These descriptions, largely derived from economic indicators, do suggest some distinguishing features of new technologies, but they have not provided a basis for evaluating a technology's potential to generate new hazards. However, if a technological hazard is defined as the consequence of exposure to materials or energy generated by a technological process or its product,[5] then industrial innovation literature can supply that conceptual basis.

According to innovation theory as presented by Abernathy and Utterback,[6] newness in a technology is indicated by a high rate of innovation. Either product or process innovation may be underway, with process innovation following behind product development. Figure 1 illustrates these cycles of high innovative activity. The path of industrial innovation can be further subdivided into three phases or patterns: the fluid, the transitional and the specific. Figure 2 shows the relationship of the rates of product and process innovation in each of the three patterns. A new technology in its earliest stages is characterized by the fluid pattern, with frequent major changes in the products under development as determined by user needs and technical inputs. In the transitional pattern, the rate of process innovation outstrips that of product innovation, with an increase in production volume. When new technologies develop into the specific pattern, they very closely resemble established industries, with product and process innovations occurring only incrementally and at great cost.

Table 1 summarizes characteristics of the three patterns which constitute the tests used to identify new technologies for the NTSHI study. Biotechnology, microelectronics, advanced materials, medical diagnostics, food technologies, and information technologies are some of the industries thus identified. From these six industries, specific examples of products or processes which generate potentially hazardous energy or materials were nominated for systematic hazard analysis.

Classifying and Rating Hazards — A Hazards Taxonomy

The CENTED hazards taxonomy[7] provides a method for analyzing technological hazards in relation to twelve hazard descriptors, and for rating them on quantitative scales specific to each descriptor. Human and nonhuman mortality, both experienced and potential, are the only outcomes considered by this taxonomy.

Hazard descriptors are grouped according to the results of factor analysis, and their ratings are consolidated to give either a "0" (non-extreme), or "1" (extreme) score for each factor. These factor scores are combined to yield a five-digit factor code for each hazard, which then may be used to compare and to rank technological hazards.

The number of extreme scores in the summary five-digit factor code, in turn, permits the assignment of a technological hazard to one of three hazard classes. Hazards (extreme in

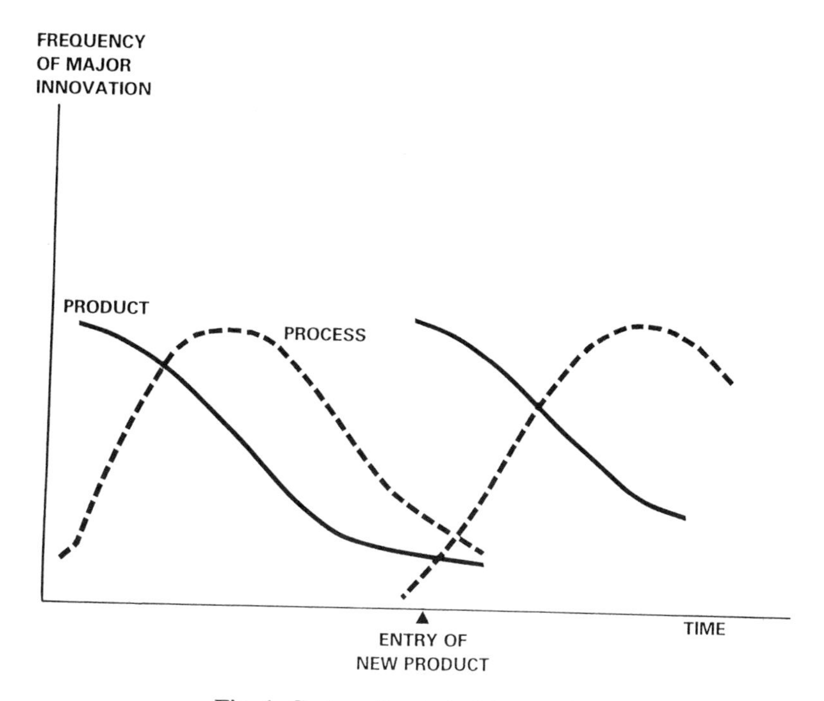

Fig. 1. Cycles of technical innovation.

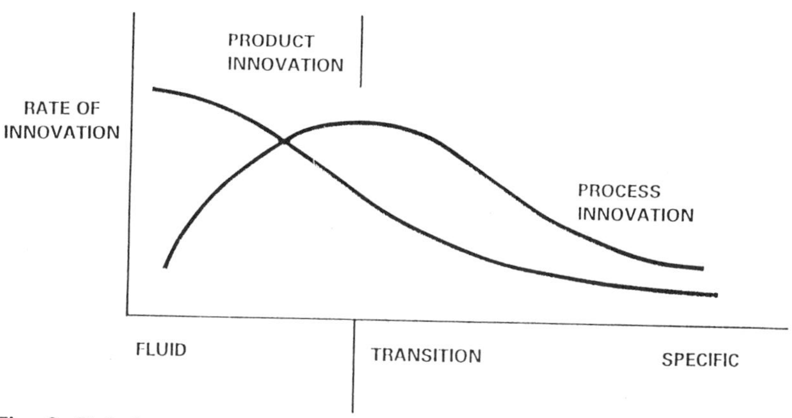

Fig. 2. Relative rates of product and process innovation in the three patterns of technical innovation.

no factor), extreme hazards (extreme in one factor), or multiple extreme hazards (extreme in more than one factor) constitute the classes of the taxonomy.

Table 2 lists the five factors of the CENTED taxonomy and their associated hazard descriptors.

A SYSTEMATIC ANALYSIS OF TEN NEW TECHNOLOGICAL HAZARDS

Ten potentially hazardous products or processes from the six new technology areas previously identified were nominated for analysis and rating using the CENTED taxonomy. While the list of hazards for this first-cut analysis could not be fully comprehensive of the

Table 1. Characteristics of the Stages of Innovation

Characteristic	Fluid	Transitional	Specific
Competitive focus	Product function	Product variation	Cost reduction
Innovative stimulus	User needs and technical inputs	Expanding technical capability	Reduce cost, improve quality
Type of innovation	Frequent changes in products	Process, required by rising volume	Incremental changes, product and process
Products	Diverse, often custom designs	At least one product with significant production volume	Standard products
Processes	Flexible, inefficient	More rigid, change occurs in major steps	Efficient, rigid
Materials	Generally available	Specialized materials may be demanded	Special materials will be demanded
Organization	Informal, entrepreneurial	Project and task groups	Emphasizes rules, structure, goals

Source: Abernathy and Utterback.

Table 2. Descriptors and Factors of the CENTED Hazards Taxonomy

Factor	Descriptor
Biocidal	Nonhuman mortality (experienced) Nonhuman mortality (potential) Intentionality
Delay	Persistence Delay Transgenerational effects
Catastrophic	Recurrence Human mortality (maximum)
Mortality	Human mortality (annual)
Global	Population at risk Concentration
Residual	Spatial extent

range of hazards associated with new technologies, there was a conscious effort to draw examples from both sides of the product/process, and material/energy designations and to represent the potential for both acute and chronic consequences of these hazards.

From biotechnology, action on an unintended target of a large-scale intentional release of genetically engineered organisms was considered.[8,9,10] From the microelectronics industry three hazards were analyzed: cancer from exposure to gallium arsenide particles;[11] acute toxicity from arsine gas exposure;[12] and clean room reproductive effects.[13] Advanced materials innovation presented three hazards for analysis: injuries from explosions or fire initiated by organometallics;[14] respiratory damage from particulates in new ceramics production;[15,16] and the thermal hazard presented by superconductors cooled with liquid nitrogen or helium.[17,18] Medical diagnostic technologies were represented by the potential mobilization of internal or external objects by magnetic resonance imaging.[19] Innovation in food technologies suggested the potential hazard of cancer from food preservation by irradiation.[20,21] Finally, in the information technologies, the hazard of cardiac effects among video display terminal (VDT) users was examined.[22,23]

Each of these new technological hazards was scored on the descriptor scales of the CENTED taxonomy, relying on expert judgment for the quantitative assessments. Table 3 lists the results of that effort for the ten hazards, giving the descriptor scores and factor code for each. Only one of the new technological hazards was classed as a multiple extreme hazard, six as extreme hazards, and three as hazards.

Comparing the Hazards of New with Established Technologies

In developing the CENTED hazards taxonomy, Hohenemser, Kates, and Slovic scored and rated ninety-three technological hazards, creating a profile of the hazards of established technologies in terms of their distribution among hazard classes and their ratings along the descriptors. This profile invites comparison with an analogous one generated by the taxonomic analysis of the ten candidate hazards of new technologies.

Figure 3 shows the distribution of the two sets of technologies among the three hazard classes. Nearly half of the hazards of established technologies fell into the least hazardous class, while the majority of new technology hazards ranked as extreme hazards. If subsequent analysis of a larger, more comprehensive data set were to reproduce this distribution, it would imply that new technologies are more likely to pose serious threats to human and nonhuman life than established technologies.

Finer distinctions between the hazards of new and established technologies may be sought by comparing differences among the individual descriptor scores earned by the two groups. This comparison unmasks the characteristics of new technologies which may be responsible for their possibly greater hazard potential. Figures 4 through 9 present the results of this comparison. The descriptor categories are grouped according to the hazard factor which they influence, with the descriptor "Spatial Extent" standing alone.

Considering first the Biocidal and Mortality factors (Figs. 4 and 7), nonhuman mortality and annual human mortality, on the whole, earned greater ratings for established technologies than for the new group. This difference may simply reflect short term experience with some of the new technologies. This hypothesis is supported by the observed greater tendency within this small sample of new technologies toward higher scores for potential nonhuman mortality and for maximum human mortality for a single hazard event (Fig. 6). This tendency, if verified by further research, may indicate that those hazards are relatively well controlled. Of course, there is also the possibility that a long latency period exists, and that the historical record has yet to reflect the true hazard potential of some new technologies. This possibility is explored further in relation to the next hazard factor, Delay, and its descriptors.

Table 3. Descriptor and Factor Codes for Ten Hazards of New Technologies

Hazard	Descriptor Score	Factor Code
rDNA—harmful release	393-869-97-1-97-9	01100*
GaAs production—particulates	363-986-31-2-64-2	01000
Clean room—reproductive effects	363-876-31-4-63-2	00010
GaAs production—arsine gas	363-546-73-1-66-5	00100
Organometallics—explosion/fire	363-213-83-1-65-4	00100
Ceramics—respiratory damage	363-986-31-2-54-2	01000
Superconductors—liquid N, He use	333-323-71-1-54-2	00000
MRI—mobilized objects	333-223-31-1-56-2	00000
Food irradiation—cancer	336-786-11-1-91-1	00001
VDTs—angina, cardiac effects	333-433-31-2-73-1	00000

*Multiple extreme hazard.

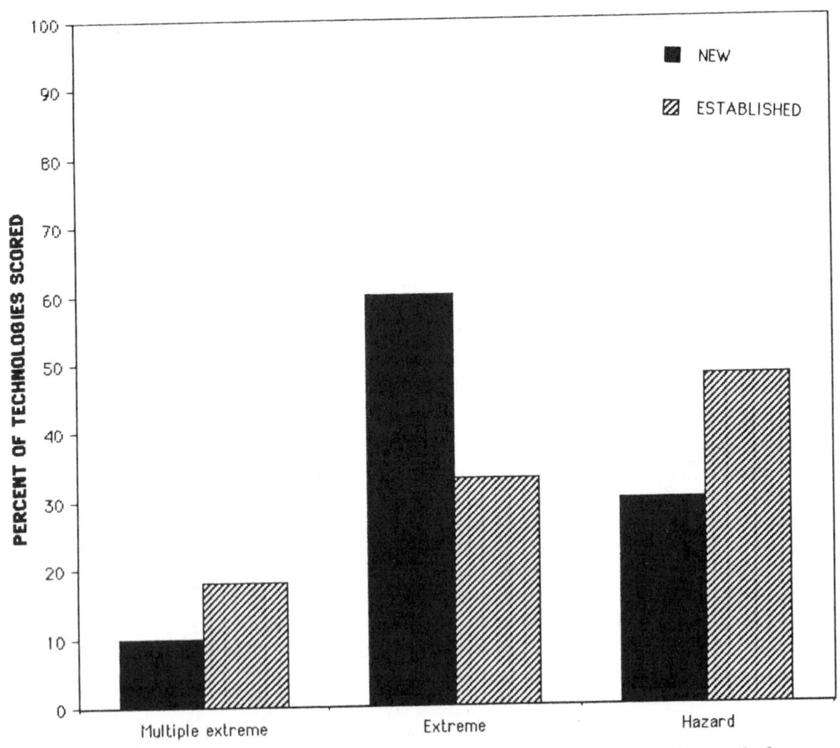

Fig. 3. Distribution of new and established technologies among hazard classes.

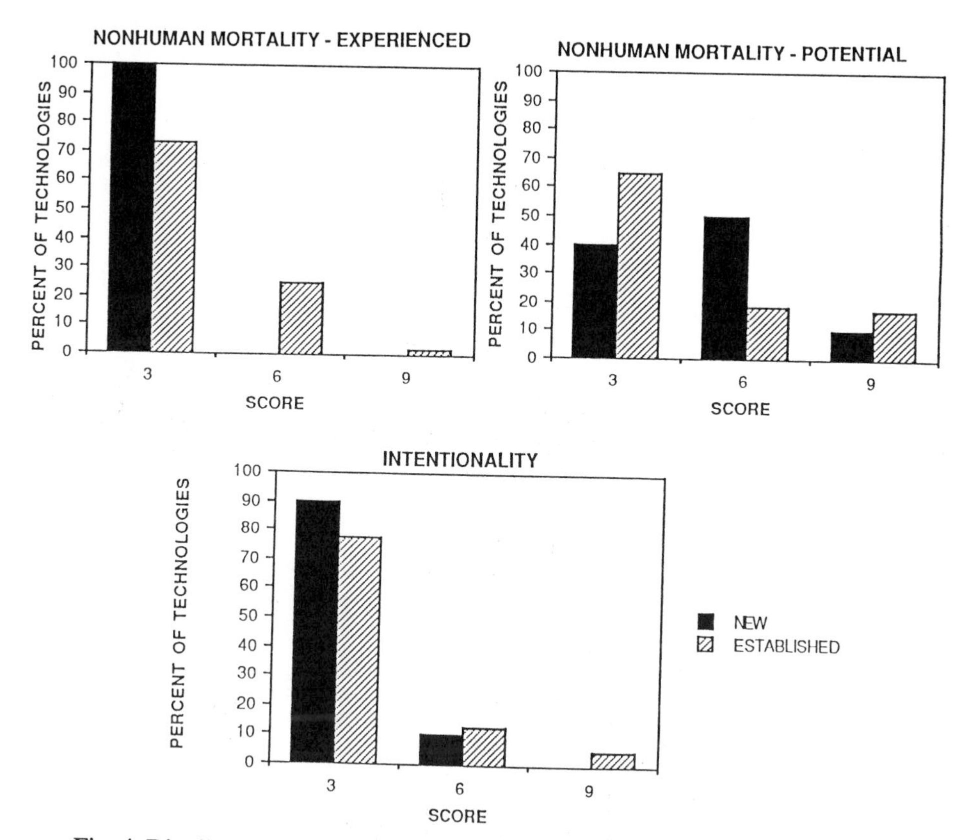

Fig. 4. Distribution of biocidal factor descriptor scores in new and in established technologies.

The Delay factor (Fig. 5) includes two descriptors which suggested greater hazard potential for new technologies. The agents released by the new technologies seemed to be more persistent in the environment than those responsible for the hazards of established technologies. Perhaps related to that persistence, the hazards of new technologies were tentatively identified as having a somewhat greater potential for transgenerational effects. Statistical significance of any of these postulated differences, of course, awaits the test of a larger study.

Examining the Catastrophic potential of technological hazards (Fig. 6), the scores for the recurrence descriptor imply that the group of ten new technologies may have generated hazard events more rarely than did the established technologies. This difference, again, may more accurately reflect the newness rather than the hazard potential of the technologies, but it does suggest an area for further research.

The potential for Global impact of technological hazards (Fig. 8) is influenced by the size of the population at risk and by the concentration of the agent released by the technology. For the small sample of new technological hazards, the population at risk tended to be smaller than that for established technologies, and the concentrations of agents generating the technological hazards also seemed to be lower for new technologies. These findings may have been influenced directly by the patterns of industrial innovation used to nominate new technologies for this analysis. The fluid and the transitional patterns do tend to focus attention on occupational hazards and low volume production processes rather than

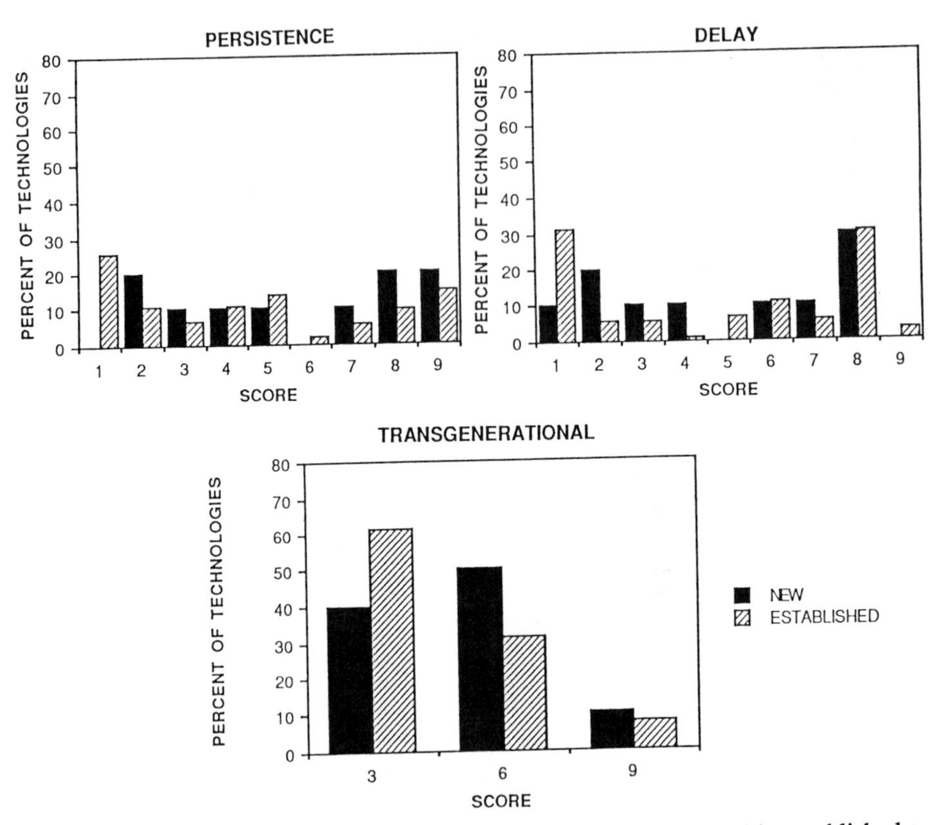

Fig. 5. Distribution of delay factor descriptor scores in new and in established technologies.

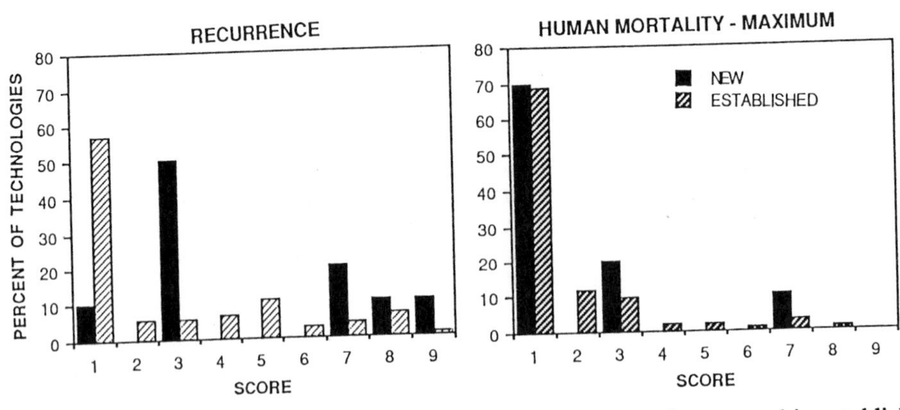

Fig. 6. Distribution of catastrophic factor descriptor scores in new and in established technologies.

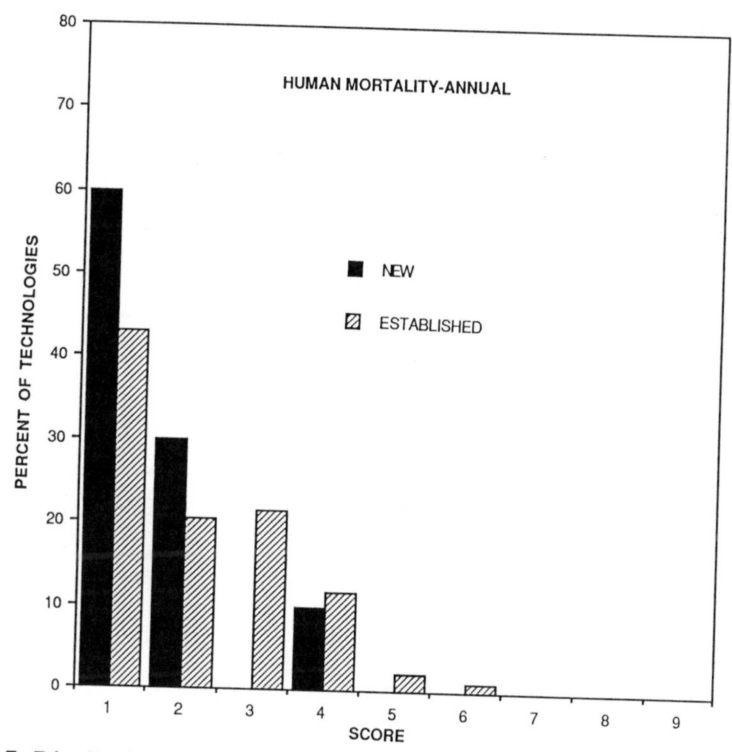

Fig. 7. Distribution of mortality factor descriptor scores in new and in established technologies.

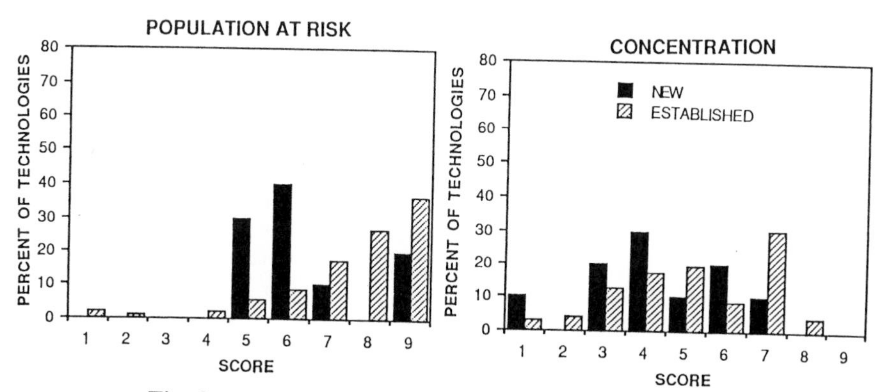

Fig. 8. Distribution of global factor descriptor scores.

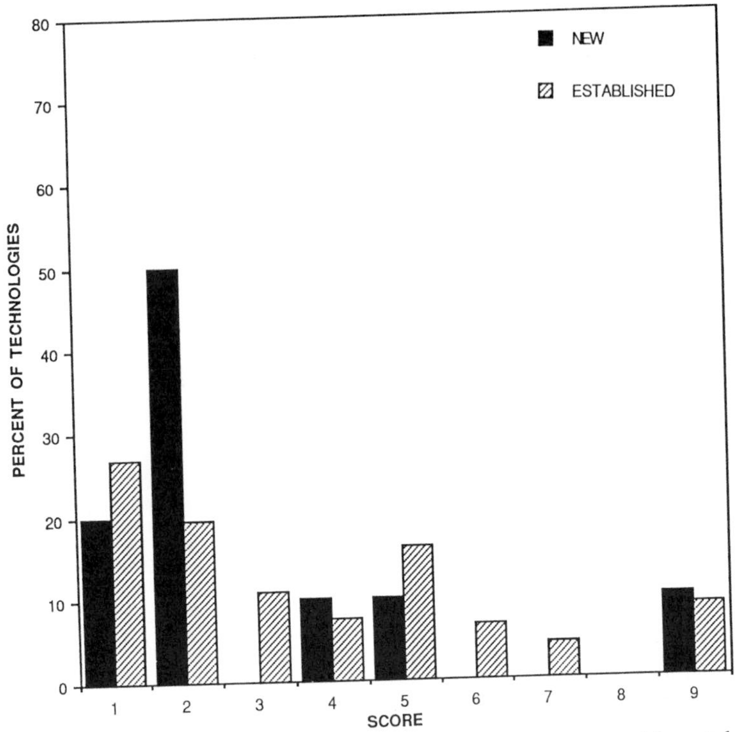

Fig. 9. Distribution of spatial extent descriptor scores in new and in established technologies.

on public health hazards and those associated with more widespread commercialization and distribution of consumer products.

A comparison of scores for the Spatial Extent descriptor (Fig. 9) implies that a greater proportion of the new technological hazards studied influenced a small area than did established technologies. This observation is compatible with the difference in production volumes possible between technologies in the fluid pattern versus those in the specific pattern of innovation, but the analysis of a broader spectrum of new technologies must be made before any clear conclusion can be drawn.

In summary, comparison of the ratings for individual descriptor scores very tentatively suggests that, for this set of new technological hazards, hazard events occurred more rarely, recorded lower mortality, exposed smaller populations within smaller areas, and released agents at lower concentrations than did the set of ninety-three hazards of established technologies. However, the potential mortality and the chance of transgenerational effects may prove to be greater for the new technological hazards in this comparison.

LIMITATIONS OF THE METHODOLOGY

Limitations of the methodology arise both from the structure of the hazards taxonomy and from the composition and size of the data set.

Since the CENTED taxonomy restricts the measure of hazard consequences solely to human and nonhuman mortality, the full range of hazards emanating from new technologies has not been addressed by this analysis. Morbidity and other outcomes need to be considered especially for occupational exposures and transgenerational effects, which may be important in emerging technologies. The structure of the CENTED taxonomy, similarly, also may tend to minimize occupational relative to public health hazards; small scale, prototypical processes relative to mature production systems; and potential hazards relative to realized ones. Repeating this analysis using other hazards taxonomies may help to clarify the bounds of these suspected limitations.

The interactive or additive effects of multiple hazards in a single technology or industry also are not addressed explicitly here. Three hazards from the microelectronics industry were scored in this analysis to explore this possibility. It is perhaps significant that across the three hazards, three of the five factors earned an extreme hazard score. Highly complex new technologies, especially in the transitional pattern with ongoing innovation in both product and process, may have enhanced potential for this type of composite hazard profile.

Identifying new technologies based on innovation theory focused attention on technologies new to the worldwide industrial scene. Technology transfer, however, does introduce new technologies into established industries. In those settings, the technology is genuinely new to that industry, corporation, or individual worker. The proposed methodology, however, does have the power to address "newness" on these levels as well, and could encompass this issue in any subsequent full scope analysis.

As has been emphasized throughout this paper, the restrictions of an admittedly small and selective data set of new technological hazards are superimposed on the potential limitations of the methodology. Any observations of the characteristics of new technological hazards derived from this prototype analysis are intended to be merely suggestive of areas requiring more extensive testing and research. A NTSHI proposal for this baseline research is under development.

CONCLUSIONS

Very preliminary results of the comparison of new with established technologies suggest that there may be some important differences in the frequency and configuration of their associated hazards. Some of those differences may arise from the characteristics of technologies with a high rate of innovation, but some may be related directly to the materials and types of energy specific to individual new technologies. The methodology described, with modification and expansion to address a broader range of hazard consequences, may be appropriate for a large scale study to test these hypotheses.

REFERENCES

1. M. J. Cooley, The New Technology-Social Impacts and Human Centered Alternatives, Milton Keynes, Open University, Technology Policy Group (1983).
2. R. R. Nelson, High Technology Policies: A Five-Nation Comparison, American Enterprise Institute for Public Policy Research, Washington, DC (1984).
3. J. X. Kasperson, On Defining High-Technology Industries, unpublished manuscript (1984).
4. G. Steed and S. Tiffin, A National Consultation on Emerging Technology, Science Council of Canada, Program on Emerging Science and Technologies, Ottawa (1986).
5. C. Hohenemser, R. E. Kasperson, and R. W. Kates, Causal Structure, in *Perilous Progress*, R. W. Kates, C. Hohenemser, and J. X. Kasperson (eds.), pp. 25-42, Westview, Boulder and London (1985).

6. W. J. Abernathy and J. M. Utterback, Patterns of Industrial Innovation, *Tech. Review* **80(7)**:41-47 (1978).
7. C. Hohenemser, R. W. Kates, and P. Slovic, A Causal Taxonomy, in *Perilous Progress*, R. W. Kates, C. Hohenemser, and J. X. Kasperson (eds.), pp. 67-89, Westview, Boulder and London (1985).
8. T. O. McGarity, Regulating Biotechnology, *Issues in Science and Technology* **1(3)**:40-56 (1985).
9. S. H. Weiss, J. J. Goedert, S. Gartner, *et al.*, Risk of Human Immunodeficiency Virus (HIV-1) Infection Among Laboratory Workers, *Science* **239**:68-71 (1988).
10. F. E. Young and H. I. Miller, Recombinant DNA Release: European Regulation, *Science* **238**:1025 (1987).
11. NIOSH, Alert: Request for Assistance in Reducing the Potential Risk of Developing Cancer from Exposure to Gallium Arsenide in the Microelectronics Industry, National Institute for Occupational Safety and Health, Cincinnati (1987).
12. J. LaDou, The Not-So-Clean Business of Making Chips, *Tech. Review*, pp. 23-36 (May/June 1984).
13. *Wall Street Journal*, p. 5, February 5, 1987.
14. L. Lewis, Chemistry's New Workhorse, *High Technology* **7(7)**:21-24 (1987).
15. H. K. Bowen, Advanced Ceramics, *Sci. Am.* **254(6)**:169-76 (1986).
16. H. K. Bowen and E. A. Thompson, New Materials in the Workplace, a conference report presented at Health and Safety of New Technologies Workplace 2000, Harvard University School of Public Health, November 13, 1986.
17. *New York Times*, Two Groups Report Substantial Gain in Research on Superconductivity, p. 1, December 31, 1986.
18. *New York Times*, Advances in Conductivity, p. D6, January 21, 1987.
19. J. E. Randall, NMR: The Best Thing Since X-Rays? *Technology Review* **91(1)**:59-65 (1988).
20. *New York Times*, Food Irradiation Fight Centers on Jersey, p. B1, November 12, 1986.
21. *New York Times*, Food Industry Eyes Irradiation Warily, p. C1, April 1, 1987.
22. W. A. Kleinschrod, The NIOSH Study of VDT Users Will Not Settle the Health-Hazard Issue, *Adm. Man.*, p. 14 (October, 1986).
23. *Wall Street Journal*, September 30, 1986.

Value-Impact Analysis of Low Temperature Overpressure Reduction Alternatives

T. V. Vo, B. G. Gore, A. J. Colburn, and E. J. Eschbach
Pacific Northwest Laboratories
Richland, WA

E. Throm
U.S. Nuclear Regulatory Commission
Washington, DC

ABSTRACT

In a study commissioned by the Nuclear Regulatory Commission (NRC), Pacific Northwest Laboratory (PNL) evaluated the costs and benefits of proposed modifications to the regulatory requirements on nuclear reactor low temperature overpressure protection (LTOP) systems. The costs and benefits were evaluated in terms of such factors as public risk and costs to industry and NRC.

Risk analyses were conducted to quantify to public risk for seven regulatory alternatives proposed as modifications of the current LTOP system or operational requirements. The Vessel Integrity Simulation Analysis (VISA) computer program and an existing risk study were used to estimate the public risk. Generic cost estimates were used to estimate the costs of industry and NRC.

The results of the risk analyses indicated that modifying the regulatory requirements could result in public risk reduction ranging up to a maximum of 2.1+04 person-rem over the remaining lifetime of the 55 plants affected. The costs associated with modification of regulatory requirements were also evaluated. Value-impact ratios calculated for the seven regulatory alternatives considered ranged from 1.0E+04 person-rem per million dollars to 500 person-rem per million dollars.

KEYWORDS: Alternatives, benefit, low temperature overpressure protection (LTOP), risk, cost

INTRODUCTION

Low temperature overpressure (LTOP) transients were identified as Generic Issue A-26 in 1978.[1] In 1979, Multi-plant Action B-04 resolved this generic issue (GI) by requiring all operating pressurized water reactors (PWRs) to implement procedures to reduce the potential for Reactor Cooling System (RCS) overpressure events and to install equipment modifications to mitigate such events.[2] Current staff requirements are stated in Standard Review Plan 5.2.2, "Overpressure Protection," and in its attached Branch

Risk Analysis, Edited by C. Zervos
Plenum Press, New York, 1991

Technical Position BTP-RSB 5-2, "Overpressure Protection of Pressurized Water Reactors While Operating at Low Temperatures."[3]

In addition to requirements for procedures and equipment, a requirement to report challenges to the Overpressure Mitigation System (OMS) via Licensee Event Reports (LERs) was also imposed. Review of challenges to the OMS since 1980,[4] including two events in which Technical Specifications pressure-temperature limits (p-T) were exceeded, led to redesignation of LTOP as a generic issue, this time as GI 94.[5] A third event in which the p-T limit curve was exceeded was identified during the course of this evaluation, which further supported redesignation of LTOP as a generic issue.

This document presents a value-impact analysis of the expected risk reduction and associated costs for the following regulatory alternatives which were proposed to resolve this generic issue.

1. Take no action. This is the base case evaluation of risks and consequences for LTOP events.
2. Prohibit operations with the RCS "water solid," except when it is depressurized and vented. Require all operating reactors to maintain a bubble of steam or noncondensible gas (N^2) in the pressurizer when the RCS is not vented.
3. Prohibit operation with the RCS water solid when either train of the OMS is out of service.
4. Prohibit operation with the RCS water solid when a high pressure safety injection pump is in service.
5. Prohibit the restart of a reactor coolant pump when the RCS is water solid.
6. Require that the pressure setpoint for automatic isolation of the Residual Heat Removal (RHR) system be raised above the setpoint for RHR safety relief valve (SRV) opening to maintain this relief path as a backup to the OMS.
7. Require the OMS system to be safety grade.

The next section of this paper summarizes the methods and results of the analysis. Summary of the results of the analysis is presented in a following section. Details of the analysis and the results of the intermediate steps can be found in the NUREG/CR-5186.[6]

METHODS AND RESULTS

This section summarizes the analysis methods and the results obtained for each of the major analysis steps.

RISK ANALYSIS METHODS

The analysis of each alternative estimated the public risk from the operation of the 63 presently operating PWRs summed over the period from the present to end-of-license (EOL). These estimates were derived by combining estimated frequencies of RCS overpressurization with calculated probabilities of reactor vessel fracture and an average radiation dose estimate.

Estimated Overpressurization Frequencies

For each alternative, an average frequency and spectrum of overpressurization were estimated for plants having each of three categories of OMSs. These categories are:

PORV	redundant relief paths through PORVs;
RHR	redundant relief paths through RHR system SRVs; and
PORV+N^2	relief through one PORV, with a bubble of steam or N^2 continuously maintained in the pressurizer.

Estimates were derived by analyzing an LER data base of 30 OMS challenge events which occurred between 1980 and 1986 to determine the frequency of challenges to the OMS, the fraction of challenges failed (unavailability), the resulting frequency of RCS overpressurization (product of challenge frequency and unavailability), and the spectrum of peak pressures expected to result when the OMS fails.

The spectrum of peak transient pressures expected when the OMS fails was determined by analyzing each event in the data base assuming OMS failure. Each LER was reviewed to determine actual plant conditions existing during the event, and NRC resident inspectors were contacted for supplementary information and to verify the authors' interpretations and expectations. This analysis incorporated the effects of alternate relief paths (through RHR SRVs for PORV category OMSs) where they existed and were not precluded by autoclosure interlocks actuated by increasing pressure.

Two fundamental assumptions were made in this analysis. First, unavailability, which was determined as the fraction of challenges for which the OMS had actually failed to prevent overpressurization, was assumed to be representative of operation with only one OMS train operable. This assumption was made because all three failure events in the data base occurred with one train out of service for maintenance (present Technical Specifications (TS) allow one train of OMS to be out of service for up to seven days).

Second, the spectrum of peak transient pressures expected after OMS failure was estimated assuming that operator action to terminate pressurization occurred three minutes after event initiation. This time is short compared to the ten minutes often assumed in safety analyses. It was selected for two reasons: the LER record included no instances where operator action required to correct a pressurization problem (primarily letdown/makeup flow imbalances) required longer than three minutes; and the authors' experience in observing simulator exercises, including operator licensing examinations, indicated that three minutes is ample time to make several attempts at event diagnosis and correction.

The overpressurization frequencies and spectra obtained from this data base analysis were used to characterize all plants having a given category of OMS. It was assumed that values remain constant between the present and EOL, so that they may be combined by simple multiplication with normalized vessel fracture probabilities summed over time.

Reactor Vessel Fracture Probability

The analysis of reactor vessel fracture probability was developed to incorporate explicitly the time dependence of increasing vessel brittleness due to increasing neutron fluence. Because embrittlement is strongly dependent on the chemistry of each individual vessel, a plant-specific analysis of vessel fracture probability (VFP) as a function of time was performed. This was possible due to the correlation of VFP with the reference temperature of the nil ductility transition (RTndt). Curves of VFP versus RTndt parameterized by peak transient pressure (PTP) were constructed via computer calculation. This information was then used along with plant-specific RTndt values (calculated from vessel chemistry and fluence as a function of time) to construct curves of VFP versus time between the present and EOL for each of the 63 operating PWRs addressed in this study.

For each of the vessels a Normalized, Integrated Vessel Fracture Probability (NIVFP) was calculated for each of three PTP values by summing (i.e., integrating) the VFP curves from the present to EOL. (The curves were normalized to one overpressurization event per year.) NIVFP values were then summed over plants having the same category of OMS.

The significance of the NIVFP for a given peak transient pressure is that, when multiplied by an estimated overpressurization frequency, the product is the vessel fracture probability integrated from the present to EOL. Thus, when a NIVFP category sum is multiplied by the average overpressurization frequency for that category, the product is the time-integrated vessel fracture probability for all plants in the category, from the present to EOL. This NIVFP information was then combined with overpressurization frequencies and pressures estimated for each of the alternatives to calculate time-integrated VFP values summed over all plants having the same category OMS, from the present to EOL, for each of the alternatives.

The key assumption which enables the separation of analysis portions is that the overpressurization frequency and spectrum remain constant over time. With this assumption it is possible to address the time behavior of vessel embrittlement due to increasing neutron fluence without requiring an inordinate amount of analysis detail.

Estimation of Public Risk

Public risk was calculated assuming an average value of radiation dose to the public per vessel fracture. This value was 50% of the value calculated for a later core melt with containment bypass, for a typical eastern site. This incorporates the assumptions that vessel fracture always causes core melt, and that the containment would be open about half of the time during operations in which an LTOP transient could occur. The resulting public risk is therefore proportional to the vessel fracture probability for all alternatives.

Risk Analysis Results

Table 1 presents total values of vessel fracture probability integrated for the present to EOL, and associated public risk values, for all seven alternatives addressed. Results of important intermediate analysis steps are also presented, with columns arranged according to the sequential multiplication steps which lead to the final results. This includes OMS challenge frequency, unavailability, spectrum of peak transient pressures, and summed values of Normalized, Integrated Vessel Fracture Probabilities for the pressures corresponding to the peak pressure spectrum. Separate analyses were carried out for plants having OMS systems employing pressure relief via PORVs, RHR SRVs, and plants which always maintain a steam or gas bubble in the pressurizer. Results are reported according to OMS category sum and the total for all 63 PWRs. Details of the analysis can be found in Ref. 6.

COST ANALYSIS OF ALTERNATIVES

In this section each of the alternatives is analyzed to determine the impact which its imposition would have on the industry and on the NRC. Both economic costs and occupational exposure to radiation are addressed. The basic framework for the analyses is that presented in the *Regulatory Analysis Guidelines*,[7] as elaborated by the *Handbook for Value Impact Assessment*.[8] Wherever possible generic cost estimation information was used.[9] All costs are escalated to 1988 dollars and rounded to the nearest hundred dollars.

Alternative 1: Take No Action

No costs are usually attributed to no action alternatives because the future costs of accidents are conventionally counted as benefits for averted costs in the assessment of alternative actions.

Alternative 2: Require an N^2 Bubble in the Pressurizer

This alternative prevents plant operation in the water solid condition by requiring that a bubble of noncondensible N^2 be maintained in the pressurizer when the plant is cooled down and the pressurizer steam bubble is collapsed. It extends the mode of operation used by B&W plants, which have PORV+N^2 category OMS systems, to plants with either PORV or RHR category OMSs.

Imposition of this alternative requires the ability to deliver large quantities of high pressure nitrogen (800 cubic feet at up to 500 psi, i.e., 10,000 scf) to the pressurizer prior to plant cooldown, and subsequently to vent it and process it through the Waste Gas system on plant heatup.

Occupational Radiation Exposure. For this alternative, the occupational radiation exposure (ORE) would occur the installation of the piping system to allow N^2 delivery directly to pressurizer and periodic maintenance and surveillance for the remaining life of the plant. This is estimated to be 341 person-rem/plant. For 55 Westinghouse and Combustion Engineering plants (W and CE plants), the total estimated ORE is 18,755 person-rem.

Industry Cost. The total industry cost is estimated to be about $601,500/plant. This cost is comprised of the following contributions.

Technical Specification Revision. Revision of the technical specifications to the plant is assumed to be routine. The cost of a routine revision of technical specifications is $17,400/plant (NUREG/CR-4627, Abstract 2.2.2).[9]

N^2 System Design, Installation and Operation. The engineering efforts associated with the installation of a N^2 system in containment are system design and definition of operations. The total effort involved is estimated at 700 staff hours for design plus 200 staff hours for operations definition. The associated cost is estimated at $48,600/plant (NUREG/CR-4627, Abstract 6.3).[9] Materials necessary to install the N^2 system include piping, hangers, wiring, instrumentation, valves and other materials. The total cost for material, procurement and distribution is estimated at $50,000/plant. Installation of the N^2 system requires pipefitters, millwrights, electricians, carpenters, and laborers. Base labor hours are estimated as follows: 200 hours pipefitters, 150 hours millwrights, 150 hours electricians, 100 hours carpenters, and 300 hours laborers. The cost estimate for installation is the sum of the product of base hours, labor productivity factor, and escalated contractor wages (NUREG/CR-4627, Abstract 6.3).[9] Installation of the N^2 system is estimated to cost $193,200/plant.

Support costs related to work performed inside containment consist of anti-contamination clothing and health physics surveillance. NUREG/CR-4627, Abstracts 2.1.5 and 2.1.6[9] provides the guidance to estimate the anti-contamination clothing and health physics surveillance costs. Anti-contamination clothing is estimated to cost $57,900/plant. Health physics surveillance is estimated to cost $19,600/plant.

Table 1. Integrated Vessel Fracture Probabilities (VFP) for the Base Case and All Alternatives

Plant Category	Challenge Frequency (yr^{-1})	Unavailability	Overpressurization Spectrum psi	Overpressurization Spectrum %	NIVFP(a) Value by Pressure	VFP Contribution by Pressure	Category Total VFP(b)	Category Average VFP per Plant per Year(c)	Public Risk(d) (p-rem)
Alternative 1 - No Action (Base Case)									
PORV	23/244 (=0.094)	2/23 (=0.087)	2500	9	3.79	2.80×10^{-3}			
			1400	9	.19	1.40×10^{-4}			
			850	13	3.7×10^{-3}	3.94×10^{-6}			
			<600	69	$<2.0\times10^{-4}$	$<1.13\times10^{-6}$	2.95×10^{-3}	3.04×10^{-6}	1.33×10^{4}
RHR	7/56 (0.125)	1/7 (=0.143)	2500	14	0.68	1.70×10^{-3}			
			850	14	9.0×10^{-4}	2.25×10^{-6}			
			<600	72	$<1.0\times10^{-4}$	$<1.29\times10^{-6}$	1.70×10^{-3}	3.76×10^{-6}	7.65×10^{3}
PORV+N2	<1/56 (<0.018)	0.087	850	5	2.0×10^{-4}	1.55×10^{-8}			
			<600	95	$<1.0\times10^{-5}$	$<1.48\times10^{-8}$	3.03×10^{-8}	1.66×10^{-10}	0.136
Overall							4.65×10^{-3} Total	2.90×10^{-6} Average	2.10×10^{4} Total
Alternative 2 - Require PZR Bubble									
PORV	15/244 (=0.061)	0.087*	<600	100	$<2.0\times10^{-4}$	1.64×10^{-6}	1.06×10^{-6}	1.10×10^{-9}	4.8
RHR	5/56 (=0.089)	0.143*	<600	100	$<1.0\times10^{-4}$	1.79×10^{-6}	1.27×10^{-6}	2.82×10^{-9}	5.7
PORV+N2	<0.018*	0.087*	850	5*	2.0×10^{-4}	1.55×10^{-8}			
			<600	95*	$<1.0\times10^{-5}$	$<1.48\times10^{-8}$	3.03×10^{-8}	1.66×10^{-10}	0.136
Overall							2.36×10^{-6} Total	1.47×10^{-9} Average	10.6 Total
Alternative 3 - 2 OMS Channels Required Operable When Water Solid									
PORV	0.094* (=0.0076)	$(2/23)^2$	2500	9*	3.79	2.43×10^{-4}			
			1400	9*	0.19	1.22×10^{-5}			
			850	13*	3.7×10^{-3}	3.43×10^{-7}			
			<600	69*	$<2.0\times10^{-4}$	$<9.83\times10^{-8}$	2.56×10^{-4}	2.64×10^{-7}	1.15×10^{3}
RHR	0.125* (=0.0204)	$(1/7)^2$	2500	14*	0.68	2.43×10^{-4}			
			850	14*	9.0×10^{-4}	3.21×10^{-7}			
			<600	72*	$<1.0\times10^{-4}$	$<1.84\times10^{-7}$	2.44×10^{-4}	5.40×10^{-7}	1.10×10^{3}
PORV+N2	<0.018*	0.087	850	5*	2.0×10^{-4}	1.55×10^{-8}			
			<600	95*	$<1.0\times10^{-5}$	$<1.48\times10^{-8}$	3.03×10^{-8}	1.66×10^{-10}	0.136
Overall							5.00×10^{-4} Total	3.12×10^{-7} Average	2.25×10^{3} Total
Alternative 4 - Remove Power from SI Pumps When Water Solid									
PORV	20/244 (=0.082)	0.087*	2500	5	3.79	1.35×10^{-3}			
			1400	10	0.19	1.35×10^{-4}			
			850	15	3.7×10^{-3}	3.96×10^{-6}			
			<600	70	$<2.0\times10^{-4}$	$<1.00\times10^{-6}$	1.49×10^{-3}	1.54×10^{-6}	6.71×10^{3}
RHR	6/56 (=0.107)	0.143*	2500	17	0.68	1.77×10^{-3}			
			850	17	9.0×10^{-4}	2.43×10^{-6}			
			<600	66	$<1.0\times10^{-4}$	$<1.01\times10^{-6}$	1.70×10^{-3}	3.76×10^{-6}	7.65×10^{3}
PORV+N2	<0.018*	0.087*	850	5*	2.0×10^{-4}	1.55×10^{-8}			
			<600	95*	$<1.0\times10^{-5}$	$<1.48\times10^{-8}$	$<3.03\times10^{-8}$	$<1.66\times10^{-10}$	0.136
Overall							3.19×10^{-3} Total	5.30×10^{-6} Average	1.44×10^{4} Total

* Same as base case, Alternative 1.

NA Not Applicable.

(a) Normalized, integrated vessel fracture probability assumes one pressurization per year to this pressure for each plant, summed from 1986 to EOL.

(b) Total, integrated vessel fracture probability summed from 1986 to EOL, assuming constant overpressurization frequency and spectrum for each plant, during all years.

(c) Reactor years from 1986 to EOL by plant category are: PORV, 969; RHR, 452, and PORV+N2, 183. Total reactor years are 1604.

(d) Core melt is assumed synonymous with reactor vessel fracture, yielding an integrated radiation dose of 4.5E+06 man-rem over 30 years when the containment is assumed open 50% of the time.

Table 1. Integrated Vessel Fracture Probabilities (VFP) for the Base Case and All Alternatives (Continued)

Plant Category	Challenge Frequency (yr^{-1})	Unavailability	Overpressurization Spectrum psi	%	NIVFP(a) Value by Pressure	VFP Contribution by Pressure	Category Total VFP(b)	Category Average VFP per Plant per Year(c)	Public Risk(d) (p-rem)
Alternative 5 - Prohibit RC Pump Operation When Water Solid									
PORV	14/244 (=0.057)	0.087*	2500	14	3.79	$2.65x10^{-3}$			
			850	21	$3.7x10^{-3}$	$3.88x10^{-6}$			
			<600	65	$<2.0x10^{-4}$	$<6.49x10^{-7}$	$2.65x10^{-3}$	$2.73x10^{-6}$	$1.19x10^{4}$
RHR	4/56 (=0.071)	0.143*	2500	25	0.68	$1.73x10^{-3}$			
			850	25	$9.0x10^{-4}$	$2.30x10^{-6}$			
			<600	50	$<1.0x10^{-4}$	$<5.10x10^{-7}$	$1.70x10^{-3}$	$3.76x10^{-6}$	$7.65x10^{3}$
PORV+N2	<0.018*	0.087*	850	5*	$2.0x10^{-4}$	$1.55x10^{-8}$			
			<600	95*	$<1.0x10^{-5}$	$<1.48x10^{-8}$	$3.03x10^{-8}$	$1.66x10^{-10}$	0.136
Overall							$4.38x10^{-3}$ Total	$2.73x10^{-6}$ Average	$1.97x10^{4}$ Total
Alternative 6 - Increase RHR Autoisolation Setpoint Above SRV Setpoint									
PORV	0.094*	0.087*	2500	9	3.79	$2.79x10^{-3}$			
			850	9	$3.7x10^{-3}$	$2.72x10^{-6}$			
			<600	82	$<2.0x10^{-4}$	$<1.34x10^{-6}$	$2.79x10^{-3}$	$2.88x10^{-6}$	$1.26x10^{4}$
RHR	0.125*	0.143*	2500	14	0.68	$1.70x10^{-3}$			
			850	14	$9.0x10^{-4}$	$2.25x10^{-6}$			
			<600	72	$<1.0x10^{-4}$	$<1.29x10^{-6}$	$1.70x10^{-3}$	$3.76x10^{-6}$	$7.65x10^{3}$
PORV+N2	<0.018*	0.087*	850	5	$2.0x10^{-4}$	$1.55x10^{-8}$			
			<600	95	$<1.0x10^{-5}$	$<1.48x10^{-8}$	$3.03x10^{-8}$	$1.66x10^{-10}$	0.136
Overall							$4.5x10^{-3}$ Total	$2.81x10^{-6}$ Average	$2.02x10^{4}$ Total
Alternative 7 - Require Safety Grade PORVs and RHR SRVs									
PORV	0.094*	0.035	2500	9*	3.79	$1.12x10^{-3}$			
			1400	9*	0.19	$5.63x10^{-5}$			
			850	13*	$3.7x10^{-3}$	$1.58x10^{-6}$			
			<600	69*	$<2.0x10^{-4}$	$<4.54x10^{-7}$	$1.18x10^{-3}$	$1.22x10^{-6}$	$5.31x10^{3}$
RHR	0.125*	0.143*	2500	14*	0.68	$1.70x10^{-3}$			
			850	14*	$9.0x10^{-4}$	$2.25x10^{-6}$			
			<600	72*	$<1.0x10^{-4}$	$<1.29x10^{-6}$	$1.70x10^{-3}$	$3.76x10^{-6}$	$7.65x10^{3}$
PORV+N2	<0.018*	0.087*	850	5*	$2.0x10^{-4}$	$1.55x10^{-8}$			
			<600	95*	$<1.0x10^{-5}$	$<1.48x10^{-8}$	$3.03x10^{-8}$	$1.66x10^{-10}$	0.136
Overall							$2.88x10^{-3}$ Total	$1.80x10^{-6}$ Average	$1.30x10^{4}$ Total

* Same as base case, Alternative 1.
NA Not Applicable.
(a) Normalized, integrated vessel fracture probability assumes one pressurization per year to this pressure for each plant, summed from 1986 to EOL.
(b) Total, integrated vessel fracture probability summed from 1986 to EOL, assuming constant overpressurization frequency and spectrum for each plant, during all years.
(c) Reactor years from 1986 to EOL by plant category are: PORV, 969; RHR, 452, and PORV+N2, 183. Total reactor years are 1604.
(d) Core melt is assumed synonymous with reactor vessel fracture, yielding an integrated radiation dose of 4.5E+06 man-rem over 30 years when the containment is assumed open 50% of the time.

Additional operating, maintenance, and testing procedures are required to support use of the N^2 system. It was estimated that two operations procedures, one maintenance procedure and three testing procedures, for a total of six additional procedures, would be necessary. The cost of the new procedures was assumed to be represented by the cost of a complex procedure revision as described in NUREG/CR-4627, Abstract 2.2.2;[9] $3,700/procedure or $22,200 total. Startup and installation testing is required to verify the system design and operability. Startup and installation testing effort is estimated at two staff-months (347 staff hours) for a cost of $18,700/plant (NUREG-CR-4627, Abstract 6.3).[9]

Given the significance of this modification it is expected that licensing support will be necessary. The licensing related effort includes FSAR change support, Technical Specification change support, as well as general coordination, 10 CFR 50.59 reviews, and resolution of system licensing problems. The licensing support effort is estimated at 1 staff-month (173 staff hours) for a cost of $9,300/plant. The QA/QC support effort for the N^2 system engineering, materials, installation, startup and installation testing, support procedure development, and licensing is estimated to be 25% (NUREG/CR-4627, Abstract 6.5[9]) of the costs associated with each activity. For the activities listed, the QA/QC cost is $104,900/plant. Although this system will be operated infrequently, training materials and initial operator training are necessary. Using the guidance of NUREG/CR-4627 (Abstract 2.2.3),[9] the cost of the training materials is $2,700/plant and the cost of the classroom training is $1,500/plant. The total training cost if $4,200/plant.

Recurring periodic inspection and system maintenance costs are estimated at $4,400/plant-year. This estimate includes planned and unplanned corrective and periodic maintenance costs, periodic inspections and surveillance testing, N^2 gas recharges attributable to this modification, and QA/QC support. The present value of this cost discounted at 10% over the average remaining life of the PORV and RHR category plants of 25 years is $39,900/plant.

It is assumed that the N^2 system can be installed during a regularly scheduled refueling outage without extending the outage. Consequently, no replacement power costs are estimated.

Waste Gas System. Engineering analysis will be needed to demonstrate that system capacities and technical specifications of the waste gas system are not exceeded. Appropriate sections of the FSAR which address waste gas system loads and applicable operating procedures must be revised. A utility 10 CFR 50.59 review will also be required. No hardware changes are expected as a result of this evaluation.

It is estimated that Engineering, Licensing and QA/QC support to update the Waste Gas system documentation will require 220 hours/plant of effort. Based on Abstract 6.3 of NUREG/CR-4627,[9] the Engineering, Licensing and QA/QC costs associated with this portion of the modification are estimated to be $1,900/plant.

It is assumed that one additional operating procedure will be necessary to guide operators on the handling of the additional waste gas load. Since a new procedure is required, the cost is estimated as a complex procedure revision

(Abstract 2.2.2, NUREG/CR-4627[9]) and is estimated to cost $3,700/plant. The total cost to evaluate the waste gas system is, therefore, $15,600/plant.

For a total of 55 plants the best estimate of the industry cost is $33 million with upper and lower bounds of $66.2 million and $16.5 million, respectively. The total industry cost is summarized in Table 2.

NRC Cost. The best estimate of the NRC cost associated with this alternative is the one-time cost of developing a routine technical specification revision and review of the licensee specific implementation program. The cost of developing the routine technical specification is $14,200/plant. Review, inspection, and evaluation of the licensee implementation is estimated to require 180 staff hours/plant (20% of the industry engineering effort). The estimated cost of the oversight is $7,500/plant (NUREG/CR-4627, Abstract 5.2[9]). Assuming that 55 plants will be impacted by this technical specification change, this results in a total NRC cost of $1.19 million, with the upper and lower bounds of $2.33 million and $0.26 million.

Alternative 3: Two Operable OMS Channels Required

This alternative would require the plants with PORV or RHR category OMSs to change their technical specifications to require both trains of the OMS to be operable while in modes 4 or 5. Action to depressurize and vent the reactor would have to be initiated within four hours. This alternative involves only a change to the wording of the technical specifications; it does not involve hardware changes.

Occupational Exposure. No additional occupational exposure is expected as a result of this change. Neither hardware failure rates of individual components nor the testing frequency will be affected by the proposed change.

Industry Cost. The industry cost associated with revision of the technical specifications of the OMS is a one-time cost which consists of developing a simple technical specification revision, and simple revisions of two operational procedures. These are estimated to be $19,300 per plant.

Replacement power costs are only estimated for plants with PORVs. The net present value of the replacement power cost is estimated to be $1,400/PORV plant, assuming a 10% discount rate and a 24-year average remaining plant life for PORV category plants. Assuming that 55 plants revise the technical specifications of their OMS, the best estimate of the total industry cost is $1.12 million, with the upper and lower bounds of $2.46 million and $0.58 million, respectively.

NRC Cost. The NRC cost associated with this option is a one-time cost consisting of the development of a simple technical specification revision. These costs are estimated to be $14,200 per plant. Assuming that 55 plants will upgrade the technical specifications of their OMS, this results in a total NRC cost in 1988 dollars of $0.78 million, with upper and lower bounds of $1.51 million and $0.41 million.

Alternative 4: Remove Power from Safety Injection Pumps When Water Solid

This alternative affects only the 55 W and CE plants. B&W plants do not operate in the water solid mode and are not susceptible to the rapid pressurization rates which result from mass addition events when the RCS is water solid.

Occupational Exposure. Revision of technical specifications and subsequent implementation are not expected to increase the affected plant occupational exposure.

Table 2. Total Industry Cost for Alternative 2 — Require an N^2 Bubble in the Pressurizer

	Total Industry Cost ($million, 1988)
Technical Specification Revision Development (routine revision)	0.96
N^2 System Engineering	2.67
N^2 System Materials	2.75
N^2 System Materials	2.75
N^2 System Installation (installation labor and support)	14.89
N^2 Additional Procedures	1.22
N^2 System Startup and Installation Test	1.03
Licensing	0.51
N^2 System QA	5.77
Initial Training	0.23
Waste Gas System Analysis	0.86
Maintenance and Periodic Inspection (present value, 10% discount over life)	2.19
Total	$33.08

Industry Cost. The best estimate of the industry cost associated with the update of the technical specifications of the safety injection system is a one-time cost which consists of developing a complex technical specification revision, complex revision of operational procedures, revision to training manuals, and training. These costs are estimated to be $54,200 per plant. Assuming that 55 plants upgrade the SI technical specifications a total one-time industry cost is $2.98 million, with upper and lower bounds of $5.97 million and $1.06 million, respectively.

NRC Cost. The best estimate of the NRC cost associated with this option is the one-time cost of developing a complex technical specification revision. This cost is estimated to be $27,400 per plant. Assuming that 55 plants will upgrade the SI technical specifications, this results in a total NRC cost in 1988 dollars of $1.51 million, with the bounds of $2.95 million and $0.78 million.

Alternative 5: Prohibit Reactor Coolant Pump Operation When Water Solid

This alternative only affects W and CE plants because B&W plants do not operate in the water solid mode and are therefore not susceptible to the rapid pressurization rates which result from energy addition events when the RCS is water solid.

Occupational Exposure. Revision to the Technical Specifications and subsequent implementation is not expected to increase the affected plant occupational exposure.

Industry Cost. The best estimate of the industry cost associated with the upgrade of reactor coolant pump operation technical specifications is a one-time cost which consists of developing a routine technical specification revision and two routine revisions of operational procedures. These costs are estimated to be $19,300 per plant. Assuming that 55 plants will upgrade the RCP operation technical specifications, a total one-time industry cost is 1.06 million, with the upper and lower bounds of $2.33 million and $0.53 million.

NRC Cost. The best estimate of the NRC cost associated with this option is the one-time cost of developing a routine technical specification revision. This cost is estimated to be $14,200 per plant. Assuming that 55 plants will upgrade the RCP Restart technical specifications, this results in a total NRC cost in 1988 dollars of $0.78 million, with upper and lower bounds of $1.51 million and $0.41 million, respectively.

Alternative 6: Increase RHR Autoisolation Setpoint Above SRV Setpoint

This alternative affects only a fraction of the W and CE plants having PORV category OMSs, because most of these plants already operate this way. It is estimated that only 14 of these plants will be affected. B&W plants do not operate in the water solid mode and therefore are not susceptible to the rapid pressurization rates which are possible when water solid. Plants with RHR category OMS are not affected, since overpressure protection attributed to the RHR SRVs could not be achieved if an interlock existed which isolated the RHR at pressures below the SRV setpoint.

Occupational Exposure. Verification of the RHRS pressure interlock setpoint change would be necessary. However, no additional occupational exposure would be incurred due to the change of RHR system pressure interlock setpoint.

Industry Cost. Industry cost associated with the revision of the automatic isolation and interlock action of the RHR system from the RCS as required in the ECCS subsystem technical specifications is a one-time cost which consists of developing routine revisions to a technical specification, an operating procedure, and a maintenance procedure. These costs are estimated to be $19,200 per plant. Assuming that 14 PORV category OMS plants will upgrade the RHR system autoisolation surveillance of the technical specifications, the total one-time industry cost is $0.26 million with upper and lower bounds of $0.51 million and $0.14 million, respectively.

NRC Cost. The best estimate of the NRC cost associated with this option is a one-time cost consisting of the development of a routine technical specification revision. This cost is estimated to be $14,500 per plant. This assumes that generic letter costs are shared among only 14 plants with PORV category OMSs under consideration. Assuming that only these plants will upgrade the RHR system autoisolation interlock surveillance specifications, this results in a total NRC cost of $0.20 million with upper and lower bounds of $0.39 million and $0.11 million, respectively.

Alternative 7: Require Safety Grade OMS

This alternative addresses only plants with PORV and RHR category OMSs because SRVs for RHR category plant are assumed to be safety grade already. B&W plants do not operate in the water solid mode and are not susceptible to the rapid pressurization rates which are possible when the RCS is water solid. This analysis develops costs for PORV category OMSs associated with environmental qualification of the PORV hardware actuation circuitry, upgrade of PORV actuation circuitry to satisfy redundancy and electrical separation criteria, and the expansion of inservice maintenance and surveillance activities.

Table 3. Total Industry Cost for Alternate 7 — Require Safety Grade OMS

	Total Industry Cost (in millions, 1988)
Technical Specification Upgrade	0.70
Maintenance Procedure Revision	0.04
Environmental Qualification	5.60
PORV Analog Circuit Design	0.60
Valve Hardware Packages	2.40
Valve Installation	0.22
Install Analog Circuit (PORV category only)	3.92
Additional Valve Testing (present value of three tests at discount rate of 10%)	0.07
Additional Analog Tests (PORV category only — present value at 10% over 24 years PORV EOL)	1.16
Replacement Power Cost (PORV category only — continuously discounted at 10% for 24 year PORV EOL)	1.68
Total for 40 plants	16.38

Occupational Exposure. The per plant total occupation dose includes replacement of two valves, installation of two additional analog circuits for PORV category plants, and three additional tests per valve. For 40 plants, the EOL industry total occupational exposure for this alternative is 891 person-rem.

Industry Cost. Costs are estimated for environmental qualification of PORV hardware and actuation circuitry packages, taking several factors into account. These include the complexity of the package to be qualified, the number of plants involved, and the number of manufacturers and valve types involved.

Cost of the OMS status upgrade will include one-time costs for technical specification revision, procedure revision, environmental qualification, PORV actuation design, hardware replacement, valve installation, PORV actuation circuit installation, valve tests, recurring analog channel tests, and replacement power costs. These costs are estimated to be $409,500 per PORV category plant. The total industry cost for this alternative is estimated to be $16.4 million, with upper and lower bounds of $30 million and $8 million, respectively. The total industry cost is summarized in Table 3.

NRC Cost. The NRC cost associated with this option is made up of the one-time cost of the development of a routine technical specification revision. This cost is $14,300 per plant. Assuming that only the 40 PORV category plants are affected by this alternative, the total NRC cost is $0.57 million, with upper and lower bounds of $1.10 million and $0.30 million, respectively.

Table 4. Summary of Risk Reduction, Occupational Exposure, Costs, and Value/Impact Ratios for Alternatives
[Affected Plants: All Operating W and CE PWR (55 plants)
Assumed Remaining Life = 26 years]

Alternative	Averted Public Risk (person-rem)	Occupational Exposure (person-rem)	Best Estimate Cost ($ Million)		Value/Impact Ratio (person-rem/$M)
			Industry	NRC	
1. Base Case	0.0	0.0	0.0	0.0	N/A
2. N_2 Bubble in Pressurizer	2.09×10^4	1.88×10^4	33.1	1.19	610
3. Two Train LTOP Operable in Modes 4 and 5 Operations	1.87×10^4	0.0	1.12	0.78	9840
4. Safety Injection System Upgrade	6.59×10^3	0.0	2.98	1.51	1470
5. Reactor Coolant Pump Restart Requirements	1.40×10^3	0.0	1.06	0.78	760
6. Increase Auto-Isolation Setpoint of the RHR System[(a)]	7.00×10^2	0.0	0.30	0.23	1320
7. OMS Safety Grade	8.00×10^3	891.0	16.4	0.57	471

[(a)]Cost is for only 14 plants since 65% of plants already have this feature. This factor is incorporated in the risk estimate through the overpressurization spectrum of Section 5.6.5.

VALUE-IMPACT RESULTS

Table 4 summarizes the results of risk reduction, occupational exposure, costs, and value/impact ratios for all alternatives. The value/impact ratio is simply the ratio of public dose averted divided by the total costs incurred. It is the figure of merit used to rank the alternatives in this value/impact analysis.

Costs were identified in the categories of Industry Implementation, Industry Operation, and NRC Implementation. No costs were identified in the categories of NRC Development or NRC Operation, and it was assumed that there would be no improvements in the categories of Regulatory Efficiency or Improvements in Knowledge resulting from imposition of any of the alternatives.

For Alternatives 3, 4, 5 and 6, costs were identified for Technical Specifications changes and for procedure modifications only, since these alternatives were selected to require only administrative changes and thus to minimize costs. Occupational radiation exposures for these alternatives were therefore zero.

Alternative 2, requiring a bubble in the pressurizer at all times, yielded the highest cost and occupational exposure estimates. Although the analysis indicated that nitrogen delivery systems and waste gas systems at most plants would have adequate capacity to supply a nitrogen bubble when needed and to process the waste gas when a steam bubble was reestablished, costs would be incurred for engineering and safety analyses required to demonstrate this. The major cost, however would result from design, purchase and installation of system components to supply the nitrogen to the pressurizer, with additional costs for maintenance, testing, QA, procedures, training, and licensing modifications. Installation in the radiation field of the pressurizer would yield significant occupational radiation doses, as would subsequent maintenance and valve testing.

Alternative 7, requiring the OMS system to be safety grade, addressed only PORV category plants, since it was assumed that RHR system SRVs already are safety grade because the RHR/LPI system is a safety system. Nevertheless, significant costs were identified for the design, environmental qualification, purchase and installation of redundant, independent, safety grade PORVs and sensing and actuation circuitry. Costs were also identified for modifications to Technical Specifications and procedures and for additional testing required for safety grade components. A small cost for replacement power when an outage was prolonged by a failed surveillance shortly before mode change was also identified.

Review of Table 4 shows that the highest value/impact ratio results from Alternative 3. It is almost seven times larger than the next highest value, for Alternative 4. It is also the only value/impact ratio which significantly exceeds 1000 person-rem per million dollars.

Alternative 2, which produces the greatest reduction of public risk, has next to the lowest value/impact ratio. This is due to the high cost of nitrogen supply system modifications required to provide a nitrogen bubble in the pressurizer when the plants are in cold shutdown. Alternative 2 also results in a significant occupational exposure due to hardware installation and to maintenance and inspection activities in the radiation field near the pressurizer. Over plant lifetime this occupational exposure almost equals the reduction in public exposure provided by this alternative.

REFERENCES

1. NUREG-0371, Task Action Plans for Generic Activities (Category A), U.S. Nuclear Regulatory Commission, Washington, DC (1978).
2. NUREG-0748, Operating Reactors Licensing Action Summary, U.S. Nuclear Regulatory Commission, Washington, DC (1984).
3. NUREG-0800, Standard Review Plan for the Review of Safety Analysis Reports for Nuclear Power Plants, Section 5.2.2: Overpressure Protection, U.S. Nuclear Regulatory Commission, Washington, DC (1981).
4. NUREG/CR-2000, Licensee Event Report Compilation, U.S. Nuclear Regulatory Commission, Washington, DC (1980-1986).
5. H. R. Denton, Schedule for Resolving and Completing Generic Issue 94 — Additional Low Temperature Overpressure Protection for Light Water Reactors, memorandum to R. M. Bernaro, U.S. Nuclear Regulatory Commission, Washington, DC (July 23, 1985).
6. B. F. Gore, T. V. Vo, A. J. Colburn, M. S. Harris, and E. J. Eschbach, Valve/Impact Analysis Generic Issue 94, Additional Low Temperature Overpressure Protection, NUREG/CR-5186, Pacific Northwest Laboratory, Richland, WA (1988).
7. NUREG/BR-0058, *Regulatory Analysis Guidelines of the U.S. Nuclear Regulatory Commission*, Rev. 1, U.S. Nuclear Regulatory Commission, Washington, DC (1984).
8. S. W. Heaberlin *et al.*, *A Handbook for Value Impact Assessment*, NUREG/CR-3568, U.S. Nuclear Regulatory Commission, Washington, DC (1983).
9. NUREG/CR-4627, Generic Cost Estimates, U.S. Nuclear Regulatory Commission, Washington, DC (1986).

Carcinogenic Risk of Benzene Derived from Animal and Human Data

Linda Tollefson, Carol B. Gable, Ronald J. Lorentzen
Robert N. Brown, and Janet A. Springer
U.S. Food and Drug Administration
Washington, DC

ABSTRACT

Benzene is widely considered to be an animal and human carcinogen but there are wide-ranging estimates of its potency. Risk assessments of benzene and human leukemia have primarily focused on exposure by inhalation over an occupational lifetime. The Food and Drug Administration (FDA) regulates benzene as a contaminant in food additives and thus is interested in the risk from lifetime exposure by the oral route. The risk from lifetime ingestion of benzene is assessed using the NTP animal gavage studies and the National Institute of Occupational Safety and Health (NIOSH) epidemiology studies, and the results are compared. The unit risks derived from the human epidemiology data for leukemia are similar to those derived from the rodent data when the animal risks are summed over all organ sites in each sex grouping. The collective unit risk values calculated from the animal data were .038 and .039 per mg/kg body weight/day exposure for male and female mice, respectively. The unit risks calculated from the human epidemiology data were .043 and .024 per mg/kg body weight/day exposure using the relative and absolute risk models, respectively.

KEYWORDS: Benzene, carcinogenicity, leukemia, relative risk model, absolute risk model

INTRODUCTION

Substantive evidence exists which indicates that benzene is carcinogenic to both laboratory animals and humans. The best evidence of benzene's carcinogenicity in humans comes from workers exposed by inhalation, while in animals the best evidence is derived from oral gavage studies. This provides something of a dilemma to the FDA in that the appropriate route of administration for assessing contamination of food or food additives by benzene is in a less appropriate species, the rodent, whereas the most appropriate species for human risk assessment was exposed by a less appropriate route, inhalation.

The most relevant animal study for quantitative risk assessment of benzene's carcinogenicity was sponsored by the National Toxicology Program (NTP) with B6C3F1 mice. There were significantly increased incidences of mice with neoplasms at several organ sites, including the lymphoreticular system, associated with administration of benzene by the oral route. There are several epidemiology studies associating benzene

Risk Analysis, Edited by C. Zervos
Plenum Press, New York, 1991

exposure by inhalation with the induction of leukemia in humans. After reviewing the epidemiology studies most useful for quantitative risk assessment, we decided that the studies performed by NIOSH provided the best data, with the exposure assessment of the NIOSH cohort done by Crump and Allen[1] the most accurate.

The FDA regulates benzene as a contaminant in food additives and therefore is interested in the potential risk from lifetime exposure to benzene by the oral route. We calculated unit risks, or potencies, from both the rodent data and human data in order to estimate upper bound risks for given exposure scenarios.

ASSESSMENT OF RISK FROM RODENT STUDIES

Benzene, in corn oil, was administered by gavage to Fischer 344 rats and B6C3F1 mice 5 days weekly for 2 years in the NTP-sponsored studies. All four sex/species groupings exhibited increased incidences of neoplasms at multiple sites. Male and female mice both appeared to be somewhat more sensitive to the effects of benzene. Therefore, unit risks from mice for each positive site were calculated. The dose levels administered were 25, 50, and 100 mg/kg bw/day, 5 days per week. The positive sites for male mice were skin, lung, lymphoreticular system, preputial gland, Hardarian gland, and Zymbal gland. For female mice, they were lung, lymphoreticular system, liver, mammary gland, ovary, and Zymbal gland.

For each of the positive sites, the low-dose level was a reasonable point on the dose-response curve to extrapolate linearly (after substracting control incidence) to calculate the unit risk used to predict upper bound lifetime risk for a given exposure. In cases where the low-dose level produced a zero incidence, the mid-dose level was used. Other seemingly more sophisticated curve-fitting techniques such as the linearized multistage model could be used to implement the linear-at-low-dose approach. Although such methods are more conservative due to the incorporation of an upper confidence limit on each site, they are also computationally elaborate and rarely give substantively different results. The FDA, generally, does not use upper confidence limits on responses from normal-sized bioassays. In this case we particularly chose not to do this because (1) if unit risks from many sites are to be summed, the conservative bias is multiplied, and (2) the human values to be used for comparison are not derived from data on which upper confidence limits are placed.

The time-averaged dose was calculated as follows: 25 mg/kg bw/day × 5 days/week × 1 week/7 days = 17.9 mg/kg bw/day and 50 mg/kg bw/day × 5 days/week × 1 week/7 days = 35.7 mg/kg bw/day.

Male Mice Unit Risks

Skin: squamous cell carcinoma incidences: 0/49, 0/48, 2/50, 3/49 (control, low, mid, and high dose, respectively). Unit Risk = (2/50)/(35.7 mg/kg bw/day) = .0011 per mg/kg/day

Lung: adenoma + adenocarcinoma incidences: 10/49, 16/48, 19/50, 21/49. Unit risk = (16/48 - 10/49)/(17.9 mg/kg/day) = .0072 per mg/kg/day.

Lymphoreticular System: lymphoma + leukemia incidences: 4/49, 10/48, 10/50. 15/49. Unit risk = (10/48 - 4/49)/(17.9 mg/kg bw/day) = .0071 per mg/kg/day.

Preputial Gland: squamous cell carcinoma + carcinoma NOS incidences: 0/21. 5/28, 19/29, 31/35. Unit risk = (5/28)/(17.9 mg/kg bw/day) = .010 per mg/kg/day.

Hardarian Gland: adenoma + carcinoma incidences: 1/49, 10/46, 13/49, 14/48. Unit risk = (10/46 - 1/49)/(17.9 mg/kg bw/day) = .011 per mg/kg/day.

Zymbal Gland: squamous cell carcinoma incidences: 0/43. 1/34. 4/40. 21/39. Unit risk = (1/34)/(17.9 mg/kg bw/day) = .0016 per mg/kg/day.

Female Mice Unit Risks

Lung: adenoma + carcinoma incidences: 4/49, 5/42, 10/50, 13/49. Unit Risk = (5/42 - 4/49)/(17.9 mg/kg bw/day) = .0021 per mg/kg/day.

Lymphoreticular System: lymphoma + leukemia incidences: 15/49, 25/45, 26/50, 22/49. Unit risk = (25/45 - 15/49)/(17.9 mg/kg bw/day) = .014 per mg/kg/day.

Liver: adenoma + carcinoma incidences: 4/49, 12/44, 13/50, 7/49. Unit risk = (12/44 - 4/49)/(17.9 mg/kg bw/day) = .011 per mg/kg/day.

Mammary Gland: carcinoma incidences: 0/49, 2/45, 5/50, 10/49. Unit risk = (2/45)/(17.9 mg/kg bw/day) = .0025 per mg/kg/day.

Carcinosarcoma incidences: 0/49, 0/45, 1/50, 4/49. Unit risk = (1/50)/(35.7 mg/kg bw/day) = 5.6E-4 per mg/kg/day.

Ovary: granulosa cell tumor + carcinoma incidences: 1/47, 1/44, 6/49, 8/48. Unit risk = (6/49 - 1/47)/(35.7 mg/kg bw/day) = .0028 per mg/kg/day.

Luteoma incidences: 0/47, 2/44, 3/49, 2/48. Unit risk = (2/44)(17.9 mg/kg bw/day) = .0026 per mg/kg/day.

Mixed cell tumor incidences: 0/47, 1/44, 12/49, 7/48. Unit risk = (1/44)(17.9 mg/kg bw/day) = .0013 per mg/kg/day.

Tubular cell tumor or carcinoma: 0/47, 0/44, 3/47, 3/48. Unit risk = (1/37)(35.6 mg/kg bw/day) = .0018 per mg/kg/day.

Zymbal Gland: squamous cell carcinoma incidences: 0/43, 0/42, 1/37, 3/31. Unit risk = (1/37)/(35.6 mg/kg bw/day) = 7.6E-4 per mg/kg/day.

If neoplasia at all of these sites are considered to be independently induced, it can be argued that unit risks for all sites should be summed. That is, each tumor type represents an independent risk. The argument against summing the unit risks is that linear extrapolation itself represents an upper bound estimate. In this case, summing the unit risks is probably not too extreme since one or two sites tend to dominate the potency estimate whereas the others contribute essentially nothing. When unit risks were estimated with the standard approach using linearity-at-low-dose of the dose response curve, the collective unit risk values were .038 and .039 per mg/kg body weight/day exposure for male and female mice, respectively.

ASSESSMENT OF RISK FROM HUMAN STUDIES

Although benzene was administered by both inhalation and gavage (ingestion) to animals, the human epidemiology studies are from industrial settings and are limited to exposure by inhalation. There are four large, well-conducted epidemiology studies associating benzene with leukemia in humans which are of potential use for quantitative risk assessment. These are, in addition to numerous case reports, most notably those by

Aksoy[2-4] and less well-controlled epidemiology studies. The four epidemiology studies of interest for risk assessment are the NIOSH series[5-7] on the Goodyear rubber hydrochloride workers, the Dow Chemical manufacturing facility study,[8,9] the Chemical Manufacturers Association study[10] of chemical workers, and the Yin *et al.* study[11] of 233 factories using benzene in China.

In 1978 Ott *et al.*[8] reported on the mortality experience of 594 men employed by the Dow Chemical Company between 1940 and 1970 and exposed to low levels of benzene as well as to other chemicals. Exposure to benzene was assessed by environmental monitoring data from 1944 to 1973 and categorized by specific jobs. Exposures in the various job categories ranged from .1 to 35 ppm (time-weighted average), and overall average exposure was approximately 5 ppm. Based on comparison with external controls (U.S. white males), 3 leukemia deaths were observed versus 0.8 expected (SMR=375, p=.047). The most important deficiencies in the Dow Chemical study when considering its use for risk assessment are the small number of workers exposed, which results in wide confidence intervals for the reported SMR, the lack of a dose response effect, the very low levels of benzene present in the facility, and the confounding factor of exposure to several other chemicals.

In a study conducted for the Chemical Manufacturers Association (CMA), Wong *et al.*[10] assessed the mortality experience of 4,602 male chemical workers from seven plants who were occupationally exposed to benzene for at least six months between 1946 and 1975 and followed through 1977. The results were compared to external controls (U.S. white males) and also to 3,074 male chemical workers from the same plants who had no known occupational exposure to benzene. Benzene exposure was assessed by dividing jobs into 34 tasks and determining the time spent at each task for every worker. Benzene concentrations for each task were based on the available industrial hygiene measurements. Some plants had few exposure estimates for the early years, and there is a possibility that workers were exposed to other chemicals at some of the plants. Each plant collected data on its own workers.

Seven leukemia deaths were observed compared with 5.96 expected based on the external controls; no leukemia deaths were observed in the internal control group. None of the leukemia deaths among the exposed workers was acute myelogenous, the type of leukemia most commonly associated with occupational exposure to benzene. When the results were analyzed by cumulative benzene exposure, there was a significant dose-response relationship between exposure in ppm-months and mortality from lymphatic and hematopoietic cancer.

Several problems were encountered in attempting to use the CMA epidemiology data for a quantitative assessment of benzene's risk for leukemia. These include the possible lack of uniformity in the collection of the data and thus a potential for bias, the lack of substantive exposure data, the lack of consistency in the methodology used for exposure assessment, and the cohort's exposure to chemicals other than benzene. Two of the original nine participating plants withdrew due to alleged difficulties in data collection, raising the suspicion that this decision was influenced by the mortality data collected. In addition, there are other concerns such as the absence of acute myelogenous leukemia cases and no leukemia deaths in the internal control group so that a relative risk could not be determined between the exposed cohort and the internal controls.

The NIOSH series of epidemiology studies concern Goodyear workers in pliofilm manufacturing (rubber hydrochloride) in three facilities at two locations in Ohio. The cohort consists entirely of white males. Infante *et al.*[5] originally analyzed the mortality experience of employees who worked between 1940 and 1959. Rinsky *et al.*[6] expanded the cohort in 1981 by including six more years, through 1965, and subsequently, through 1978.

Ten broad exposure classes were associated with specific job titles, and then job-exposure matrices were constructed which linked an average annual benzene exposure with each class. Actual industrial hygiene data were used, when available, for both locations. When no data were available, Rinsky interpolated between available previous and subsequent values. In addition, few data were available for location 2, so the location 1 benzene concentrations were used because the processes and job assignments were identical at the two locations. These procedures have been extensively critiqued, primarily citing that exposures were underestimated (and therefore risk would be overestimated). Location 1 had no data prior t0 1946, no company data available for 1951 through 1963, and only 15 benzene concentration levels from four different days for the years 1946 to 1950. In 1963, the company began to measure benzene levels but did so infrequently: there was an average of 2.3 surveys per year from 1963 to 1971. Location 2, which had the majority of the leukemia deaths, had two plants. Plant 1 had three sample points, all determined in a survey on one day in 1948. Plant 2 had one survey done "around 1957." Therefore, there was no sampling data for 27 of 29 years of operation at location 2.

At the International Symposium on Benzene Metabolism, Toxicity, and Carcinogenesis in March, 1988, Rinsky responded extensively to the criticism that the NIOSH epidemiology study relied on very incomplete environmental monitoring data. Although few measurements were made, as described above, those made were considered to be quite accurate, and other information is available which supports Rinsky's interpolation procedures. Most importantly, an exhaustive survey was performed on the various tasks performed at the two locations and the then-current benzene levels (at the time of the survey—all plants are now closed). The results showed that the jobs were identical and that the procedure of using location 1 benzene concentrations for location 2 was justified.

The 1981 Rinsky *et al.*[6] study found eight deaths from leukemia among the exposed workers, all either myelocytic or monocytic in cell type, whereas only 1.81 deaths were expected based on rates for U.S. white males (SMR=442). A subanalysis of workers exposed to benzene for more than five years gave an SMR = 2100. The excess of leukemia deaths remained significant when mortality was examined at the two locations separately.

In 1987 S. N. Yin *et al.*[11] published the results of a retrospective cohort study of leukemia in benzene workers. The mortality experience of 28,460 exposed workers from 233 factories in 12 cities in China was compared with 28,267 control workers from 83 factories not using benzene in the same cities. The benzene factories were involved in painting, shoe-making, rubber synthesis, leather, adhesive, and organic synthesis. The subjects had worked in these factories for at least six months between January 1, 1972 and December 31, 1981. Both cohorts (exposed and control) were followed through 1981 so that 178,556 person-years were obtained for the benzene cohort and 199,201 for the control cohort. There were 25 cases of leukemia in the exposed cohort compared with four cases in the control cohort, resulting in an SMR = 625. Five additional cases of leukemia, all among the living, were also found in the exposed cohort.

Benzene concentrations in the factories were assessed from factory records; the mean levels varied from 10 to 1000 mg per cubic meter with the majority in the range of 50-500 mg per cubic meter (about 16 to 160 ppm). Additional data on this cohort was presented at the March 1988, International Symposium on Benzene Metabolism, Toxicity, and Carcinogenesis by Dr. Yin. The most interesting finding was a statistically significant excess of lung cancer among the males in the exposed cohort after controlling for smoking. The National Cancer Institute is now collaborating with the Chinese investigators in an expansion of this study.

There are several problems with this study if it is to be considered for quantitative risk assessment. The time between the beginning of exposure (1972) to the end of follow-up

(1981) is too brief to justify confidence that a substantial portion of the leukemia cases has been ascertained. In addition, information on the methodologies employed for exposure assessment and the actual age-specific exposure and response data are not yet available. Moreover, the complexities due to the diversity of factories and cities in the study must be considered.

Currently, the results of the NIOSH studies[5-7] are the most appropriate epidemiology data to use for a quantitative risk assessment of benzene's leukemogenicity. All the epidemiology studies have some weakness in their design and/or conduction. However, the NIOSH studies have been extensively scrutinized and critiqued and the important criticisms have been answered sufficiently well to retain confidence in the results. Both the Ott *et al.*[8] (Dow Chemical) and the Wong *et al.*[10] (CMA) studies are confounded by exposure to other chemicals, and more substantive information is needed on the Chinese study before we can confidently use the results for risk assessment. The NIOSH study is the most reliable and most informative for purposes of determining the potency of benzene. This study dominates the estimates of potency among the American studies, primarily because of its higher exposures, more reliable estimates of exposure and large cohort size.

On September 11, 1987, the Occupational Safety and Health Administration (OSHA) published its final rule lowering the standard for occupational exposure to benzene to an eight-hour time-weighted average of 1 ppm and a short-term exposure limit of 5 ppm (Fed. Reg. 52:CF34460). Crump and Allen[1] performed a detailed risk analysis for OSHA to support this rulemaking, using several alternative data sets and exposure scenarios. Among these alternatives was a reassessment of the NIOSH cohort exposure data. For our analysis we used Crump and Allen's exposure assessment of the NIOSH cohort which began exposure in 1950 and was followed through 1978. Although the industrial plants were operating between 1940-1950, exposure measurements do not exist prior to 1946. There has been debate about whether the 1946 exposures should be assumed constant back to 1940,[6] or whether the much higher 1940 maximum tolerance levels should be use.[1] Taking into consideration the six years of missing data and their minor effects upon potency estimated by either approach, we feel it is sufficient to use the NIOSH data from 1950 to 1978. These data are reproduced in Table 1.

An important choice to make among the alternatives offered by Crump and Allen in their risk assessment for OSHA is whether to stress their relative or absolute risk models. The relative risk model expresses age-specific cancer incidence as the ratio of the risk of the exposed to the risk of the unexposed, i.e., the Standardized Mortality Ratio (SMR). The absolute risk model expresses the age-specific cancer risk as the excess risk added above background. Both these models fall within the conceptual framework of the classical linear-at-low-dose models used for extrapolating animal data. However, neither the relative nor the absolute model of Crump and Allen is entirely satisfactory with regard to multistage theory. Nevertheless, the limitations are not severely restrictive, and we shall utilize both models in our benzene risk assessment until alternative multistage-derived models are available.

The two models used by Crump and Allen[1] to express age-specific incidence E_i are the absolute and relative risk linear models. The age-specific incidence in Crump and Allen's relative risk model can be written as:

$$E_i = E_{bi}a[1+bd_{ci}] , \tag{1}$$

where a is the factor which allows the study cohort background tumor rate to differ from that of the reference population, b is the potency, d_{ci} is the cumulative dose up to the beginning of the ith age interval, and E_{bi} is the background age-specific leukemia incidence of the general population in the ith age interval. Crump and Allen's absolute risk model expresses age-specific incidence as:

Table 1. Observed and Expected Leukemias in NIOSH Cohort by Cumulative Benzene Exposure 1950-1978 Followup[a]

Cumulative Exposure in ppm-years (average)	Observed	Expected	SMR	Person-Years
0-5 (1.29)	2	1.11	180	16890
5-20 (11.0)	0	0.52	0	7092
20-80 (42.2)	0	0.50	0	6591
80-200 (129.0)	0	0.31	0	3557
200-1000 (421.0)	5	0.32	1560	3075
1000+ (1489)	1	0.049	2040	396

[a]See Table 6, Crump and Allen.[1]

$$E_i = E_{bi} + (a+bd_{ci})Y_i \,, \tag{2}$$

where a is the factor which allows the study cohort background tumor rate to differ from that of the reference population, b is the potency (distinct from the relative risk b factor), d_{ci} is the cumulative exposure to the beginning of the ith age interval, Y_i is the person-years of exposure within the ith age interval, and E_{bi} represents the background population's age-specific incidence.

A simple fitting of the absolute risk model $E_i = E_{bi} + (a+bd_{ci})Y_i$ to the NIOSH cohort 1950-1978 data results in an estimate for the potency b = 2.06E-6 (Fig. 1) using a value for the background adjustment factor $a = 0$ (i.e., the cohort's background age-specific response rate is estimated to be the same as that of the reference population). Fitting the relative risk model results in an estimate for ab = .019 (Fig. 2) with a = .87. Because b and a are interdependent and a is close to 1, we set a = 1; therefore, b = .019.

Using the 1976 leukemia mortality rates for white males and their 18-interval summation formula, Crump and Allen[1] estimated that the background lifetime white male leukemia mortality rate is .00797. Using the same interval summation, without using Crump's special approximation for the 18th interval, we obtained a background lifetime leukemia mortality rate = .0078. Because our estimate is similar to Crump's, we dispensed with his 18th interval adjustment in the 85+ age group for the sake of computational convenience.

Using a hypothetical work-life exposure scenario of 40 years exposure at 10 ppm beginning at age 20, we calculated excess risk using the NIOSH epidemiology data. Using the relative risk model with b = .019, we estimated 48 excess leukemia deaths predicted per 1000 workers. Using the absolute risk model with b = 2.06E-6, we estimated 24 excess

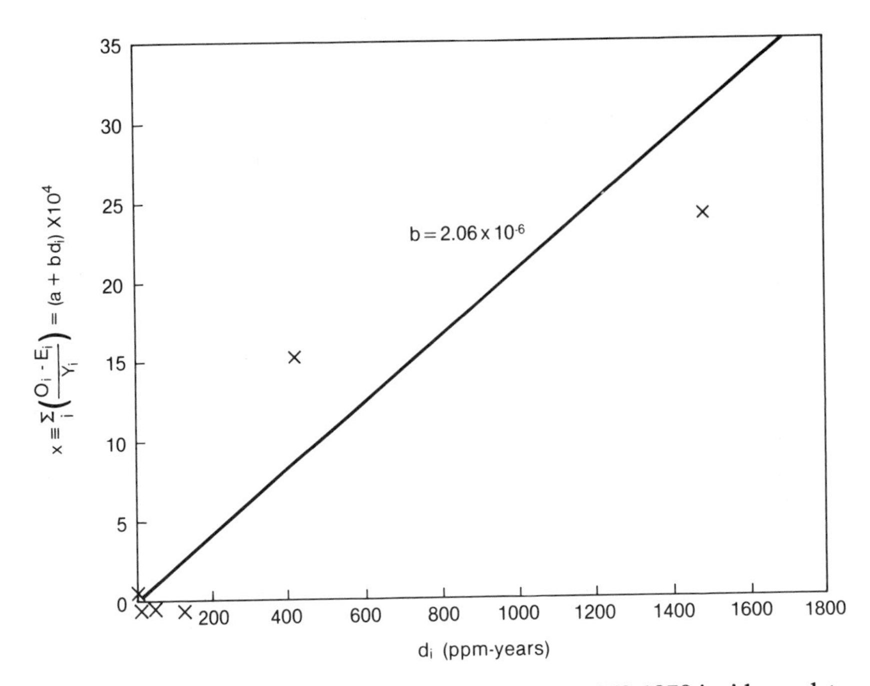

Fig. 1. Absolute risk model with NIOSH Cohort 1950-1978 incidence data.

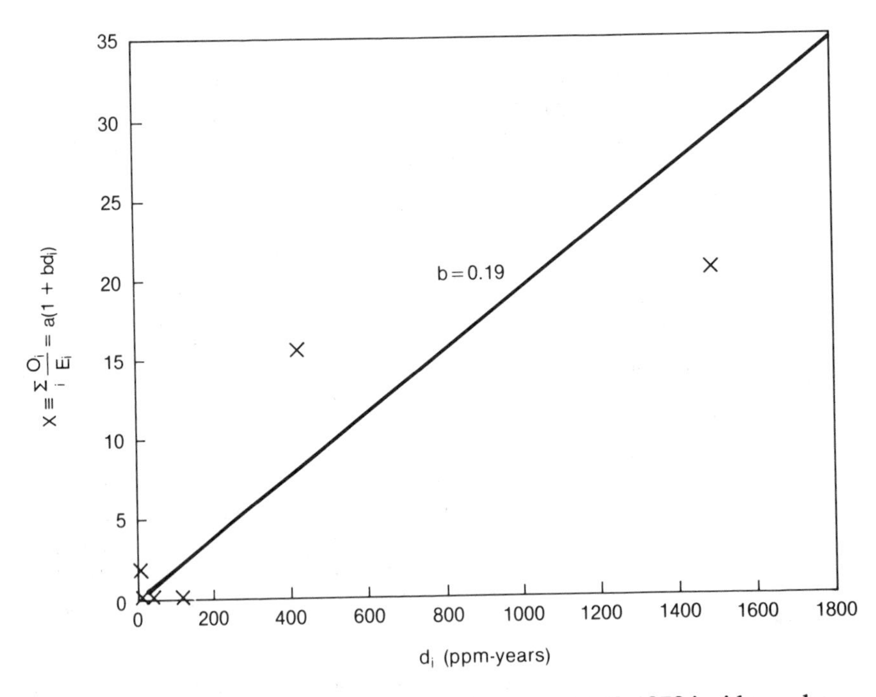

Fig. 2. Relative risk model with NIOSH Cohort 1950-1978 incidence data.

leukemia deaths predicted per 1000 workers. Therefore, at high human exposures of 10 ppm benzene for 40 years, the relative risk model is about twice as conservative as the absolute risk model.

Since potential model nonlinearities may produce different ratios of excess risk at low doses compared with high doses, we recalculated the excess risk at .1 ppm, a 100-fold lower dose. We obtained .24 excess leukemia deaths predicted per 1000 workers from the absolute risk model, as would be expected by dividing the predicted 24 excess tumors by 100. Applying the relative risk model, we obtained .51 excess leukemia deaths predicted per 1000 workers compared with .48 expected by dividing the predicted 48 excess tumors by 100. These computations show that both models of excess risk are virtually linear below 10 ppm. Therefore, the approximate twofold ratio between the two models also appears to hold below 10 ppm.

Since FDA is interested in excess risks from lifetime exposures beginning at birth, we adjusted the risks obtained above from the occupational exposure scenario (40 years beginning at age 20) to the situation where 1 ppm benzene in air for a normal work period, i.e., 8 hours per day, 5 days per week, 50 weeks per year, was encountered for a hypothetical entire lifetime. Using the relative risk model, 9.0 excess leukemia deaths are predicted per 1000 people. Using the absolute risk model, 5.0 excess leukemia deaths are predicted per 1000 people.

To consider the risk to a person exposed continuously since birth, rather than only during normal working house, the 1 ppm dose of benzene in air must be converted to continuous exposure:

$$1 \text{ ppm benzene} \times \frac{8 \text{ hours}}{24 \text{ hours}} \times \frac{5 \text{ days}}{7 \text{ days}} \times \frac{50 \text{ weeks}}{52 \text{ weeks}} = .23 \text{ ppm benzene}$$

This dose, .23 ppm benzene in air, inhaled daily for a lifetime, is equivalent to 1 ppm exposure over a normal work period for a lifetime. However, FDA is interested in benzene as a contaminant in food additives, and so the risk from ingested rather than inhaled benzene must be assessed. The workers in the occupational inhalation studies were inhaling low doses of benzene. We will assume that at such doses all the benzene will be absorbed and metabolized, thus allowing a value for systemic dose to be estimated. The systemic nature of leukemia allows the inference that the body burden of benzene is a reasonable measure of dose. The body burden of benzene in mg/kg ingested can then be calculated as follows:

Assuming that a person engaging in moderate activity has a respiratory rate of 12 liters per minute, he/she would be exposed to approximately 12 liters per minute × 1440 min/day = 1.73E4 liters of air per day. Using 1 mole weight in grams = 24.5 liters at room temperature and one atmosphere pressure, and the molecular weight of benzene = 78, 24.5 liters of benzene = 78 g. Thus,

$$\frac{1 \text{ molecule benzene}}{10^6 \text{ molecule air}} \times \frac{78 \text{ g}}{24.5 \text{ l}} \times \frac{1000 \text{ mg}}{1 \text{ g}} \times \frac{1.73^4}{60 \text{ kg day}}$$

$$= .92 \text{ mg/kg/day benzene} \ .$$

Therefore, the lifetime daily time-averaged dose, .23 ppm benzene inhaled, is equivalent to

$$.23 \text{ ppm benzene inhaled} \times \frac{.92 \text{ mg/kg/day benzene}}{1 \text{ ppm benzene ingested}}$$

$$= 21 \text{ mg/kg/day benzene} \ .$$

This amount of benzene ingested daily from birth throughout life would result in 9.0 excess leukemia deaths predicted per 1000 people using the relative risk model and in 5.0 excess leukemia deaths per 1000 people using the absolute risk model. To determine the potency, or unit risk, of benzene, we next divide the incidence by the dose, as follows:

$$\text{Relative Risk Model: } \frac{.0090}{.21 \text{ mg/kg}} = .043 \text{ per mg/kg/day.}$$

$$\text{Absolute Risk Model: } \frac{.0050}{.21 \text{ mg/kg}} = .024 \text{ per mg/kg/day.}$$

DISCUSSION

The unit risks derived from the human epidemiology data for leukemia are quite similar to those derived from the rodent data when the animal risks are summed over all organ sites in each sex grouping. This is somewhat surprising because of the many potential sources of bias which arise when comparing risk assessments derived from rodent and human studies. Human studies are subject to many more uncertainties and uncontrolled variables than are more tightly controlled experimental situations which occur among genetically homogeneous animals. Generally, rodents are exposed to high concentrations of a suspect carcinogen at constant dose levels. This is unlike the typical human exposure scenario of intermittent, varying exposures to a substance over a lifetime and is equally dissimilar to an occupational exposure of continuous low levels of the chemical. Moreover, currently there are no mechanisms to predict the large individual variation in human response to carcinogens which is frequently seen.

To avoid bias during the quantitative comparison of human and animal risks, it is helpful to apply the same mathematical extrapolation model to both humans and animals. Neither the relative risk nor absolute risk model is completely satisfactory for describing age-specific incidence in humans or for consistently comparing human studies to animal studies.[12] However, given only a twofold difference in prediction between the models in this case, we realize that this is more a theoretical than practical issue and we will emphasize the relative risk model because it is the more conservative of the two.

There are additional reasons for emphasizing the results from the more conservative model. First, since actual human age-specific leukemia mortality rates follow ever-increasing powers of time into old age, and since the observed human occupational exposures were limited to middle-age exposures, it is possible that lifetime excess leukemia mortality rates in humans may be larger than assumed by the absolute risk model. This would appear to be the case regardless of the biological stage affected by benzene. Second, limited evidence from Hoel[13] suggests that benzene acts primarily as a late-stage carcinogen. This may imply that the absolute risk model applied to middle-age occupational exposures would tend to underestimate actual risks from lifetime exposures. Third, if benzene is an early-stage carcinogen, as other evidence indicates,[14] then early-life exposure may also result in a higher risk than implied by the absolute risk model applied to middle-age occupational exposure. Fourth, since the model was limited to mortality data and we would like to account for the combined excess morbidity and mortality effects of benzene exposure, we prefer a risk estimate moderately greater than that implied by the absolute risk model.

REFERENCES

1. K. S. Crump and B. C. Allen, Quantitative Estimates of Risk of Leukemia from Occupational Exposure to Benzene, Occupational Safety and Health Administration, Docket H-059 B, Exhibit 152 (May 1984).

2. M. Aksoy, K. Dincol, S. Erdem, and G. Dincol, Acute Leukemia Due to Chronic Exposure to Benzene, *Am. J. Med.* **52**:160-166 (1972).
3. M. Aksoy, S. Erdem, G. Erdogan, and G. Dincol, Acute Leukemia in Two Generations Following Chronic Exposure to Benzene, *Hum. Heredity* **24**:70-74 (1974).
4. M. Aksoy, S. Erdem, and G. Dincol, Leukemia in Shoe-Workers Exposed Chronically to Benzene, *Blood* **44(6)**:837-841 (1974).
5. P. E. Infante, R. A. Rinsky, J. K. Wagoner, and R. J. Young, Leukemia in Benzene Workers, *Lancet* **2**:76-78 (1977).
6. R. A. Rinsky, R. J. Young, and A. B. Smith, Leukemia in Benzene Workers, *Am. J. Ind. Med.* **2**:217-245 (1981).
7. R. A. Rinsky, A. B. Smith, R. Hornung, T. G. Filloon, R. J. Young, A. H. Okun, and P. J. Landrigan, Benzene and Leukemia: An Epidemiologic Risk Assessment, *N. Engl. J. Med.* **316**:1044-1050 (1987).
8. M. G. Ott, J. C. Townsend, W. A. Fishbeck, and R. A. Langner, Mortality Among Individuals Occupationally Exposed to Benzene, *Arch. Environ. Health* **33**:3-10 (1978).
9. C. G. Bond, E. A. McLaren, C. L. Baldwin, and R. R. Cook, An Update of Mortality Among Chemical Workers Exposed to Benzene, *Arch. Environ. Health* **43**:685-91 (1986).
10. O. Wong, L. Kheifets, S. R. Larson, D. Cass, M. H. Doleman, G. Gawn, and A. Ruppenstein, An Industry-Wide Mortality Study of Chemical Workers Occupationally Exposed to Benzene, Environmental Health Associates, Inc., submitted to Chemical Manufacturers Association, unpublished, Berkeley, CA (December 8, 1983).
11. S. N. Yin, G. L. Li, F. D. Tain, Z. I. Fu, C. Jin, Y. J. Chen, S. J. Luo, P. A. Ye, J. Z. Zhang, G. C. Wang, X. C. Zhang, H. N. Wu, and Q. C. Zhong, Leukemia in Benzene Workers: A Retrospective Cohort Study, *Br. J. Ind. Med.* **44**:124-128 (1987).
12. R. N. Brown, C. B. Gable, L. K. Tollefson, J. S. Springer, and R. L. Lorentzen, Unifying Human and Animal Cancer Risk Assessments Using Multistage Incidence Models: Relative vs. Absolute Risk, presentation at SRA Annual Meeting, Washington, DC (1988).
13. D. G. Hoel, The Impact of Occupational Exposure Patterns on Quantitative Risk Estimation, in *Risk Quantitation and Regulatory Policy*, D. G. Hoel, R. A. Merrill, and F. P. Perera, eds., Banbury Report No. 19, pp. 105-118, Cold Spring Harbor Laboratory (1985).
14. E. P. Cronkite, R. T. Drew, T. Inoue, and J. E. Bullis, Benzene Hematotoxicity and Leukemogenesis, *Am. J. Ind. Med.* **7**:446-456 (1985).

Risk and Consent[a]

Mary R. English
University of Tennessee
Knoxville, TN

ABSTRACT

Today's risks are often technological risks, and consent to these risks is often sought by government agencies or industries. But what does it mean to consent to a risk? This paper begins by alluding to some of the ambiguities inherent in this question. It then proposes that even if consent is direct and voluntary (as opposed to indirect or coerced), a number of important issues remain: (1) whether the consent can be revoked; (2) what counts as informed consent; (3) whether the consent is explicit; (4) whether the consent is conflicted; and (5) what motivates the consent. After examining these issues, the paper concludes by discussing whether consent—even consent that is revocable, informed, explicit, unconflicted, and rationally motivated—always provides sufficient ethical grounds for the imposition of risk.

KEYWORDS: Risk, consent, volunteerism, ethics, hardship

INTRODUCTION

> "Illinois Low-Level Radioactive Waste Facility will be Good for the Local Economy . . . Already Benefits Gained Include: $400,000 unrestricted grants, $100,000 impact evaluation and assistance grants, $50,000 siting review grants, four-year scholarship to local students, new jobs for local residents"
>
> Illinois Department of Nuclear Safety,
> advertisement, *Wayne County Press*,
> Nov. 3, 1988, p. 6

> "the people should . . . not allow themselves to be swayed by the rosy promises. Vote your true feelings, as to whether you want to allow yourselves and all future generations to become Guards over an untested, maybe

---

a. The ideas developed here first appeared in Mary R. English, "Getting to 1993: Policies and Values in Low-Level Radioactive Waste Management" (July 1988) in *Ethical and Value Issues in Radioactive Waste Management* (report to the National Science Foundation's Ethics and Values in Science and Technology Program under Grant No. R11-8419118, E. William Colglazier, Principal Investigator). I have benefited from comments on those ideas by Clark Bullard, E. William Colglazier, Roger Kasperson, Steve Rayner, William Read, and especially John Hardwig—but perhaps insufficiently, as they might attest.

Risk Analysis, Edited by C. Zervos
Plenum Press, New York, 1991

dangerous facility, that could become known as the largest Mausoleum in the world."

Charles E. Smith, letter to the editor,
Wayne County Press, Nov. 3, 1988, p. 4

Government and industry are finding it more and more difficult to impose risky technologies on an unwilling public. Increasingly, the public's consent is being sought. But what counts as consent? That is the question I wish to consider here. In doing so, there is a lot that I will not consider.

First, I will concentrate on direct consent. I will not examine indirect forms of consent, such as (1) consent that may be extrapolated from people's marketplace actions (consent by revealed preference), (2) consent that may be extrapolated from a survey of people's attitudes (consent by expressed preference), and (3) consent that may be taken for granted, based either upon an initial voluntary act such as deciding to join a group or upon continuing to accept a group's benefits (hypothetical consent).[b] I will allude to hypothetical consent, but only in passing.

Second, I will only be talking about situations where direct consent is feasible—e.g., toxic waste facilities and nuclear power plants. I will not be talking about technologies whose risks are diffuse—e.g., chlorofluorocarbons and coal-fired power plants.

Technologies can be characterized according to three variables: the technology's reach, or effects, across space, its reach across time, and its complexity, including the complexity of information required to manage it and predict its effects.[c] If, for analytical purposes, these characteristics are treated as dichotomous variables (long or short spatial reach, long or short temporal reach, complex or simple technology), this produces eight logical possibilities. Direct consent is, in theory, appropriate for only two of them: the technology may be simple or complex but the spatial and temporal reach must be short. Otherwise, centralized decisions are better adapted to increase the likelihood that the preferences and well-being of those not immediately present but potentially affected will be taken into account.[d]

However, the interesting cases are those where the technology is complex, not simple. And complex technologies, including those with short spatial reaches, tend to have long reaches into the future. While centralized decisions for all technologies with long reaches might be preferable, imposing a complex technology often is not politically feasible when the spatial reach is short. Those immediately affected may insist upon their right to grant or withhold consent, and if that right is not honored, they may enforce it through political opposition or protracted battles in the courts. Thus direct consent is often necessary

---

b. For a discussion of these forms of consent, see Douglas MacLean, Risk and Consent: Philosophical Issues for Centralized Decisions, in *Values at Risk*, D. MacLean, ed., Rowman and Allanheld, Totowa, NJ (1986). Closely related to hypothetical consent is the nonconsent model, where a calculus of rational values on behalf of the group as a whole is considered more important than the consent of the group's members. The difference between the two is one of emphasis, for if one remains a member of the group and continues to benefit from it, one's hypothetical consent might also be assumed.

c. This typology was developed by Clark Bullard. See Clark W. Bullard, Management and Control of Modern Technologies, *Technology in Society* **10**:205-232 (1988).

d. This position necessarily rejects the argument that, because future persons are indeterminate in number and in their values, present persons have no duties to them. If this were the case, then direct consent would be appropriate. However, this position does not require going to the opposite extreme—i.e., the argument that future persons have rights corresponding to present persons' duties to them. Even without those corresponding rights, the present persons' duties would still suggest that the direct consent of those immediately affected is not sufficient when the fortunes of future as well as present persons are at stake. This point is developed in the conclusion.

for complex technologies with short spatial reaches, even if (and sometimes especially if) they have long reaches into the future.[e]

Third, I will not try to define precisely what counts as "consent." Defining consent raises a number of difficult issues, especially when groups are involved. There is the problem of representation: of who can consent to what on behalf of whom. This is a problem inherent in all groups except those that are both democratic and fully participatory. And for all groups, representative and nonrepresentative, there are at least two other potential problems: (1) the problem of divided opinion—of what counts as consent when there is a lack of unanimity; and (2) the problem of weighting—of whether each person's opinion on an issue should count equally if the issue affects some much more than others. These problems raise important procedural questions, but I will not go into them here.

Finally, I will not deal extensively with the type of question on which consent is being sought. On the one hand, the question at issue might primarily concern tangible outcomes; on the other hand, it might focus on the process by which a decision is reached, with the outcome of the process treated as only secondarily important. In either case, the notion of "consent to a question" is an artificial construct. In fact, it is likely that the question will not be self-contained; instead, it will involve a domain of issues and incremental decisions.

I will begin by taking an admittedly circumscribed look at some characteristics of direct consent. I will then consider possible motives for direct consent and the ethical implications of these motives.

DIRECT CONSENT: WHAT IS IT?

Consent — even if it is neither indirect nor coerced[f] — can leave a number of issues unresolved.

Revocability

One may consent to a prospective risk because of prospective benefits. If the benefits are not realized, however, one may feel that the risk should not have been imposed (regardless of whether the risk is realized by exposure or damage). For example, a nuclear power plant may bring with it the expectation of jobs at the facility and of related commercial and industrial development. If these expectations are not fulfilled, the host community may feel cheated, even though no explicit promises were made.[g]

Thus, direct consent leaves open the issue of revocability—of whether ex ante consent can be withdrawn if conditions turn out to be different than anticipated, or even if they turn out to be as anticipated. Ex ante consent presents especially difficult problems on matters involving future generations, where one generation is consenting not only for itself but also for its successors. Apart from the issue of whether the future generations' interests

---

e. Local people often think of themselves as guardians of their localities, and to many of them, "future generations" means their descendants. This is especially true in rural areas, where, because of their relatively sparse populations, risky facilities tend to be sited. While this personalized interpretation of "future generations" ignores in- and out-migration, it has a rational basis in the felt (and sometimes lived) ties of place and kinship.

f. Coercion can run the gamut from direct control to manipulation. I use the term narrowly here, leaving open the possibility of manipulation.

g. See Joseph B. Hughey, John W. Lounsbury, Eric Sundstrom, and Thomas J. Mattingly, Jr., Changing Expectations: A Longitudinal Study of Community Attitudes Toward a Nuclear Power Plant, *American Journal of Community Psychology* **11(6)**:655-672 (1983).

should be discounted, and if so at what rate, there remains the issue of whether subsequent generations can, practically and morally, withdraw the consent of their predecessors—as well as the issue of whether their predecessors can consent for them.

Informed Consent

There is also, of course, the issue of whether the consent is informed, and of what that means. "Informed consent" raises important epistemological questions about what constitutes adequate information and whom it must come from. If a principle of epistemic autonomy is used, then one must verify for oneself all of the relevant "facts" in order to consider oneself truly informed. With many of today's risk situations, especially those involving complex technologies, this is difficult to do. If, however, a principle of epistemic dependence is used, then one will choose to trust the experts rather than one's own ill-formed opinions.[h] But which experts?

Increasingly, when consent to a risky facility is sought, those proposing the facility give the prospective host grants for their "independent technical review"—i.e., in order to allow them to hire their own experts. But controversy often arises over such issues as which political or geographic boundaries should be used to define "the host," what the size of the grant should be and whether the grant can be used for adversarial purposes or to redo studies already performed by the proposers. And, more fundamentally, controversy among competing camps of experts, each with their own assumptions, theoretical models, and styles of argument, is likely to remain unresolved.[i]

Explicit Consent

Even if consent to a risk is informed (and putting aside what that means), it still may not be explicit: one may appear to go along with something by not saying no, even if offered the opportunity. This is a weak form of actual consent, and it leaves unclear whether full acquiescence is being given or whether judgment is being reserved. Because it is ambiguous, inexplicit consent is particularly susceptible to revocation at any time.

Unconflicted Consent

Another form of ambiguous consent is conflicted consent—one may explicitly agree to do X but still not be sure that X is acceptable. As long as these reservations are not expressed (perhaps even, by repression, to oneself), then the consent will appear to be unambiguous. The conflict may be due to contingencies (if Y happens, then I don't want X), in which case it can be cleared up either by taking care of the contingencies (e.g., through guarantees that Y won't happen)[j] or by allowing for the revocability of X if Y does happen.

The conflict may, however, be due to conflict over X itself—over X's anticipated costs and benefits. This conflict can be resolved only by changing either the assessment of the cost/benefit ratio or the ratio itself. Thus, those seeking to site a risky technology might need to "up the ante" to help ensure unconflicted consent, and even that might not be sufficient if the prospective host continues to have reservations about contingent conditions.

---

h. See John Hardwig, Epistemic Dependence, *Journal of Philosophy* 82(7) (1985).

i. See Sheldon J. Reaven, How Sure is Sure Enough: How and Why Stakeholders Differ on Repository Scientific Issues, in *Ethical and Value Issues in Radioactive Waste Management*, op. cit.

j. For example, attempts are being made to promote the development of "inherently safe" nuclear power reactors—i.e., reactors designed to eliminate the possibility of a core meltdown without relying on either mechanical or human intervention. See, e.g., Jack N. Barkenbus, Joint Development of an Inherently Safe Nuclear Reactor, Policy Brief, The Johns Hopkins Foreign Policy Institute, November 1988.

But even if the consent is unconflicted as well as explicit and "informed," questions remain about what has motivated the consent.

MOTIVES FOR CONSENT

Douglas MacLean has proposed that, as each model of indirect consent moves further away from actual consent, the role of rationality—i.e., of justification by appeals to rational values—becomes more important.[k] Thus, less justification is needed for centralized decisions based on expressed preference than on revealed preference; on revealed preference than on hypothetical consent; and on hypothetical consent than on nonconsent.

While I agree with MacLean's analysis, I would contend that the role of rational values in the instance of direct consent should not be minimized. Unless A (the party seeking consent) is convinced that the decision of B (the party whose consent is being sought) is based not only on full information but also on rational values, A is not justified in accepting B's consent.[l] What, though, counts as "rational values?"

"Rational" is, of course, a loaded term, as is "values." Taking values to mean principles as well as interests, rationality cannot be reduced to the calculus of costs and benefits that, according to classical economics, the "rationally self-interested" man would perform. Rationality will include that calculus, but the net result may still be countervailed by principles. This complicates things, for while it may be difficult to assess whether B's interests are rational, it is even harder to assess the rationality of his principles. What standards should be used to assess the rationality of both?

Three rational motives for consent—apart from the obvious one of a cost/benefit comparison—come to mind:

1. *Consent from Obligation.* B believes (and has good reason to believe) that he is best-suited to do the job. He therefore feels he has an obligation to A to consent.[m]

2. *Consent from Promise.* B has said he will do the job; therefore, when the time comes he does it. Consent from promise is related to hypothetical consent in that both suggest an ex ante consent actualized in the future. With hypothetical consent, however, the consent is to the institution, whereas with consent from promise the consent is to the issue at hand.

3. *Consent from Love or Patriotism.* B's overriding concern is for the well-being of A; to promote that well-being B consents and perhaps volunteers to do things that may not be in his own self-interest (if that self-interest is narrowly construed to exclude

---

k. Douglas MacLean, Risk and Consent: Philosophical Issues for Centralized Decisions, op. cit., p. 22.

l. Baruch Fischhoff makes a similar although more restricted point when he says: "In order to interpret the choice of the risky option as an act of informed consent, the other party must be able to claim that it has constituted the individual's optimal choice." Baruch Fischhoff, Cognitive and Institutional Barriers to 'Informed Consent', in *To Breathe Freely*, p. 184, Mary Gibson, ed., Rowman & Allanheld, Totowa, NJ (1985). Fischhoff explains (p. 170) that for a decision to be considered optimal, the individual must choose the course of action that is in his or her best interests, exploiting fully the available evidence. He defines "best interests" as whatever consequences the decision maker considers to be important.

m. During the early days of the search for a high-level radioactive waste repository, a Utah newspaper editorial commented that "neither Utah nor any other state can properly refuse to bear the nuclear waste burden once it (the repository site) has been established to the best of human conditions. However, the honor of making such a sacrifice . . . must confer on the luckless lamb the honor of knowing first-hand that the duty couldn't have been just as well assigned elsewhere." *Salt Lake City Tribune*, April 24, 1981. For a discussion of the context of this comment, see E. William Colglazier and Remi B. Langum, Policy Conflicts in the Process for Siting Nuclear Waste Repositories, *Annual Review of Energy 1988* **13**:317-357.

A's well-being). Consent from patriotism is promoted by seeing others do the same thing and by times of extremity. The feelings that inspire this type of consent may come naturally, or they may be evoked by manipulation.[n]

Of these motives for consent, the first two are from principle, although principles of different sorts. Consent from obligation is grounded in an evidential principle (that of who is best suited), whereas consent from promise is grounded in a procedural principle (that of commitment to process). The third motive, consent from love or patriotism, is derived from a mixture of both principle and interest. In a given situation, more than one motive may come into play at any one time—for example, one may promise to do a task out of a sense of obligation, as the person best-suited; and one may volunteer for, say, the army out of both patriotism and the desire for paid training and travel. Thus either more than one principle or both principles and interests may be at work.

People sometimes hesitate to take advantage of these motives, especially the first and third—perhaps because their altruism does not conform to conventional views about human nature. Conversely, to the extent that B's motive for consent is grounded in interests, A may feel more that he is on sound ethical ground in negotiating an offer with B and more comfortable with B's consent. Negotiation and compromise in conflicts over interests are more common and mutually acceptable than negotiation and compromise in conflicts over principles.[o] Furthermore, especially in a pluralistic culture such as ours, interests are more likely to be shared than are principles (everyone wants the same primary goods).

This suggests another motive for consent—one that is tacitly being emphasized by the A's in their searches for places to locate facilities perceived as risky. This is consent from hardship. B is in dire economic straits; he'll consent to A's offer even if the offer is low and the risks are high, in order to alleviate his immediate condition. Unlike the three motives described above, this does focus on a straightforward calculation of costs and benefits, but it is a calculation all too familiar to some, e.g., Appalachian coal miners. Because of need, the value placed on the benefits is inflated and the actual or potential costs are discounted. Thus it might take a guarantee of $10 million per year to persuade an affluent rural county to take a toxic waste disposal facility (if they could be persuaded at all), but $1 million per year might suffice for a poor county.

Because extreme need is the ultimate, distilled form of interest, A can be all the more confident that B's consent is rational if it is motivated by hardship. A may then feel especially secure that he is on sound ethical grounds in negotiating an offer with B. But should A feel more comfortable with that offer and B's consent to it, if the consent is from hardship? I will conclude by proposing that, under some theories of justice, A should not.

CONCLUSION

Especially if B's consent is motivated by hardship, A may have a responsibility to produce his own justification for his offer and B's consent to it by doing an independent calculation of costs and benefits, not merely using B's. This does not mean that B's calculation is not rational; it may be very rational, given his situation. But his situation is one of financial hardship, and financial hardship often leads to "knowledge hardship"—i.e., to a lack of expertise in acquiring and analyzing information and in bargaining. In other

n. Feminist ethical theory has pointed out that love or caring as a motive for consent is both potent and vulnerable to manipulation.

o. See, e.g., Martin P. Golding, The Nature of Compromise: A Preliminary Inquiry, and Theodore M. Benditt, Compromising Interests and Principles, in *Compromise in Ethics, Law, and Politics*, pp. 3-37, J. Roland Pennock and John W. Chapman, eds., NOMOS XXI, University Press, New York (1979).

words, if B is financially disadvantaged, it is likely that he also will have a relative inability to bargain and to extract safety concessions. Thus consent motivated by hardship does not spring from a free, informed choice; instead it is internally coerced and is likely to be ill-informed. While rational for B, it would not be rational if his position were not decisively shaped by hardship.

Given B's financial and knowledge hardship, is it just for A, in negotiating his offer, to take advantage of B's situation and derive his own justification from that situation? That depends on the theory of justice to which A subscribes. It might be just under a free-market theory,[p] and it would be just under act utilitarianism, if the net benefits to society exceeded the net costs. However, it would not be just under rule utilitarianism or "justice as fairness" as espoused by John Rawls[q] and as practiced by our society in other instances (e.g., the minimum wage law).

Instead, "justice as fairness" would dictate setting the terms of the offer either (1) by using a Rawlsian "veil of ignorance"—i.e., by determining how much it would take to get B to accept if all the possible B's did not know their stations in life,[r] or (2) by using Rawls' difference principle—i.e., by setting the terms so that the net benefit B derives by consenting is greater than the net benefit others better off than he derive by having him accept. Neither approach is wholly plausible if taken alone: the first, because the relative stations in life are known, and the second because the net benefits of others would be virtually impossible to calculate.[s] However, taken together they suggest the need for widespread discussions about what a fair minimum offer would be—discussions that should occur well before any identification of technically suitable hosts.

This approach might be considered paternalistic, but it would be paternalism in the benign sense—that of exceeding others' expectations.[t] Another recourse is open to A: A can refuse to accept consent motivated by hardship. This, however, would be paternalism in a much more objectionable sense—that of making decisions for others that don't coincide with their judgments of their own best interests. I thus am advocating, not that A reject consent motivated by hardship, but that A make independent, non-market determinations of what counts as a "fair" offer.

---

p. See, e.g., Robert Nozick, *Anarchy, State, and Utopia*, Basic Books, New York (1974). Nozick argues for a minimal state limited largely to providing protection for its citizens. However, in his chapter on "Prohibition, Compensation, and Risk" (pp. 54-87), he suggests that if a party (X) is put at significant risk by the activity of another (Y) and that activity is productive, either in that it benefits both or in that it benefits Y for reasons that don't have the do with an "abstention bribe" from X, then two fair recourses are available. Y can go ahead with the activity but must compensate X for being put at significant risk, or X can prohibit the activity but must compensate Y if Y is disadvantaged by the prohibition, in the sense of being made worse off as compared with others. Nozick calls this the "principle of compensation." It appears that this principle would apply only if there is one possible X. If there is more than one, than it appears that Nozick's theory would argue for a free-market approach.

q. John Rawls, *A Theory of Justice*, Belknap Press, Cambridge, MA (1971).

r. This is a very free use of the "veil of ignorance" concept. Rawls intended it in a more restricted sense, as a condition that only existed prior to the generation of his two fundamental principles of justice.

s. Economic models for valuing changes such as the "willingness to pay" and "willingness to accept" frameworks might be appropriate in theory, but they are not without problems and would be extremely difficult to apply.

t. This assumes that the societally-established offer will result in a better deal for B than any deal that he could negotiate with A. Given the "veil of ignorance" and "difference principle" to be used in developing the offer, this is a reasonable assumption, especially if one also assumes that, all other things being equal, A would otherwise have sought the lowest bidder. If it turned out that the negotiated offer would have been better for B than the societally-established one, it still could be argued that the latter is fairer, taking A's welfare as well as B's into consideration.

It could be objected that the intent of the non-market determination of a "fair" offer is to make the offer sufficiently good to attract even the non-needy, and that if this intent is realized, then others motivated by greed rather than need may compete with B, and B may lose out. This is, in theory at least, a reasonable objection. It could be answered either (1) by giving preference to hardship cases (all other things being equal), or (2) by application of the "difference principle," such that the better off B is, the less handsome the offer is. With the first approach, the offer is relatively firm; with the second, it is on a sliding scale based on hardship. But the effect of either is likely to be the same: only hardship cases will both apply and be considered.

Apart from ethical considerations, A has other good reasons for not profiting from consent motivated by hardship. Hardship is perhaps the least stable motive for consent, since the hardship conditions can change. This leaves open the possibility that B will feel at some future point that "I've been had," leading, at a minimum, to resentment and political alienation. It also raises two related issues referred to above: the issue of revocability of consent and the issue of the responsibility of both A and B to future generations.

The domain of consent to a technology—even one of short spatial reach—involves a range of issues: the need for the technology, including who will use it and for what purposes, its safety, and cost and liability considerations. The issue of consent to a technology is thus inextricably connected with the problem of continuing uncertainty, insofar as the technology's safety or benefits accruing from it cannot be absolutely guaranteed. And uncertainty extending into the future suggests that B is consenting to something, not simply on his own behalf, but for future generations as well.

Thus, with technologies having a long temporal reach, what starts as direct consent becomes hypothetical consent, especially if revocability is not possible. This suggests an additional reason for A's not accepting consent motivated by hardship at face value, without doing an independent calculation of costs and benefits. Even if A demurs at the paternalism to B implied by doing such an independent calculation, A must, to justify the hypothetical consent of future generations, assume a paternalistic role with respect to B's successors, especially because B, out of hardship, may not be able to serve a fiduciary role on their behalf.

And even if the technology is of short temporal reach, affecting only B, A can reject the role of paternalism only if he is willing to alter B's station in fundamental ways, so that B is an equal among equals and is not consenting to a raw deal out of hardship. Unless A is both willing and able to undertake a fundamental redistribution of wealth and power, benign paternalism is, under a "justice as fairness" concept, his only recourse.

Risk Analysis Issues in Developing Countries

Masahisa Nakamura
Lake Biwa Research Institute
Shiga Prefecture, Japan

Tomitaro Sueishi
Osaka University
Osaka, Japan

ABSTRACT

Developing countries are faced with a growing number of risks, particularly those arising from proliferation of chemicals and from the use of highly sophisticated industrial technologies. As these risks often defy conventional managerial approaches, scientists and government officials in developing countries have shown great interest in risk assessment and risk management methodologies based on experiences in developed countries. These methodologies could prove useful in dealing with a variety of risks. However, there are fundamental differences between developed and developing countries in priorities and in the way risks are handled. We summarize below some of the important risk analysis issues in developing countries and highlight possible disparities in risk concepts and risk management approaches between them and developed countries.

KEYWORDS: Risk analysis, developing countries, chemicals, risk comparisons, primary and secondary risks

INTRODUCTION: GROWING INTEREST IN RISK ANALYSIS IN DEVELOPING COUNTRIES

We live in a risky world. Judging by the rapidly growing body of literature, particularly in the United States, it appears our world is becoming saturated with newly identified risks of all kinds. Other developed countries have also become very risk-conscious, and now risk-related studies are beginning to attract attention in many developing countries. The interest in risk is likely to grow in developing countries just as rapidly as it has in the developed countries.

Air, water, and solid waste pollution have long been known to be extremely serious in many urban and industrial population centers in developing countries. But health risks from pollution have become increasingly difficult to identify and manage, particularly those due to the rapidly growing number of newly introduced chemicals. The amount of toxic substances inhaled or ingested by urban dwellers has been found, in general, to be far in excess of tolerances to the extent of posing serious health risks.[1]

The trend toward viewing risks as omnipresent has obviously been accelerated by the Bhopal chemical plant accident and the explosion of liquid natural gas containers in downtown Mexico City. Both accidents killed large numbers of the local population. It has also been accelerated by natural calamities in developing countries which often result in a large number of casualties, as in the cases of deadly carbon dioxide poisoning at Lake Nyos, earthquakes in Managua, and floods in Bangladesh. Nuclear reactor failures and accidents such as those experienced at Three Mile Island and Chernobyl have also accelerated the trend toward extreme concern for such risks in developing countries.

Concomitant to this trend toward increased concern about risky events, international organizations including UN agencies and regional collaboration bodies (WHO, FAO, UNEP, OECD, etc.) have been actively involved in the promotion of risk analysis, particularly with respect to risks associated with potent as well as latent exposures to chemicals. Some of the priority programs actively promoted by these organizations are concerned with risks due to the use of pesticides, chemical accidents, and hazardous waste management.

The number of occurrences of risky incidents in developing countries is indeed increasing, and analyses produced thus far will be extremely useful for developed countries. However, in general, developing countries face risks differently than developed countries. Their approaches to risky events, therefore, must also be different, and thus priority setting in the management of risks requires elaboration from many different perspectives.

The papers presented at the Second U.S.-Japan Workshop on Risk Assessment and Risk Management[2-7] and other similar reports[8] were reviewed. The following is a review and discussion of some priority areas requiring consideration in developing countries. It highlights potentially useful approaches to risk assessment and risk management there. It focuses specifically on the countries represented in the aforementioned workshop.

PERCEIVED NEEDS FOR RISK CONSIDERATIONS: SUMMARY OF SITUATION ANALYSIS

Conventional Environmental and Natural Hazards

According to a WHO survey[9] of the status of national environmental pollution control programs in 1984,[9] the degree to which countries in the midst of moderate-to-rapid industrial development meet pollution control requirements depends strongly on their level of industrialization (Table 1). This implies that types of environmental hazards and risk considerations differ according to the level of industrialization and to the country's capability of meeting pollution control requirements.

The environmental health risks identified were common among the represented countries, particularly with respect to pollution of air, water, and soil. The unavoidable by-products of developmental activities in the urban centers continue to be of major concern to most of the developing countries in the region. For example, the largest number of complaints received by Malaysian environmental agencies pertained to air pollution (80%), 55% of which had an industrial origin. Similarly, a significant portion of air pollution in Korea is caused by industrial activities such as chemical manufacturing, metallurgical operations, and petroleum refining, and by general fugitive emissions associated with various manufacturing operations. Risks from pathogenic microorganisms and acute chemical poisoning in solid and liquid waste are gradually becoming less important than chronic risks from the accumulation of low level chemical contaminants. Such risks will be discussed in the next section.

Table 1. Distribution of Countries According to Their Level of Development and Their Environmental Pollution Control Performance

Pollution control Activity Indicators	Highly Industrialized Countries	Moderately To Rapidly Industrializing Countries	Countries With Low Development Activity
Most Requirements Met	31	10	0
Some Requirements Met	0	29	9
Few Or No Requirements Met	0	20	67

Other concerns of high priority, particularly in countries heavily dependent on utilization of natural resources for economic development, are aspects of resource degradation, such as deforestation and forest fires, soil erosion, loss of terrestrial habitat, reduction in wildlife species, and irreversible damage to marine ecosystems, including the destruction of mangrove (Indonesia, Malaysia, Thailand and Philippines). The rate of deforestation in Thailand, for example, is estimated to be 10 million rai per annum (1.6 million ha per annum). In the Philippines, the forest coverage has been reduced to 35% of the total land as compared to more than 55% in 1950. Deforestation, as well as the risk of forest fires due to shifting agriculture, prevails in the vast island regions of Sumatra, Kalimantan, Selawesi, Irian Jaya, and Nusa Tenggara in Indonesia. In their lending policies the international development banks take into consideration the protection of forests and reforestation of denuded land, an indication of the significance of the problem.

Emerging Concern for Risks from the Use of Marketed Chemicals

By far the most significant health risks causing increasing concerns are chemical risks. They assume a variety of forms. According to the workshop papers, the priority chemical risks and the degree of preparedness for risk management differ even among the countries represented in the workshop. Some of the fragmentary statistics presented in the workshop highlighted the chemical risks in these countries. For example, in the Republic of Korea, a country undergoing extremely rapid industrialization, there were 10,000 chemicals in use in 1983, of which 8300 were imported. Currently only 385 chemicals are classified as toxic, requiring permits.

In the Philippines, efforts are currently underway to develop an inventory of toxic chemicals and to conduct policy studies on the regulation of toxic and hazardous substances. In Indonesia, the use of non-biodegradable chlorinated hydrocarbon pesticides such as DDT, BHC and PCP is prohibited. Finally, the amount of hazardous wastes produced in China is estimated to be around 40 million tons.

The number of chemicals used varies between countries, but it is estimated that the more developed countries use up to a million chemicals or mixtures of chemicals. Many are potential health risks because they are not controlled adequately. Among them, pesticides such as DDT, Chlordane, Heptachlor, Dieldrin, Paraquat, Aldrin, 2,4,5-T, BHC, Lindane, Endrin, 2,4-D, and Endosulfan constitute the most important group because they are known to be hazardous, bioaccumulating and carcinogenic. They are potentially too detrimental to human health and ecosystems to justify their use for the control of pests and weeds and have been banned in many developed countries. They are sold freely in developing countries, mostly because of a lack of adequate control. Developed countries producing excess amounts of such pesticides are blamed for dumping them in developing countries, taking advantage of the lack of legal controls on importation of specific products.[10,11]

Although information is limited, it is believed that there are many instances of reported and unreported pesticide overexposure and misuse accidents in developing countries. Some—estimated between 0.2 and 10%—involve fatalities. According to WHO statistics, fatalities are on the order of 5000 per year, but the figure excludes cancers, miscarriages, deformed babies and still births resulting from the use of pesticides. Deaths are due to inadequate pesticide regulations, illiteracy, lack of awareness, and general apathy of the authorities, as well as the shortage of manpower capable of managing programs for safe handling, transport, and application of these often deadly chemicals.

Risks Facing the Underserved and Underequipped Population

One important aspect of chemical safety often overlooked is the effects of toxic chemicals on the most vulnerable segments of a country's population, e.g., farmers, farm laborers, women, and children. From the occupational health point of view, farmers and laborers need greater protection from direct exposure to hazardous chemicals. They need to be instructed in proper handling of such chemicals. According to Travis and Covello,[12] women and children need special attention because of the following reasons:

1. Women and children are relatively more sensitive to the effects of toxic substances. In some instances children might be in double jeopardy, being subject both to the direct reproductive health effects of a toxicant and to the teratogenic effects of maternal intoxication.
2. Health effects are likely to result from chronic exposures, creating problems for adequate monitoring and corrective action.
3. Sociodemographic factors associated with age and sex roles may affect significantly occupational and home-based exposures to toxic substances.
4. Women represent a valuable human resource in world development, and implementation of regulatory and safety standards will often require the active support of women.

There are a number of endemic diseases known or suspected to have an environmental chemical etiology.[9] Fluorosis, a vision disorder, and the Kashin-Beck disease are examples. Many are only rarely reported because of inadequate surveillance programs in most developing countries. Often cases are mistakenly assigned to pathogenic or genetic causes, and frequently patients are referred to improper treatment.

Risks from Wrongly Released Hazardous Materials

Accidents involving chemical manufacturing equipment, storage facilities, and chemical transport vehicles are another source of chemical hazards. Often in developing countries accident prevention measures are seriously inadequate, and when an accident occurs the consequences can be devastating to the entire ecosystem surrounding the accident site for miles because of the lack of emergency procedures.

Many developing countries have yet to enact legislation concerning the storage, transport, use, and disposal of chemicals, including agricultural chemicals. In addition to the fragmentation of responsibility for the management of chemicals, the absence of adequate laws hampers the establishment of well coordinated and comprehensive national chemical safety programs, making public health and environmental protection even more difficult.

A subject of growing concern in developing countries is the management of toxic and hazardous wastes. Industries such as petrochemical production, fertilizer manufacturing and electroplating produce wastes toxic to the environmental biota and to human health. Similarly, some industrial operations such as mines and smelters, like hazardous waste disposal sites, produce localized hazardous environmental pollution and become serious health threats to the local residents. Most developing countries are still struggling with the safe disposal of municipal wastes. Few have the resources to implement the regulatory and technological management provisions for the safe disposal of hazardous wastes.

Exposure to radioactive materials used in energy production, agriculture, and medicine is also of great concern to developing countries. Unlike chemicals, all radioactive materials are presumably placed under strict control by appropriate authorities. In particular, there are well established international standards on the allowable levels of exposure to radioactivity for medical treatment. The standards may not be difficult to adhere to as long as x-ray examinations and other radiation therapies are professionally conducted. On the other hand, it is often difficult to institute strict control over the handling and eventual disposal of radioactive waste from hospitals, research institutions, and mining operations. Accidental exposures from improperly handled or misplaced radioactive materials have also been reported. The risks involving possible breakdowns of nuclear power generation facilities are studied extensively in many developed countries, particularly in connection with past failures of various magnitudes, including the Three-Mile Island and Chernobyl cases. Only very limited capabilities exist in developing countries with regard to assessment and management of risks due to failures of technologically complex facilities such as nuclear energy plants.

DISPARITIES IN RISK ANALYSIS BETWEEN DEVELOPED AND DEVELOPING COUNTRIES

Environmental and health risk issues facing developing countries have been reviewed. The next step is to see if developing countries are up to the task of dealing with the risk issues in a manner similar to what has been proposed so far in developed countries. This is a difficult task for the following reasons.

First, risk analysis is an attractive aid in deciding the extent to which a society should depend on potentially risky products or situations. Decisions involve trade-offs between the risks, costs, and expected benefits. Risk analysis assumes that there exists a solution to the risk/benefit conflict satisfying society's requirements, that risks can be assessed with reasonable accuracy and that they can be controlled and managed. To control risk, resources must be mobilized for developing proper institutional structures and adequately functional management systems responsible for implementing risk management measures. Such basic assumptions do not necessarily hold for most of the risky situations that prevail in developing countries. Often they do not hold even for risky situations in developed countries.

There are other difficulties. Even in developed countries, neither the definitions of risk assessment and management terms, nor the scopes of the processes are standardized.[13] Thus it is difficult to make generalized but definite statements. It is likely that a wide array of issues will continue to surface in the risk analysis field, and standardization of risk analysis methods will continue to be confined only within specific subject areas even in developed countries.

Second, the importance of separating risk assessment and risk management, one of the prerequisites for conducting scientific analysis of risks, may not be recognized as strongly in many developing countries. In such countries, priority risk considerations are concerned with potent (e.g., pathogenic microorganisms) and apparent (e.g., operational failures) risks rather than latent (e.g., low level chronic chemical exposures) risk. The information required for the assessment of the former risks is obtained in the course of risk management in the field, while the evaluation of risk in the latter case involves risk assessment independent of the mode of risk management. Some attempts have been made in the past to address this problem.

RISK ANALYSIS LIMITATIONS IN DEVELOPING COUNTRIES

Examining water pollution prevention schemes, Lumbers and Jowitt[14] focused on some of the subtleties of conducting risk analysis in developing countries. They identified three broad levels of uncertainties that militate against any straightforward and definite resolution of a problem.

1. Uncertainties in describing the resource system to be controlled (pollution control facilities).
2. Uncertainties in efficiency and reliability of the particular engineering or other measures to be used (treatment system to be employed).
3. Uncertainties during operation of the prevention scheme, and institutional and financial failures (breakdowns and mismanagement).

In addition, Lumbers and Jowitt categorized risks as primary and secondary. The former are targeted to be reduced immediately (e.g., by chlorination for control of pathogens or by control of trace organic and heavy metal concentrations) The latter are risks associated with the implementation of the scheme for reduction of primary risks (e.g., trihalomethane formation, breakdown of a chlorinator or failure of a reporting system).

In general, risk analysis efforts in developing countries are concentrated on reducing difficulties in defining and assessing primary risks and their causal relationships.

Table 2 shows comparisons of the differences between developed and developing countries in dealing with primary and secondary risks. Pathogenic organisms and chemical contaminants are used as examples.

In most developed countries, latent (chemical) and transient risks are of greatest concern. Risks from pathogenic organisms do exist under certain circumstances, but they are generally confined within the capabilities of existing treatment technology and management provisions. They are generally considered to be under control and the associated mortality rates are negligible. Risk analyses, therefore, are directed toward establishing a firm scientific basis for dose-response relationships at low exposure levels and toward developing more reliable approaches for assessing the probability of occurrence of transient phenomena such as equipment failures and other accidents.

In most developing countries, on the other hand, concern is greatest for potent pathogen risks stemming particularly from inadequate management. Perhaps the reason is not because latent chemical risks are not significant in magnitude, but because their magnitudes are not fully appreciated and because acute adverse impacts from prevalent waterborne disease epidemics are much more conspicuous. Precise risk assessments required to determine carcinogenic potential, for example, are of theoretical interest only to many water supply personnel in developing countries. The magnitude of latent health risks is masked by high mortality rates from waterborne diseases caused by inadequate facilities

Table 2. Management of Health Risks from Biological and Chemical Contaminants in Drinking Water

Risks	Developed Countries	Developing Countries
Primary		
Pathogenic contamination (potent)	Negligibly small	Significant
Chemical contamination (latent)	Becoming increasingly serious	Estimated to be serious but not thoroughly known
Secondary		
Poor management of risk information	Infrequent	Frequent due to poor surveillance systems
Unexpected transient phenomena (e.g., equipment failure)	Infrequent	Frequent due to difficulties in poor equipment maintenance and operator training
Mobilization of resources for risk management	Increasing, particularly for controlling chemical risks	Grossly inadequate both for biological and chemical risks

and poor operation and maintenance practices. The risks from inadequate water supplies and sanitation are obvious, and assessment of their magnitudes is carried out only on an informal and ad hoc basis.

Aside from the emphasis on potent rather than latent risks, there are other limitations on risk analysis in many developing countries. There are perennial shortages of financial and human resources and severe lack of risk management skills, particularly with respect to the development of realistic systems of managing information, institutional development, and personnel. Successful development of such systems requires, among other things, simplicity in information management, familiarity in operational management, and accountability in institutional coordination.

Simplicity. The framework of analyses must be simple and within the limitations of the resources available to the health and environmental institutions in developing countries. This is not so much because of limited institutional capabilities, but rather because risk-cost-benefit trade-offs are often much more straightforward. Acceptable levels of risk depend not on preference but on basic needs instead.

Familiarity. Risk analyses must be placed in a framework familiar both in concept and in practice to conventional regulatory activities in health and environmental agencies. Most risks are old problems with new names. Existing control frameworks are not irrelevant to the emerging awareness of newly identified risks. These frameworks need to be made appropriately functional.

Accountability. Due to diffuse sociocultural orientation and awareness, a reasonable degree of accountability in health and environmental activities is difficult to achieve in many developing countries. This lack of accountability frequently leads to easy breakdowns of communication links, and what appears to be preventable marginal risks in developed countries could become risks of serious magnitude in developing countries.

OUTSTANDING RISK ANALYSIS ISSUES IN DEVELOPING COUNTRIES

Approaches to risk analysis differ according to priorities and of resources which can be mobilized for risk management. Full assessment of chemical risks, for example, requires manpower and financial resources beyond what most developing countries can afford to mobilize. Options available for management of hazardous wastes are likely to be limited in many developing countries because of institutional and technological inadequacies. For risk assessments, developing countries usually depend on developed countries. For risk management they are necessarily limited in scope and in extensiveness.

International organizations have been searching for ways to assist developing countries to deal with environmental and health risks, taking into account local realities. Their efforts include information consolidation and dissemination, development of human resources, strengthening of institutional capabilities, and collaborative research. Listed below are some of the major categories of issues identified in the course of these efforts.

Determination of the Magnitude of Risks. There are on-going but limited efforts to establish the magnitudes of the various risks faced by the developing countries. Generally such magnitudes are not yet fully established.

Socio-economic Development Status and Recognition of Risk. Risks are relative. What may be regarded as risky in developed countries may not necessarily be regarded as such in developing countries. Many of the transboundary risk issues are closely linked to the differences in the recognition of risks.

Political Will. Control of environmental and health risks is dependent on the overall national policy framework which reflects the political will of the country. Since political will is generally much more responsive to short term needs, the long term and latent risks are often underestimated and/or overlooked despite concerns by ordinary citizens. Under such circumstances, international organizations could play crucial roles in drawing political commitments to the development of appropriate national programs.

Use of Existing Institutional Frameworks. It is difficult for most developing countries to mobilize resources to establish new programs for risk analysis. Modification of existing institutional frameworks and introduction of appropriate legislative measures are essential and realistic initial steps for dealing with priority risks.

Dealing with Multimedial Risks. Most risks are multimedial in nature. It is, therefore, almost impossible to have a single agency responsible for all environmental and health risks. Intersectoral coordination is often critical for risk management. Fragmentation of responsibilities is one of the major barriers to establishing effective risk management programs in developing countries.

Appropriate Technology and Risks. Risks associated with chemicals, for example, are often due to by-products of imported commodities. Risk management options may include the importation of less risky commodities or technologies.

The strong initiatives of international organizations such as WHO, FAO, UNEP and OECD have brought about significant improvements in the dissemination of essential information on risks and risk analysis procedures. Collation of scientific facts and authoritative statements of international scientific groups, standardizing of national decisions, and integration of environmental management policy with international trade and development policy are high priority activities at the international level.

But a great deal needs to be accomplished at the bilateral level as well, particularly in view of the fact that actual transfer of risks occurs directly between the risk-generator and the risk-taker countries. Among examples of such cases are the transfer of risky commodities (e.g., the movement of banned pesticides from developed countries to developing countries) transfer of risky technologies (e.g., nuclear power generation or manufacture of highly toxic chemicals such as methyl iso-cyanate) or even the transfer of technologies perceived to be novice and risky in developing countries (e.g. food irradiation).

Self-imposed regulation by the exporting countries may not be very reassuring to the importing countries. However, overemphasis on international rather than bilateral agreements may diminish the incentives for the exporting countries themselves to take initiatives to prevent transnational transfer of unwarranted risks.

SUMMARY AND CONCLUSIONS

Developing countries face a large number of health and environmental risks. Many are old problems with new names and will continue to be handled within the context of such measures as pollution control, environmental management, and resource conservation. Others defy conventional perceptions and conventional management approaches. The magnitudes of the latter have not yet been fully assessed, and systems for their management have also not yet been established. Concern for them will have to be addressed properly, and emerging problems must be handled with whatever resources and tools are made available by developed countries or international organizations.

There are some fundamental differences between developed and developing countries with respect to the concept of risk. They originate from many sources, including different priority concerns, different resource limitations, and different management structures and capabilities. The consequences of such differences have not yet been fully addressed.

Hasty transfers of risk analysis frameworks from developed to developing countries may not be realistic. To meet the requirements and constraints of developing countries, risk analysis methodologies must be adapted. It will take some time before suitably tailored methodologies begin to make tangible impacts on the assessment and management of risks prevalent in developing countries.

REFERENCES

1. World Health Organization (WHO) and United Nations Environment Programme (UNEP), Global Pollution and Health—Results of Health-Related Environmental Monitoring, GEMS/WHO, Geneva, Switzerland (1987).
2. Bakar Jaafar Abu, Environmental Risk Management in Malaysia, in Proceedings of the 2nd U.S.-Japan Workshop on Risk Management, Suita-Osaka, Japan (1987).
3. B. H. Cho, Country Report: Republic of Korea, in Proceedings of the 2nd U.S.-Japan Workshop on Risk Management, Suita-Osaka, Japan (1987).
4. C. P. B. Caludio, Risk Assessment and Management: The Philippine Case, in Proceedings of the 2nd U.S.-Japan Workshop on Risk Management, Suita-Osaka, Japan (1987).
5. Herman Haeruman, Jr., Environmental Risk Management in Indonesia, in Proceedings of the 2nd U.S.-Japan Workshop on Risk Management, Suita-Osaka, Japan (1987).

6. Yusheng Liu, The State-of-the-Art of Risk Analysis and Management in China, in Proceedings of the 2nd U.S.-Japan Workshop on Risk Management, Suita-Osaka (1987).
7. Setamanit Surin, Development, Environmental Risks and Management in Thailand, in Proceedings of the 2nd U.S.-Japan Workshop on Risk Management, Suita-Osaka, Japan (1987).
8. A. V. Whyte and I. Burton, *Environmental Risk Assessment, SCOPE 15*, John Wiley & Sons, New York (1980).
9. World Health Organization, Control of Environmental Health Hazards, A WHO Strategy for Technical Cooperation with Member States, WHO, Geneva, Switzerland (1987).
10. Gaik Sim Foo, The Pesticide Poisoning Report, A Survey of Some Asian Countries, in International Organization of Consumers Unions, Penang, Malaysia (1985).
11. Alam Malaysia Sahbat (Friends of the Earth), Pesticide Dilemma in the Third World—A Case Study of Malaysia, Penang, Malaysia (1984).
12. C. C. Travis and V. Covello, Risks of Toxic Substances in Developing Countries: Implications for Women and Children, a paper obtained from the authors (undated).
13. E. W. Lawless, Risk Assessment Methodology for Hazardous Waste Management, presented at the Workshop on Risk Assessment of Hazardous Chemicals in Developing Countries (1987).
14. J. P. Lumbers and P. W. Jowitt, Risk Analysis in the Planning Design and Operational Control of Water Pollution Prevention Schemes—A Perspective, *Water Science and Technology* **13**:27-34 (1981).

Risk Assessment — Science or Fiction?

Wayne Tusa and David Lipsky
Dynamac Corporation
Fort Lee, NJ

ABSTRACT

This paper is designed to focus on whether or not the conservative bias typically employed in completing risk assessments in the environmental arena results in risk assessment conclusions that are generally realistic or potentially unsuited for decision making purposes. The paper discusses the concept of risk assessment and how it is intended to be applied to contamination issues at specific sites, describes the various inputs to the risk evaluation process and discusses how the risk assessment process is inherently conservative due to the assumptions typically used to estimate health risks. The paper then gives examples of how practitioners in the field are utilizing overly conservative input assumptions relating to source definitions, pathway availability estimates, exposure estimates, etc., resulting in overly conservative risk conclusions. Practical suggestions are also made with respect to improving input assumptions, dealing with data uncertainties and utilizing sensitivity analysis to improve input assumptions and remedy selection processes.

KEYWORDS: Risk assessment, risk guidance, sensitivity analysis

INTRODUCTION

The use of risk assessment as a site-specific decision-making tool has increased dramatically in the past few years. Risk assessment methods are now commonly used to evaluate potential remedies under the federal Superfund program (Publ. No. 96-510 as amended by Publ. No. 99-499), to evaluate siting and air pollution control issues for proposed resource recovery facilities, and to evaluate design requirements for new or expanded land disposal facilities. More recently, as the potential usefulness of risk assessment techniques has been increasingly recognized, risk assessment methods are being applied to an even broader array of site specific issues—such as evaluating the acceptability of proposed manufacturing facility expansions, assessing potential liabilities due to the transfer of contaminated real estate and selecting remedies for underground storage tank leaks.

Notwithstanding the particular application, the objective of any site-specific risk assessment is to provide input for decisions relating to the acceptability of a proposed project or a project modification from a health risk or environmental impact perspective. In this context, the application of risk assessment typically consists of a sequence of specific analytical steps. In the first step, the database on the proposed project is evaluated to identify all potential sources of contaminants and the relative quantity and availability of those contaminants. Indicator chemicals, i.e., those contaminants that by virtue of their availability, mobility, or toxicity pose the highest potential risks, are often selected to model the potential risks posed by the project.

In the second step, the potential for migration of the selected indicator chemicals is assessed for each migration pathway of potential significance—typically including direct contact, air, surface water and groundwater. The availability of each pathway is evaluated and/or modeled to assess the potential extent and rate of transport of identified contaminants.

In the third step, the presence of potential receptors that might be affected by contaminants migrating in available pathways is evaluated. Depending on site-specific factors, this analysis may include the identification of existing human and/or environmental receptors, potentially including sensitive receptors, and the development of projections for future receptor populations.

In the fourth step, the degree of existing or potential exposure is assessed. In this analysis, measured or modeled concentrations and measured or anticipated exposure durations at receptor points are translated into estimated doses due to direct contact, inhalation or ingestion.

In the fifth step, baseline carcinogenic and noncarcinogenic risks are typically estimated for each indicator chemical for each potential pathway. In some cases, effects to environmental receptors may also be estimated.

Depending on the specific issues at hand, the final step may consist of an evaluation of the acceptability of a proposed project from a risk or impact perspective, an analysis of the relative risks posed by a project being considered for several locations, or an analysis of various engineering alternatives being considered to reduce the risks associated with a specific project located at an existing site. In the first case, the baseline risks estimated for a proposed facility or facility expansion are assessed to assist in determining whether unacceptably high health or environmental impacts might occur should the proposed project be completed. In the second case, the risks posed by a project at various locations are estimated to assist in making siting decisions. In the third case, the levels of residual risks posed after implementation of various engineering alternatives are assessed to assist in making design decisions. In all cases, this last step should include an analysis, at a sufficient level of detail, which would permit comparison of the relative advantages and disadvantages of each risk management option, including the baseline risks posed by the project and the residual risks posed by the various design alternatives.

Regardless of the issues being considered, it should be clear that the types of decisions being made have significant impacts on both the project sponsors and the potentially affected communities. From a societal perspective, adequate protection of the environment and human health is paramount. Balanced with this basic need, however, must be adequate consideration of the community's infrastructure needs, e.g., providing sufficient job opportunities, having access to appropriate waste treatment and disposal facilities, or providing public access to areas previously unsuitable due to past contamination problems. In most cases, constructing and operating facilities to meet societal needs results in some increase in risk. Balancing the associated risks and benefits typically involves making or adjusting public or private investment decisions that may involve up to tens of millions of dollars in capital and/or operating expenses. Unfortunately it is very clear that risk assessment, as currently practiced, does not often provide the kind of rational input needed to adequately support of cost-effective risk management decisions.

ANALYSIS

In reaching the above conclusion, the authors completed an informal review of a large number of site-specific risk assessments prepared for projects of various types during the last three years. These risk assessments were completed by a variety of practitioners under a number of state and federal regulatory programs. A large proportion of these risk assessments were obtained in 1987 via a Freedom of Information Act request directed to various USEPA CERCLA/SARA program offices.

The results of this review were not encouraging for the following reasons.

- There was very little consistency in formats or procedures even for risk assessments completed under the same regulatory program.

- Most risk assessments were prepared after the data collection program was designed or completed; thus, they were based on data often insufficient data to adequately define input terms. Consequently, risk assessment practitioners were forced to rely on modeled or projected concentrations in lieu of measured exposure concentrations.

- While many risk assessments were intended to be quantitative, most used arbitrary input values to define potential sources, pathways and/or receptors, often resulting in unsupportable exposure estimates. Frequently, arbitrary input values were supported on the basis of equally subjective referencing techniques.

- Typically, the lack of experimental data also led to the selection of input terms that were clearly improbable given the actual conditions at the site under consideration. Most importantly, exposure assumptions were almost always extremely conservative. For example, instead of assessing impacts on receptors utilizing existing wells, receptors were often assumed to be consuming drinking water for seventy years from as yet nonexisting wells located in the most highly contaminated portion of the groundwater plume being assessed.

- Very few risk assessments successfully separated background risks due to existing levels of indicator contaminants from the incremental risks posed by anticipated releases from the project under consideration.

- Very few risk assessments provided useful information on both the magnitude and probability of the risks being estimated. In this context, the most common flaws included lack of consideration of the probability of risks being incurred and the size of the receptor populations potentially being affected.

- Most risk assessments tended to present the risk and/or impact conclusions conclusively, rather than as probabilities or ranges.

- Very few risk assessments incorporated comprehensive discussions of the analytical uncertainties and/or the implications of those uncertainties on the risk assessment conclusions. Similarly, very few risk assessments successfully described the toxicological uncertainties associated with translating projected exposures into quantitative risk estimates.

- Potential impacts on non-human receptors tended to be ignored or evaluated in an even more subjective manner than human health risks.

- Environmental standards or criteria were very often arbitrarily utilized to assess the acceptability of baseline risks. Numerical air, water and groundwater standards or criteria—which were developed for entirely different regulatory purposes often using significantly different exposure scenarios—were often directly compared to measured or extrapolated exposure concentrations.

- Most risk assessments were not structured or designed to facilitate comparison of risk management options, such as alternative engineering or remedial designs. Thus, in most cases the evaluation of baseline risks was not useful in assessing the potential reduction in residual risks associated with various remedial options.

- Similarly, very few risk assessments provided risk reduction analyses assessing the residual risks associated with implementation of the various engineering alternatives. Thus the potential use of risk/benefit analysis approaches for evaluating the reduction in risks potentially achievable with increasing resource investments was essentially eliminated.

SUPPORTING EXAMPLES

To illustrate the above comments further, the following provides a summary of the types of unrealistic assumptions commonly found in many risk assessments.

Input Term	Typical Unrealistic Input Assumptions
• Source Terms	• Maximum measured concentrations were utilized to assess exposures;
	• Contaminants were assumed to be available even though chemical data would suggest that contaminants are generally not mobile;
	• Contaminants were assumed to be available to receptors even though their quantities at the source were not sufficient to result in migration and exposure over long periods;
	• The more toxic end products associated with existing contaminants, such as vinyl chloride, were selected as indicator chemicals even though no evidence of chemical transformation was available.
• Pathway Terms	• Quantity and rates of transport of contaminants through air, surface water or groundwater pathways were estimated without consideration of dilution, dispersion or absorption;
	• Dramatically conservative input terms were used in transport models;
	• Groundwater pathways were assumed to be available even though site hydrogeology was not conducive to groundwater flow.
• Receptor Terms	• Existing receptors were presumed exposed despite changed behavior or the completion of interim remedies;
	• Hypothetical receptors often were selected to model existing exposures (i.e. trespassers) without consideration of actual site conditions limiting the potential for such exposures;
	• Future receptors were arbitrarily selected and presumed exposed to worst case concentrations without regard for the actual potential for such receptors to exist;

- Sensitive receptor populations were used to assess risks without adequate consideration of the actual risks to typical receptors.

- Exposure Terms
  - Dramatically conservative input terms were often used to estimate direct contact, ingestion and inhalation dosages and/or exposures;
  - Lifetime durations were automatically assumed for workers, local residents and other receptors.

DETAILED CASE HISTORY

A recently completed risk assessment for a resource recovery facility provides an example of the range of risk conclusions that can result if assumptions are selected arbitrarily without due consideration of actual site conditions.

In 1988, a risk assessment was prepared by a state contractor for a 150 ton per day mass burn resource recovery facility. The resource recovery facility, which was to be located within a small city of approximately 40,000 situated immediately adjacent to a large river, was to be equipped with a dry acid gas scrubber and fabric filter pollution control equipment. This equipment ensemble is regarded by many as best available control technology (BACT).

The risk assessment consisted of a well written multipathway exposure analysis which addressed the risks associated with multiple exposures resulting from particulate and gaseous emissions and the consequent dispersion and deposition of selected contaminants. Included was an analysis of the potential risks associated with various exposure pathways, such as fish consumption, soil ingestion, meat and vegetable consumption, and breast milk consumption.

For the purposes of this analysis, the consequence of utilizing a variety of input terms for the "avid sports fisherman receptor group" will be reviewed since it was this group that the contractor identified as having the highest risks. It was hypothesized that such an individual would ingest up to 30 grams of fish per day caught exclusively from one shallow backwater pool underlying worst-case concentrations in the air resulting from stack emissions from the proposed facility.

The risk assessment was performed using a fugacity model as described by Mackay *et al.* Based on the state contractor's model, referred to herein as the Fuga(1) model, it was estimated that the lifetime excess dioxin-related cancer risk for the avid sports fishermen group was 5.1×10^{-4}. Since these projected risks were significantly higher than similarly projected risks for much larger facilities, an independent contractor was retained by the project sponsor to review the risk assessment. In conducting this review, this contractor attempted to demonstrate the extent to which the risk conclusions of the Fuga(1) model were sensitive to several key input parameters. He utilized the same basic model as Fuga(1) but with more realistic assumptions, referred to herein as the Fuga(2) approach.

As summarized in Fig. 1, both approaches made a number of common assumptions relating to various input terms, including dioxin toxic equivalent emission rates, the area and depth of the potentially impacted backwater pool, and the quantity of fish consumed by an avid sports fisherman per day. Both approaches also assumed the same cancer potency factor for 2,3,7,8-TCDD toxic equivalents, although Fuga(2) noted that EPA was critically reviewing this number. Fuga(2) also accepted, for comparison purposes, that the avid sports fisherman group actually existed and that fish resided in the most impacted portion of the backwater pool for their entire lifetime (a highly conservative assumption).

Source:

- Source term for dioxin emission rates the same
- All dioxins assumed emitted bound to particulates

Pathway:

- All risk assessments used same air dispersion modeling
- Particulate bound dioxins settle onto 10,000,000 M^2 backwater pool
- Pool 0.67-m deep

Receptor:

- Avid sports fisherman consumes 30 grams of fish per day
- 100% of fish consumed by avid sports fishermen are trapped from most impacted backwater pool
- Fish reside in most impacted backwater pool for 100% of their lifetime

Risk:

- All approaches assumed same cancer potency factor for 2,3,7,8-TCDD toxic equivalents

Fig. 1. Common assumptions.

Analysis of the Fuga(1) risk assessment indicated that the risk conclusions were highly sensitive to several input parameters, including the estimate of the rate of dioxin deposition into the backwater pool and the depth of the sediment mixing zone. For example, to calculate the dioxin contribution to the backwater pool, the Fuga(1) model assumed that a 10,000,000 square meter backwater pool was overlain by a column of air containing the maximum concentration of particulate-bound dioxins projected by the air modeling study. Not only did no such pool exist in the study area, but the area of maximum dioxin concentrations as estimated in the air model was also much smaller.

Another key parameter was the selection of the depth of the sediment on the bottom of the backwater pool. The state contractor assumed that dioxins entering the backwater pool reached equilibrium with the sediments being deposited each year (approximately 0.2 cm/yr). Not only was this figure very low according to most references, it also ignored the existence of significant quantities of sediment already deposited on the river bottom.

The impact of using worst-case inputs as compared to more plausible input parameters is demonstrated in Fig. 2. Revised inputs included the assumptions that the backwater pool underlies a column of "average case" air and that the actively available depth of sediment is 3 cm/yr. Making no other changes to the Fuga(1) model, the lifetime excess cancer risks decreases from 5.1×10^{-4} to 8×10^{-6}, approximately two orders of magnitude. A similar analysis for several of the other conservative input assumptions in Fuga(1), such as the assumption that dioxins chemically bound to particulates are reasonably mobile in water and sediments, that avid fishermen will fish from only one backwater pool for their entire life, and that fish feed and reside for their entire lives only in the maximally impacted portions of the river, indicates that the actual risks posed by the

	Fuga(1)	Fuga(2)
Source		
- Dioxin concentrations in air (pg/m^3) over entire backwater pool	Worst (.011)	Avg. (.002)
- Dioxins entering backwater pool are in equilibrium with sediment	yes	yes
- Dioxins bound to particulates able to exert intrinsic fugacity	yes	yes
Pathway		
- Sediment mixing zone (cm/yr)	0.2	3.0
- Organic carbon content of sediment	2%	2%
Receptor		
- Biomagnification factor	12	12
Risk		
- Estimated lifetime excess dioxin cancer risk (10^{-4}) for avid sports fishermen	5.1	0.06

Fig. 2. Comparison of two approaches.

the proposed facility are much lower than originally projected and that the input assumptions in Fuga(1) were clearly implausible.

IMPLICATIONS

Given the above examples, it is very clear that different risk assessment assumptions can readily result in risk estimates that differ by orders of magnitude. Unfortunately the societal consequences of scientifically unsupportable risk conclusions can be very significant. Throughout the USA, many proposed projects are being delayed and/or canceled due to inaccurate representations of the risks posed by specific projects and/or the lack of risk communication which place the anticipated risks in proper perspective. The types of projects apparently most severely affected to date have been solid and hazardous waste management facilities. However, to some extent almost any project involving chemicals or wastes of any type is being affected. Even in those instances in which projects are approved and permits to construct are received, very significant cost penalties are being incurred, often in direct response to unrealistic risk estimates.

The increments of risks typically considered acceptable by regulatory agencies are quite small and range from 10^{-5} (one in 100,000) to 10^{-7} (one in 10,000,000). At many locations, the public's perception of what constitutes an acceptable level of risk is often much more stringent—with zero risk remedies typically receiving strong public support. From a project perspective, this range of "potentially acceptable risk increments" often translates into a broad array of alternative designs and costs. For example, if the increments on the X-axis of Fig. 3 were to represent expenditures of $5 million to remedy an existing contaminated site, then for this hypothetical example, reducing the risks to 10^{-5} would require an expenditure of $5 million. Reducing risks to 10^{-7} for this same site would cost $30 million. Obviously then, even relatively small overestimates in the baseline risks and/or underestimates of the reduction of residual risks achievable by various remedial alternatives can lead to dramatically increased resource commitments, i.e., costs which would not be reasonable to incur if more realistic and scientifically supportable risk estimates had been originally provided.

CONCLUSIONS

Many risk assessments appear to be highly subjective, dramatically overestimate baseline risks, and are not structured or organized to support the risk management decision process. The implications of this statement are that many site-specific risk assessments directly contribute to inappropriate public alarm, the delay or cancellation of some projects that are needed from a societal perspective and inappropriately increased costs for many projects that are actually implemented. This appears to be occurring for several reasons.

- The relative complexity of the issues being assessed.
- The lack of more comprehensive protocols, procedures and/or guidelines for risk assessments and the lack of consistency in applying risk assessment methodologies even within specific regulatory programs.
- The lack of emphasis on obtaining the specific data needed for realistic estimates of the various risk assessment input terms.
- The apparent lack of understanding on the part of many practitioners that risks can only occur if there really is a source of contaminants, if those contaminants can really migrate in at least one environmental media, and if receptors are actually exposed to concentrations which would result in health or environmental impacts.
- The apparent lack of understanding on the part of many practitioners that risks are defined by both the potential magnitude of a hazard and the probability of that hazard occurring.
- The lack of emphasis on accurate communication of the risk assessment conclusions with respect to key input assumptions and the resulting uncertainties.
- The lack of understanding on the part of many risk assessors of the remedial alternative issues at hand such that each risk assessment is not designed to assist in making specific siting, permitting, design and/or remedial engineering decisions.
- The recent emergence of the risk assessment field, which has led to a rapid increase in the number of risk assessment practitioners, many of whom have relatively little risk assessment training or experience.

RECOMMENDATIONS

What can a risk practitioner do to reduce the subjectiveness of his or her risk conclusions and to improve the utility of each risk assessment to support the risk management decision process?

First of all, the risk assessor must become involved in the risk management process as early as possible. Ideally, a qualitative risk evaluation should be completed to eliminate those risk scenarios of limited potential consequences and to focus the site investigation and risk management process on exposure pathways posing potentially unacceptable risks. At

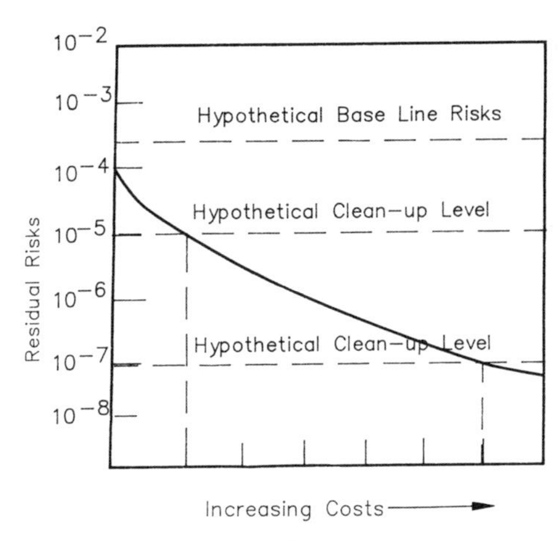

Fig. 3. Risk reduction versus costs.

the same time, the initial data collection process should be explicitly focused on collecting those data which will be necessary to evaluate baseline risks and/or to assess the risks associated with the array of potential design alternatives.

The risk practitioner should then use the results of the data collection process to verify the accuracy of the initial risk hypotheses, to evaluate the need for any additional data, to further refine the problem definition, and/or to measure rather than model potential exposures. Finally, the practitioner should consider what risk assessment techniques would be most conducive to evaluating the risk management alternatives.

With the above complete, the risk practitioner should try to develop an estimate of the potential risks by inputting source, pathway and receptor terms that duplicate to the maximum extent the exposures likely to occur under existing and/or future site conditions.

The results of the baseline risk analysis should then be tested to evaluate which input parameters have the most impact on the baseline risk conclusions. The basis for these input parameters should then be re-examined to assess how realistic those values actually are.

With this information in hand, the risk practitioner should then deliberately test the baseline conclusions developed above by utilizing less probable (i.e. worst-case) assumptions. The results of this analysis, if completed in concert with an evaluation of the probability of occurrence of these more conservative scenarios, will provide both a sensitivity check on the original risk estimate as well as an evaluation of the range of risks to which receptors might be exposed.

Using the same risk methodology employed above, the risk practitioner should evaluate the reduction in risks potentially available via implementation of the various remedial options using realistic reductions in source terms, pathway terms and receptor terms based upon the anticipated performance of the various risk management options.

Once the above analyses have been completed, the risk practitioner should attempt to place the estimated risks in perspective. In this context, several approaches are possible. These might include, for example, comparing estimated risk increments to background risks posed by existing levels of the same contaminants, comparing estimated risks increments from the project to other similar projects, or comparing risks increments from the proposed project to the risks posed by alternative projects or approaches.

In summary, each risk practitioner must insist on using documented facts to the maximum extent possible to define input terms, must insist on employing rational analytical techniques to project exposures and risks and must not lose sight of the ultimate goal of the risk assessment process—to assist in making realistic and cost-effective risk management decisions relating to the need for, acceptability of and required safety features of real world projects reflecting real world needs. To the extent that each practitioner is successful in applying the scientific method in meeting these goals, risk assessment will be increasingly perceived as a useful scientific tool rather than the fiction that many currently perceive it to be.

Reducing Uncertainty in Risk Assessment: Exposure Assessment

Susan Hunter Youngren
ENVIRON Corporation
Washington, DC

Robert G. Tardiff
Versar Corporation
Springfield, VA

ABSTRACT

Major uncertainties exist in the assessment of health risks associated with complex mixtures to which humans are exposed through numerous routes (e.g., hazardous waste sites). These uncertainties are derived from processes that contain limitations in source characteristics, in toxicity and exposure information, and in the evaluate of their significance to human health. This paper examines one source of uncertainty (quantity and duration of dose—a part of the exposure assessment process) and evaluates the relative impact on the confidence in risk estimates from directly measuring exposure versus relying on seemingly reasonable assumptions to characterize exposure. Two case studies of multi-chemical/multi-media risk assessments (for hazardous waste sites) illustrate the complexity of exposure assumptions and relate quantitatively the relative value of characterizing the same exposures through direct measurements of dose and duration.

KEYWORDS: Exposure assessment, uncertainty, risk assessment, hazardous waste site

INTRODUCTION

Public health risk assessment has become an increasingly important tool used in decisions on remedial measures, at hazardous waste sites, having major economic proportions. Risk assessment is the process of estimating, under actual and hypothetical conditions of exposure, the likelihood of adverse health outcomes to diverse populations. The scientific community recognizes that this process is rife with unknowns; individual risk assessments contain diverse uncertainties—some of enormous proportions—that stem largely from the absence of vital information and the consequent reliance on inference. This paper focuses on exposure assessment, particularly exposures associated with substances likely to reach humans through complex means, its inherent uncertainty, and a method for

Risk Analysis, Edited by C. Zervos
Plenum Press, New York, 1991

reducing uncertainty. An increased understanding of the source and nature of the uncertainty will aid in focusing data acquisition to accomplish the greater reduction in uncertainty and in defining the degree of confidence in the estimates of risk.

A general discussion of exposure assessment is followed by two case study analyses that highlight the uncertainty inherent in this step of risk assessment and present practical approaches to reducing such uncertainty.

EXPOSURE ASSESSMENT

Exposure assessment describes the nature and size of the population receiving a dose of the substance of interest and ascertaining the magnitude and duration of their exposure. Exposure refers to contact between a person and either the environmental media (e.g., air, water, soil, diet) containing the chemical of concern or direct contact with the chemical (e.g., a spill onto the skin).

Some exposures can be assessed directly. For instance, cosmetics applied directly to the skin can be measured; drugs ingested in pill form can be counted; the concentration of food additives can be analyzed and the quantity of food consumed can be measured directly. It is preferable to obtain physical measures of direct exposures to increase assurance of the accuracy of the measure of delivered chemical dose.

Assessing indirect exposures, by contrast, is much more complex for it entails investigation of numerous possible environmental pathways that link a chemical at its source(s) to the possible point(s) at which people will be exposed. An illustration is that of a substance present at a waste site (e.g., a landfill) that may be volatilized, transformed in part by sunlight, and inhaled as a mixture of parent and by-products. The same substance may simultaneously migrate to an underground aquifer, which serves as a source of irrigation and drinking water, be converted in part by soil microorganisms, and be incorporated in the diet, tap water, and bathing water of humans.

For convenience, we consider this as a four step process. The first step identifies the source and its strength, while the second step identifies the media of concern through which the substance moves and by which it can be modified. In the third step, the concentrations of the chemicals of concern are estimated in each media, from either sampling and analysis of the contaminated media or through mathematical modeling. The latter may project past, present, and future concentrations and changes in chemical form. Translation of concentrations in media (exposure) to human dose for an exposed population is the fourth step. These dose estimates the product of the quantitative assessment of the exposure, which are then used in part to assess the probability of harm (that is, risk) to an individual or group of individuals (the population).

All four steps contain elements of uncertainty from estimating the initial strength at the source to assumptions used in estimating the dose. In most assessments, no attempts are made to reduce the uncertainty. Sometimes they are merely identified, while in other cases the magnitude of uncertainty is described. However, we have identified a method to reduce uncertainty which uses a sensitivity analysis to determine critical assumptions for which further data should be acquired if possible. Acquiring data to refine our estimates of the most critical parameters gives us the greatest reduction in uncertainty in our final assessment.

Each of these steps is explained in further detail below. Two case studies are then presented that illustrate practical application of the exposure assessment process, examples of data uncertainties, and methods for reducing such uncertainties.

FOUR STEPS OF EXPOSURE ASSESSMENT

Source and Quantity of Chemicals of Interest

We begin an exposure assessment by listing all possible sources of environmental exposure in detail. The points at which the chemical enters the environment are identified, along with estimated rates of entry. For each relevant source, the quantities of the chemical on, in, or released to the transporting media are estimated. This source information requires sufficient detail to determine the size and nature of the release: location of the source; amount of the chemical present or being released as a function of time for each relevant medium of exposure; physical characteristics of the source; and the physical and chemical form of the chemical.

Pathways from Source to Humans

For indirect exposures, an exposure assessment considers the environmental pathways that link the releases of chemicals at their sources to the settings within which the populations at risk are actually exposed. These pathways involve one or more environmental media, i.e., air, water, soil, and biota.

Estimations of Concentrations of Chemicals of Interest

Quantifying the concentration of chemicals of interest is relatively difficult compared to determining the sources of contaminants. Source characteristics and strengths are all related to some type of physical measurement. Direct measurement is the preferred method. An example of this is stack emissions, which can be computed from direct measurement of gas flow rates and the stack gas concentrations. Direct measurement through actual sampling of the affected media provides only the concentration at that specific time and location. Levels at other locations and times must be inferred.

A second method is a materials balance approach, which depends on measurement and inference. That is, if a measured amount is known to be entering a source, then by inferring the loss among other environmental media or other fates (e.g., chemical transformation, destruction), we can estimate the amount leaving the source.

Simple and complex mathematical models are also used for estimating releases of chemicals from their sources. They are usually derived from basic physical and chemical principles that are established under idealized circumstances but may have only limited application to actual situations. Models based on knowledge of emissions of a similar type or calibrated from measured values can be used to estimate concentrations at other places and times. These models take into account known chemical transformations and other changes such as degradation or absorption to soil.

Translation of Exposure to Human Dose

Chemical concentration in a specified medium does not describe the amount that enters and is retained by the body. At environmental levels, the amount of substances that reaches an internal organ is directly related to the probability of injury. Numerous physiological processes influence the dose that may be achieved at susceptible sites in the body. Thus to estimate dose from environmental levels is a complex process, some elements of which are described below.

For chemicals, dose is the amount of a substance taken into the body per unit body weight per unit time. The usual expression of chemical dose is mg contaminant/kg body weight/day. Several factors affect the extent of exposure, including the duration of exposure, the route(s) of exposure, the amount of contaminant absorbed into the body by each route, and the characteristics of the population exposed.

The method for estimating dose depends in part on the route of exposure. For example, to calculate dose from ingestion of water, it is necessary to know the concentration of the contaminant in the water, the amount of water a person ingests, the amount of contaminant absorbed from the gastrointestinal tract after ingestion (gastrointestinal absorption factor), and the weight of the person. For substances that are either inhaled or that pass through the skin, different factors (e.g., skin penetration rates, inhalation absorption factors, breathing rate, etc.) determine dose.

Two characteristics of the exposed population need to be considered in an exposure assessment: demographics and activity. The composition of the population will determine certain physiological parameters that affect exposure. For example, the body weight and breathing rate of an adult male, adult female, and child differ substantially. The type of people in the exposed population may also determine their activities and may, therefore, affect their extent of exposure. Children, for example, are more likely to play in, or eat, dirt than are adults.

The dose estimates for each route of exposure are then calculated based on route-specific data and assumptions. These estimates are calculated in a manner similar to that described in the USEPA Superfund Public Health Evaluation Manual[1] and the Superfund Exposure Assessment Manual.[2] They are in the following form:

$$LADD = \frac{C \cdot IF}{BW \cdot L}$$

where,

LADD = lifetime average daily dose received through each route of exposure, mg/kg/day;

C = concentration of contaminant in a specific medium, mg/kg in soil, mg/l in water, mg/m^3 in air;

IF = human intake factors, based on the specific assumptions for each route, including duration and absorption;

BW = body weight, kg; and

L = lifetime, lifetime-days.

The estimated dose from each route of exposure is calculated. In addition, the total dose, assumed to be all of the doses added together, is presented, as it is quite probable that a person could be exposed by several routes during his exposure.

METHODS FOR REDUCING UNCERTAINTY

One method for reducing uncertainty in exposure assessment entails acquiring additional data. However, it is necessary to determine which is critical data (i.e., if additional information can be obtained, what data set(s) will have the greatest impact on the precision of the dose estimate) and acquiring additional data. A sensitivity analysis performed on the assumptions used in each pathway allows one to determine which assumptions have the greatest impact on total dose. However, as a practical decision, every assumption cannot be examined if there are a multitude of possible pathways. Thus, the "critical" pathway (the one appearing to make the largest contribution to dose) is chosen. To ensure a complete analysis, the pathways which have a dose estimate within one order of magnitude of the critical pathway are also included in the sensitivity analysis. Even though one may be sacrificing the remote possibility of excluding an important assumption, this approach increases the efficiency of the analysis.

Next, a sensitivity analysis is performed on the various assumptions for each selected pathway. The percentage change from the initial total dose to the estimated dose after changing various assumptions is calculated.

The next step is to determine if the data used to replace an assumption are capable of being acquired within reason. Data acquisition can occur through two means: 1) literature search, and 2) observation. For example, it may be difficult to measure exactly how much time children actually playing in a certain area. However, laboratory studies can be designed to determine route-specific absorption efficiency.

Then, the analysis examines the cost of acquiring the data which includes not only the monetary cost, but also the time needed to acquire the data. These are site-specific questions that can only be answered after a complete analysis of the cost of the original outcome versus the cost of data acquisition plus the cost of a new outcome after inclusion of additional data.

These points are quantitatively illustrated in the following case studies.

CASE STUDY I: EXPOSURE IN A MARSHLAND

Source and Quantity of Chemicals of Interest

The first case study is an assessment of the potential public health risks associated with contamination migrating off-site from an industrial facility designated as a Superfund site. As a result of past disposal practices at the facility, the underlying groundwater was contaminated and was discharging chemicals into a nearby marshland. The marshland adjoins a river and is situated in a public parkland adjacent to a residential community. The focus of the risk assessment was several scenarios to assess potential public health risks associated with exposure in the marshland.

Pathways from Source to Humans

Exposure of humans to contaminants in the marsh was judged to be limited as there were no organized or supervised recreational uses of this area, but it was considered reasonable to assume that children exploring in the area could find the marsh an inviting place to play. Potential exposure for a child between the ages of six to twelve (using a nine-year-old child as an average) was estimated. It was assumed that children younger than six years of age are unlikely to be found playing away from home unattended. A number of exposure scenarios were considered.

Exposure via the following routes were modeled:

1. contaminants in marsh soil, as a result of unintentional soil ingestion and dermal absorption;
2. contaminants in surface water, as a result of unintentional water ingestion and dermal absorption; and
3. contaminants in air, as a result of inhalation of volatile organic chemicals.

Scenarios were constructed that accounted for the duration of exposure, route of exposure, and the amount of chemical absorbed in the body, as well as the characteristics of the exposed population.

Estimation of Concentration of Chemicals of Interest

The contaminants identified in the marsh were comprised largely of volatile organic chemicals, as well as base/neutral extractable compounds. Because of the large number of chemicals associated with the site, a subset of "indicator" chemicals was selected. Selection of indicator chemicals are generally made on the basis of toxicity, concentration, and mobility of the chemicals. In this analysis, the major contaminants selected included benzene, chlorobenzene, chloroform, tetrachloroethylene, and trichloroethylene. Surface water and sediment data were available to characterize the nature of contamination. A major unknown in the assessment was the concentration of chemicals in the air above the marsh. This exposure pathway was of particular concern since several of the chemicals identified in the marshland waters were highly volatile and could potentially be inhaled by children playing in the marsh. Therefore, an air model (the box model) was developed to determine air concentrations above the marsh based on surface water data. This model was further validated through an air and surface water sampling program.

Translation of Exposure to Human Dose

Information on actual conditions of exposure at the marshland area was not readily available. To estimate the dose, it was necessary to develop specific exposure scenarios which modeled potential human exposure at these areas. Assumptions were made concerning specific factors relating to contact with soil, water, and air.

Certain assumptions are the same in each exposure route. It was assumed that during the period of exposure (ages six to twelve) a child could conceivably play in the marsh 180 times (e.g., 2 times a week during the 15 warmer weeks of the year, for the six years of possible exposure). In addition, each exposure period was assumed to be for 2 hours.

Soil Ingestion. In modeling incidental ingestion of contaminated soil and sediment, three factors require consideration: (1) the rate of soil ingestion; (2) the period of time over which soil ingestion occurs; and (3) the efficiency of gastrointestinal absorption for the contaminant contained on the soil.

In EPA's Air Quality Criteria for Lead,[3] the authors suggest a soil ingestion value of 100 mg soil/day for children. This is based on a study by Lepow *et al.*,[4,5] who estimated soil ingestion values from measurements of soil on hands and observations of mouthing behavior of young children. The Superfund Exposure Assessment Manual[2] suggests an overall average soil ingestion value of 100 mg/day. Other estimates for children over five range from 50 mg/day (most probable estimate) to 250 mg/day (worst-case estimate).[6] For this analysis, it was assumed that a nine-year-old child could potentially ingest 100 mg of soil each time he played in the marsh. The estimates of the amount of soil ingested per day apply to days when exposure is assumed to occur.

Specific information on gastrointestinal absorption efficiency of the contaminant from the ingested soil is often unavailable. Thus to be conservative, it was assumed that 100% of ingested contaminants would be absorbed from the soil by the gastrointestinal tract.

Soil Dermal. Dermal exposure to contaminants in soil may occur when the skin comes in contact with contaminated soil. Four factors were taken into account when evaluating this potential route of exposure: (1) the skin surface area exposed to the soil; (2) the amount of soil deposited on the skin; (3) the period of time over which exposure occurs; and (4) the extent to which chemicals adsorbed to the soil are subsequently absorbed through the skin.

The amount of skin exposed to soil is an estimate based on the expected activities and types of clothing worn during the exposure period. The amount of skin exposed to soil is also influenced by the weather. For example, during warm weather seasons, it is possible that a child would wear less clothing than in colder times. In this case, it was assumed that a child could expose his face and neck, two-thirds of his upper limbs, and one-half of his lower limbs (i.e., wearing a short-sleeved shirt and short pants) to the soil and sediment each time he played in the area.

The amount of soil deposited on the skin was derived from deposition levels reported in the literature and modifications based on potential activities during the exposure period. A review of the methods used for measurement and estimation in a number of studies on the amount of soil deposition suggested that the methodology used by Roels *et al.*[7] is the most effective for estimating soil deposition levels for a child playing in soil or sediment. Roels collected samples of dust and dirt from children's school playgrounds and compared these values to lead levels on the children's hands. Deposition levels were estimated to be 0.8 and 1.7 mg/cm^2 for girls and boys, respectively. The range of values in the literature are from 0.056 mg/cm^2 (indoor levels) to 3.5 mg/cm^2 (outdoor levels).[8] For this assessment, a value of 1.25 mg/cm^2 (the average of Roels et al.[7]) was used. The estimates of soil deposition apply to days when exposure is assumed to occur.

Dermal absorption of contaminants from soil depends on the adsorption of the contaminant to soil, the degree of desorption and skin contact, and the ability of the contaminant to penetrate the skin and enter the blood stream. Dermal absorption was assumed to be less than 100% because of the barrier provided by the skin. Few chemicals have been tested for dermal absorption from soil. Dermal absorption from soil was assumed to be 1% of the concentration present in the soil on the skin surface for chemicals with a high octanol/water coefficient, (log Kow greater than 4), based on a conservative estimate derived from dermal absorption data obtained by Poiger and Schlatter.[9] Dermal absorption data for all other chemicals was assumed to be 10%, unless additional chemical-specific information on dermal absorption was available.

Water Ingestion. In modeling incidental ingestion of contaminated water, three factors, similar to those used in modeling ingested soil, were considered: (1) the rate of water ingestion, (2) the period of time over which water ingestion occurred, and (3) the gastrointestinal absorption efficiency of the contaminant from the ingested water.

Specific information on the amount of water a child might ingest while playing in the marsh was not known. It was assumed that a child could ingest 50 ml of water by scooping up a handful from the marsh water each time he played in the marsh. As with the soil, the estimates of the amount of water ingested per day apply to days when exposure is assumed to occur.

Specific information on gastrointestinal absorption efficiency of the contaminant from ingested water is often unavailable. Thus to be conservative, it was assumed that 100% of ingested contaminants would be absorbed from the water by the gastrointestinal tract.

Water Dermal. Dermal exposure to contaminants in water may occur when the skin comes in contact with contaminated water. Three factors were taken into account when evaluating this potential route of exposure: (1) the skin surface area exposed to the water, (2) the duration of the exposure, and (3) the extent to which chemicals in the water are subsequently absorbed through the skin.

As with dermal exposure to soil, the amount of skin exposed to water is an estimate based on the expected activities, types of clothing worn and weather during the exposure period. It was again assumed that a child could expose his face and neck, two-thirds of his upper limbs, and one-half of his lower limbs (i.e., wearing a short-sleeved shirt and short pants) to the water (as he did to the soil and sediment) each time he played in the area.

Generally, only un-ionized lipid-soluble compounds are absorbed significantly through the skin. This is not only reflected in the permeability coefficient, which is primarily a function of the diffusional and partitioning properties of the chemical, but also can be related to the thickness of the skin and the relative portions of aqueous-phase and lipid-phase in the stratum corneum of the skin.[10] Empirical correlations between the dermal permeability rate and the octanol/water coefficient (Kow), have been developed from existing data to allow estimation of the permeability coefficients for a wide range of compounds.[11,12] A coefficient (in cm/hr) based on the equation: $0.005 \times [1 + (Kow)0.65]$[13] was used in these estimations.

Vapor Inhalation. Inhalation of vapors from chemicals volatilizing from the marshland water was of concern. Factors that were considered when evaluating this route of exposure are (1) the volume of air inspired, (2) the duration of the exposure, and (3) the extent to which the chemicals in the inhaled air are absorbed in the lung.

The volume of air inspired is dependent upon the physiologic characteristics of the individuals. A standard inhalation rate of 0.625 m3/hr was used (which assumes 8 hours of light activity, 8 hours of rest, and 8 hours nonoccupational activity). The duration of exposure is assumed to be the entire time a child is playing in the marsh.

Specific information on inhalation absorption efficiency of the contaminant is often unavailable. Thus to be conservative, it was assumed that 100% of inhaled contaminants would be absorbed in the lungs.

Quantitative Analysis

The dose estimates for each route of exposure are then calculated based on the above assumptions. The route-specific equations are shown in Fig. 1.

The estimated dose from each route of exposure are presented in Table 1. In addition, the total dose (all of the doses added together) is presented, as it is quite probable that a child playing in the marsh could be exposed by all the routes during his time in the marsh.

Method for Reducing Uncertainty

A method to reduce uncertainty entails determining critical assumptions for which additional data can be acquired. To accomplish this the critical pathway if first chosen after examination of dose estimates based on the current assumptions and data. The critical pathway is that with the greatest dose estimate, in this case vapor inhalation (Table 1). Following the rule to choose a secondary critical pathway(s) (less than one order of magnitude different), dermal exposure from water would also be of interest.

Next, a sensitivity analysis was performed on the various assumptions for these pathways. The levels in the sensitivity analysis are based on the range of values for each assumption. These values may be from the literature (e.g., soil ingestion rates ranged from 50 to 250 mg/day) or site-specific evaluation (e.g., the number of hours a child might play in the marsh each time could range from 1 to 4 hours). The percentage change from the initial total dose to the estimated dose after changing various assumptions was calculated. Changing the amount of time in the marsh has the greatest effect on the total dose estimates. Reducing the percentage of chemicals absorbed through inhalation from a conservative 100% to 10% also significantly affected the dose estimates.

Soil Ingestion

$$LADD_{si} = \frac{C_s \cdot I_{si} \cdot T_{si} \cdot A_{gi}}{BW \cdot L}$$

where

$LADD_{si}$ = lifetime average daily dose received through ingestion of soil, mg/kg/day
C_s = concentration of contaminant in soil, mg/kg
I_{si} = ingestion rate of soil, mg/day
T_{si} = exposure period, days/life
A_{gi} = gastrointestinal absorption factor, dimensionless
BW = body weight, kg
L = days per lifetime, days/life

Soil Dermal

$$LADD_{sd} = \frac{C_s \cdot SA_{sd} \cdot DP_{sd} \cdot T_{sd} \cdot A_{sd}}{BW \cdot L}$$

where

$LADD_{sd}$ = lifetime average daily dose received through dermal absorption from soil, mg/kg/day
C_s = concentration of contaminant in soil, mg/kg
SA_{sd} = surface area of skin exposed to soil, cm^2
DP_{sd} = deposition rate of soil, $mg/cm^2 day$
T_{sd} = exposure period, days/life
A_{sd} = dermal absorption from soil, dimensionless
BW = body weight, kg
L = days per lifetime, days/life

Water Ingestion

$$LADD_{wi} = \frac{C_s \cdot I_{wi} \cdot T_{wi} \cdot A_{gi}}{BW \cdot L}$$

where

$LADD_{wi}$ = lifetime average daily dose received through ingestion of water, mg/kg/day
C_w = concentration of contaminant in water, mg/l
I_{wi} = ingestion rate of water, l/day
T_{wi} = exposure period, days/life
A_{gi} = gastrointestinal absorption factor, dimensionless
BW = body weight, kg
L = days per lifetime, days/life

Water Dermal

$$LADD_{wd} = \frac{C_w \cdot SA_{wd} \cdot T_{wd} \cdot P_{wd}}{BW \cdot L \cdot 1000}$$

where

$LADD_{wd}$ = lifetime average daily dose received through dermal absorption from water, mg/kg/day
C_w = concentration of contaminant in water, mg/l
SA_{wd} = surface area of skin exposed to soil, cm^2
T_{wd} = exposure period, hours/life
P_{wd} = permeability coefficient, cm/hr
BW = body weight, kg
L = days per lifetime, days/life

Vapor Inhalation

$$LADD_{vi} = \frac{C_a \cdot R_{vi} \cdot T_{vi} \cdot A_{vi}}{BW \cdot L}$$

where

$LADD_{vi}$ = lifetime average daily dose received through inhalation of vapors, mg/kg/day
C_a = concentration of contaminant in air, mg/m^3
R_{vi} = inspiration rate, m^3/hr
T_{vi} = exposure period, hours/life
A_{vi} = inhalation absorption factor, dimensionless
BW = body weight, kg
L = days in lifetime, days/life

Fig. 1. Route specific dose equations.

Table 1. Case Study 1: Dose Estimates

Route	Dose (mg/kg/day)
Water Ingestion	5.68×10^{-8}
Water Dermal	1.43×10^{-4}
Soil Ingestion	1.14×10^{-7}
Soil Dermal	4.41×10^{-7}
Vapor Inhalation	1.42×10^{-3}
TOTAL DOSE	1.56×10^{-3}

The next step examined whether the additional critical data identified can be acquired within reason to replace the assumption(s). For example, it may be difficult to determine exactly how much time children actually spend in the marsh playing. However, laboratory studies can be designed to determine inhalation absorption efficiency.

One must then determine whether the cost of acquiring the data can be justified, but there is adequate time to acquire the data. These are site-specific questions that can only be answered after a complete analysis of the cost of the original outcome versus the cost of data acquisition plus the cost of a new outcome after inclusion of additional data. In this case, the time frame would not allow for additional laboratory tests, however time was spent in the marsh and the nearby community to determine if children actually played in the marsh and to what extent. It was learned that the original estimates were reasonable and further study was deemed unnecessary.

CASE STUDY II: EXPOSURE FROM DOMESTIC USE OF CONTAMINATED WATER

Source and Quantity of Chemicals of Interest

The second case study is a risk assessment which evaluated the potential risks created by off-site migration of contaminants from a former industrial landfill. The landfill is bounded by a river, a residential community, and the industrial facility. As a result of former disposal practices, the upper aquifer of the ground water is contaminated. This aquifer flows under the residential area. Thus, the focus of the risk assessment was an evaluation of the potential risks to the population from exposure to contaminants in the residential area.

Pathways from Source to Humans

Exposure to humans on the landfill itself was considered to be negligible as it was a fenced, secure property. However, the residential community abutting the landfill used well water from the upper aquifer as their primary source of water. Residents of all ages live in this area, so a composite population was considered, comprised of an adult male (average of ages eighteen to seventy), an adult female (average of ages eighteen to seventy-seven), a fifteen-year-old teenager (average of ages twelve to eighteen), a nine-year-old child (average of ages six to twelve), and a four-year-old child (average of ages two to six).

The following exposure scenarios were modeled:

1. contaminants in well water, as a result of water ingestion and dermal absorption while showering; and
2. contaminants in air, as a result of inhalation of organic chemicals which volatilize from water during showering.

Scenarios were constructed which accounted for the duration of exposure, route of exposure, and the amount of chemical absorbed in the body, as well as the characteristics of the exposed population.

Estimations of Concentrations of Chemicals of Interest

The contaminants identified in the ground water were comprised largely of volatile organic chemicals. Because of the large number of chemicals associated with the site, a subset of "indicator" chemicals was again selected based on the toxicity, concentration, and mobility of the chemicals. In this analysis, the major contaminants selected included benzene, bis(2-chloroethyl)ether, chlorobenzene, 1,1-dichloroethylene, phenol, tetrachloroethylene, toluene, trichloroethylene, and vinyl chloride.

Translation of Exposure to Human Dose

To estimate the dose, it was necessary to develop specific exposure scenarios which modeled potential human exposure in the community. Assumptions were made concerning specific factors relating to contact with water and air.

Certain assumptions are the same for each route of exposure. A lifetime of exposure was assumed with daily use of the water (i.e., 365 days a year for 52 years for the adult male; 365 days a year for 58 years for the adult female; 365 days a year for 6 years for the teenager; 365 days a year for 6 years for the older child; and, 365 days a year for 4 years for the younger child).

[The factors in modeling the three routes of exposure (water ingestion, dermal absorption from water, and vapor inhalation) are identical to Case Study 1. However, values for specific factors are different and are discussed below.]

Water Ingestion. The amount of water a person might ingest on a daily basis has been estimated by various sources.[14,15,16] The most frequently used daily consumption figure is 2 liters a day for adults and one liter a day for children.[1]

Dermal Water. The amount of skin exposed to water is an estimate based on the expected activities and types of clothing worn during the exposure period. Thus for bathing and showering, it is assumed that no clothing is worn and the total body surface area is exposed.

Vapor Inhalation. The volume of air inspired is dependent upon the physiologic characteristics of the individuals. A standard inhalation rate was used for each specific age group. The duration of exposure is assumed to be the entire time a person is in the shower (15 minutes per day).[2]

Quantitative Analysis

The dose estimates for each route of exposure are calculated based on the above assumptions and those described in Case Study 1. The route-specific equations were provided in Fig. 1.

The estimated lifetime dose from each route of exposure are presented on Table 2. In addition, the total dose (all of the doses added together) is presented, as it is quite probable that a person using a domestic source of water would ingest and shower with water from the same source during his entire lifetime.

Method for Reducing Uncertainty

Using the method described previously, the critical pathway was determined to be vapor inhalation (Table 2) with a secondary critical pathway of water ingestion.

A sensitivity analysis performed on the various assumptions for these pathways showed that the most critical assumption is the time spent in the shower. Secondarily, inhalation absorption efficiency was also significant.

It would be difficult to acquire more precise data on the amount of time spent in the shower; however, as discussed previously inhalation absorption efficiency information may be obtainable.

Finally there is the a cost-benefit analysis. Will the cost of acquiring the data be justified and is there adequate time to acquire the data? These are site-specific questions that can only be answered after a complete analysis as discussed in Case Study 1.

SUMMARY

In almost all risk assessments, risk assessors are required to go beyond available data and make inferences about risks expected from conditions of exposure for which direct evidence of risk cannot now be collected. In fact, a major conclusion of the NAS report on risk assessment[17] was that "the basic problem in risk assessment is the sparseness and uncertainty of the scientific knowledge." When scientific uncertainty is encountered in a risk assessment, an assumption is used to fill the information gap. As a matter of conservative public health policy, EPA and other regulatory agencies prefer to err on the side of overestimating risk when addressing such uncertainty, in order to protect public health. This is generally accomplished in the exposure assessment step by incorporating conservative assumptions which represent the upper-bound of reasonably foreseeable exposures into the risk assessment process. However, if a number of conservative assumptions are used, the estimate of exposure may be overly conservative and even improbable due to the additive effect of combining assumptions in the same scenario. To prevent this, we try to gather additional data in order to reduce this upper bound assumption to a more reasonable estimate. This raises the question, "If additional scientific data is to be gathered, what data will critically affect the outcome?"

We suggest answering that question by performing a sensitivity analysis on the critical pathway(s) to determine the critical assumptions. Three issues must be addressed: (1) how can the data be acquired — through a literature search, a controlled setting analysis, or a noncontrolled setting analysis; (2) will the time-frame for the project allow the additional data acquisition; and (3) a cost-benefit analysis. If these issues can be addressed satisfactorily, a compelling argument should be made to obtain the additional data which can be used to reduce uncertainty. The reduction of uncertainty will lead to more confidence in the risk estimates and a firmer foundation for public policy decisions.

Table 2. Case Study 2: Dose Estimates

Route	Dose (mg/kg/day)
Water Ingestion	1.26×10^{-6}
Water Dermal	5.32×10^{-8}
Vapor Inhalation	6.58×10^{-6}
TOTAL DOSE	7.89×10^{-6}

REFERENCES

1. U.S. Environmental Protection Agency (USEPA), Superfund Public Health Evaluation Manual, Office of Emergency and Remedial Response, Washington, D.C., EPA-540/1-86-060 (1986).
2. U.S. Environmental Protection Agency (USEPA), Superfund Exposure Assessment Manual, Pre-publication Edition, Office of Remedial Response, Washington, D.C., EPA/540/1- 88/001 (1988).
3. U.S. Environmental Protection Agency (USEPA), Air Quality Criteria for Lead, External Review Draft, EPA-600/8-83-028B (1984).
4. M. L. Lepow, L. Bruckman, R. A. Burino, S. Markowitz, M. Gillette, and J. Kapish, Role of Airborne Lead in Increased Body Burden of Lead in Hartford Children, *Environ. Health Perspect.* **7**:99-102 (1974).
5. M. L. Lepow, L. Bruckman, M. Gillette, S. Markowitz, R. Robino, and J. Kapish, Investigations Into Sources of Lead in the Environment of Urban Children, *Environ. Res.* **10**:415-426 (1975).
6. P. LaGoy, Estimated Soil Ingestion Rates for Use in Risk Assessments, *Risk Analysis* **7(3)**:355-359 (1987).
7. H. A. Roels, J. P. Buchet, R. R. Lauwerys, P. Braux, F. Claeys-Thoreau, A. Lafontaine, and G. Verduyn, Exposure to Lead by the Oral and Pulmonary Routes of Children Living in the Vicinity of a Primary Lead Smelter, *Environ. Res.* **22**:81-94 (1980).
8. John Hawley, Assessment of Health Risk from Exposure to Contaminated Soil, *Risk Analysis* **5**:289-302 (1985)
9. H. Poiger, and C. Schlatter, Influence of Solvents and Adsorbants on Dermal and Intestinal Absorption of TCDD, *Fd. Cosmet. Toxicol.* **18**:477-481 (1980).
10. R. J. Scheuplein, Permeability of Skin, in *Handbook of Physiology — Section 9: Reactions to Environmental Agents*, American Physiological Society, Bethesda, MD (1977).
11. M. S. Roberts, R. A. Anderson, and J. Swarbrick, Permeability of Human Epidermis to Phenolic Compounds, *J. Pharm. Pharmac.* **29**:677-683 (1977).
12. R. J. Scheuplein and I. H. Blank, Mechanism of Percutaneous Absorption: IV. Penetration of Nonelectrolytes (Alcohols) from Aqueous Solutions and from Pure Liquids, *J. Invest. Dermat.* **60**:286-296 (1973).
13. ENVIRON, Dermal Absorption of Chemicals from Potable Water, prepared for Dynamac Corporation and Office of Drinking Water, U.S. Environmental Protection Agency (September 1987).

14. International Commission on Radiological Protection (ICRP), *Report of the Task Group on Reference Man*, ICRP Publication No. 23, Pergamon Press, New York (1984).
15. M. E. Gillies and H. V. Paulin, Variability of Mineral Intakes from Drinking Water: A Possible Explanation for the Controversy Over the Relationship of Water Quality to Cardiovascular Disease, *Intl. J. Epidem.* **12**:45-50 (1985).
16. J. B. Andelman, Inhalation Exposure in the Home to Volatile Organic Contaminants of Drinking Water, *Sci. Tot. Environ.* **47**:443-460 (1985).
17. National Research Council (NRC), Risk Assessment in the Federal Government: Managing the Process, National Academy Press, Washington, D.C. (1983).

The Role of Risk Analysis in Protecting Computer Hardware, Software and Information

Diane M. Gifford
Severn, MD

ABSTRACT

With organizations becoming increasingly dependent on the use of computers to accomplish their objectives, the need to protect computer resources takes on greater importance. A computer security risk analysis is perhaps the most effective approach in determining how much protection already exists in computer systems and how much protection is required.

The primary purpose for conducting a computer security risk analysis is to evaluate the risk to computer hardware, software and information, and to identify the most cost-effective countermeasures for reducing the risk to these assets. This paper presents the basic computer security risk analysis model currently being used. The model consists of asset identification and valuation, threat analysis, probability forecasting, vulnerability analysis, potential loss evaluation, countermeasure selection, and cost benefit analysis. Problems with this model, as well as possible solutions, are identified. The use of automated risk analysis tools may alleviate some of the problems. The issue of whether to use a quantitative or qualitative approach is also addressed.

KEYWORDS: Computer, risk analysis, software, hardware, information

INTRODUCTION

With organizations becoming increasingly dependent on the use of computers to accomplish their mission, the need to protect computer hardware, software and information takes on critical importance. A risk analysis is perhaps the most effective approach in determining how much protection already exists in computer systems and how much protection is required.

Within the emerging field of computer security, work is well underway in applying risk analysis concepts traditionally used in other disciplines, to decrease the risk to computer resources.

The purpose of this paper is to present the underlying concepts of the general computer security risk analysis model currently in use. Specific applications of risk analysis methodologies do deviate somewhat from this model, but they all appear to have similarities with the presented model. This paper also discusses the need for conducting such a risk analysis. You do not need to be an expert in computers or computer security to conduct a computer security risk analysis. If you have valuable computer assets, or if you consider the information you process, store or transmit using your computer to be valuable, you would no doubt benefit from conducting a risk analysis to protect these resources.

BACKGROUND

The field of computer security is still in the early stages of development. The possibility of damage by threats, such as natural disasters, sabotage and poor management practices, were not a major concern to most computer managers in the past. In fact, many organizations proudly displayed their computer resources as showpieces in easily accessible areas. Now, the trend is moving in the opposite direction: most organizations restrict access to their computer resources, recognizing that this asset needs protection from threats just like any other valuable resource.

Due to the increase in the number of crimes involving computers, the emphasis on computer security is now receiving more attention. There are many organizations today that would be severely crippled if their computers and, perhaps more significantly, the information contained within their databases, were damaged, whether this occurred through an accident or by deliberate, malicious action.[1] Individuals referred to as "Hackers," penetrators of computers for esoteric reasons, are now gaining public attention and are frequently looked on as heroes. There are others who, for less esoteric reasons, heist hundreds of thousands of dollars from businesses by intrusion and misuse of computer assets. The literature suggests significantly more computer crime exists than is reported.[2] Even when computer crimes have been detected, many have gone unreported due to potential for embarrassment to the organization. The reality is that outsiders, like hackers are much less likely to cause computer problems than are data errors and omissions, dishonest or disgruntled employees, a failure of administrative controls, or water damage.[3] With the increased awareness of the need for computer security, has come the need for a method to assess the impact of potential threats on organizations supported by computer systems. Risk analysis is one such method.[4]

There are a number of other methods that pertain to the inspection, evaluation or testing of the security of computer systems, specifically penetration attempts, security audits, checklists and questionnaires. However, none of them can take the place of a risk analysis because their purposes are different. They do not consider the following key elements:[4]

1. The damage that may result from an unfavorable event, or threat.
2. The likelihood of such an event occurring.

Unlike traditional, interdisciplinary risk analyses which deal with concrete consequences (such as money or lives lost), often computer security concerns are diffuse and intangible (e.g., military advantage, competitive advantage, privacy protection). Asset values are more difficult to assess, since data can be an ambiguous asset whose value varies significantly over time and by use. And perhaps more so than in other areas, operational priorities, put real-world constraints on what computer security measure will be used. Until recently, the computer security community concentrated largely on either technical or administrative solutions without paying a great deal of attention to exposure assessment, risk characterization (including uncertainty), or weighing of alternative solutions.[3]

AREAS OF IMPACT TO COMPUTER HARDWARE, SOFTWARE AND INFORMATION

It is important to recognize how the computer hardware, software or information of an organization may be harmed or misused. There are four ways that assets can suffer loss; they are frequently referred to as "impact areas":[5]

1. *Destruction.* Destruction takes place through unauthorized actions that result in deprivation, which may include either total destruction or theft.
2. *Modification.* Unauthorized modification occurs when the asset has been changed in some way, and usually the value of the asset is diminished.
3. *Disclosure.* Unauthorized disclosures, which apply only to the asset of information, include disclosures of trade secrets, Privacy Act information, sensitive data, etc.
4. *Denial of Service.* Denial of service results in a computer resource being made unavailable to an authorized user, and is usually temporary in nature.

The four impact areas demonstrate the need to properly protect an organization's computer resources. It is important to note that although all of these impacts may occur deliberately, some may occur accidentally. For example, an authorized user may accidentally modify or even destroy a computer asset, like a software program. The organization needs to protect against both accidental and intentional acts.

OVERVIEW OF THE RISK ANALYSIS MODEL

Although there are a variety of computer security risk analysis methodologies currently in use, each one somewhat different from the other, this paper presents the general concepts and typical sequence representative of most methodologies. This general model consists of the following steps:

1. asset identification and valuation,
2. threat analysis,
3. probability forecasting,
4. vulnerability analysis,
5. potential loss calculation,
6. countermeasure selection, and
7. recommendation to management.

These seven steps do not necessarily have to occur in this sequence. Additionally, two steps may be combined into one. For example, some methodologies do not conduct a discrete vulnerability analysis, Step 4, but combine the same concepts of Step 4 within their threat analysis, Step 2.

Step 1

The first step in a computer security risk analysis is asset identification and valuation. An inventory of all computer resources is required, including hardware, software and information. Office furniture, buildings, personnel and other resources dedicated for use in supporting the computer systems may also be included in the inventory. Frequently, organizations have such an inventory in existence for the tangible resources. However, information is rarely identified as an asset. This must be done to properly conduct a computer security risk analysis.

Once the inventory of computer assets is complete, the current value of the assets need to be identified. Typically, replacement cost is used. Asset valuation is usually calculated by identifying the replacement or reconstruction costs for hardware, software and information.

The importance of information can be assessed by detailed interviews or questionnaires directed at the owners and users of the information. They should be asked to state what the effect on the organization would be if the data were to be disclosed, modified, made unavailable (loss of service), or destroyed.[6]

Step 2

The second step, threat analysis, is perhaps the most important phase of a computer risk assessment. Without accurately determining specific threats to the organization's computer resources, the remainder of the risk analysis would be invalid. A thorough investigation of all possible threats is the crux of a risk assessment. Threats are typically identified by reviewing historical information about the organization and interviewing organization personnel, typically operations managers, or those most knowledgeable of existing and potential threats. Some examples of threats to computer resources[7] are:

Alteration of hardware/software/information
Building structural failure
Enemy overrun/civil disorder
Environmental control failure
Fire
Hardware instability
Improper marking and handling
Intentional denial of hardware, software or information
Misuse of computer resources
Natural disasters
Poor management practices
Sabotage
Software design flaws
Telecommunications failure
Theft
Unauthorized access
Unauthorized data entry error
Unauthorized disclosure
Unintentional operator error
Unintentional programmer error

Step 3

Probability forecasting, the third step of a risk analysis, involves estimating the probability of each threat occurring. This prediction of the likelihood is necessary to calculate the expected loss dollar values for each computer resource during later steps of the risk analysis. Although estimating threat probabilities is somewhat subjective in nature, it is a necessary requirement of the computer risk analysis process. Without it, a threat with a high likelihood of occurrence, such as a programmer error, would not be distinguished from a threat with a low likelihood of occurrence, such as a hurricane in California. Typically, interviews are conducted by the risk analysis team with individuals in the organization who are considered expert in their knowledge of the particular threat in question. The probability of a threat taking place should be expressed as an annual probability; the number of occurrences of the threat per year (e.g., one act of vandalism every ten years is a 0.1 annual probability). The annual probabilities may be grouped by severity of impact: total loss, major loss, or minor loss. Developing threat probabilities is an area in which you should lean heavily on the experience of operations managers and the expertise of consultants.[8]

Estimates of threat likelihoods are hard to elicit and validate; nevertheless, the risk analysis community has already made some important progress in the area of uncertainty by using probability distributions to quantity uncertainty about exposures and severity of efforts. There is very little case data available on which to base estimates or assessments; and computer security personnel have long bemoaned the fact that estimates of threats are hard to elicit and very hard to justify; there is not enough historical data.[3]

Step 4

The fourth step, vulnerability analysis, encompasses a review of to what degree the computer resources are vulnerable to each specific threat. Countermeasures, or protective features, already in place are identified, and their effectiveness in protecting the each computer resource is assessed. The degree of vulnerability for each computer asset is identified. Examples of vulnerabilities to computer hardware, software and information include:

Inadequate or unreliable air-conditioning, heating or ventilation
Application software design weakness
Inadequate or nonexistent audit procedures
Inadequate or nonexistent backup
Insecure, unstructured or nonexistent data management
Ineffective error detection and correction provisions
Inadequate fire protection
Inappropriate geographical location
Lack of management support for security
Incompetent, disloyal or unreliable personnel
Unreliable electric power source
Inadequate or nonexistent risk management

Step 5

Potential loss calculation, the fifth step, incorporates information gathered in the previous four steps. Often the potential losses of computer resources are intangible — related to national defense, corporate goodwill, or other non-monetary assets. Unlike traditional risk analysis problems, computer security problems tend to often lie in a relatively uncharted area, that of diffuse risks from adversarial sources, where the objects at risk and the nature of the risk may be diffuse and where the source of the risk may be a malevolent adversary (see Ref. 3, p. 156).

In potential loss calculation, losses are typically calculated using an annualized dollar figure, called annual loss expectancy (ALE). Perhaps the easiest way to describe how to calculate an ALE is by working through an example. Suppose that ten microcomputers cost a total of $25,000. Assume that the threat probability of total destruction by fire is estimated at once in twenty-five years; i.e., 0.04. Using the annual loss expectancy formula:

$$\text{ALE} = \text{Asset Value} \times \text{Threat Probability} = \$25{,}000 \times 0.04 = \$1{,}000$$

After the ALEs are calculated, threats are usually prioritized based on the ALEs. However, the reasonableness of the ALEs must be reviewed and caution must be exercised, particularly in cases where the probability of the threats may be low, but the dollar loss of the assets may be high. For example, the probability of an earthquake occurring in Florida may be 0.001, and the value of an organization's computer resources may be $100,000,000.

An ALE of $100,000 may give the appearance of an area that needs significant protection, when in reality the chance of the threat occurring is negligible.

Step 6

For proper countermeasure selection, Step 6, information from the five previous steps is assimilated and used. Countermeasures may be viewed in terms of their security objectives. Preventive-type countermeasures attempt to eliminate vulnerabilities by denying a path for a threat to attack. If total elimination is impossible, the vulnerabilities is at least controlled or monitored so when a threat attempt occurs, an alarm is sounded. Countermeasures designed to alert security personnel to an attempted or actual breach of security are referred to as deterrence or detection countermeasures. Recovery countermeasures are designed to minimize the impact associated with either short-term or long-term unavailability of resources by speeding up the return of computer services to a workable level.[8] It is helpful consider the following classifications and examples of countermeasures to assist in the selection process:[5]

Organizational measures (appointing a security officer)
Administrative measures (keeping a badge list)
Personnel selection and training (conducting background investigations of new employees)
Physical access control (locks, intruder alarms)
Environmental control (uninterruptable power, air conditioning, heating, ventilation)
Disaster control (protection from fire, water damage, building collapse)
Communications security (scramblers, encryption, "sweeping" for electronic eaves-dropping devices)
Computer security (secure operating systems, password control)

Countermeasures may require an investment ranging from no cost to prohibitive cost. Therefore, during the process of countermeasure selection, a cost/benefit analysis should be conducted to determine which countermeasures provide the most cost-effective protection against threats for the least cost, using the ALE information from Step 5.

Step 7

Finally, Step 7 consists of presenting recommendations to management. According to FIPS PUB 65,[4] the results of a risk analysis provide management with information on which to base decisions, e.g., whether it is best to prevent the occurrence of a situation, to contain the effect it may have, or to simply recognize that a potential for loss exists.

Management determines which risks are acceptable. For those that are not currently acceptable, management decides which of the alternatives will be implemented and approves the resources required to purchase, design or develop them.[8]

The first time a computer security risk analysis is conducted, a significant investment of time and manpower resources is required. Subsequent risk analyses build on and use previous risk analysis information, and therefore require significantly less of an investment. It is important to note that the same computer system used in a different environment or to process different kinds of information, will probably be vulnerable to different threats. Thoroughness and attention to situation specifics, is essential in conducting a computer security risk analysis.

QUANTITATIVE VS. QUALITATIVE RISK ANALYSIS

The primary reason for conducting a computer security risk analysis is to prevent the loss of computer resources and to provide management with a basis for comparing the resources that will be required for adequate protection of those resources. In most organizations, public or private, the bottom line generally relates to dollars. An argument against using the quantitative approach is the amount of time and resources required to conduct a quantitative risk analysis.

Methodologies that use qualitative statements of loss generally require a smaller commitment of time and manpower. The problem is in comparing potential loss with the cost to implement countermeasures to reduce that loss. For example, if the cost of a particular loss is considered high and the cost to reduce the loss is low or medium, what is the level of resources required to decrease the risk? Probably the best use of a qualitative risk analysis is to identify where the major problems are, and then utilize a quantitative approach to determine a more exact statement of loss for the major problem areas.[8]

BENEFITS

An organization reaps a number of benefits as a result of conducting a computer security risk analysis, such as:

1. The organization maintains an up-to-date list of its computer hardware, software and information, and the current value of those resources.

2. The organization has identified specific threats and the probability of those threats causing harm to valuable computer resources.

3. The organization has determined how vulnerable its computer resources are to threats and the effectiveness of countermeasures currently in place.

4. The organization has determined which additional countermeasures, if any, are needed, and which ones would be most cost-effective to implement relative to the degree of risk.

5. An increase in computer security awareness at all organizational levels, from management through operations, of the need to protect computer hardware, software and information.

PROBLEM AREAS

Along with the benefits of conducting a computer security risk analysis, there are several significant problem areas:

1. The major resource required is manpower. Many man-months of work may be necessary to conduct a risk analysis for an organization with a large number of computer resources, such as an organization with numerous mainframe computers networked together, located in different geographical areas.

2. Since little historical data exists, most of the information about threat and threat probabilities is acquired by interviewing knowledgeable individuals within the organization. Identifying threat probabilities leaves room for variance and subjectivity, depending on which individual is interviewed.

3. If management decides to take no action on the results of a risk analysis, it could be perceived by those involved in conducting the risk analysis, that their time and efforts have been wasted.

POSSIBLE SOLUTIONS

1. There are a number of automated computer security risk analysis packages commercially available today. These packages reduce the amount of time required to conduct a risk analysis, particularly for organizations with a great many computer assets. Interviews within the organization still need to be conducted to determine specific threats and threat probabilities. However, a significant amount of manpower and time is saved by using an automated package.

2. To more accurately reflect the uncertainty of estimating threat probabilities, frequency distributions may be used in place of discrete probability values. A discrete value, such as $p = 0.05$, implies some degree of precision, while a range, such as 0.03 to 0.09, reflects some degree of uncertainty. With regard to threats that have little or no associated historical data, it may be more appropriate to use a range of probability or a frequency distribution, versus a discrete value.

3. One approach to decrease the time required to conduct a computer security risk analysis is to use a combination of quantitative and qualitative techniques. Traditionally in computer security risk analysis, the quantitative approach has been employed. The critics of this approach say that it is too time-consuming; when the risk analysis is complete, the information resulting from the risk analysis may be obsolete. Some say that an organization may have acquired new computer resources or they may be processing more sensitive kinds of information. On the other hand, use of a qualitative approach, which takes less time, has been criticized for its lack of precision and the results not being presented to management in a form that management can relate to, i.e., dollar values. The idea of combining both qualitative and quantitative techniques has gained more interest. For example, a preliminary qualitative analysis could identify and prioritize the threats and vulnerabilities. Then a quantitative approach could be used to focus on the most valuable computer resources, threats most likely to occur, and the most effective countermeasures to be used.

4. It is imperative to have management support prior to conducting a risk analysis. A meeting should be scheduled to explain the need to conduct such a risk analysis, the benefits, as well as the organizational resources required. It is advisable to meet again with management in the middle of the risk analysis, after the threats and vulnerabilities have been identified. This meeting will not only provide management with the current status of the risk analysis, but management will have the opportunity to provide emphasis on threats perceived as important from a management perspective. A final meeting with management, with the results of the risk analysis in a format that management can readily understand, is essential.

CONCLUSION

The use of risk analysis for protecting computer hardware, software and information is gaining a significant role in the arena of computer security. As a result of conducting a computer security risk analysis, the most cost-effective countermeasures are identified. A risk analysis helps an organization avoid unnecessary spending on security features that may not be needed. A heightened awareness of computer security, a requirement to maintain an up-to-date list of computer resources and their dollar values, a determination of threat and threat probabilities, also result. The field of computer security risk analysis is still in the early stages of development. It is expected that greater emphasis will be placed on the use of qualitative techniques, in conjunction with the quantitative approaches already in existence, as well as an increased interest in using automated risk analysis packages.

REFERENCES

1. D. Barber, Some Thoughts on Security and Related Issues, *Information Age* **5(3)**:157 (1983).
2. J. Bloombecker, How to Recognize the Computer Criminal, *Information Age* **4(4)**:195 (1982).
3. L. J. Hoffman, Risk Analysis and Computer Security: Bridging the Cultural Gap, Proceedings of the Ninth National Computer Security Conference, pp. 156-159 (1986).
4. National Bureau of Standards, *Guidelines for Automatic Data Processing Risk Analysis*, FIPS PUB 65, Gaithersburg, MD (1979).
5. J. M. Carroll, *Managing Risk*, Butterworth Publisher, Stoneham, MA (1984).
6. R. H. Moses, Risk Analysis and Management in Practice for the UK Government, Proceedings for the Tenth National Computer Security Conference, pp. 104-105 (1986).
7. D. M. Gifford, Identification of Threats and Estimation of Threat Frequencies to Computer Assets at the Naval Postgraduate School, Master's Thesis, Naval Postgraduate School, Monterey, CA (1985).
8. Datapro Risk Analysis: Section Guide, Datapro Research Corporation, Delran, NJ (1988).

Methodology for Calculating Reactor Vessel Fracture Probability Integrated Over Plant Lifetime

B. G. Gore, T. V. Vo, and A. J. Colburn
Pacific Northwest Laboratories
Richland, WA

E. Throm
U.S. Nuclear Regulatory Commission
Washington, DC

ABSTRACT

A methodology is presented for estimating the public risk integrated from now until the end-of-license (EOL) for low temperature overpressurization transients at pressurized water reactors. This methodology has been applied to estimate the reduction of public risk expected to result from several alternative regulatory strategies proposed to resolve the US Nuclear Regulatory Commission Generic Issue 94, "Additional Low Pressure Overpressure Protection for Light Water Reactors." Of concern is the rapid pressure increase of systems which are "water solid" (lacking a bubble of steam or gas) when high pressure pumps start or when temperature is rapidly increased, combined with recent failures of pressure relief mechanisms.

Two proposed alternatives were shown to reduce public risk greatly. Eliminating the present allowance that one of the two required, trains of pressure relief may be out of service for up to seven days, yielded a 92% reduction of risk. Requiring that a bubble of steam or noncondensible gas be maintained in the system at all times yielded a risk reduction of greater than 99% (resulting from much slower pressurization if relief fails, allowing more time for operator intervention).

A value/impact analysis of the proposed alternatives is presented in a companion paper presented at this conference. The requirement of redundant-train operability is shown to be considerably more cost effective than the other alternatives.

KEYWORDS: Neutron embrittlement, weld embrittlement, value/impact, RTndt (reference temperature of the nil ductility transition), generic issue, fluence

INTRODUCTION

In this paper we present a method for performing the value/impact analysis of several regulatory alternatives that have been proposed to resolve the U.S. Nuclear Regulatory

Commission (NRC) Generic Issue 94 (GI94) entitled "Additional Low-Pressure Overpressure Protection for Light-Water Reactors." The results obtained with this method, i.e., the public risk estimates for each of the alternatives and for the no-action base case, are also presented. In a companion paper,[1] expected costs to the nuclear industry and to the NRC are developed and compared with this associated risk reduction for each alternative. Thus, these two papers present both the method and the results of the value/impact analysis of GI 94.

In 1978 the NRC identified LTOP transients as Generic Issue A-26.[2] In 1979 Multiplant Action B-04 resolved this generic issue by requiring all operating pressurized water reactors (PWR) to implement procedures to reduce the potential for reactor cooling system (RCS) overpressure events and to install equipment modifications to mitigate such events.[3] Current NRC staff requirements are stated in Standard Review Plan 5.2.2, "Overpressure Protection," and in its attached Branch Technical Position BTP-RSB 5-2, "Overpressure Protection of Pressurized Water Reactors While Operating at Low Temperatures."[4] Analyses performed in this study indicate that imposition of the 1979 requirements resulted in a reduction of the plant-lifetime public risk from the 63 operating PWRs by a factor of about 100.

In addition to procedural and equipment specifications, the regulations of 1979 included a requirement to report challenges to the overpressure mitigation system (OMS) via Licensee Event Reports (LER). Review of challenges to the OMS since 1980,[5] including two events in which pressure-temperature (p-T) limits exceeded technical specifications, led to redesignation of LTOP as a generic issue, this time as GI 94. A third event in which the p-T limit curve was exceeded was identified during the course of this evaluation, which further supported redesignation of LTOP as a generic issue.

Below are the seven regulatory alternatives that this method was developed to evaluate:

1. Take no action. This is the base case evaluation of risks and consequences for LTOP events.
2. Prohibit operations with the reactor cooling system (RCS) "water solid" except when it is depressurized and vented. Require all operating reactors to maintain a bubble of steam or noncondensible gas (N_2) in the pressurizer when the RCS is not vented.
3. Prohibit operation with the RCS water solid when either train of the OMS is out of service.
4. Prohibit operation with the RCS water solid when a high pressure safety injection pump is in service.
5. Prohibit the restart of a reactor coolant pump when the RCS is water solid.
6. Require that the pressure setpoint for automatic isolation of the residual heat removal (RHR) system be raised above the setpoint for RHR safety relief valve (SRV) opening, to maintain this relief path as a backup to the OMS.
7. Require the OMS system to be safety grade.

RISK ASSESSMENT OVERVIEW

For each alternative, the public risks from the operation of the 63 presently operating PWRs, expressed in person-rems, were estimated by summation over the period covering from the present to the EOL. These estimates combined estimated frequencies of RCS overpressurization, calculated probabilities of reactor vessel fracture, and an average public radiation dose estimate per vessel fracture.

OMS Categories and Plant Groupings

Review of the OMSs for operating PWRs showed that there are three basic categories of OMS. Most plants (32 Westinghouse and 8 Combustion Engineering) use redundant pilot operated relief valves (PORV) for overpressure mitigation. These are referred to as PORV category OMS. The next largest group of plants used redundant SRVs in the RHR system (9 Westinghouse and 6 Combustion Engineering). These are referred to as RHR category OMS. The third group of 8 plants, by Babcock and Wilcox, maintain a steam or N_2 bubble in the pressurizer at all times. These are referred to as PORV+N_2 category OMS.

Data Base of OMS Challenge Events

Between January 1980 and December 1986, 63 PWRs logged 356 reactor years of commercial operation. Plants with PORV, RHR, and PORV+N_2 category OMS logged 244, 56, and 56 reactor years, respectively.[5] During this period, there were 30 OMS challenges (23 in the PORV category and 7 in the RHR category). In three cases (2 PORV, 1 RHR), as a result of OMS failure, RCS pressure exceeded the p-T limit curve described in the technical specifications (Appendix G curve).

The above information was developed from searching the LER data base using the Sequence Coding and Search System and from Phung[6] and Lanning.[7]

The challenges were driven by the addition of mass, energy (heat), or a combination of the two. Significantly, in all three overpressurization events, the p-T curve was exceeded when one of the OMS trains was unavailable due to maintenance. Review of the data base shows a marked correlation between data for PORV and RHR category plants. Specifically, compared to plants in the RHR category, plants in the PORV category are two to three times as numerous and have roughly two to three times as many challenge events, overpressurization events, and reactor years of operation. Data for each category of OMS were analyzed separately.

Overpressurization Frequencies and Spectra

For each alternative other than the no-action base case (Alternative 1), the data base was reanalyzed to determine which challenge events would have been eliminated by the proposed regulatory requirement (if it had been in effect), and how the outcome of remaining events would have been changed. Thus, for the various alternatives, there resulted different estimates of OMS challenge frequency, unavailability, overpressurization frequency, and peak pressure spectrum.

For PORV and RHR category OMS, unavailability was determined as the fraction of challenges for which the OMS had actually failed to prevent overpressurization. This unavailability is actually representative of operation with only one OMS train operable, since all three failure events in the data base occurred with one train out of service for maintenance. Present technical specifications allow one train of OMS to be out of service for up to seven days. This is a long time when compared with the time required for plant startup, when most challenge events can be expected as system surveillances are conducted and systems are returned to service. Consequently, from a safety analysis perspective, the present operability requirements and unavailability data must be considered to be representative of a single-train OMS.

The data base contained no challenge (or overpressurization) events for PORV+N_2 category OMS. Consequently, PORV+N_2 category OMS unavailability was assumed to be equal to the unavailability for PORV category OMSs. Since PORV+N_2 category OMS utilize only one PORV, this assumption incorporates the conclusion discussed above, that the calculated unavailability of PORV category OMS is characteristic of single-train OMS operation.

The same unavailability values were used for all the alternatives except Alternatives 3 and 7. For Alternative 3, the base case unavailability is squared since independent failure of two channels is required. For Alternative 7, the unavailability of PORV category OMSs is estimated to be reduced due to installation of an improved system.

The spectrum of peak transient pressures expected when the OMS fails was determined by analyzing each event in the data base assuming that the OMS failed. Each LER was reviewed to determine actual plant conditions existing during the event, and NRC resident inspectors were contacted for supplemental information and to verify interpretations and expectations made by Pacific Northwest Laboratory (PNL). This analysis incorporated the effects of alternate relief paths (through RHR SRVs for PORV category OMSs) where they existed and were not precluded by autoclosure interlocks actuated by increasing pressure. Actual pump shutoff heads, flow imbalances, temperature differences, and relief capacities existing during the event were used in the analysis of these hypothetical overpressurization events.

A key assumption used in deriving the pressure spectrum was that operator action to terminate pressurization occurred three minutes after event initiation. This time is short when compared with the 10 minutes often assumed in safety analyses. The three-minute time period was selected for two reasons. First, the LER record included no instances where operator action necessary to correct a pressurization problem (primarily letdown/makeup flow imbalances) required longer than three minutes. Second, PNL's experience in observing simulator exercises, including operator licensing examinations, indicated that three minutes is ample time to make several attempts at event diagnosis and correction. This assumption that pressurization was terminated three minutes after event initiation clearly makes this a "best-estimate" as opposed to "worst-case" analysis.

The overpressurization frequencies and spectra obtained from this data base analysis were used to characterize all plants having a given category of OMS. It was assumed that values remain constant between the present and EOL, so that they may be combined by simple multiplication with vessel fracture probabilities (VFP) summed over time.

Reactor Vessel Fracture Probabilities

The analysis of reactor VFPs was developed to incorporate explicitly the exponential increase in vessel brittleness that occurs with increasing neutron fluence. The following paragraphs summarize key aspects of the methods used to accomplish this analysis. Because the rate of vessel embrittlement is strongly dependent on the chemistry of each individual vessel, a plant-specific analysis of VFP as a function of time was performed. Plant-specific information on vessel chemistry and fluence was used to determine the reference temperature of the nil ductility transition (RTndt) as a function of time between the present and EOL for each of the 63 operating PWRs addressed in the study.

The RTndt information was used to determine the fracture probability for each vessel as a function of time for each of three peak transient pressures (PTP). This was accomplished by specifying a representative "standard LTOP transient" and using representative vessel geometry to calculate curves of VFP versus RTndt parameterized by PTP. From this information, curves of VFP versus time were constructed for each of the 63 vessels, for each of three overpressure values. These curves are normalized to an overpressurization frequency of one per year, since the VFP plotted for each year corresponds to one overpressure event.

For each of the 63 vessels, a normalized (to unit overpressurization frequency), integrated (over time and plants in the category) vessel fracture probability (NIVFP) was calculated by summing (i.e., integrating) the normalized fracture probability values from the present to EOL. This was done for each of the three PTPs. The NIVFP values were then summed over plants having the same OMS category.

The significance of the NIVFP for a given PTP is that, when multiplied by an estimated overpressurization frequency, the product is the VFP integrated from the present to EOL. Thus, when a NIVFP category sum is multiplied by the average overpressurization frequency for that category, the product is the time-integrated VFP for all plants in the category from the present to EOL. A power-law interpolation scheme was developed to allow determination of category sum NIVFP values for intermediate PTPs. This enabled determination of category sum NIVFP values that corresponded to pressures identified in the OMS challenge data base analyses for the various alternatives. With this information, a true category sum integrated VFP was calculated by multiplying the overpressurization frequency times the matrix product of the pressure spectrum fraction, and then multiplying that product with the corresponding category sum NIVFP value for that pressure.

The key assumption that enables this separation of analysis portions is that the overpressurization frequency and spectrum remain constant over time. With this assumption it is possible to address the time behavior of vessel embrittlement with increasing neutron fluence without requiring an inordinate amount of analytical details.

Correlation of Risk with Vessel Fracture Probability

Reactor vessel failure was assumed to result in core damage due to loss of core cooling with a probability of one. The results of an analysis performed by Brookhaven National Laboratory[8] were adopted for direct application in this study. That analysis assumed a late core melt into open containment at a typical eastern site, with risk reduced by 50% due to the assumption that the containment would only be open 50% of the time. The public radiation dose resulting over a 30-year period from this analysis is 4.5×10^6 person-rem per vessel fracture. This value was used for all plants in the study. The resulting public risk is therefore proportional to VFP for all alternatives.

CALCULATION OF REACTOR VESSEL FRACTURE PROBABILITY

The Vessel Integrity Simulation Analysis (VISA) code[9] was used to calculate the probability of reactor VFP resulting from overpressurization due to failure of the OMS. The VISA code performs a deterministic fracture mechanics analysis for a temperature and pressure transient, yielding stress intensity factors and temperatures throughout the vessel wall as a function of time during the transient. It then performs a Monte Carlo simulation, randomly sampling flaw-depth and vessel-toughness values to estimate the probability of vessel fracture. Required inputs to the code for each calculation include information on vessel geometry, material properties such as chemical constituents, vessel neutron fluence, and such information on the transient such as the temperature and pressure history to which the vessel is subjected.

Since this study addresses 63 different reactor vessels from the present to EOL and over a significant range of possible temperature and pressure excursions, a very large number of VISA calculations could be required. However, Monte Carlo simulations are time consuming and expensive to run. Consequently, an approach was developed that allowed the necessary number of VISA calculations to be bounded using reasonable, but conservative, assumptions to reduce the number of variables that had to be considered.

There are two main features of the methodology that was developed. First, a "Standard LTOP Transient" was defined to fix the temperature and pressure parameters that had to be considered. Second, the RTndt, which incorporates the multiple effects of chemical composition and fluence into a single parameter, was used to characterize the properties of the reactor vessels for each of the 63 PWRs addressed in this study.

The calculations performed by the VISA code defined a family of curves of VFP versus RTndt. These curves were parameterized according to the peak pressure achieved in the overpressure transient. The VFP of any specific vessel at any time during its lifetime could then be obtained from the curves, given the RTndt of the vessel at the time in question and the PTP achieved. This approach is based on the fact that, over a wide range of vessel compositions and neutron fluence values, the VFP is directly correlated with the RTndt of the vessel.

Standard LTOP Transient

OMS challenges and subsequent overpressurization events can occur during heatup or cooldown, at temperatures from ambient to several hundred degrees Fahrenheit. They are characteristically rather rapidly evolving transients and can be rapidly mitigated by operators once they are recognized to be in progress. They are usually associated with water-solid operation, when there is no steam or N_2 bubble in the pressurizer. The magnitude of the stresses encountered during an overpressurization transient is greatest on the inner wall of the vessel, and higher during cooldown, when contraction of the cooler inner wall adds to the tensile hoop stresses caused by pressure in the vessel, than during heatup.

A worst-case overpressurization transient would occur during cooldown, at as low a temperature as is expected in the reactor building. This was not selected for the standard transient, however, because overpressurization transients are far more likely during heatup than during cooldown. During cooldown, the operators are taking systems off line, securing pumps used for high pressure injection, securing RCS pumps that circulate primary coolant through the steam generators, and opening the valves isolating the RCS from the RHR system that provides additional cooling and relief valve protection. During heatup, systems are being actuated and pumps started that have the capability of pressurizing the system either directly or by circulating primary coolant through a steam generator which is hotter than the coolant in the reactor vessel (which has been cooled by the RHR system coolers). Most overpressurization transients occur in connection with these latter activities.

The standard overpressurization transient was therefore defined as a heatup transient, occurring at a temperature of 120°F, during a heatup of 25 degrees per hour. This temperature of occurrence is lower than that at which the reactor head may be removed at many plants, and it is in the range where radioactive decay heating might balance heat losses from the system. It therefore represents a reasonable limiting temperature for a heatup transient.

RTndt Characterization of Fracture Probability

New reactor pressure vessels have a high fracture toughness which degrades with neutron irradiation. This degradation depends on both the neutron fluence that the vessel receives and on the chemical constituents that it contains. The higher the copper and nickel content, the greater the embrittlement caused by a given neutron fluence. This effect is often greatest in weld material, which may contain elevated levels of these impurities. The RTndt captures the combined effects of these factors in a single parameter that is related to the probability of fracture of the vessel.

Fracture probabilities calculated for vessels having the same RTndt are similar, despite significant differences in chemical content and neutron fluence. This is of considerable importance to this analysis because extensive efforts have been devoted in other NRC-sponsored work to the calculation of RTndt values for operating reactors. In particular, Regulatory Guide 1.99, Revision 2, presents a table of EOL RTndt values for 61 operating PWRs.

The approach used to calculate the fracture probabilities for all operating reactors was based on the assumption that fracture probability depends only on RTndt value, and that any differences due to specifics of vessel composition or construction are less than the statistical errors of the VISA calculations. Having made this assumption, it is only necessary to use VISA to calculate parametric curves of fracture probability versus RTndt, from which the fracture probability may be read once the RTndt value is obtained from other sources. Since a spectrum of peak pressures may result from overpressurization transients, a family of curves must be plotted spanning the range of possible overpressure events.

The VFP increases rapidly with RTndt. Conversely, the number of simulations necessary to estimate VFP increases rapidly with decreasing RTndt and pressure. VISA calculations were performed for RTndt values from a maximum of 320°F, slightly above the maximum EOL value predicted for operating reactors, down to 110°F. This was sufficient for use in identifying the shape of the curves, and it spans several decades of probability.

Curves of VFP versus RTndt are presented in Fig. 1. The curves are seen to be roughly exponential over much of the range of interest, as is indicated by the linearity of the semi-log plots. However, they deviate from exponential as high values of RTndt and pressure are reached, since VFP cannot exceed unity.

NORMALIZED, INTEGRATED VESSEL FRACTURE PROBABILITIES

Plant-specific values of VFP as a function of time were determined assuming a unit annual overpressurization frequency to a specific pressure. This normalized VFP was then integrated from the present to EOL. The resulting NIVFP represents the probability of vessel fracture between the present and EOL if the vessel were subjected to one overpressurization per year to the giver pressure. These NIVFP values were then summed over the plants in each of the three categories of LTOP systems (PORV, RHR, and PORV+N_2). NIVFP values have been calculated for specific PTPs of 2500, 1500, and 700 psi, and values are presented for all plants, as are LTOP category sums. A method for interpolating between overpressure values, which can be used either for individual plants or for category sums, is presented.

This information was used to calculate the actual integrated VFP for each alternative by incorporating the overpressurization frequency and spectrum for each OMS category. This was done by multiplying the category sum for each pressure listed in the spectrum times the product of the overpressurization frequency and the fraction of overpressurizations to the pressure. The resulting values were then summed over the spectrum, giving the actual integrated VFP.

The calculation of NIVFP begins with the curves of VFP verses RTndt presented in Fig. 1 for PTPs of 2500, 1500, and 700 psi. For each operating PWR, RTndt was determined as a function of time for the operating period from January 1, 1986 to EOL. Using the curve of VFP versus RTndt and the values of RTndt at specific times during plant life, graphs of VFP versus time were prepared for each value of PTP. This was done for each plant. VFP summed over plant lifetime was obtained by integrating each curve

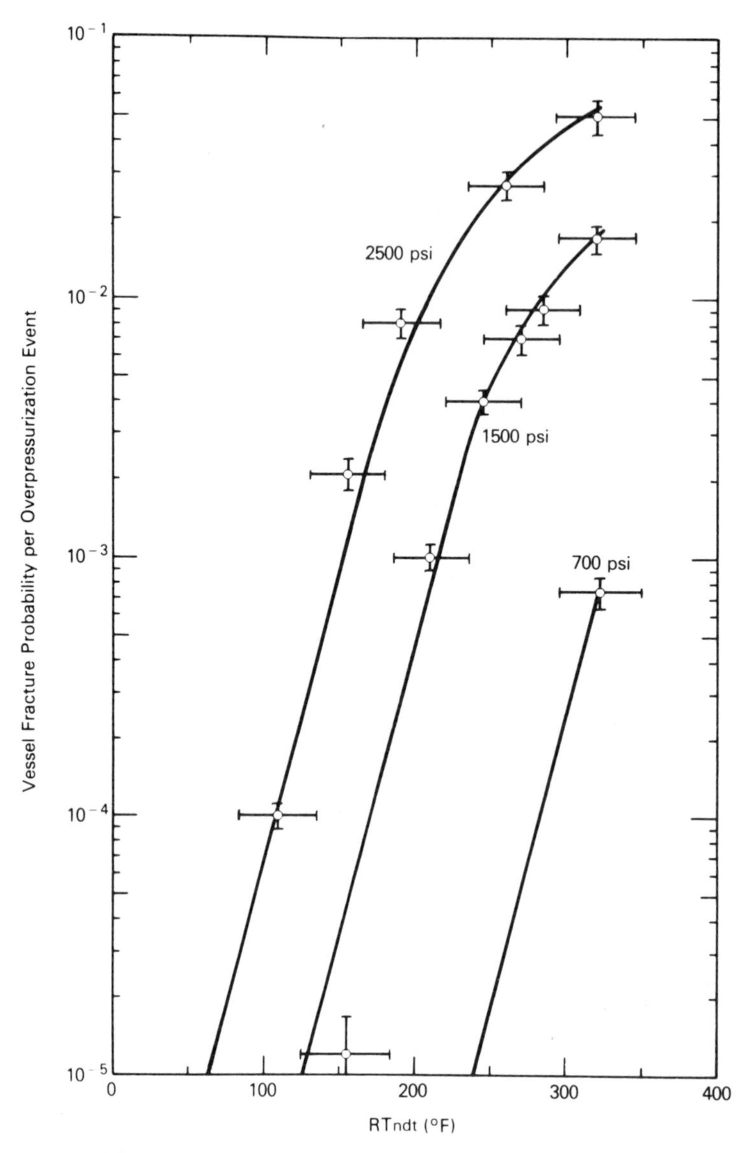

Fig. 1. Values of VFP as a function of RTndt and PTP.

between January 1986 and EOL. To facilitate the integration process, each curve was approximated by an exponential function of time (i.e., a straight line on a semi-log plot). This procedure fit the data well near EOL. In the majority of cases, this procedure resulted in an overprediction of VFP values at earlier times (i.e., when VFP values are smaller and contribute less to the sum). It was demonstrated that the overprediction of integrated VFP does not exceed 10% for any individual plant. The total overprediction is estimated to be considerably less than 10%, because plants with high RTndt (i.e., (190°F and up) have less structure in their VFP versus time plots and also contribute a higher percentage to the overall VFP than do plants with smaller values of RTndt.

Construction and Integration of Plant-Specific VFP Versus Time Plots

This calculation was done with the method of Regulatory Guide 1.99, Revision 2,[10] which provides for estimating RTndt given reactor vessel chemistry, fluence, and initial RTndt values. Values for chemistry factors, fluence at January 1986 and at EOL, and the initial value of RTndt [i.e., RTndt (0)] were provided by the NRC. This information was then used in calculating RTndt as a function of time over plant life.

A linear fluence variation with time was assumed between January 1986 and EOL, and the equation relating fluence as function of time was established for each plant. Fluence was then calculated at five-year intervals from January 1986 to EOL. The change of RTndt with fluence (F) was calculated as the product of the chemistry factor and a fluence factor (FF), which is given by:

$$FF = (F/10^{19})^{(0.28 - 0.10 \, \text{Log}_{10}(F/10^{19}))}$$

These RTndt values were then used along with Fig. 1 to plot curves of VFP versus time from January 1986 to EOL. For each plant, each RTndt value was used to determine corresponding VFPs from Fig. 1 (for PTPs of 2500, 1500, 700 psi). This resulted in a graph of VFP versus time for each pressure for each plant in the data base.

In general, these curves are reasonably well approximated by a straight line on a semi-log plot near EOL, where VFP values are greatest. This indicated that they might be approximated by an exponential function, which could be integrated analytically to provide NIVFP values. However, most of the curves deviated from a straight line for the first 5 to 10 years of reactor operation after January 1986.

Figures 2 and 3 present the VFP versus time curves for two plants along with the exponential approximations that were evaluated. These are examples of minimum and maximum curve structure.

For simple exponential integration, a straight line was drawn through the data points near EOL on the VFP versus time plots and extrapolated back to January 1986. An exponential curve of the form:

$$P(t) = Ce^{at}$$

was assumed for each straight line, and the constants were determined using the end points at January 1986 (projected) and EOL. This curve was then mathematically integrated from January 1986 to EOL to yield an integrated VFP over the plant life.

This method was used to calculate the areas under the VFP versus time curves for each plant in the data base. The results of this effort for all plants are summarized by plant OMS category in Table 1.

Interpolation of Integrated VFP Values with Varying Pressures

Overpressurization spectra included PTP values differing in some cases from the 2500, 1500, and 700 psi values used in the NIVFP analysis. Consequently a scheme was developed that allows interpolation with pressure between category sum values of NIVFP.

Study of the data determined that the relationship between NIVFP and PTP is close to linear on a log-log plot. This is true for category sum values and also for individual plant results.

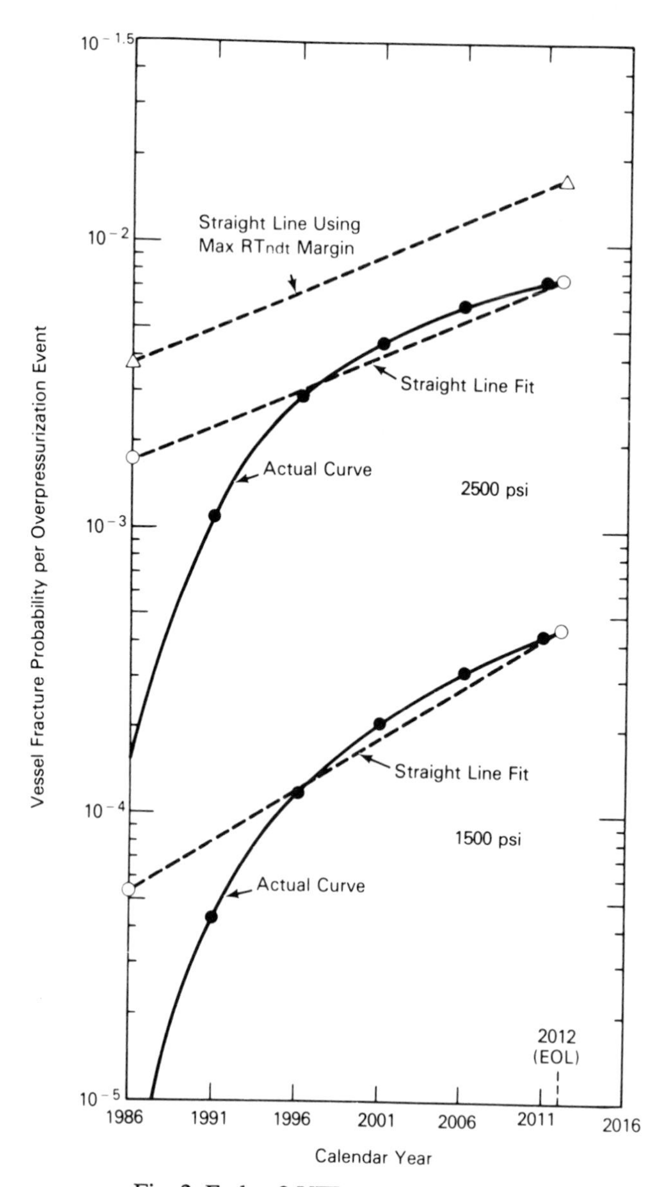

Fig. 2. Farley 2 VFP versus time curves.

NIVFP values for intermediate PTP values were calculated assuming a relationship of the following form:

$$\text{NIVFP} = cp^d$$

where c and d are constants determined by fitting this curve (log-log straight line) to values calculated for pressures of 2500, 1500, and 700 psi.

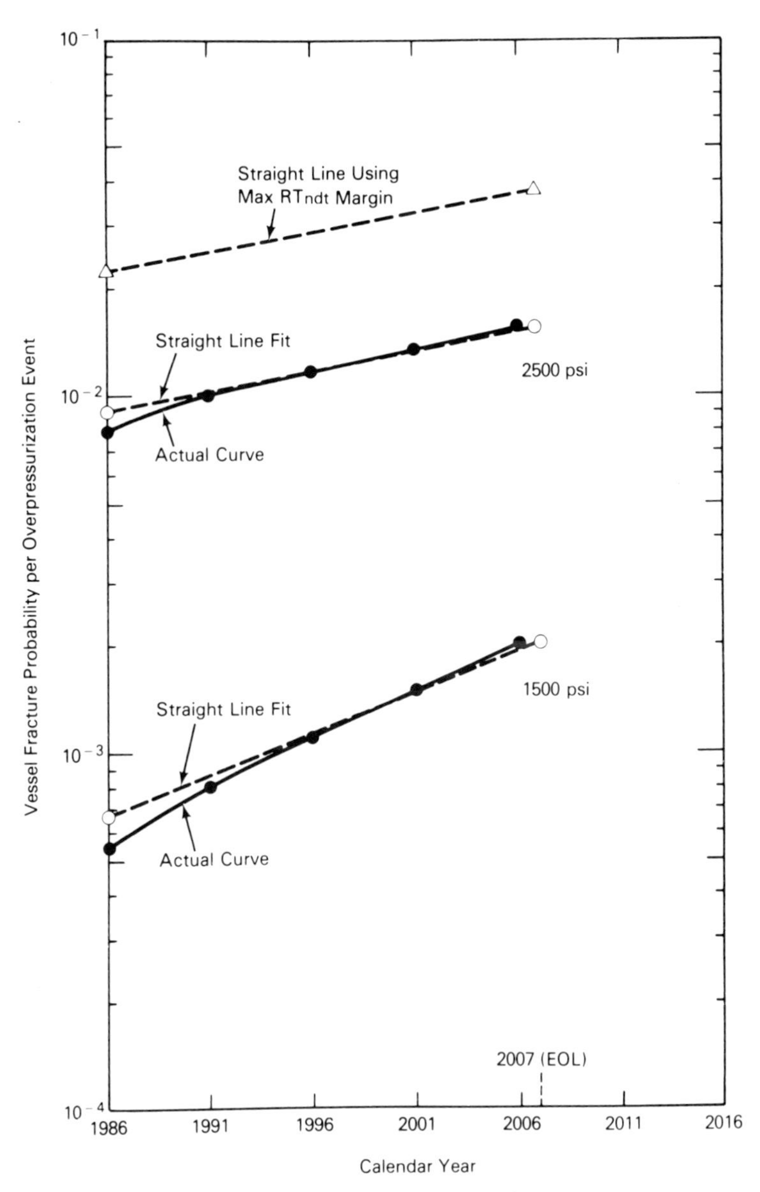

Fig. 3. Turkey Point 3 VFP versus time curves.

RESULTS OF THE RISK ANALYSIS

Table 2 presents the results of the risk analysis for the base case and all the alternatives. It also summarizes the inputs to each calculation. The calculation proceeds from left to right for each row of the table. Additional explanation is provided by the footnotes to the table.

For each alternative, the table presents analyses for plants with PORV, RHR, and PORV+N_2 category OMS, in successive rows. Finally an "Overall" category is presented in which the total integrated VFP values for all three categories are summed, and an overall VFP average per plant, per year is calculated (using the plant year total from Footnote 3 in

Table 1. Reactor VFP, Assuming One Overpressure Event Per Plant Per Year Through EOL

	Category: PORV	1986 Fracture Probability per Event					EOL Fracture Probability per Event					Integrated Fracture Probability		
EOL	Plant Name	ϕ ($\times 10^{19}$)	RTndt	2500	1500	700	ϕ ($\times 10^{19}$)	RTndt	2500	1500	700	2500	1500	700
2014	Calvert Cliffs 1	1.133	165	1.9E-3	7.6E-5	1.8E-7	5.373	245	2.2E-2	4.0E-3	1.4E-5	3.67E-1	5.33E-2	1.40E-4
2016	Calvert Cliffs 2	1.1008	118	1.7E-4	6.6E-6	<1.0E-7	5.330	163	1.8E-3	7.2E-5	1.6E-7	3.00E-2	1.18E-3	1.33E-6
2008	Fort Calhoun 1	1.090	177	3.5E-3	1.5E-4	3.5E-7	2.880	236	1.85E-2	2.9E-3	8.4E-6	2.46E-1	2.63E-2	6.85E-5
2008	Main Yankee 1	0.590	131	3.2E-4	1.3E-5	<1.0E-7	1.470	186	5.0E-3	2.3E-4	5.6E-7	4.74E-2	1.98E-3	4.06E-6
2010	Millstone 2	0.810	72	1.6E-5	5.8E-7	<1.0E-7	4.320	131	3.3E-4	1.3E-5	<1.0E-7	3.71E-3	1.46E-4	<1.00E-7
2007	Palisades	1.290	174	3.0E-3	1.2E-4	2.9E-7	4.100	223	1.4E-2	1.7E-3	4.2E-6	2.01E-1	1.71E-2	4.14E-5
2010	St. Lucie 1	0.339	85	3.1E-5	1.1E-6	<1.0E-7	1.680	173	2.9E-3	1.2E-4	2.6E-7	2.14E-2	8.59E-4	8.47E-7
2023	St. Lucie 2	0.306	72	1.6E-5	5.7E-7	<1.0E-7	4.790	138	4.7E-4	1.8E-5	<1.0E-7	9.01E-5	3.31E-4	<1.00E-7
2010	Beaver Valley 1	0.600	149	8.4E-4	3.3E-5	<1.0E-7	4.500	223	1.4E-2	1.6E-3	3.9E-6	2.06E-1	1.64E-2	4.02E-5
2024	Catawba 1	N/A	0	<1.0E-7	<1.0E-7	<1.0E-7	N/A	<50	<1.0E-7	<1.0E-7	<1.0E-7	<1.00E-7	<1.00E-7	<1.00E-7
2024	Catawba 2	0.0	33	<1.0E-7	<1.0E-7	<1.0E-7	2.100	86	3.2E-5	1.2E-6	<1.0E-7	7.19E-4	2.71E-5	<1.00E-7
2009	D.C. Cook 1	0.490	119	1.8E-4	6.8E-6	<1.0E-7	1.660	194	6.4E-3	3.5E-4	8.2E-7	5.69E-2	2.65E-3	5.54E-6
2009	D.C. Cook 2	0.324	133	3.7E-4	1.4E-5	<1.0E-7	1.360	176	3.4E-3	1.40E-4	3.1E-7	3.97E-2	1.60E-3	2.76E-6
2008	Diablo Canyon 1	0.090	36	<1.0E-7	<1.0E-7	<1.0E-7	1.540	204	8.4E-3	5.9E-4	1.4E-6	6.81E-2	3.47E-3	7.20E-6
2010	Diablo Canyon 2	0.0	67	1.2E-5	4.4E-7	<1.0E-7	1.490	178	3.7E-3	1.5E-4	3.5E-7	3.56E-2	1.45E-3	2.24E-6
2004	Haddem Neck	2.830	77	2.0E-5	7.5E-7	<1.0E-7	5.670	93	4.6E-5	1.7E-6	<1.0E-7	6.09E-4	2.17E-5	<1.00E-7
2006	Indian Point 2	0.381	150	8.8E-4	3.5E-5	<1.0E-7	0.889	187	5.2E-3	2.4E-4	5.6E-7	5.79E-2	2.42E-3	4.96E-6
2009	Indian Point 3	0.273	178	3.5E-3	1.5E-4	3.5E-7	1.020	235	1.8E-2	2.8E-3	7.5E-6	2.58E-1	2.68E-2	6.89E-5
2013	McGuire 1	0.270	67	1.2E-5	4.4E-7	<1.0E-7	2.890	190	5.6E-3	2.8E-4	6.6E-7	4.54E-2	2.08E-3	4.67E-6
2013	McGuire 2	0.270	75	1.8E-5	6.7E-7	<1.0E-7	2.900	154	1.1E-3	4.3E-5	<1.0E-7	1.22E-2	4.64E-4	<1.00E-7
2011	North Anna 1	0.740	143	6.1E-4	2.4E-5	<1.0E-7	3.110	187	5.4E-3	2.4E-4	5.6E-7	7.71E-2	3.18E-3	7.00E-6
2011	North Anna 2	0.530	135	4.1E-4	1.6E-5	<1.0E-7	3.400	183	4.2E-3	2.0E-4	4.5E-7	6.09E-2	2.61E-3	5.46E-6
2010	Point Beach 1	0.810	159	1.4E-3	5.6E-5	1.2E-7	2.100	203	8.4E-3	5.6E-4	1.3E-6	1.18E-1	6.41E-3	1.43E-5
2013	Point Beach 2	1.300	193	6.0E-3	3.3E-4	7.8E-7	3.500	239	2.0E-2	3.2E-3	9.3E-6	3.70E-1	4.44E-2	1.14E-4
2008	Prairie Island 1	1.530	85	3.1E-5	1.1E-6	<1.0E-7	9.750	115	1.4E-4	5.5E-6	<1.0E-7	2.30E-3	8.80E-5	<1.00E-7
2008	Prairie Island 2	1.460	104	8.2E-5	3.1E-6	<1.0E-7	9.750	142	5.8E-4	2.3E-5	<1.0E-7	8.63E-3	3.33E-4	<1.00E-7
2006	R.E. Ginna	1.300	181	4.0E-3	1.8E-4	4.1E-7	2.900	217	1.2E-2	1.2E-3	2.8E-6	1.61E-1	1.24E-2	2.86E-5
2007	H.B. Robinson 2	0.918	156	1.2E-3	4.8E-5	1.1E-7	1.760	196	6.8E-3	3.9E-4	9.2E-7	8.48E-2	3.72E-3	8.92E-6
2008	Salem 1	0.390	164	1.8E-3	7.3E-5	1.6E-7	1.460	222	1.45E-2	1.5E-3	3.7E-6	1.86E-1	1.34E-2	3.26E-5
2008	Salem 2	0.130	34	<1.0E-7	<1.0E-7	<1.0E-7	1.010	136	4.3E-4	1.7E-5	<1.0E-7	4.30E-3	1.66E-4	<1.00E-7

continued

Table 1. Continued.

EOL	Category: PORV	1986 Fracture Probability per Event					EOL Fracture Probability per Event					Integrated Fracture Probability		
	Plant Name	ϕ (x10^{19})	RTndt	2500	1500	700	ϕ (x10^{19})	RTndt	2500	1500	700	2500	1500	700
2004	San Onofre 1	3.730	178	3.7E-3	1.5E-4	3.5E-7	9.985	194	6.2E-3	3.5E-4	8.2E-7	9.45E-2	4.82E-3	1.11E-5
2010	Sequoyah 1	0.268	115	1.4E-4	5.5E-6	<1.0E-7	3.010	191	5.8E-3	3.0E-4	7.0E-7	6.78E-2	3.02E-3	6.22E-6
2010	Sequoyah 2	0.231	67	1.2E-5	4.4E-7	<1.0E-7	3.010	132	3.5E-4	1.3E-5	<1.0E-7	4.04E-3	1.54E-4	<1.00E-7
2008	Surry 1	0.182	122	2.1E-4	8.0E-6	<1.0E-7	0.571	187	5.0E-3	2.4E-4	5.6E-7	4.30E-2	1.85E-3	3.69E-6
2008	Surry 2	0.203	106	9.0E-5	3.4E-6	<1.0E-7	0.627	160	1.5E-3	5.9E-5	1.3E-7	1.34E-2	5.29E-4	2.39E-7
2011	Trojan	0.387	97	5.7E-5	2.1E-6	<1.0E-7	2.890	162	1.6E-3	6.5E-5	1.5E-7	1.78E-2	6.94E-4	6.45E-7
2007	Turkey Pt 3	1.270	202	8.0E-3	5.4E-4	1.3E-6	2.150	227	1.55E-2	2.0E-3	4.9E-6	2.52E-1	2.54E-2	6.11E-5
2007	Turkey Pt 4	1.270	202	8.0E-3	5.4E-4	1.3E-6	2.150	227	1.55E-2	2.0E-3	4.9E-6	2.52E-1	2.54E-2	6.11E-5
2011	Zion 1	0.443	163	1.7E-3	6.9E-5	1.5E-7	1.470	233	1.7E-2	2.5E-3	6.8E-6	2.38E-1	2.20E-2	5.61E-5
2008	Zion 2	0.141	103	7.7E-5	2.9E-6	<1.0E-7	0.626	183	4.4E-3	2.0E-4	4.5E-7	3.31E-2	1.41E-3	2.29E-6
											TOTAL FP-PORV	**3.79**	**0.331**	**8.06E-4**

PORV - TOTAL RX YEAR (1986 EOL) = 969

Total assuming one event per year at each pressure for each plant.

continued

Table 1. Continued.

EOL	Category: PORV Plant Name	1986 Fracture Probability per Event ϕ (x10^{19})	RTndt	2500	1500	700	EOL Fracture Probability per Event ϕ (x10^{19})	RTndt	2500	1500	700	Integrated Fracture Probability 2500	1500	700
2012	Farley 2	0.590	117	1.6E-4	6.1E-6	<1.0E-7	5.040	199	7.5E-3	4.6E-4	1.1E-6	1.02E-1	4.93E-3	1.06E-5
2012	ANO-2	0.640	78	2.4E-5	8.2E-7	<1.0E-7	4.380	120	1.8E-4	7.0E-6	<1.0E-7	1.31E-3	1.07E-4	<1.00E-7
2024	Palo Verde 1	0.0	30	<1.0E-7	<1.0E-7	<1.0E-7	6.300	94	4.8E-5	1.9E-6	<1.0E-7	1.20E-3	4.83E-5	<1.00E-7
2025	Palo Verde 2	N/A	0	<1.0E-7	<1.0E-7	<1.0E-7	N/A	<50	<1.0E-7	<1.0E-7	<1.0E-7	<1.00E-7	<1.00E-7	<1.00E-7
2013	San Onofre 2	0.180	51	5.2E-6	1.9E-7	<1.0E-7	3.680	103	7.4E-5	2.9E-6	<1.0E-7	1.22E-3	4.66E-5	<1.00E-7
2013	San Onofre 3	0.120	57	7.2E-6	2.6E-7	<1.0E-7	3.680	90	4.0E-5	1.5E-6	<1.0E-7	7.53E-4	2.80E-5	<1.00E-7
2012	Farley 1	0.840	108	1.0E-4	3.8E-6	<1.0E-7	5.040	152	9.8E-4	3.9E-5	<1.0E-7	1.41E-2	5.65E-4	<1.00E-7
2013	Kewaunee	1.250	177	3.6E-3	1.4E-4	3.3E-7	4.600	247	2.3E-2	4.2E-3	1.4E-5	3.89E-1	6.02E-2	1.53E-4
2013	Summer	0.300	74	1.7E-5	6.4E-7	<1.0E-7	4.780	121	2.0E-4	7.6E-6	<1.0E-7	3.14E-3	1.20E-4	<1.00E-7
1997	Yankee Rowe	1.584	200	7.6E-3	4.8E-4	1.1E-6	2.337	215	1.13E-2	1.1E-3	2.6E-6	1.03E-1	8.22E-3	1.92E-5
2024	Waterford 3	0.0	22	<1.0E-7	<1.0E-7	<1.0E-7	3.680	49	<1.0E-7	<1.0E-7	<1.0E-7	<1.00E-7	<1.00E-7	<1.00E-7
2024	Byron 1	0.0	40	<1.0E-7	<1.0E-7	<1.0E-7	2.800	79	2.2E-5	8.3E-7	<1.0E-7	5.74E-4	2.15E-5	<1.00E-7
2024	Callaway 1	0.110	72	1.6E-5	5.7E-7	<1.0E-7	3.630	118	1.7E-4	6.4E-6	<1.0E-7	4.18E-3	1.58E-4	<1.00E-7
2010	Millstone 3	N/A	0	<1.0E-7	<1.0E-7	<1.0E-7	N/A	<50	<1.0E-7	<1.0E-7	<1.0E-7	<1.00E-7	<1.00E-7	<1.00E-7
2025	Wolf Creek	0.030	50	5.0E-6	1.8E-7	<1.0E-7	3.140	97	5.7E-5	2.1E-6	<1.0E-7	1.50E-3	5.63E-5	<1.00E-7
									TOTAL FP-RHR			**0.623**	**0.0746**	**1.83E-4**
														RHR - TOTAL RX YEAR (1986 EOL) = 452
2008	ANO-1	0.280	128	2.8E-4	1.2E-5	<1.0E-7	0.860	188	5.4E-3	2.8E-4	6.4E-7	5.06E-2	2.26E-3	4.15E-6
2008	Crystal River 3	0.200	120	1.8E-4	7.4E-6	<1.0E-7	0.720	191	5.6E-3	3.0E-4	7.2E-7	4.70E-2	2.17E-3	4.57E-6
2007	Oconnee 1	0.300	123	2.2E-4	8.4E-6	<1.0E-7	0.970	183	4.2E-3	1.9E-4	4.6E-7	3.72E-2	1.81E-3	3.28E-6
2013	Oconnee 2	0.321	153	1.0E-3	4.2E-5	<1.0E-7	1.060	226	1.5E-2	1.9E-3	4.8E-7	2.06E-1	1.65E-2	1.08E-5
2007	Oconnee 3	0.390	128	2.7E-4	1.1E-5	<1.0E-7	1.600	195	6.4E-3	3.7E-4	9.0E-7	6.81E-2	3.15E-3	6.96E-6
2008	Rancho Seco 1	0.260	134	3.7E-4	1.5E-5	<1.0E-7	0.690	189	5.4E-3	2.9E-4	6.9E-7	5.25E-2	2.39E-3	4.55E-6
2008	TMI - 1	0.170	119	1.7E-4	6.8E-6	<1.0E-7	0.643	196	7.0E-3	4.2E-4	9.4E-7	5.94E-2	2.85E-3	5.46E-6
2011	Davis Besse	0.240	111	1.2E-4	4.4E-6	<1.0E-7	1.300	193	6.0E-3	3.2E-4	8.0E-7	5.89E-2	2.71E-3	6.10E-6
									TOTAL FP-PORV + N_2			**0.580**	**3.38E-2**	**4.59E-5**
														PORV + N_2 - TOTAL RX YEAR (1986 EOL) = 183

Table 2. Integrated VFPs for the Base Case and All Alternatives

Plant Category	Challenge Frequency (yr^{-1})	Unavail.	Overpressurization Spectrum psi	Overpressurization Spectrum %	NIVFP[1] Value by Pressure	VFP Contribution by Pressure	Category Total VFP[2]	Category Average VFP per Plant per Year[3]	Public Risk[4] (p-rem)	Factor of Improvement Over Base Case[5]	Reduction of Public Risk[6] (p-rem)
Alternative 1 - No Action (Base Case)											
PORV	23/244	2/23	2500	9	3.79	$2.80x10^{-3}$					
	(=0.094)	(=0.087)	1400	9	.19	$1.40x10^{-4}$					
			850	13	$3.7x10^{-3}$	$3.94x10^{-6}$					
			<600	69	$<2.0x10^{-4}$	$<1.13x10^{-6}$	$2.95x10^{-3}$	$3.04x10^{-6}$	$1.33x10^{4}$	NA	NA
RHR	7/56	1/7	2500	14	.68	$1.70x10^{-3}$					
	(0.125)	(=0.143)	850	14	$9.0x10^{-4}$	$2.25x10^{-6}$					
			<600	72	$<1.0x10^{-4}$	$<1.29x10^{-6}$	$1.70x10^{-3}$	$3.76x10^{-6}$	$7.65x10^{3}$	NA	NA
PORV+N2	<1/56	0.087	850	5	$2.0x10^{-4}$	$1.55x10^{-8}$					
	(<0.018)		<600	95	$<1.0x10^{-5}$	$<1.48x10^{-8}$	$3.03x10^{-8}$	$1.66x10^{-10}$	0.136	NA	NA
Overall							$4.65x10^{-3}$ Total	$2.90x10^{-6}$ Average	$2.10x10^{4}$ Total	NA	NA
Alternative 2 - Require PZR Bubble											
PORV	15/244 (=0.061)	0.087*	<600	100	$<2.0x10^{-4}$	$1.64x10^{-6}$	$1.06x10^{-6}$	$1.10x10^{-9}$	4.8	2800	$1.33x10^{4}$
RHR	5/56 (=0.089)	0.143*	<600	100	$<1.0x10^{-4}$	$1.79x10^{-6}$	$1.27x10^{-6}$	$2.82x10^{-9}$	5.7	1340	$7.55x10^{3}$
PORV+N2	<0.018*	0.087*	850	5*	$2.0x10^{-4}$	$1.55x10^{-8}$					
			<600	95*	$<1.0x10^{-5}$	$<1.48x10^{-8}$	$3.03x10^{-8}$	$1.66x10^{-10}$	0.136	1.0	0.0
Overall							$2.36x10^{-6}$ Total	$1.47x10^{-9}$ Average	10.6 Total	1980 Overall	$2.09x10^{4}$ Overall

continued

Table 2. Continued.

Plant Category	Challenge Frequency (yr^{-1})	Unavail.	Overpressurization Spectrum psi	Overpressurization Spectrum %	NIVFP(1) Value by Pressure	VFP Contribution by Pressure	Category Total VFP(2)	Category Average VFP per Plant, per Year(3)	Public Risk(4) (p-rem)	Factor of Improvement Over Base Case(5)	Reduction of Public Risk(6) (p-rem)
Alternative 3 - 2 OMS Channels Required Operable When Water Solid											
PORV	0.094*	$(2/23)^2$	2500	9*	3.79	2.43×10^{-4}					
		(=0.0076)	1400	9*	.19	1.22×10^{-5}					
			850	13*	3.7×10^{-3}	3.43×10^{-7}					
			<600	69*	$<2.0\times10^{-4}$	$<9.83\times10^{-8}$	2.56×10^{-4}	2.64×10^{-7}	1.15×10^{3}	11.5	1.22×10^{4}
RHR	0.125*	$(1/7)^2$	2500	14*	.68	2.43×10^{-4}					
		(=0.0204)	850	14*	9.0×10^{-4}	3.21×10^{-7}					
			<600	72*	$<1.0\times10^{-4}$	$<1.84\times10^{-7}$	2.44×10^{-4}	5.40×10^{-7}	1.10×10^{3}	7.0	6.46×10^{3}
PORV+N2	<0.018*	0.087	850	5*	2.0×10^{-4}	1.55×10^{-8}					
			<600	95*	$<1.0\times10^{-5}$	$<1.48\times10^{-8}$	3.03×10^{-8}	1.66×10^{-10}	0.136	1.0	0.0
Overall							5.00×10^{-4} Total	3.12×10^{-7} Average	2.25×10^{3} Total	9.3 Overall	1.87×10^{4} Overall
Alternative 4 - Remove Power from SI Pumps When Water Solid											
PORV	20/244	0.087*	2500	5	3.79	1.35×10^{-3}					
	(=0.082)		1400	10	.19	1.35×10^{-4}					
			850	15	3.7×10^{-3}	3.96×10^{-6}					
			<600	70	$<2.0\times10^{-4}$	$<1.00\times10^{-6}$	1.49×10^{-3}	1.54×10^{-6}	6.71×10^{3}	2.0	6.59×10^{3}
RHR	6/56	0.143*	2500	17	.68	1.77×10^{-3}					
	(=0.107)		850	17	9.0×10^{-4}	2.43×10^{-6}					
			<600	66	$<1.0\times10^{-4}$	$<1.01\times10^{-6}$	1.70×10^{-3}	3.76×10^{-6}	7.65×10^{3}	1.0	0.0
PORV+N2	<0.018*	0.087*	850	5*	2.0×10^{-4}	1.55×10^{-8}					
			<600	95*	$<1.0\times10^{-5}$	$<1.48\times10^{-8}$	$<3.03\times10^{-8}$	$<1.66\times10^{-10}$	0.136	1.0	0.0
Overall							3.19×10^{-3}	1.99×10^{-6}	1.44×10^{4}	1.5	6.59×10^{3}

Table 2. Continued.

Plant Category	Challenge Frequency (yr^{-1})	Unavail.	Overpressurization Spectrum psi	%	NIVFP(1) Value by Pressure	VFP Contribution by Pressure	Category Total VFP(2)	Category Average VFP per Plant, per Year(3)	Public Risk(4) (p-rem)	Factor of Improvement Over Base Case(5)	Reduction of Public Risk(6) (p-rem)
Alternative 5 - Prohibit RC Pump Operation When Water Solid											
PORV	14/244	0.087*	2500	14	3.79	$2.65x10^{-3}$					
	(=0.057)		850	21	$3.7x10^{-3}$	$3.88x10^{-6}$					
			<600	65	$<2.0x10^{-4}$	$<6.49x10^{-7}$	$2.65x10^{-3}$	$2.73x10^{-6}$	$1.19x10^{4}$	1.1	$1.40x10^{3}$
RHR	4/56	0.143*	2500	25	.68	$1.73x10^{-3}$					
	(=0.071)		850	25	$9.0x10^{-4}$	$2.30x10^{-6}$					
			<600	50	$<1.0x10^{-4}$	$<5.10x10^{-7}$	$1.70x10^{-3}$	$3.76x10^{-6}$	$7.65x10^{3}$	1.0	0.0
PORV+N2	<0.018*	0.087*	850	5*	$2.0x10^{-4}$	$1.55x10^{-8}$					
			<600	95*	$<1.0x10^{-5}$	$<1.48x10^{-8}$	$3.03x10^{-8}$	$1.66x10^{-10}$	0.136	1.0	0.0
Overall							$4.38x10^{-3}$ Total	$2.73x10^{-6}$ Average	$1.97x10^{4}$ Total	1.06 Overall	$1.40x10^{3}$ Overall
Alternative 6 - Increase RHR Autoisolation Setpoint Above SRV Setpoint											
PORV	0.094*	0.087*	2500	9	3.79	$2.79x10^{-3}$					
			850	9	$3.7x10^{-3}$	$2.72x10^{-6}$					
			<600	82	$<2.0x10^{-4}$	$<1.34x10^{-6}$	$2.79x10^{-3}$	$2.88x10^{-6}$	$1.26x10^{4}$	1.1	700
RHR	0.125*	0.143*	2500	14	.68	$1.70x10^{-3}$					
			850	14	$9.0x10^{-4}$	$2.25x10^{-6}$					
			<600	72	$<1.0x10^{-4}$	$<1.29x10^{-6}$	$1.70x10^{-3}$	$3.76x10^{-6}$	$7.65x10^{3}$	1.0	0.0
PORV+N2	<0.018*	0.087*	850	5	$2.0x10^{-4}$	$1.55x10^{-8}$					
			<600	95	$<1.0x10^{-5}$	$<1.48x10^{-8}$	$3.03x10^{-8}$	$1.66x10^{-10}$	0.136	1.0	0.0
Overall							$4.5x10^{-3}$ Total	$2.81x10^{-6}$ Average	$2.02x10^{4}$ Total	1.04 Overall	700 Overall

continued

Table 2. Continued.

Plant Category	Challenge Frequency (yr^{-1})	Unavail.	Overpressurization Spectrum psi	%	NIVFP[1] Value by Pressure	VFP Contribution by Pressure	Category Total VFP[2]	Category Average VFP per Plant, per Year[3]	Public Risk[4] (p-rem)	Factor of Improvement Over Base Case[5]	Reduction of Public Risk[6] (p-rem)
Alternative 7 - Require Safety Grade PORVs and RHR SRVs											
PORV	0.094*	0.035	2500	9*	3.79	1.12×10^{-3}					
			1400	9*	.19	5.63×10^{-5}					
			850	13*	3.7×10^{-3}	1.58×10^{-6}					
			<600	69*	$<2.0\times10^{-4}$	$<4.54\times10^{-7}$	1.18×10^{-3}	1.22×10^{-6}	5.31×10^{3}	2.5	7.99×10^{3}
RHR	0.125*	0.143*	2500	14*	.68	1.70×10^{-3}					
			850	14*	9.0×10^{-4}	2.25×10^{-6}					
			<600	72*	$<1.0\times10^{-4}$	$<1.29\times10^{-6}$	1.70×10^{-3}	3.76×10^{-6}	7.65×10^{3}	1.0	0.0
PORV+N2	<0.018*	0.087*	850	5*	2.0×10^{-4}	1.55×10^{-8}					
			<600	95*	$<1.0\times10^{-5}$	$<1.48\times10^{-8}$	3.03×10^{-8}	1.66×10^{-10}	0.136	1.0	0.0
Overall							2.88×10^{-3} Total	1.80×10^{-6} Average	1.30×10^{4} Total	1.62 Overall	8.00×10^{3} Overall

* Same as base case, Alternative 1.

NA Not Applicable.

(1) Normalized, integrated vessel fracture probability assumes one pressurization per year to this pressure for each plant, summed from 1986 to EOL.

(2) Total, integrated vessel fracture probability summed from 1986 to EOL, assuming constant overpressurization frequency and spectrum for each plant, during all years.

(3) Reactor years from 1986 to EOL by plant category are: PORV, 969; RHR, 452, and PORV+N2, 183. Total reactor years are 1604.

(4) Core melt is assumed synonymous with reactor vessel fracture, yielding an integrated radiation dose of 4.5E+06 man-rem over 30 years when the containment is assumed open 50% of the time.

(5) Ratio of total VFP or total risk for the base case divided by total VFP or total risk for the alternative.

(6) Difference between risk for the base case and for the alternative.

the table). Public risk is likewise summed for the categories. An overall factor of improvement over the base case is calculated by dividing the base case overall total integrated VFP value or public risk value by the corresponding value for the alternative. The overall reduction of public risk is also presented for each alternative.

A review of column 10 of Table 2 shows that Alternatives 2 and 3 would reduce the public risk by factors of roughly 2000 and 10, respectively. The remaining alternatives would reduce public risk by less than a factor of 2.

The large reduction of risk estimated for Alternative 2 results from the greatly reduced rate of pressurization resulting when a bubble is maintained in the pressurizer (as opposed to water-solid operations). With a pressurizer bubble, the pressures achieved during the three-minute delay assumed in the analysis before operators terminate the transient are considerably lower than for water-solid operation.

Although the risk reduction factor estimated for Alternative 3 is smaller than for Alternative 2, Alternative 3 would nevertheless yield a reduction of 92%. This reduction results from eliminating the present technical specification action statement allowing one train of the OMS to be out of service for up to seven days, which has effectively reduced the OMS to a single-train system from a safety analysis perspective (all three overpressurization events in the data base used to calculate system unavailability occurred with one train out of service for maintenance).

REFERENCES

1. T. V. Vo, B. F. Gore, A. J. Colburn, E. J. Eschbach, and E. Throm, Value-Impact Analysis of Low Temperature Overpressure Reduction Alternatives, in Proceedings of the 1988 Annual Meeting of the Society for Risk Analysis, McLean, VA, October 30 - November 2, 1988.
2. U.S. Nuclear Regulatory Commission (NRC), Task Action Plans for Generic Activities (Category A), NUREG-0371, Washington, DC (1978).
3. U.S. Nuclear Regulatory Commission (NRC), Operating Reactors Licensing Action Summary, NUREG-0748, Washington, DC (1984).
4. U.S. Nuclear Regulatory Commission (NRC), Standard Review Plan for the Review of Safety Analysis Reports for Nuclear Power Plants, NUREG-0800, Section 5.2.2, Overpressure Protection, Washington, DC (1981).
5. U.S. Nuclear Regulatory Commission (NRC), Licensee Event Report Compilation, NUREG-2000, Washington, DC (1980 with addenda through 1986).
6. D. L. Phung, Pressure Vessel Thermal Shock at U.S. Pressurized Water Reactors: Events and Precursors, 1963 - 1981, NUREG/CR-2789, U.S. Nuclear Regulatory Commission, Washington, DC (1983).
7. W. D. Lanning, Low Temperature Overpressure Events at Turkey Point Unit 4, AEOD Case Study, U.S. Nuclear Regulatory Commission, Washington, DC (1984).
8. C. J. Hsu, K. Perkins, and R. Youngblood, Estimation of Risk Reduction from Improved PORV Reliability in PWRs, NUREG/CR-4999, Brookhaven National Laboratory, Upton, NY (1987).
9. F. A. Simonen and K. I. Johnson, VISA-II—A Computer Code for Predicting the Probability of Reactor Pressure Vessel Failures, NUREG/CR-4486, U.S. Nuclear Regulatory Commission, Washington, DC (1986).
10. U.S. Nuclear Regulatory Commission (NRC), Effects of Residual Elements in Predicting Radiation Damage to Reactor Vessel Materials, Regulatory Guide 1.99, Revision 2, Washington, DC (1988).

An Analysis of the Structure of Chemical Accidents in the U.S. for Local Emergency Response Planning

James Cummings-Saxton, Marc Benoff, and Amy J. Barad
Industrial Economics, Inc.
Cambridge, MA

Samuel J. Ratick
Clark University
Worcester, MA

Frederick W. Talcott
U.S. Environmental Protection Agency
Washington, DC

ABSTRACT

This paper presents the results of a comprehensive analysis of over 11,000 accidents involving toxic chemicals in the United States from 1980 to 1986. This analysis is accomplished using the Acute Hazardous Events Data Base (AHE/DB) which was developed by the authors under sponsorship of the U.S. Environmental Protection Agency to provide supportive information for community emergency response planning activities. Each accident coded into the data base is characterized according to whether: the accident occurred at a fixed facility or in-transit; the type of facility at which the accident occurred; the causes and contributing circumstances of the release; the resultant end effects of the accident; among others. Special attention is paid to the more serious events, including over 1000 events that led to more than 300 deaths and 11,000 injuries, and slightly less than 900 events that resulted in the evacuation of approximately one-half million people. The paper also provides a discussion of how this information is being used to help set priorities for local emergency response planning including the analysis of the types of releases associated with specific chemicals or groups of chemicals, and the nature of releases at specific types of facilities, such as production, distribution, and storage facilities.

KEYWORDS: Chemical spills, accidental releases, acute hazardous events, emergency response planning

THE DEVELOPMENT OF THE ACUTE HAZARDOUS EVENTS DATA BASE

Historical Context

Activities in the United States in response to the perceived growing potential for catastrophic chemical accidents have rapidly evolved in the aftermath of the tragic accident at Bhopal, India. The U.S. has passed broad and encompassing legislation related to local emergency response planning for chemical accidents. The legislation is designed to prompt communities to gather pertinent information from organizations that produce, use, and store chemicals and to mandate the nationwide development of local emergency-response plans for dealing with acute chemical events. The U.S. Environmental Protection Agency (EPA) has been designated as a lead agency for this effort. The Acute Hazardous Events Data Base (AHE/DB) was developed for the U.S. EPA by the authors, with significant assistance from a number of other government and industry professionals, to provide a historical perspective on previous chemical accidents and to provide an analytical framework for evaluating information generated in the evolving emergency-response planning process.[1-3]

In the reauthorization of the Comprehensive Environmental Response, Compensation, and Liability Act (CERCLA) in October 1986 (enacted as Public Law 99-499 and called the Superfund Amendments and Reauthorization Act, SARA), EPA and other agencies were instructed to assist communities in their planning for response to chemical-related accidents. These provisions were contained in Title III of the law, designated as the Emergency Planning and Community Right-To-Know (CRTK) section. The CRTK provisions direct each state to organize a system of Local Emergency Planning Committees (LEPCs) to coordinate the local emergency-response efforts, and to establish a State Emergency Response Commission (SERC) to coordinate the efforts of all the LEPCs. The legislation also calls for a tiered reporting procedure for facilities that produce, store, or handle acutely toxic chemicals. These reporting procedures include requirements for such facilities to provide the LEPCs with Material Safety Data Sheets (MSDSs) and other chemical-related information for those chemicals appearing on a general list of chemicals issued by EPA, and to provide additional detailed information on specific chemicals upon request by the LEPCs.

The AHE/DB has been one component of EPA's ongoing effort to support the nationwide emergency-response planning effort. The initial AHE/DB, developed in 1985, contained 3,121 event records, which through data sampling represented 6,928 events.[2,3] Since 1985, the AHE/DB has been substantially expanded and adapted for use in support of Title I and Title III of SARA. The principal enhancements were to increase the number of records and to augment the AHE/DB with supportive data bases containing information on the chemicals and companies involved in the reported events.

Methodology

Because EPA's primary interest has been focused on events similar in some ways to the accident in Bhopal, several criteria were used to screen event data for inclusion in the AHE/DB. Emphasis was placed on incidents that had acute hazard potential, with incidents resulting in deaths, injuries, or evacuations given highest priority. Events that resulted in releases of hazardous chemicals were given priority, and those that released petroleum related and other miscellaneous substances were not included. Priority also was given to incidents involving air releases of chemicals. Events releasing large quantities of chemicals were given priority, while events involving releases of less than one pound of material were not included.

The methodology employed in the development of the AHE/DB has been to convert available information from a large number of different kinds of accidental releases into a form convenient for summary and analysis. We found that no one data source was sufficiently comprehensive either in its breadth or its depth to supply the overall perspective on accidental releases in the U.S. Thus, we adopted the approach of: (1) accessing large numbers of records from several different kinds of data sources; (2) screening out irrelevant or duplicate records; (3) taking a sample of certain categories of records; and (4) coding the information into a computerized data base. The coding process involves the organization and characterization of the descriptive information contained in the original sources into a consistent set of categories that enable the generation of summary statistics and cross-tabulations.

Because the AHE/DB is comprised of data that are taken from many different contributing sources and restructured into a single consistent format, comment sections are used in the coding form to maintain information that does not fit the coding scheme, thereby preventing the loss of important unique accident information. The comment information is usually a verbatim transcription of the text included in the record of the contributing source, and this is often quite terse. In other cases, the coders entered precis of more extensive records. The original 1985 coding format was re-organized and expanded during development of the 1988 version of the AHE/DB. The choice of new categories that were added and the re-coding of the existing data from the original AHE/DB were made possible by reviewing data contained in the comment fields.

Current Status

The 1988 version of the AHE/DB contains 6,305 records, which through sampling represent 11,048 separate chemical accidents. These data come from 41 sources. National sources include the National Response Center (7,555 events), United Press International and Associated Press (286 events), and DOT's Hazardous Materials Information System (171 events). Other sources include EPA's Region 7 (510 events), 26 daily newspapers (340 events), and six offices of five state governments (1,855 events). AHE/DB records encompass the period from before 1980 to 1987. However, the major data gathering effort focused on the five-year period from 1982 to 1986. The AHE/DB contains an average of 2,100 events per year for that period, ranging from 1,515 events for 1982 to 2,638 events for 1984.

In addition to the coded information on reported chemical accidents, two additional data bases have been developed to augment the accident information by detailing attributes of the facilities at which these accidents have occurred and the properties of the chemicals involved.

The Company/Facility (COMFAC) Data Base contains information on facilities involved in the AHE/DB events. This information includes: facility name, address, unique hierarchical identifier containing the three-digit zip code for the facility and an indication of any parent/subsidiary relationships, and four-digit Standard Industrial Classification (SIC) for that facility. All facilities in COMFAC were classified into one of five categories: primary producers (facilities that produce chemicals); secondary producers (facilities that use the chemicals to produce another product); distributors; end users; and waste-related activities.

The Chemical (CHEM) Data Base contains information on the chemicals involved in the events in the AHE/DB. This information includes: chemical name, Chemical Abstracts Service (CAS) number, four-digit SIC of the originating industry, commodity or specialty chemical designation, and production characteristics. In addition, CHEM contains chemical property information such as: toxicity data, including "Immediately Dangerous to Life and Health" (IDLH) concentrations; physical characteristics, including vapor pressure, boiling point, melting point, and air half-life estimates; and hazard ranking information, including National Fire Protection Association reactivity and flammability rankings. CHEM also identifies whether or not the chemical is listed under RCRA, CERCLA, or SARA (Titles 302 and 313).

Figure 1 graphically displays the representative sources of information accessed in developing the AHE/DB and its ancillary data bases, COMFAC and CHEM.

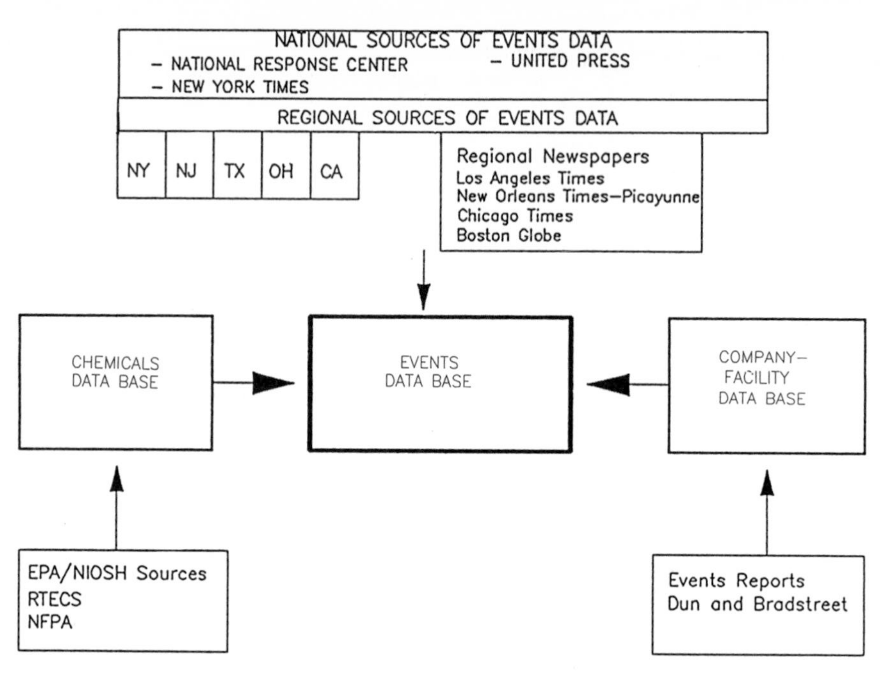

Fig. 1. AHE/DB system's three interconnecting data bases.

SUMMARY ANALYSIS OF THE MORE SEVERE EVENTS

Each of the original records coded into the data base was examined for indications of human casualties. In most cases, the record unambiguously indicated whether or not the event led to deaths or injuries. Altogether, injuries were reported in 9.2 percent of the events, and fatalities in 1.1 percent of the events. Another 8.4 percent of the records indicated injuries as unknown, and 6.0 percent of the records listed deaths as unknown. Although some other records in the data base may represent events that involved injuries or deaths, it was not possible to estimate the degree of under-reporting without follow-up on event reports.

Limitations of the Data

Some cautions are necessary in interpreting the reported casualty data:

- *Reported Deaths or Injuries:* Only a few of the events in this study have been independently verified, either by EPA or its contractors. Thus, one should interpret these data as "deaths or injuries reported by one or more of the contributing sources."

- *Causation:* Direct evidence of causation rarely exists in the contributing sources of these records. Some of the deaths or injuries reported to have occurred in association with a particular event may not, in fact, have been caused by the event. For example, some casualties may have been caused by a triggering accident that released a substance into the environment (e.g., injuries to a truck driver which were caused by a collision and not the succeeding exposure to released materials.) Whenever possible, deaths explicitly resulting from a collision were removed from the data base. However, it is not possible to identify how many of the deaths and injuries remaining in the data base fall within this type of situation.

- *Range of Severity:* Although some records indicate in detail the type and severity of the reported injuries, most records do not. To categorize the severity of injuries for these records where possible, we coded whether or not the injured parties were hospitalized. This then served as a surrogate for injury severity. While this categorization provides some resolution of the question of severity, it should be noted that not all data sources provided information on hospitalizations and not all hospitalizations are necessarily serious. Thus, even in the case of hospitalizations an individual "injury" could range from temporary respiratory or eye irritation treated on-site to critical injury leading to prolonged hospital treatment.

- *Numbers:* Some of the source records provide counts of injuries that suggested precision, whereas others (explicitly or implicitly) were approximate counts. If the source provided a number, it was recorded, but sometimes it was necessary to translate phrases such as "about 50" into specific numbers. Thus, the accuracy of the individual records composing the data base is highly variable.

Although there is understandable interest in making nationwide estimates of deaths and injuries, the study was not designed with that purpose in mind. Rather, the objective was to understand better the nature, causes, and effects of accidental releases.

Summary Results

Altogether, 309 deaths and 11,341 injuries are reported in the AHE/DB. Among the 6,567 injuries whose severity could be estimated, 1,587 injuries required hospitalization. Fire and explosion played a larger relative role among the subset of events involving deaths and/or injuries (D/I) than in the general type of event. In fact, fire/explosion was reported as the cause of nearly one-fifth of the D/I events, but of only five percent of all events. Equipment failure, in contrast, was the reported cause of less than one-third of the D/I events, but of nearly one-half of all events. Operator error was reported as the accident cause with equal frequency among D/I events and all events—approximately one-fifth of each.

Transportation related incidents play a slightly larger role in death/injury events than they do in all events — 37 percent versus 29 percent. Among in-transit events, truck transport represents a significantly increased share (66 percent versus 49 percent) and rail transport a decreased share (28 percent versus 44 percent) for events resulting in deaths/injuries as compared to all in-transit events.

Industry sectors were identified for the responsible parties in 84 percent of the 1,045 events reporting deaths and/or injuries by assigning 4-digit Standard Industrial Classification (SIC) codes. Sources for assigning SIC codes included the Dun & Bradstreet Reference Book and identifying information in the event records. Five industry groups were classified: *Primary Producers*, including Chemical and Allied Products and Petroleum Refining and Allied Products (SICs 28 and 29); *Secondary Producers*, including all other manufacturing sectors (SICs 20 to 39, except 28 and 29); *Distributors*, those firms involved in transporting, storing, and distributing chemical products (SICs 40 to 47, 50 to 51); *End Users*, including residential and commercial users (SICs 01 to 17, 48, 49 except 495, and 52 to 99); and *Waste Disposal* (SIC 495).

Events involving fatalities occur most frequently at primary producers. These facilities account for 39 percent of reported events involving death. End-users and secondary producers rank second and third in responsibility for fatalities, accounting for 18 percent and 15 percent of the death events, respectively. When the broader class of severe events, i.e., D/I events, is considered, however, distributors are found to account for the largest share, representing 31 percent of the total. Primary producers rank second in responsibility for D/I events, accounting for 26 percent of such events.

Primary producers again rank first with regard to number of injuries — 3,377 injuries occur at such facilities, representing 30 percent of the total. Distributors rise to the second rank when injuries are considered, accounting for 25 percent, and secondary producers account for 17 percent. End users and waste disposers account for 9 percent and less than 1 percent of the injuries, respectively. Eighteen percent occur at facilities of unknown type.

Evacuations occurred in 855 of the total 11,048 events in the AHE/DB. Half of the remaining events did not have associated evacuations, and for an almost equal number of events it was not known whether an evacuation took place. The 29 media sources (26 newspapers, 2 wire services, and 1 trade journal) contributed 54 percent of the total number of evacuation records. In the 419 events for which the number of evacuees was identified, the total number of people evacuated was 464,677.

Injuries were associated with 40 percent of the evacuation events compared to only 9 percent of all events. Deaths were associated with 5 percent of the evacuation events compared to 1 percent of all events. For some of the evacuation events it was possible to distinguish between workers and non-workers evacuated. Of the 335,323 people evacuated in those events, 308,183 (92 percent) were residents and 27,140 (8 percent) were workers.

Distributors and primary producers account for the majority of evacuations. End users and secondary producers account for the next largest shares. Compared to their frequency of involvement in all events, distributors and end users have a higher frequency and primary producers a lower frequency of involvement in evacuation events. The rates for secondary producers and waste related are the same for all events and evacuation events.

CONCLUSIONS

The type of information contained in the AHE/DB and its ancillary data bases provides a historical context for assessing the accidental release potential of specific chemicals and/or types of facilities. The following tasks are representative of the type of emergency planning activities that the AHE/DB can support:

- for certain chemicals, a sufficiently large number of events are included in the AHE/DB that the overall modes of behavior of the type discussed in the preceding section can be assessed for the specific chemical;
- the general nature of releases can be assessed for the different types of facilities — severity, frequency, location, type of chemical, etc.;
- the behavior of similar types of chemicals can be assessed, with the nature of the similarity being defined by the user, e.g., in terms of toxicity, storage configuration, or other characteristics; and
- states or regions can assess behavior in their areas vis-a-vis that of similar chemicals in similar facilities in other states or regions (or the overall national pattern), and thereby place in perspective the nature and frequency of the events reported to them; this perspective can include adjusting for the relative level of chemical and manufacturing activity in that state or region and then seeing how their statistics compare to others similarly adjusted — such analysis may shed light on performance at the plant level and/or on the reporting system.

All analysis of this type and that discussed in the preceding section will increase in robustness as additional data are entered into the AHE/DB.

REFERENCES

1. J. Cummings-Saxton *et al.*, Accidental Chemical Releases and Local Emergency Response: Analysis Using the Acute Hazardous Events Data Base, *Industrial Crisis Quarterly* **2**:1 (1988).
2. J. Cummings-Saxton, S. J. Ratick, and F. W. Talcott, The Structure of Accidental Releases in the U.S.: The Acute Hazardous Events Data Base, Boston University, *The Bulletin of the Center for Energy and Environment* **3**:1 (1987).
3. Industrial Economics, Acute Hazardous Events Data Base, Report to the U.S. Environmental Protection Agency (1989).

Evaluation of a Risk-Bounding Approach for Setting Environmental Priorities

Thomas H. Walker
Industrial Economics, Inc.
Cambridge, MA

Ellen Tohn
Jellinek, Schwartz, Connolly, and Freshman, Inc.
Washington, DC

ABSTRACT

This paper explains how comparative risk analysis can help decision makers set environmental management priorities. We believe that "screening level" techniques, based on readily available data and methods, can characterize the relative magnitude of the health risks and economic damages posed by environmental problems. This hypothesis was recently tested as part of the EPA's Environmental Strategies Project in Denver, Colorado. The problems analyzed for metro-Denver included indoor and outdoor air pollutants, drinking water quality, releases from hazardous waste management sites, surface water pollution, and exposures to lead in the environment. We used risk as a common denominator to evaluate problems with dissimilar characteristics. The results helped local decision makers identify problems deserving priority attention. Given the current levels of public and private dollars that are spent on environmental protection, we believe that conducting comparative risk analysis to set priorities may be a wise use of public funds.

KEYWORDS: Environmental priorities, Denver Environmental Strategies Project (ESP), risk bounding, hazardous waste

INTRODUCTION

Today local environmental priority setting is more important than ever before. Over the past several decades we have made major strides in reducing environmental pollution through the implementation of such federal statutes as the Clean Water Act, the Clean Air Act, and the Resource Conservation and Recovery Act. The environmental problems that remain are different in nature than the problems that justified the passage of such federal legislation. Today's environmental problems vary more widely among localities and are often difficult to observe (i.e., ground-water contamination from toxics at levels that we could not even detect a decade ago). Environmental priorities are no longer obvious. This paper describes our effort to use risk information to help local decision makers in Denver, Colorado identify their top environmental priorities.

Risk Analysis, Edited by C. Zervos
Plenum Press, New York, 1991

BACKGROUND ON THE DENVER ENVIRONMENTAL STRATEGIES PROJECT

During the 1980's, the Environmental Protection Agency's (EPA's) Office of Policy Analysis undertook a series of comparative risk projects. The purpose of these projects was to help decision makers direct their limited resources towards problems where the greatest improvements in public health and environmental quality could be achieved. One comparative risk project was carried out at the national level—EPA's 1987 "Unfinished Business: Comparative Risk Assessment of Environmental Problems"—while four other projects were completed at the local level. The Denver Environmental Strategies Project (ESP) was the last of the local comparative risk projects.

The Denver ESP began in 1986 and is now nearing its conclusion. Fundamental to the project was the development of a "risk-bounding" methodology. The development and implementation of this methodology laid the foundation for priority setting. The risk-bounding analysis took approximately one year to complete.

A second integral aspect of the project was the formation of an ESP advisory committee composed of local environmental officials, representatives of businesses, and representatives of environmental groups. The committee was divided into five workgroups to evaluate the following twelve environmental problems:

1. airborne particulate matter;
2. ozone;
3. air toxics;
4. indoor radon;
5. environmental tobacco smoke;
6. environmental lead (e.g., lead in drinking water, lead paint, and lead-bearing dust);
7. drinking water toxics;
8. active municipal landfills;
9. underground storage tanks;
10. active hazardous waste treatment, storage, and disposal facilities;
11. Superfund sites; and
12. surface water contamination.

The committee and its workgroups reviewed the proposed risk-bounding methodology, evaluated the results of the risk-based analysis of individual environmental problems, and interpreted the results of the comparative risk conclusions suggested by the risk-bounding to set their own environmental priorities. Table 1 provides a list of the possible health effects associated with each of the twelve problems.

DENVER RISK-BOUNDING METHODOLOGY

Overview

A primary goal of the Denver ESP risk-based analyses was to generate estimates of the range of potential human health risk associated with local environmental problems and to make these estimates available to members of the ESP Advisory Committee in the early stages of the project. Because of the limited resources available to conduct these assessments, we were forced to rely exclusively on previously developed assessment methods and on existing data.

The risk-based analyses that were conducted for the ESP are substantially different in scope and emphasis from risk assessments designed to support regulatory development and from analyses performed to evaluate the risks at an individual Superfund site. In general, they are significantly less detailed, do not focus on the development of "best" estimates of actual or expected risks, and have not been peer reviewed to the extent required for many EPA efforts.

For the majority of environmental problems, the data we relied on were not adequate to support an analysis of the most likely levels of adverse effects. To perform such an assessment would have required detailed information on the probability distributions of those factors with the greatest influence on environmental risks and damages. While such information could be developed, this was far beyond the budget and time frame for the study. The available information, however, was adequate to support an analysis of upper and lower bounds on the hazards attributable to the majority of the environmental problems under consideration. For this reason, the relatively simple goal of trying to distinguish problems based on comparisons of upper and lower bounds was selected as the method most likely to yield useful risk and damage information to the ESP Advisory Committee members. We refer to this method as "risk bounding."

Under the risk-bounding approach we estimated upper and lower bounds on the health and, where possible, economic effects, for the twelve environmental issues identified above. These estimates were designed to be conservative (i.e., most experts would agree that the actual hazards are likely to fall somewhere between the upper and lower bounds). By comparing the upper bound for each problem with the lower bounds for the others, we hoped to identify those problems that, under almost any reasonable conditions, could be said to pose greater risk than others.[a]

Analytic Methods

Four types of analytic approaches, tailored to make the best use of available data, were selected to support the risk-bounding effort.[b]

First, whenever data were available to support such an approach, we applied EPA approved health risk assessment methods to monitored pollutant concentrations in metro-Denver in order to estimate potential risks.[c] Under this heading were the analyses of indoor radon (ESP, 1987), Superfund sites (IEc, 1988b), air toxics (Versar, 1987), and drinking water toxics including lead (Woodward-Clyde, 1988; Hagler Bailly, 1988). For all four of these environmental problems, recent Denver area monitoring data were available, as were EPA approved cancer potency factors or Reference Doses for non-carcinogens.

Second, the analyses of health effects attributable to airborne particulates and ozone relied on recently completed epidemiological studies relating adverse health effects to air pollution concentrations (Hagler Bailly, 1988). Application of the epidemiological data to monitored pollutant concentrations in Denver yields estimates of the potential aggregate annual incidence of adverse health effects. Individual risks were calculated by dividing the potential aggregate incidence by estimates of the exposed population.

Third, the analyses of hazardous waste treatment facilities (TSDFs), underground storage tanks (USTs), and active municipal landfills are based on an evaluation of

---

a. For example, if the upper bound estimates for cancer cases attributable to Superfund sites is less than the lower bound estimate for lung cancers caused by radon exposures, we would be confident in concluding that radon is likely to pose the more serious cancer threat.

b. A careful reading of the background documents providing the details of the individual studies will reveal that in some cases the approaches cannot be categorized as cleanly as is done here. A certain amount of hybridization does occur where complete data are not available to fully implement the preferred approach. However, for purposes of this overview, the categories provide an indication of primary mode of analysis.

c. A full list of the issues covered and definitions of the measures of health and economic effects is included in Table 1.

Table 1. Human Health and Economic Damages Considered for Metro-Denver Environmental Problems

Problem	Effect	Description
OUTDOOR AIR POLLUTANTS		
Particulates	Health	o Fatalities. o Emergency room visits (ERV) to treat adverse health effects resulting from exposure to particulates. o Restricted activity days (RAD): days when human activities are restricted because of illness or adverse health effects attributable to particulates.
	Economic	o Materials damage: costs to households of cleaning and maintaining soiled materials. o Visibility losses: the dollar value that individuals place on improving visibility.
Ozone	Health	o Asthma: number of individual asthma attacks caused by exposure to ozone. o Respiratory restricted activity days (RRAD): days when human activities are restricted because of ozone-induced respiratory illness. o Eye irritation.
	Economic	o Materials damage: costs to tire manufacturers and tire retreading firms of using additives, preservatives and/or reformulations to prevent tire damage from ozone.
Air Toxics	Health	o A range of cancers resulting from exposure to volatile organics and metals (including benzene, chloroform, chromium and arsenic).
INDOOR AIR POLLUTANTS		
Radon	Health	o Lung cancer.
Passive Smoking	Health	o Lung cancer.
DRINKING WATER TOXICS	Health	o Cancers from exposure to metals and organics.
LEAD	Health	o Blood FEP: disruption of blood cell synthesis and function in adults and children. o Fetal: developmental effects to the fetus, such as growth retardation and neurological damage. o Reproductive: potential infertility in men. o Renal: kidney damage resulting in kidney dysfunction in adults. o Neurological: reduction in (1) learning ability in children, and (2) sensory and motor nerve function in adults. o Anemia in children. o Hypertension in men. o Hypertension in men leading to heart attack. o Death resulting from hypertension-induced heart attack in men.

Table 1. (Continued)

Problem	Effect	Description
HAZARDOUS WASTE AND MATERIALS		
Waste Treatment Facilities	Health	o Cancer (leukemia) from exposure to benzene-contaminated well water. o Non-cancer effects from exposure to lead-contaminated well water (see list of those effects under Lead Drinking Water problem).
Active Municipal Landfills	Health	o Cancers from exposure to solvents and metals in contaminated well water. o Lead-induced non-carcinogenic effects from exposure to contaminated well water (see list of these effects under Lead Drinking Water problem).
Underground Storage Tanks	Health	o Cancer (leukemia) from exposure to household air contaminated with benzene.
"Superfund" Sites	Health	o Lung cancer from exposure to radon-contaminated air, and a variety of other cancers from exposure to contaminated well water. o Non-carcinogenic effects from exposure to contaminated soil and well water.
SURFACE WATER QUALITY	Economic	o Lost recreational opportunities (LRO): the dollar value of recreation activities not occurring because of reduced surface water quality.

Source: See bibliography of references at end of this paper.

individual risks at representative facilities under hypothetical upper and lower bound risk scenarios (IEc, 1988a). These upper and lower bound scenarios were developed using local expert judgment about the range of environmental conditions likely to exist in the Denver area for the three types of facilities. Population risks were calculated by applying the individual risk estimates for the representative facility to estimates of the exposed population around each currently operating facility of that type in the study area.

Fourth, there are three analyses that do not fit well into either of the three categories discussed above. Our estimates of potential individual cancer risks from environmental tobacco smoke (ETS) are based on national estimates developed by EPA. The population risks were derived by multiplying national individual risks by estimates of the exposed population in metro-Denver (Repace, 1985). The analysis of the damages resulting from poor surface water quality is based on an economic assessment of the value of reduced recreational opportunities on major water bodies in metro-Denver (Hagler Bailly, 1987b). Estimates of risks posed by lead paint and dust were developed by scaling results from Baltimore based on demographic and housing age data for Denver.

Limitations

The risk-bounding methodology developed for the Denver ESP is subject to a variety of limitations that influence the interpretation and use of the results. In particular, the reader should be aware of four key issues.

First, the methodology generally does not yield results that are indicative of the most likely level of hazard posed by environmental pollutants. Upper bounds are only representative of extreme worst cases. While we are aware that these worst cases are unlikely to occur, their use allows us to draw fairly strong conclusions when the worst case for one problem poses a lesser hazard than the lower bound for another.

Recognition of this characteristic of the methodology is particularly important in reviewing the results of analyses based on the "representative" sites approach discussed above (e.g., USTs, TSDFs, active municipal landfills). In these analyses we selected facilities with fairly typical facility configurations and wastes. We then applied pessimistic environmental and exposure assumptions to generate the worst case risk estimates. In these scenarios, the resulting upper bound risk estimates are not indicative of the most likely level of risks for the existing facilities.

The impact of this first limitation is a tendency to reduce our ability to differentiate between environmental problems. In all likelihood, the estimated risk ranges are wider than is actually the case. A refined approach based on a more realistic range of risks might permit finer resolution in the ranking of environmental hazards.

A second important limitation of the risk bounding approach stems from our inability to analyze certain important hazards that could influence policy makers' overall ranking of the issues. For example, the comparisons discussed in this report do not take into account acute risks resulting from releases of toxics to air or groundwater. Recent events such as Bhopal have demonstrated that such releases can have catastrophic consequences, yet data and methods were not available to assess their potential impact in metro-Denver. For similar reasons, the analyses also do not consider degradation of aquatic and terrestrial ecosystems or the health impacts of carbon monoxide. Furthermore, we have not addressed the economic damages that might occur if remedial measures were taken to reduce the likelihood of adverse health effects. For example, if users of contaminated drinking water switched to bottled water or drilled new wells, they might incur substantial economic costs. For potential sources such as leaking underground storage tanks, such costs might be quite significant.

Overall, this second limitation implies that the reader should view the results of the comparative assessment as a starting point for evaluating the hazards posed by environmental problems in Denver. The initial hazard rankings suggested by the risk-bounding results should be adjusted qualitatively to take into account factors that could not be considered more rigorously in the analyses.

A third possible limitation of our approach relates to the techniques used to generate the lower bound risks for each problem. In general, lower bounds always assume that at least some exposure to toxic pollutants will take place and that exposure to pollutants at these low concentrations will result in some, usually very small, health risk. There are scenarios, however, were such exposure assumptions may still overstate the level of health risk. For example, considerable uncertainty exists about whether airborne particulates are actually the cause of adverse health effects observed in areas with high particulate levels. Uncertainty about the causal relationship implies that our lower bound might be too high.

The implication of this limitation is that for issues where the reader believes that the lower bounds are too high, he or she may wish to evaluate whether a lower risk estimate would change the ranking. We believe that this problem is of greatest concern for the analysis of particulates.

Finally, a fourth limitation derives from our inability to generate a range of potential risk for certain issues such as air toxics and environmental lead. For issues where worst case upper bounds could not be developed, "strong" relative risk conclusions generally cannot be drawn. If the reader has some qualitative sense of the range of risks for these issues, he or she might wish to reconsider the relative hazard ranking of these issues.

In summary, the major limitations of the comparative risk methodology suggest that conclusions about the relative hazards of environmental problems should be taken as an initial starting point rather than an answer to the question "what are metro-Denver's environmental priorities?" Policy makers should adjust the rankings developed from the analytic work conducted for the ESP to reflect their conclusions about the impact of the four limitations discussed above.

COMPARISON OF HUMAN HEALTH RISKS AND ECONOMIC DAMAGES

The comparison of the risks and damages caused by metro-Denver's environmental problems must account for fundamental difficulties inherent in comparing results from different studies. Foremost among these is that risks and damages were assessed using measures of harm that differ in both the type and severity of effects. Given the variety of potential health and economic effects, direct comparison of the number of adverse effects or the magnitude of individual effects may be misleading. For example, although ozone potentially causes a large number of cases of eye irritation relative to the number of premature deaths associated with airborne particulates, it is obviously inappropriate to conclude that ozone is a more severe environmental problem. Instead, both the type and severity of the effects should be considered in any ranking of issues.

In view of this problem, we limit our comparisons to issues that pose relatively similar types of hazards. This results in the following three general comparisons:

1. cancers and other fatal health effects,
2. non-fatal effects of non-carcinogens, and
3. economic damages.

Information about the timing of environmental risks and damages is also an important aspect of any comparisons among the issues. For example, in some cases releases of hazardous waste may not affect metro-Denver residents until far in the future while air pollution is likely to have a more immediate impact. While our results do not explicitly take into account timing, the implications of timing are addressed as part of our discussion of the relative severity of each issue.

Finally, in evaluating the severity of environmental problems, it is important to consider individual as well as aggregate population effects. In the past, numerous pollutants have been regulated because they posed relatively high risks to a small number of individuals, even though in aggregate they resulted in a relatively small number of adverse effects. A recent analysis of federal environmental rulemakings illustrates the importance accorded to individual risks. This study reviewed 132 recent regulatory decisions for which either individual or population risk information was available to decision makers. The authors concluded that even when aggregate impacts are small, agencies regulate when the lifetime risks to an individual are expected to exceed 1 in 1000 for serious adverse health effects such as cancer. Furthermore, these agencies often choose to regulate even when individual risks are at lower levels (Travis *et al.*, 1987). Because of the importance of individual risk, this report compares estimates of health and economic impacts to individuals as well as the total ("population") effects in metro-Denver.

Potential Cancer and Non-Cancer Effects Causing Premature Death

Population Impacts. The extent to which the total impacts of metro-Denver's environmental problems can be differentiated from one another is illustrated in Fig. 1, which graphically summarizes for each problem the range of human health risks posed by pollutants causing either (1) carcinogenic effects or (2) non-carcinogenic but fatal health effects. Examination of this figure indicates that radon, environmental tobacco smoke ("passive smoking") and particulates are likely to be the primary sources of cancer and fatal non-cancer effects. The total number of potential adverse health effects posed by each of these issues is substantially greater than the upper bound for risks from drinking water, the next largest potential source of aggregate adverse effects.

While the results indicate that radon, environmental tobacco smoke and particulates are associated with the greatest number of estimated cancer and fatal non-cancer health effects, a ranking of the other problems is more difficult because of the overlap in the risk ranges. However, two other groupings of issues are possible. The total incidence of potential adverse effects from exposure to lead, air toxics, and drinking water toxics are relatively similar. All are less risky than indoor air pollutants and particulates but generally more risky than the other issues plotted on the graph.

There is also some overlap between estimates for these three issues and the upper end of the risk ranges for Superfund sites and waste treatment facilities. However, the relatively low likelihood of worst cases for the two types of waste management facilities suggests that these issues are of lesser concern than air toxics and drinking water problems. In addition, the worst case risks for Superfund sites and waste management facilities are unlikely to occur until sometime in the future, while exposures to contaminated drinking water, air toxics and lead are happening now. Overall, the waste management activities (waste treatment facilities, Superfund sites, USTs and active municipal landfills) constitute a third group with ranges for total adverse health effects that are generally lower than those for the other two categories, and with health effects that are more likely to occur in the future than in the present.

Within each of the three groupings discussed above, overlap of the risk ranges makes further distinctions between the issues difficult. While some conclusions might be drawn based on the more probable outcomes, we believe such conclusions are not merited given the uncertainties in the analyses.

An important caveat to these conclusions relates to the potential for particulate-induced health effects. The epidemiological studies on which our estimates are based were conducted in cities that may differ significantly from Denver in terms of the size and composition of particulate matter. As a result there is considerable uncertainty as to whether the adverse health effects predicted by the particulates epidemiological model would actually occur in metro-Denver. Exposure to particulates might be a lesser public health problem than predicted by the analysis conducted for the Denver ESP.

Individual Effects. Comparison of the cancer and fatal non-cancer health effects illustrated in Fig. 1 indicates several important conclusions about individual risks. Under worst case assumptions, each of Denver's major environmental problems could result in lifetime individual risks in excess of 1 in 10,000. As indicated in the review of federal regulatory decisions cited above, risks at these levels often have formed the basis for decisions to further reduce environmental releases.

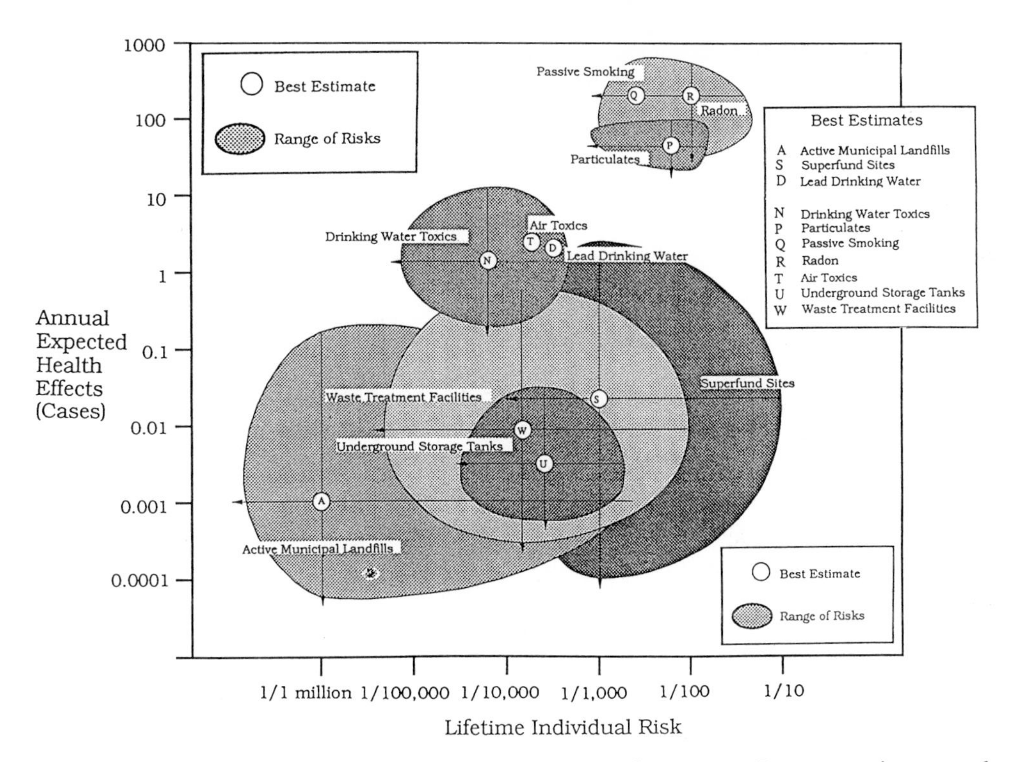

Fig. 1. Cancer and fatal non-cancer health risks from metro-Denver environmental problems.

Our analysis also suggests, however, that individual risks are likely to be considerably higher for certain problems than for others. The likely lower bounds on individual risks for radon, environmental tobacco smoke and particulates are greater than the upper bounds on the risks for drinking water and overlap only slightly with the upper bounds for active municipal landfills and underground storage tanks. In addition, these individual risks are higher than those for possible premature deaths caused by lead exposures. As a result, we are reasonably confident that indoor air pollutants (radon, environmental tobacco smoke) and particulates pose greater individual risks than these other sources of environmental contamination.

Much less can be said about the individual risks for waste treatment facilities and Superfund sites. The range of potential individual risks for these types of sites is very broad. Furthermore, there is considerable uncertainty about when these risks would be likely to occur. In some cases, exposures might only take place in the future. Thus, while individual risks as high as those for radon and particulates are possible, so are risks as low as the lowest individual risks expected for any issue. More precise estimates of the individual risks that are likely to result from exposures near these types of sites were impossible to determine using the data and methods available for the background analyses.

The high degree of uncertainty in the risk estimates for Superfund sites and waste treatment facilities complicates the relative ranking for issues other than particulates and indoor air pollutants. Highly risk averse regulators might consider the environmental problems with the highest worst case risks to pose the most severe problems, regardless of the timing of these risks. However, little is currently known about the probability or timing of these worst case risks. On the other hand, rankings based on more probable outcomes are suspect due to the lack of precision in these estimates. Given these uncertainties, we conclude that little can be said about the ranking of cancer and fatal non-cancer individual risks other than that indoor air and particulate risks appear generally higher than those caused by the other issues.

As in the case of the aggregate risks, the most important caveat to these results relates to the risks posed by particulates. Individual risks for particulates may be overstated by the epidemiological model used in the ESP analyses. While it is fair to conclude that individual risks potentially might be high, there is significantly more uncertainty about this conclusion than there is for the other high individual risk issues.

OTHER NON-CANCER HEALTH EFFECTS AND ECONOMIC DAMAGES

In addition to cancer and fatal non-cancer health effects, we also considered a variety of other health and economic impacts. For the health effects analysis we considered both population and individual health effects from exposure to environmental lead (lead in drinking water, lead paint, lead dust), particulate matter and ozone. In terms of both population and individual effects, environmental lead poses the greatest risks. This conclusion weighs both the magnitude and severity of the health effects. For example, while exposure to ozone and particulates results in a very large number of adverse health effects, these effects we judged to be less severe, (e.g., eye irritation from exposure to ozone) than the types of health effects caused by exposure to lead paint and dust (e.g., neurological damage).

The economic effects considered included materials damage and visibility reductions associated with ambient levels of particulate matter and ozone and reduced recreational opportunities due to surface water contamination. For both aggregate and individual economic impacts, it was difficult to differentiate between the three issues because of overlap in the estimates. However, if damages from visibility reductions and materials damages caused by particulates are added together, it is reasonable to conclude that air pollution imposes greater damages than those due to reduced surface water recreational opportunities.

CONCLUSIONS

To assess the usefulness of the risk bounding methodology developed for the Denver ESP study, we evaluated three questions.

1. *Is risk bounding an effective technique for differentiating among environmental problems?*

   A review of the Denver risk bounding results suggests three interesting insights about when the application of this methodology will be most fruitful. First, the risk bounding approach did provide useful insights when applied to aggregate effects. For example, the risk of lung cancer attributable to radon and environmental tobacco smoke both appears to be substantially greater even in the lower bound scenarios, than the risk associated with issues such as hazardous waste management. These differences are largely attributable to the substantial variation in the size of the potentially exposed population for each issue. Because large differences in the size of the potentially exposed population are quite common, we believe the risk-bounding methodology developed for this study can yield interesting insights with respect to the total number of health effects caused by various environmental problems.

Second, risk bounding was not particularly useful for differentiating among issues based on individual risks. Estimates of individual risks are highly site specific and for virtually all the environmental problems analyzed can range over many orders of magnitude. As a result, considerable overlap almost always exists between the ranges for different issues making it virtually impossible to categorically conclude that one issue poses greater individual risks than another. Since these conditions are likely to be representative of individual risks for most environmental problems, we believe the risk-bounding method is generally less useful for distinguishing among environmental problems based on an analysis of upper and lower bounds of individual risks.

Third, we are unable to draw any strong conclusions about the usefulness of the method for comparing economic effects of environmental pollution. Our metro-Denver work included economic analysis of only three problems—materials damage and visibility reduction due to air pollution and lost recreational opportunities resulting from poor surface water quality. While the differences between the surface water economic losses and the combined air pollution losses appear significant, we do not believe the analysis of such a small number of issues is adequate for drawing any conclusions about the overall utility of the methodology.

2. *Can risk bounding help local decisionmakers set environmental priorities?*

In Denver, the results of the risk bounding analysis helped local decision makers identify several major environmental issues that were not receiving adequate attention given the relative magnitude of their potential impacts. By highlighting the importance of lead, radon, environmental tobacco smoke, and particulate matter, the study elevated these issues relative to other issues that were previously considered to be the predominant threats to public health and the environment (e.g., hazardous waste sites and carbon monoxide). ESP advisory committee members are currently discussing how these results should change their environmental priorities in Denver.

3. *Is risk bounding a cost-effective approach for evaluating local environmental priorities?*

The development and implementation of the Denver risk bounding methodology cost approximately $250,000 and took roughly one year to complete. The cost of the study appears relatively modest when compared to the benefits derived from identifying several key environmental problems that are not being adequately addressed by ongoing regulatory efforts. For example, in the case of radon, if the study ultimately results in actions that reduce the estimated 200 annual lung cancers by as little as one case, the study will have paid for itself many times over. Considering the additional reductions in health and economic effects that could result from increasing the priority given to radon, lead, environmental tobacco smoke, and particulates, implementation of the risk-bounding approach appears to be a highly cost effective investment of local environmental planning resources.

REFERENCES/BIBLIOGRAPHY

Studies prepared for the Environmental Strategies Project for Metro-Denver:

Hagler, Bailly, and Co., 1988, Ambient Particulate Matter and Ozone Benefit Analysis for Denver, draft report prepared for Environmental Strategies Project for Metro-Denver, U.S. Environmental Protection Agency.

Hagler, Bailly and Co., 1987a, The Health Effects Associated with Lead in Gasoline and Drinking Water in Metro-Denver, draft report prepared for Environmental Strategies Project for Metro-Denver, U.S. Environmental Protection Agency.
Hagler, Bailly and Co., 1987b, Recreation Benefits from Water Quality Improvements in Metro-Denver: Background Analysis, draft report prepared for Environmental Strategies Project for Metro-Denver, U.S. Environmental Protection Agency.
Industrial Economics, Incorporated, 1988a, Potential Human Health Risks and Economic Damages from Management of Non-Superfund Wastes in Metro-Denver, draft report prepared for Environmental Strategies Project for Metro-Denver, U.S. Environmental Protection Agency.
Industrial Economics, Incorporated, 1988b, Potential Human Health Risks and Natural Resource Damages from Metro-Denver 'Superfund' Sites, draft Report prepared for Environmental Strategies Project for Metro-Denver, U.S. Environmental Protection Agency.
Travis *et al.*, 1987, Cancer Risk Management: A Review of 132 Federal Regulatory Decisions, *Environmental Science and Technology* **21(5)**.
U.S. Environmental Protection Agency, Environmental Strategies Project for Metro-Denver (ESP), 1987a, Summary Table of Indoor Air Risks, draft report.
U.S. Environmental Protection Agency, Environmental Strategies Project for Metro-Denver (ESP), 1987b, Summary of Indoor Radon Issues and Risk Results, draft report.
Versar, Inc., 1987, Denver Risk Analysis for Toxic Air Pollutants, draft report prepared for Environmental Strategies Project for Metro-Denver, U.S. Environmental Protection Agency.
Woodward-Clyde Consultants, 1988, Screening Level Risk Assessment of Four Drinking Water Systems in Metro-Denver, draft report prepared for Environmental Strategies Project for Metro-Denver, U.S. Environmental Protection Agency.

Other References

Applied Decision Analysis (ADA), 1987, A Site Ranking Panel Evaluation of the Relative Risks Posed by Twenty Superfund Sites.
Holguin, A. H., *et al.*, 1985, The Effects of Ozone on Asthmatics in the Houston Area, in AI(Evaluation of the Scientific Basis for Ozone/Oxidants Standards), Si Duk Lee, ed., Transactions of an APCA International Specialty Conference, Houston, Texas, Air Pollution Control Association, Pittsburgh, PA.
Levin, R., 1987, Reducing Lead in Drinking Water: A Benefit Analysis, Revised Draft Final Report, U.S. Environmental Protection Agency, EPA-230-09-86-019, Washington, DC.
Manuel, E. H., R. L. Horst, K. M. Brennan, W. N. Laven, M. C. Duff, and J. K. Tapiero, 1982, Benefits Analysis of Alternate Secondary National Ambient Air Quality Standards for Sulfur Dioxide and Total Suspended Particulates, Final Report to the U.S. EPA Office of Air Quality Planning and Standards Research Triangle Park, NC.
Ostro, B. D., March 1987, Air Pollution and Morbidity Revisited: A Specification Test, *Journal of Environmental Economics and Management.*
Ozkaynak, H., and G. Thurston, 1987, Association Between 1980 U.S. Mortality Rates and Alternative Measures of Airborne Particle Concentration, *Risk Analysis* **7**:449-461.
Portney, P. R., and J. Mullahy, 1986, Urban Air Quality and Acute Respiratory Illness, *Journal of Urban Economics* **20**:21-38.
Repace, J. L., and A. H. Lowrey, 1985, A Quantitative Analysis of Lung Cancer Risks from Passive Smoking, *Environment International* **II**:3-22.
Rowe, R. D., L. G. Chestnut, D. P. Peterson, C. Miller, R. M. Adams, W. R. Oliver, and H. Hogo, 1986, The Benefits of Air Pollution Control in California, Report to California Air Resources Board by Energy and Resource Consultants, Inc., Boulder, CO.
Samet, J. M., Y. Bishop, F. E. Speizer, J. D. Spengler, and B. G. Ferris, 1981, The Relationship Bewtween Our Pollution and Emergency Room Visits in An Industrial Community, *Journal of the Air Pollution Control Association* **31**:236-40.

Schwartz, J., H. Pitcher, R. Levin, B. Ostro, and A. Nichols, 1985, Costs and Benefits of Reducing Lead in Gasoline: Final Regulatory Impact Analysis, U.S. EPA, Office of Policy Analysis.
Stankunas, A. R., F. H. Haynie, and D. Rae, 1982, Economic Analysis of Oxidant Damage to Rubber Tires, unpublished.
U.S. Environmental Protection Agency, 1979, Protecting Visibility: An EPA Report to Congress, EPA-450/5-79-008, Office of Air Quality Planning and Standards Research, Triangle Park, NC.
U.S. Environmental Protection Agency, Criteria for Particulate Matter and Sulfur Oxides, EPA-600/8-82-029a, Research Triangle Park, NC.
U.S. Environmental Protection Agency, 1983, Air Quality Criteria for Ozone and Other Photochemical Oxidants, Office of Research and Development.
U.S. Environmental Protection Agency, 1984, Regulatory Impact Analysis on the National Ambient Air Quality Standards for Particulate Matter, Research Triangle Park, NC.
Whittemore, A. S., and E. L. Korn, 1980, Asthma and Air Pollution in the Los Angeles Area, *American Journal of Public Health* **70**:687-696.

Other Reading Material

Bureau of Economic Analysis, 1988, Gross State Product by Industry, 1963-86, Survey of Current Business.
The Conservation Foundation, Groundwater Protection, Washington, DC.
The Conservation Foundation, 1987, State-By-State Environmental Data Summaries.
Development Planning and Research Associates, Inc. (DPRA), 1985, Biennial Report Summary.
Legislative Commission on Toxic Substances and Hazardous Wastes, 1987, Hazardous Waste Facility Siting: A National Survey.
Management Associates, Inc., 1986, Siting Hazardous Waste Facilities.
Outlook for Hazardous Waste Facilities: A Nationwide Perspective, 1985-1988, *The Hazardous Waste Consultant*, March/April.
RCRA Permitting Staff, 1988, Regions 2, 3, 4, 5, 6, 7, 10, Personal Communication, August.
Society of Industrial and Office Realtors, 1988 Guide to Industrial and Office Real Estate Markets, Washington, DC.
U.S. Advisory Commission of Intergovernmental Relations (ACIR), 1987, Significant Features of Fiscal Federalism, December.
U.S. Department of Commerce, 1986, Bureau of the Census, State and Metropolitan Area Data Book, Washington, DC.
U.S. Department of Commerce, 1988, Bureau of the Census, Statistical Abstract of the United States, Washington, DC.
U.S. Environmental Protection Agency, 1986, EPA Survey of Treatment, Storage, Disposal, and Recycling Facilities.
U.S. Environmental Protection Agency, 1988, Hazardous Waste Data Management System (HWDMS).
U.S. Environmental Protection Agency, Office of Emergency and Remedial Response, 1988, National Priorities List.
U.S. Environmental Protection Agency, 1985, Robert S. Kerr Environmental Research Laboratory, DRASTIC: A Standardized System for Evaluating Ground Water Pollution Potential Using Hydrogeologic Settings.
U.S. Government Accounting Office, 1988, Hazardous Waste: Future Availability of and Need for Treatment Capacity Are Unknown.

Impact of Aging on Availability and Spares

R. W. Hockenbury and R. F. Kirchner
Rensselaer Polytechnic Institute
Troy, NY

J. K. Rothert, R. J. Schmidt, and F. O. Cietek
Northeast Utilities Service Co.
Hartford, CT

ABSTRACT

The effects of time-dependent, increasing (aging) failure rates on component and system availability and reliability are presented. There are significant implications of aging for component design, materials selection, application, in-service inspection and maintenance. The prediction of reliability and availability has always been challenging due to uncertainties in the data. Vesely and others have now demonstrated that in many cases, failure rates can increase with time. This time dependence varies with system environment and maintenance practices. In this paper, the primary objective is to predict system availability and the spare component inventory, recognizing that component failure rates should not be accepted as constant. The components of concern are major in size and cost (i.e. large pumps, motors). Only catastrophic failures are considered, or those requiring essentially complete replacement. Thus, if no spare is available, serious losses in plant operational time will occur. Calculations have been done for single components and typical system configurations including constant and time-dependent failure rates, with and without spare components. Significant changes in the predicted availability and likelihood for needing spares are seen. These differences occur at both early and later times due to the basic difference in the calculation of failure rates when the aging fraction is taken into account.

KEYWORDS: Aging, hazard function, spares, availability, risk

INTRODUCTION: RELIABILITY AND AVAILABILITY

Catastrophic failures of large, costly components in plants used for power generation or chemical processing can result in excessive downtimes. Usually this type of component is not readily available from the manufacturer and must be purchased, constructed and delivered to the buyer. Alternatively, the purchase of spare components can be considered on a cost-benefit basis. Such considerations then involve component failure rate, Mean-Time-To-Failures (MTTF), Mean-Time-To-Install (MTTI) and Mean-Time-To-Deliver (MTTD). Component reliability and availability, and system reliability and availability have to be evaluated to compare the benefits of increased availability vs. the costs of stocking spare components. These costs involve several financial factors such as capital costs, present worth factors, storage and other details relevant to company policy. This paper focuses on the reliability and availability aspects of the spare component question. The comparison between spare-no spare availability can be expressed in terms of Megawatt-hours (MWH), or the dollar cost of replacement power or the change in risk for power generation plants. For other installations, availability can be equated to production efficiency or other terms.

This paper focuses on the reliability and availability aspects of the spare component question. The component failure rate and the effect of aging, in particular, are studied.

BASIC RELIABILITY THEORY

The probability density function for times-to-failure, $f(t)$, is

$$f(t) = z(t) \exp\left[-\int_o^t z(t')dt'\right] \tag{1}$$

where $z(t)$ is the hazard function. When $z(t)$ is constant and equal to λ, the times-to-failure are said to be exponentially distributed. That is, $f(t)$ is:

$$f(t) = \lambda \exp\left[-\lambda t\right] . \tag{2}$$

The reliability, $R(t)$ is then:

$$R(t) = \exp\left[-\lambda t\right] . \tag{3}$$

The MTTF is the inverse of the failure rate:

$$\mathrm{MTTF} = 1/\lambda . \tag{4}$$

The component availability A can be written:

$$A = \frac{\mathrm{MTTF}}{\mathrm{MTTF} + \mathrm{MTTR}} , \tag{5}$$

where the Mean-Time-To-Restore (MTTR) is used rather than specifically indicating the presence of a spare at this point.

A system may be capable of operating in several states corresponding to, for example, 100% capacity, partial capacity and zero capacity. The equivalent availability (EA) is defined as the sum over all states of the product of state availability A_i times state capacity C_i.

$$EA = \sum_{i=1}^{n} A_i C_i , \tag{6}$$

where a total of n states are assumed.

Thus EA is the capacity in each state weighted by the probability of being in that state. For reliable systems, partial capacity states are less likely than the 100% capacity state. This weighted capacity can be used as a figure of merit to measure power generation increases or losses in terms of Megawatt hours (MWH) or their dollar equivalent.

The Weibull probability density function for times-to-failure may be considered when the hazard function is not constant. For example, the failure rate may be decreasing in a "break-in" period or increasing with time due to aging effects. The hazard function $z(t)$ corresponding to the Weibull distribution is:

$$z(t) = \frac{\beta}{\alpha}\left(\frac{t}{\alpha}\right)^{\beta-1} . \tag{7}$$

The Weibull probability density function is:

$$f(t) = \frac{\beta}{\alpha}\left(\frac{t}{\alpha}\right)^{\beta-1} \exp\left[-\left(\frac{t}{\alpha}\right)^{\beta}\right] . \tag{8}$$

For this case, the reliability $R(t)$ is:

$$R(t) = \exp\left[-\left(\frac{t}{\alpha}\right)^{\beta}\right] . \tag{9}$$

The first moment of the Weibull can be found by integration:

$$\text{Mean} = \int_o^\infty t' f(t') dt' , \tag{10}$$

or for later reference in this paper:

$$\text{Mean} = \int_o^\infty R(t') dt' , \tag{11}$$

Substituting for the Weibull form in either Eq. (10) or Eq. (11), the mean is found to be:

$$\text{Mean} = \alpha\Gamma\left(\frac{\beta+1}{\beta}\right) . \tag{12}$$

The change in reliability P_{us} from year $(n-1)$ to year (n) is:

$$P_{us} = R(n-1) - R(n) . \tag{13}$$

The reliability $R(t)$ is complementary to the cumulative probability distribution $p(t)$:

$$p(t) = \int_o^t f(t') dt' = 1 - R(t) . \tag{14}$$

Thus P_{us} can be expressed as

$$P_{us} = p(n) - p(n-1) . \tag{15}$$

Green and Bourne[1] interpret the right-hand side of Eq. (15) as the limiting ratio of variate values (times-to-failure, in this case) in year $(n-1)$ to year (n) to the total number of all possible variate values. Thus P_{us} is the probability of surviving to year (n-1) and failing in the following year.

Until recently, most analyses led to constant hazard rates and exponentially distributed times-to-failure as in Eq. (2) above.

AGING EFFECT AND RELIABILITY ANALYSIS

Extensive date analysis programs by Meale and Satterwhite,[2,3] and Subudhi *et al.*[4] have determined that significant aging effects are observed in certain components in nuclear power plant systems. Aging failure modes include wearout, vibration, corrosion and other phenomena which shorten the expected life of a component.

Vesely Linear Aging Failure Rate Model

Vesely[5] has developed a linear aging failure rate model and illustrated the effects of aging on component and system unavailability. In the work by Vesely and in the present paper, it is assumed that the degradation effects of aging are not corrected during maintenance. Thus the hazard rate increases with time. Simultaneous failure modes generally exist consisting of random failure and aging modes. The constant failure rate is denoted by λ_0 while the hazard rate due to the time dependent aging effect is symbolized by $\lambda(t)$.

In this paper, the term failure rate will be used to refer to situations where the hazard rate is constant [$z(t) = \lambda$]. Hazard rate or hazard function will refer to a time-dependent process as defined by Green and Bourne[1] and others.

In Vesely's notation, the overall hazard rate λ_T is:

$$\lambda_T = \lambda_o + \lambda_1(t) + \lambda_2(t) + \ldots \quad , \tag{16}$$

where several aging hazard functions [$\lambda_i(t)$] are allowed. Vesely derives a linear model for $\lambda_i(t)$ assuming that the degradation effects follow a Poisson process and that the deterioration accumulates in an independent fashion. For a constant portion and one aging mode, Vesely shows that:

$$\lambda(t) = at \qquad a = \text{aging rate}$$
$$t = \text{time} \tag{17}$$

The aging rate (a) is found by Vesely from the fraction of failures due to aging, f_A, the average age, T_A, over which the failures occur and the fraction of failures due to random causes, ($1-f_A$). The aging rate is shown to be:

$$a = \frac{f_A \, \lambda_o}{1 - f_A \, T_A} \quad . \tag{18}$$

Examples of the aging fractions found by Meale and Satterwhite[2] are given in Table 1. This table illustrates the variation of aging fraction vs. system type. Also shown are the 95% confidence intervals for these aging fractions. The differences in aging fractions, for the components listed, result from differences in the conditions of each application such as water chemistry, temperature and frequency of use.

Identifying the hazard function $z(t)$ with λ_T in Eq. 17 and using the general relationship:

$$R(t) = \exp\left[-\int_o^t z(t')dt'\right] \quad . \tag{19}$$

Substituting and integrating:

$$R(t) = \exp\left[-\int_o^t \left(\lambda_o + at'\right)dt'\right] \quad . \tag{20}$$

Table 1. Aging Fraction vs. System[2]
Uncertainty Study: Statistical System Dependence Related to Aging

Component	Aging Fraction	95% Confidence Interval	Systems
Instrumentation-Switch	0.06	(0.04, 0.10)	RHR,HPIS
	0.20	(0.17, 0.23)	SWS,RPS,1E
Instrumentation-Transmitter	0.55	(0.49, 0.60)	RPS,MFW
	0.03	(0.02, 0.05)	AFW,HPIS,RHR
Pump	0.60	(0.55, 0.65)	SBL,CCW,1E,SWS
	0.31	(0.26, 0.37)	MFW,RHR,HPIS,AFW
Supports	0.37	(0.21, 0.56)	HPIS
	0.12	(0.07, 0.18)	MFW,RHR
Valve	0.54	(0.52, 0.57)	1E,SWS,MFW,AFW
	0.37	(0.34, 0.41)	RHR,CCW,HPIS,SBL

The reliability $R(t)$ for the hazard function in Eq. (17) is then:

$$R(t) = \exp\left[-\left(\lambda_o t + \frac{at^2}{2}\right)\right] . \tag{21}$$

and the cumulative probability of failure by time t, $F(t)$, is:

$$F(t) = 1 - \exp\left[-\left(\lambda_o t + \frac{at^2}{2}\right)\right] . \tag{22}$$

Thus, reliability predictions can be made, based on experience, for similar applications.

An Alternate Approach

An alternate method for predicting reliability parameters has been proposed recently.[6,7] Based on the observations from the extensive data analyses cited above and Vesely's aging models, it appears that the use of Nelson's[8] Weibull analysis technique may contribute to the data analysis.

The conditions relating to the consideration of Nelson's method are:

a. zero or a small number of failures
b. evidence of a time-varying failure rate (aging)
c. justification for a choice of a shape parameter of the Weibull distribution
d. multiply censored data.

All of the above conditions apply to the problem at hand, namely, to predict the reliability and likelihood for requiring spare components.

The shape parameter β in Eq. (7) is assumed to be known from experience or from other information. In any case, sensitivity tests can be made later. For a linear aging model, the shape parameter β is equal to 2. For random failure (constant failure rate), β is of course equal to unity.

The scale parameter α is estimated by Nelson:

$$a = \left[\frac{\sum_{i-1}^{n} T_i^{\beta}}{r} \right]^{\frac{1}{\beta}} , \tag{23}$$

where

r = number of failures, i==1, ...n

T_i = times-in-service and times-to-failure.

For zero or r failures, the lower $C\%$ confidence limit is:

$$\underset{\sim}{\alpha} = \hat{\alpha} \left[\frac{2r}{\chi^2(C; 2r+2)} \right]^{\frac{1}{\beta}} \text{ for } r \geq 1 , \tag{24}$$

or

$$\underset{\sim}{\alpha} = \alpha \left[\frac{2\sum_{i-1}^{n} T_i^{\beta}}{\chi^2(C; 2r+2)} \right]^{\frac{1}{\beta}} \text{ for } r \geq 0 , \tag{25}$$

where χ^2 (C; $2r$ + 2) is the Cth percentile of the chi-square distribution with ($2r$ + 2) degrees of freedom.

The data in Table 2 have been used for illustrative purposes to estimate the scale parameter α. Table 2 shows one aging failure, one random failure and three times-in-service. The aging failure is to be regarded as censoring of random failure data and vice versa. Taking β as one for the random failure, r = 1, the 5%, 50%, and 95% estimates are obtained. For β equal to unity, the inverse of alpha (50%) is the constant λ_o (see Eq. (7)):

$$\lambda_o = 2.71 \times 10(-6) \text{ per hour} . \tag{26}$$

Similarly, assuming beta is two corresponding to the linear aging model, alpha estimates are obtained. With beta equal to two, the hazard function Eq. (7) becomes:

$$(t) = \frac{2t}{\alpha^2} = 4.01t \times 10(-11) \text{ per } (\text{hour})^2 , \tag{27}$$

where the 50% confidence alpha value has been used. Combining Eqs. (26) and (27), the total is then:

$$z_T(t) = \lambda_o + \frac{2t}{\alpha^2} . \tag{28}$$

Finally, treating both failures as random and calculating the resulting constant failure rate λ_C in Table 2:

$$\lambda_C = 4.34 \times 10(-6) \text{ per hour} . \tag{29}$$

Table 2. Failure Data Analysis
WEIBULL PARAMETERS

Random Failures	Aging Failures
BETA= 1	BETA= 2
ALPHA-L=129787.1	ALPHA-L=132407.7
ALPHA-M=368766.4	ALPHA-M=223189.2
ALPHA-H=1734760.	ALPHA-H=484080.2
HAZARD FUNCT. = 2.71E-06	HAZARD FUNCT.=4.01 T E-11

Weibull Parameters Constant Failure Rate

All Failures
BETA= 1
ALPHA-L=97830.0
ALPHA-M=230651.6
ALPHA-H=751024.3
HAZARD FUNCT. = 4.34E-06

This failure rate will be used for comparison purposes later.

Next, integrating $z_T(t)$ in Eq. 28:

$$\int_o^t z_t(t')dt' = \lambda_o t + \frac{t^2}{\alpha^2} \ , \tag{30}$$

and the reliability $R(t)$ is:

$$R(t) = \exp\left[-\left(\lambda_o t + \frac{t^2}{\alpha^2}\right)\right] \ . \tag{31}$$

The estimates of alpha at various confidence levels can be used in Eq. 31 to find corresponding estimates of the reliability.

Note that beta and alpha can be updated as additional data become available accommodating changes in beta, if warranted.

For the availability and equivalent availability calculations in the present work, the Mean-Time-To (first)—Failure is used since we are concerned with catastrophic, non-repairable failures. The Mean-Time-To-Failure is found from:

$$\text{MTTF} = \int_o^\infty R(t')dt' \ . \tag{32}$$

Substituting from Eq. 30, we find:

$$\mathrm{MTTF} = \left[\alpha \exp\left(\frac{\lambda_o^2 \alpha^2}{4} \right) \right] \int_{\frac{\lambda_o \alpha}{2}}^{\infty} \exp\left(-y^2\right) dy \ , \tag{33}$$

and alternately:

$$\mathrm{MTTF} = \left[\frac{\sqrt{\Pi}\alpha}{2} \exp\left(\frac{\lambda_o^2 \alpha^2}{4} \right) \right] \left[1 - 2 \int_o^{\frac{\lambda_o \alpha}{\sqrt{2}}} \frac{e - \frac{t^2}{2}}{\sqrt{2\Pi}} dt \right] . \tag{34}$$

APPLICATIONS

The methods in the preceding section have been implemented mainly in the form from Nelson's approach, Eq. 26 through 34. The sample data in Table 2 have been used for the basic parameters. The following have been calculated:

a. Component reliability
b. System reliability for a two-of-three logic configuration
c. System reliability for a three-of-three logic configuration
d. P_{us} for each system in (b) and (c)
e. Component availability and equivalent availability
f. System equivalent availability for (b) and (c)

All calculations were carried out for both the constant failure rate in Eq. 29 and the time-dependent case in Eq. 30.

Figure 1 shows component reliability for the constant failure rate (Eq. (29)) and the time-dependent case (Eq. (31)) over a twenty-year period. For the time-dependent case, three curves are shown corresponding to the three values of alpha in Table 2. Note that the constant rate overestimates the reliability (for the 50% estimate of alpha in Eq. 31) after about nine years for these particular values.

In Fig. 2, the system reliability for both the constant and time-dependent situations is shown for both system configurations. The crossover in reliability is seen in both systems. Also, more visible in this figure, is seen the higher reliability for small values of time for the time-dependent case. This is present in Fig. 1 as well but more difficult to see.

The quantity P_{us} is shown in Fig. 3 for the two-of-three system. The time-dependent case predicts higher values of Pus with the maximum occurring later in time than for the constant rate. The three-of-three system exhibits a different behavior as seen in Fig. 4.

The component availability (repeating Eq. 5) for the two conditions of spare-no spare is:

$$A = \frac{\mathrm{MTTF}}{\mathrm{MTTF} + \mathrm{MTTR}} \ ,$$

where now the values of MTTF are taken from Eq. 4 for the constant rate and from Eq. (33) or Eq. (34) for the time-dependent case. The MTTR is selected as MTTI if a spare is assumed to be onsite and as (MTTI + MTTD) if no spare is onsite. Values of MTTI equal to 36 hours and MTTD of 1344 hours were assumed.

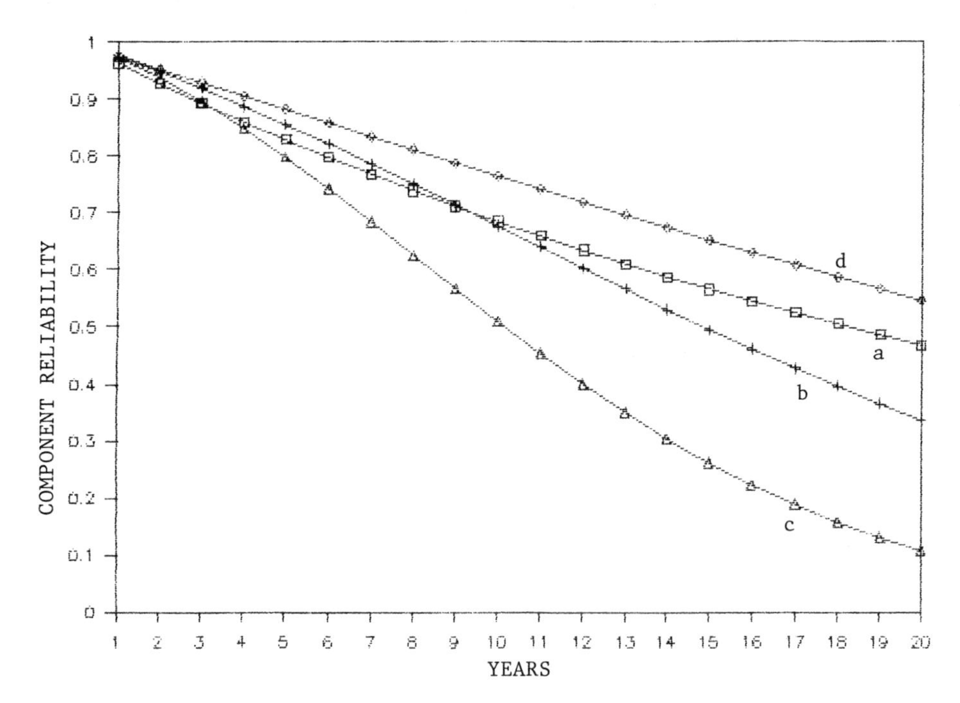

Fig. 1. Component reliability vs. time for (a) constant failure rate, (b) alpha-50%, (c) alpha-5%, (d) alpha-95% time-dependent cases. (See Table 2).

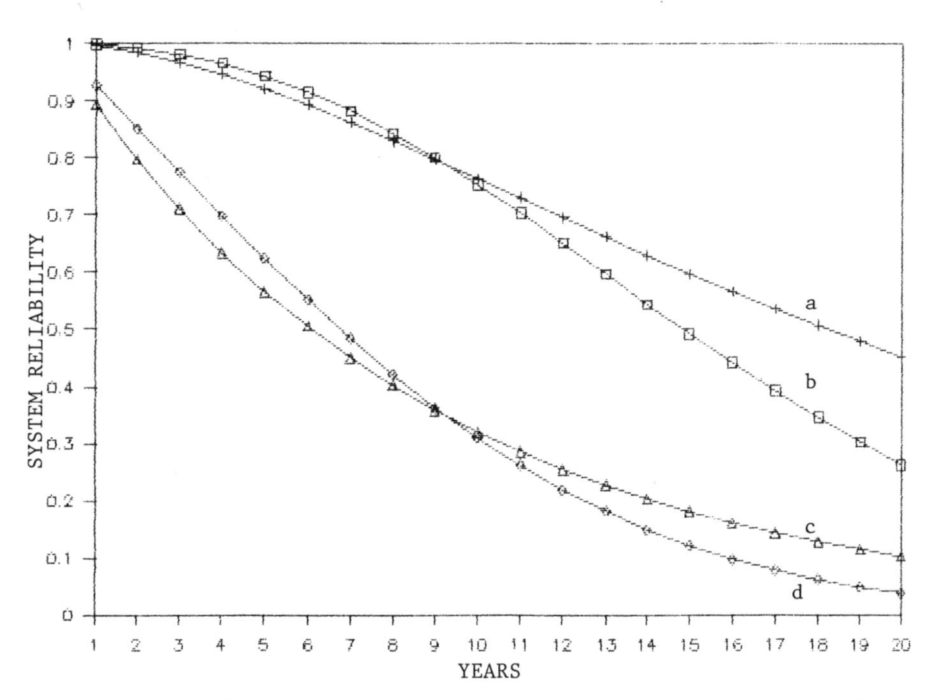

Fig. 2. Reliability for two-of-three system (a) constant failure rate, (b) time-dependent case and three-of-three system, (c) constant failure rate and (d) time-dependent case.

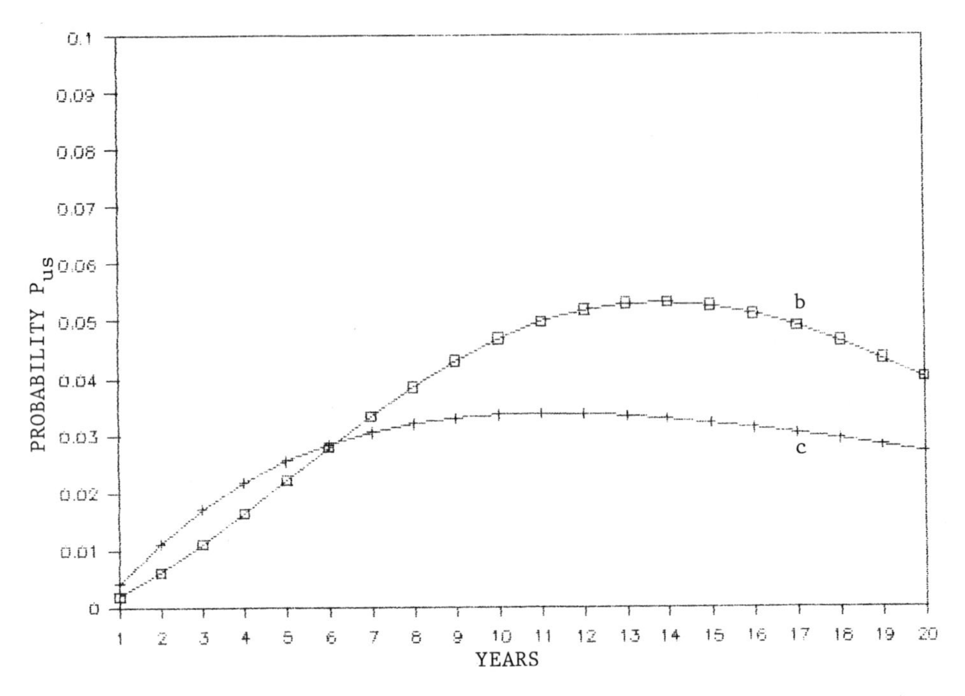

Fig. 3. Probability P_{us} for two-of-three system for (a) constant failure rate and (b) time-dependent case.

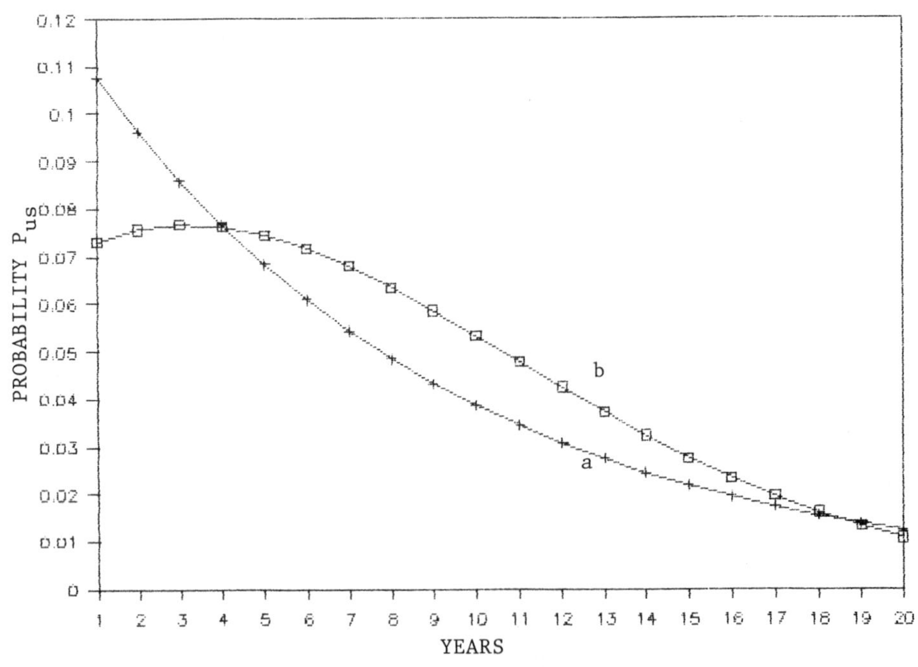

Fig. 4. Probability P_{us} for three-of-three system for (a) constant failure rate and (b) time-dependent case.

Table 3 contains the results of the component availability calculations for the spare-no spare conditions. As expected, the availability is lower when the time-dependent (aging) rate is used. The presence of a spare onsite, of course, increases the availability as seen in columns 3 and 4.

The equivalent availability was calculated for the two-of-three and three-of-three systems for the spare-no spare assumptions. The equivalent availability, from Eq. 6, for the two-of-three system is:

$$EA = A^3 + 3A^2 (1-A) + 3(0.5) A (1-A)^2 \tag{35}$$

In Eq. (35), the coefficient 0.50 refers to the capacity of the system state in which only one component is functioning. The other working states have capacities of 1.0. For the three-of-three system:

$$EA = A^3 + 3(0.66)A^2 (1-A) + 3(0.33) A (1-A)^2 \tag{36}$$

where the coefficients 0.66 and 0.33 refer to the capacities of the states with two and one working components, respectively. (Different component capacities were used for the systems.) Using the component availabilities in Eq. 35 and 36, the results for the spare-no spare conditions are given in Table 4.

OBSERVATIONS AND CONCLUSIONS

The approaches to the calculation of the overall hazard function by Vesely and by the Nelson method can be compared. The features of Vesely's model include:

a. Direct use of the aging fraction obtained by Meale and Satterwhite[2] to find the random (constant) failure rate from existing data bases and the aging rate (a).

b. Adjustment of (a) to the appropriate average age of the components and to the application environment of interest.

c. Extendable to nonlinear and dependent aging mechanisms.

The characteristics of the Nelson approach are:

a. The choice of beta, the shape parameter, must be determined from analysis of basic failure date or, as in the present case, from the same source, Meale and Satterwhite.[2]

b. The determination of beta is also based on identification of the root causes of failure, if one starts from the raw data.

c. The statistics or uncertainty in the estimates of the hazard function are incorporated into the analysis through the calculation of alpha.

The choice of approach might depend on the resources at hand or on time restrictions. Further experience with both methods will be helpful.

Comparisons of the equivalent availability (*EA*) for the two system configurations were made including the factors of:

a. Constant failure rate (4.34 × 10(–6) per hour, Table 2) vs. that derived from the time-dependent (aging) hazard function in Eqs. 28 and 31. See Table 2 also.

b. Spare vs. no spare present onsite.

Table 3. Results of the Component Availability Calculations for the Spare-No Spare Conditions

Parameters

Mean-Time-To-Install = 36 hours
Mean-Time-To-Deliver = 1344 hours
Time-Dependent MTTF = 144955 hours
Constant Rate MTTF = 230415 hours

Component Availability

Constant No Spare	Time-dep. No Spare	Constant With Spare	Time-dep. With Spare
0.9940046	0.990570	0.999844	0.999752

Table 4. System Equivalent Availability

	No Spare		With Spare	
	Constant	Time-dep.	Constant	Time-dep.
Two-of-Three System	0.999947	0.9998670	0.9999999	0.9999999
Three-of-Three System	0.993928	0.990384	0.999841	0.999747

c. Megawatt hours (MWH) generated and dollar equivalents.

d. Sensitivity to failure rate.

The changes in equivalent availability, MWH and dollars-equivalent vs. factors (a), (b), and (d) may be considered measures of risk. The sensitivity to failure rate is of value for assessing the priority of data collection and evaluation programs.

Detailed cost-benefit calculations involve capital costs, interest charges, storage charges, present worth and other details specific to the company. It is of interest to make some estimate or indication of the gain in equivalent availability related to spares and to the sensitivity to failure rate. In order to do this, the following equation was used, realizing that it is an arbitrary approach, which however can be modified by others to better suit their applications:

$$\text{Dollar-equivalent} = [dEA]\,[MW]\,[HRS]\,[C] \tag{37}$$

where

dEA = gain in EA due to spare
MW = peak power 1000 Megawatts assumed
HRS = number of hours assumed, for 20 years here
C = an industry-overall "guess" of $30/MWH for the cost of replacement power.

Table 5. Increase in Equivalent Availability With Spare
(Dollar-Equivalent in Millions)

	Two-of-Three		Three-of-Three	
	Constant	Time-dep.	Constant	Time-dep.
Alpha-5%	\$0.25M	\$1.41M	\$28.4M	\$66.9M
Alpha-50%	\$0.25M	\$0.63M	\$28.4M	\$44.9M
Alpha-95%	\$0.25M	\$0.25M	\$28.4M	\$28.0M

In Table 5, the increase in equivalent availability given in spare component onsite (vs. no spare) is listed for both systems and for both types of failure rates (see (a) above). The sensitivity to failure rate is calculated here by using the three values of alpha from Table 2 in Eq. 34. The increase in *EA* is shown in terms of dollars as found from Eq. (37). It can be seen that as expected, the two-of-three system being more reliable, shows less benefit due to a spare, remembering that different component capacities were used. The gain for the three-of-three system is strikingly larger than that for the two-of-three system.

Also, the assumption of a constant failure rate consistently underestimates the benefit for most of the cases examined here, for all values of alpha. The gain in *EA* is seen to vary by factors of two to five, depending on alpha. Other parameters in the hazard function (Eq. (28)) could also be varied to fully explore the sensitivity.

Only the possible gains are estimated here, using assumed constants in Eq. (37). It is possible to change the calculations to an annual basis or to MWH, if desired. The net benefit in *EA* can only be evaluated after assessing overall costs; this is beyond the scope of the present work.

The behavior of P_{us} vs. time was affected by the inclusion of aging as seen in Fig. 3 and 4. These figures show how the probability of needing a spare varies with time. Note that this probability goes through a maximum for the time-dependent hazard function for both systems considered. In all cases here, P_{us} eventually decreases with time reflecting the relative likelihood of failure.

The impact of aging, with the associated increasing failure rate, definitely affects the predicted reliability and thus cost-benefit determinations. The calculations shown here assumed that degradation due to aging effects was not corrected over the long time span considered. Although this may be overly conservative, this view does reveal the significance of aging for some components and systems.

The risks in this application have been defined in terms of gains in equivalent availability for the spare component vs. no spare condition. This risk was expressed roughly in dollar-equivalent cost of replacement power. A measure of priority for better knowledge of failure rates was also demonstrated here in terms of this risk. It would seem that more work in these areas would be very beneficial.

REFERENCES

1. A. Green and A. Bourne, *Reliability Technology,* Wiley-Interscience, NY (1972).
2. B. M. Meale and D. G. Satterwhite, An Aging Failure Survey of Light Water Reactor Safety Systems and Components, NUREG/CR-4747, Vol. 1 (1987).

3. B. M. Meale and D. G. Satterwhite, An Aging Failure Survey of Light Water Reactor Safety Systems and Components, NUREG/CR-4747, Vol. 2 (1988).
4. M. Subudhi, E. L. Burns, and J. A. Taylor, Operating Experience and Aging-Seismic Assessment of Electric Motors, NUREG/CR-4156 (1985).
5. W. E. Vesely, Risk Evaluations of Aging Phenomena: The Linear Aging Reliability Model and Its Extensions, NUREG/CR-4769, EGG-2476 (1987).
6. R. W. Hockenbury, R. F. Kirchner, J. K. Rothert, and R. J. Schmidt, Failure Data Analysis Including Aging Effects, Int'l. Nuc. Power Plant Aging Symposium, Bethesda, MD, August 1988.
7. R. W. Hockenbury and R. F. Kirchner, General Methodology for the Calculation of Availability Gain-Based Spare Parts Inventory, Final Report to Northeast Utilities, Oct. 1988, unpub.
8. W. Nelson, Weibull Analysis of Reliability Data with Few or No Failures, *J. Quality Tech.* **17(3)**:140 (July 1985).

Evaluation of Risk Assessment as Evidence for Decision Making[a]

S. P. Proctor, G. Marchant, and M. S. Baram
Boston University School of Public Health and School of Law
Boston, MA

ABSTRACT

The process of risk assessment has the potential to improve the factual component of health risk decision making in several forums (e.g. regulatory agencies, courts, workers compensation boards, etc.). However, the use of RA as evidence for decision making must be consistent with forum rules which govern the admissibility and value of scientific evidence. Risk assessment is a analytical tool utilized quantitatively to estimate public health risks. By its nature, there are definite weaknesses is using the process as evidence for risk decision making. The information database in RA is not complete; it involves uncertainty due to limited data available and from unresolved methodological issues which together create areas of conflict where scientific judgments or policy decisions must be made.

The focus in Part I of this project is to categorize those areas of inferences and scientific policy decisions in the RA process that require evaluation by those who utilize RA as evidence for decision making. A summary of the preliminary results of our analysis of the regulatory agency forum is presented in a matrix format. Part II provides a review of the judicial review practices regarding agency risk assessments. In conclusion, recommendations of specific principles for reasoned decision making in the federal agency forum will be made.

KEYWORDS: Risk assessment, decision making, judicial review, scientific peer review

PART I. IDENTIFICATION OF SCIENTIFIC ISSUES IN THE RA PROCESS

To understand and illuminate the areas in quantitative Risk Assessment where inferences and judgments have to be made due to scientific uncertainties, an analysis of studies by the National Research Council,[1] United States General Accounting Office,[2] and

a. This research has been supported by National Science Foundation grant No. SES 8618746, "Development of a conceptual framework for evaluating risk assessment as evidence for risk decision making."

the Office of Technology Assessment[3] was made to categorize certain scientific areas requiring attention when addressing the use of RA as evidence in decision making. An analysis of inference components identified by the National Research Council's Committee on the Institutional Means for Assessment of Risks to Public Health, the scientific components presented as criteria for evaluating the adequacy of the Federal RA process in the GAO study, and of agency carcinogen assessment policies presented in the OTA study was made. On review, these components were grouped into 10 categories defined by the type of scientific or policy issue addressed (Table 1).

The first 5 deal with the type and interpretation of scientific studies that are utilized primarily in the hazard identification and dose-response assessment steps in the process:

1. The first issue is the relative weight of different types of studies, epidemiological, animal bioassay, short-term tests, structure activity relationships, as positive evidence for carcinogenicity. Which types of positive studies are considered to be most indicative of human carcinogenicity from environmental chemical exposures?

2. The second issue is evaluation of the statistics indicative of a positive study. Does the study demonstrate a level of statistical significance and is the method of study analysis an appropriate measure of significance?

3. The third issue is an evaluation of the quality and validity of the studies' designs. This category involves the interpretation of studies which may have used the maximum tolerated dose, utilized historical control data or involved a different route of dose administration than would be expected in the human setting. Do these research techniques meet the proper scientific principles for demonstrating a measure of human carcinogenicity?[4]

4. The fourth issue is an evaluation of the comparability between studies when there are conflicting results. What is the importance of valid negative studies and how should conflicting animal study results or conflicting animal and human study results be interpreted?

5. The fifth issue is an evaluation of the choice of endpoints measured. How should the use of data with results indicating an increase in benign tumors be evaluated?

   The next 2 categories are concerned with judgments which must be made on (i) the "frontiers of scientific knowledge" and (ii) "trans-science"[5] issues of extrapolation; "issues which hang on the answers to questions which can be asked of science and yet which cannot be answered by science."[6]

6. The sixth issue is an assessment of the conformity of the modeling assumptions, and other physiologic and environmental mechanisms, made with respect to known scientific rationale.

7. The seventh issue is evaluating the appropriateness of the extrapolation used and the choice of adjustment factors in extrapolation from animal data to predicting human responses.

   The last three categories involve the recognition and presentation of uncertainties inherent in different aspects of the process.

8. The eighth issue involves a general attention to the evaluation of human variabilities in assessing health effects. How best to extrapolate from one section of the population to the general population?

9. The ninth issue is the evaluation and the presentation of the uncertainties in the quantitative estimates of exposure dose, potency, and risk characterization.

10. The tenth issue is presentation and evaluation of the qualitative uncertainties in the process of characterizing the risk.

Table 1. Categories of Scientific Criteria Issues Requiring Evaluation in Risk Assessment

Issues of Best Evidence

1. Criteria for defining relative weight of different types of positive studies.
2. Criteria for defining what appropriate measure of statistical significance is required to indicate a positive study.
3. Criteria for defining the quality and validity of a positive study's structure and design.
4. Criteria for evaluating the degree of comparability between studies when they provide conflicting results.
5. Criteria for determining the appropriate choice of study endpoints and their measurement of specific health effects.

Trans-Scientific Issues

6. Criteria for the qualitative decision regarding the disease causation model, and about physiologic and/or environmental mechanisms, when scientific knowledge is not available.
7. Criteria for determining the quantitative extrapolation model and the adjustment factors to utilize when extrapolating from high to low dose and from animals to humans.

Issues of the Presentation of Uncertainties

8. Attention to human variability in estimating health risks.
9. Criteria for defining the choice of best estimate of exposure dose, potency, and risk characterization, and for presenting the quantitative uncertainties surrounding those estimates.
10. Criteria for the presentation of the qualitative uncertainties inherent in the risk assessment process.

Comparison of Scientific Criteria Practices Across the Federal Regulatory Agencies: EPA, OSHA and FDA

The different agencies respond to these issues in contrasting manners as identified by analysis of available regulatory forum documentation.[3,7-10] A tension exists between the need for formalization and for flexibility in the presentation of agency "rules" on risk assessment. Summary of agency practices concerning the 10 criteria issues reveals that (i) the choice of conservatism in the face of uncertain data and (ii) reliance on peer review decisions representing the guise of "good scientific judgment," serve as the deferring statements in the risk assessment process.

The risk assessment process provides an estimate of health risk based on evaluation of available scientific evidence and of modeling constructs designed to provide estimates when scientific knowledge is not available or possible, hence its use of causal criteria draws from the capacity and limits of science and statistics.[11] Inferences from uncertain data and decisions on scientific policy are inherent in the risk assessment process.

As discussed earlier, the process of risk assessment has the potential to improve the factual component of health risk decision making in several forums. It has the potential to do so by pointing out the areas of uncertainties which require further study or pointing out areas where for further analysis on the impact of policy judgments is needed. Three recommendations are prescribed below to improve the factual component of risk assessment process:

1. Attention should be made of the uncertainties inherent throughout the process so that as more scientific data becomes available, the information can be utilized to improve the characterization of risk. If no disclosure of the uncertainty is made in describing the initial assessment of risk, then it becomes difficult to appropriately input new information.

2. Flexibility should be maintained in practice, but guidelines should be devised and followed so that others can follow the process to insure the comprehensiveness and validity of the risk assessment. Newer additional information from pharmacokinetics, DNA adduct monitoring and mechanistic distinctions will require the risk assessment community to think about the inferences made and may possibly alter the accepted inferential choices. The consequences of changing points of view will have to be evaluated and explained.

   For example, the recently considered change in the numerical estimate for the potency of dioxin (specifically 2,3,7,8-tetrachlorodibenzo-p-dioxin or TCDD) by the EPA[12] has provoked controversy about the use of risk assessment as evidence in decision making. It has called for, by a number of scientists in editorial comments, the need to articulate igorous scientific standards for the evaluation of both 'new' as well as currently accepted risk assessment approaches; and to recognize the consequences, both to science and to policy, of over- or under-estimating risks.[13-15]

3. The risk assessment process should have built in methods and financing to obtain or sanction studies to fill in data gaps about new chemicals, chemical mixtures, and other health effects besides cancer. "The failure to require meaningful information on new chemicals and the overreliance on models rather than on monitoring have resulted in a void of information in calculating human exposure."[16] It is critical, especially when evaluating chemicals for which there is lesser quality and quantity of study evidence, that their health risks not be passed over. If so, this infers that chemicals with less weighty evidence can be considered less risky than those with more positive, stronger evidence.[17]

   Risk assessment is a dynamic science by nature. It should not be viewed as existing in a vacuum, but as demanding constant interaction with the scientific, legal and political arenas in which it operates.

PART II: PRINCIPLES FOR DECIDING RISK ASSESSMENT ISSUES

This section of the paper will discuss how risk assessment practitioners, risk managers, policy makers in government agencies, and reviewing courts should decide the risk assessment issues identified in Part I. A set of five principles will be proposed that parties involved in the risk assessment process can use to ensure the reasonableness of risk assessment decisions.

Unlimited discretion by federal agencies in making risk assessment decisions is incompatible with our political culture and sound management practices. Some form of external quality control is needed to guard against sloppy or inadequate risk assessments, or even worse, the deliberate manipulation of risk assessment choices and results to reach a pre-selected conclusion.

The two major mechanisms for oversight of agency risk assessments are the political process and judicial review. Since federal agencies are not directly accountable to the electorate, the political process must act on agencies through either the White House or Congress. However, neither of these institutions have the resources, time, or political inclination to review agency risk assessments on a case-by-case basis. Direct intervention by Congress or the White House will therefore be limited to rare cases of grievous abuses of discretion by agencies. Furthermore, the effectiveness of political oversight will often be limited by the "opacity" of many risk assessments with respect to the assumptions used and the uncertainties involved. Accordingly, judicial review will usually be the primary mechanism for external quality control of agency risk assessments.

Judicial Review of Agency Risk Assessments

Agency risk assessments often form the evidentiary basis supporting proposed regulations for protecting public health or the environment. It is not surprising, therefore, that legal challenges to proposed regulations by industry, trade unions, and environmental organizations often focus on the adequacy and sufficiency of the agency's risk assessment. An agency's treatment of controversial and difficult risk assessment issues, such as those outlined in the first part of this paper, is often a tempting target for legal challenges by parties opposed to the proposed regulation.

The Supreme Court's landmark *Vermont Yankee* decision prohibited reviewing courts from requiring additional agency procedures beyond those specified by the relevant enabling statute and the Administrative Procedure Act.[18] Consequently, judicial review has since necessarily focused primarily on the substantive rather than the procedural aspects of agency risk assessments.

Substantive judicial review of risk assessment controversies usually involves two general criteria, which one court has described as the "consistency" and "reasonableness" requirements.[19] The consistency standard requires the agency to make risk assessment choices consistent with the enabling statute; while the reasonableness standard requires the agency's risk assessment to meet some minimal standard of rationality.

During the late 1970s and early 1980s, most courts relied primarily on the consistency standard when reviewing agency regulations based on risk assessments. Many of the statutes were new, and hence controversies such as whether risk assessments should be based on the most sensitive individuals in the population,[20] or whether conservative assumptions could be used,[21] were often resolved by looking for evidence of Congressional intent in the wording and legislative history of the newly enacted statutes. Given their areas of experience and expertise, judges were more comfortable interpreting statutory language than trying to evaluate the scientific adequacy of complex risk assessment choices.

However, the prominence of the consistency principle for judicial review has recently been declining. As the case law has developed and the courts have interpreted the meaning of key statutory phrases, the number of cases turning on legal issues of statutory interpretation, rather than the reasonableness of agency findings, have diminished.[22] Furthermore, the recent Supreme Court decision in *Chevron v. NRDC* requires the courts to give much greater deference to the statutory interpretations adopted by agencies.[23]

As the court's role in reviewing the procedures and statutory interpretations used by federal agencies has been limited, judicial review of risk assessments has increasingly focused on the "reasonableness" standard. No rules of evidence apply to control the quality of particular pieces of evidence in an agency's rulemaking record,[24] so courts must evaluate whether the record as a whole provides "substantial evidence" for the agency's findings or is not "arbitrary and capricious." However, the criteria for determining whether an agency risk assessment is supported by substantial evidence or is not arbitrary and capricious are amorphous and ill-defined.

While many types of agency findings can be supported by empirically verifiable facts, risk assessment controversies usually involve science policy and trans-scientific issues not amenable to proof. Agency decisions on the risk assessment issues identified in Part I often involve assumptions and "quasi-legislative" policy choices for which the conventional criteria such as "clearly erroneous" do not apply. Accordingly, it is very difficult to elucidate clear criteria for evaluating the reasonableness of these types of agency findings. As a result, courts frequently decide the reasonableness of an agency finding with only a conclusory statement that sheds little light on the criteria the court used in reaching its decision.[25]

Without a clear definition of the meaning of the reasonableness standard for risk assessment issues, the minimal evidentiary requirements needed to uphold an agency finding are uncertain. From an examination of cases involving judicial review of agency risk assessments, two problems emerge from this uncertainty. First, there is considerable inconsistency between the holdings in different cases. Second, the appropriate level of deference to an agency's findings is unclear. Each of these two problems is discussed below.

1. Inconsistent Holdings. Because there are no clear criteria for courts to use in assessing the reasonableness of an agency's risk assessment finding, courts often apply inconsistent standards and reach contradictory holdings. For example, the Supreme court's review of OSHA's proposed benzene standard held that an agency's findings must meet a "more likely than not" test;[26] while other courts have held that an agency's findings need not be supported by the preponderance of evidence.[27] Courts have also differed on whether the agency or challenger has the burden of proof.[28]

Judicial disagreement on the requirements of the substantive review standard translate into contradictory holdings on specific risk assessment issues. Examples are numerous. At least one court has suggested that an assumption of no threshold below which no harm occurs is of "questionable validity,"[29] while other courts have held that the no-threshold assumption is supported by substantial evidence.[30] The holdings of at least two cases suggest that an agency cannot use data on the health effects from high exposure levels as probative evidence of health risks at lower exposures.[31] Yet, many other cases have upheld the agency's use of high exposure studies to estimate risks at lower levels.[32] As a final example, the Fifth Circuit Court of Appeals invalidated an OSHA rule because the agency made an error that overestimated the number of lives that would be saved by the proposed standard;[33] while the D.C. Circuit upheld a different regulation even though OSHA made an even greater miscalculation of lives saved.[34]

These contradictory outcomes result in incoherence, unfairness, and unpredictability. They have also prompted some observers to cynically suggest that judicial review of risk assessments is driven primarily by the individual judge's view of the merits of the agency's rulemaking.[35]

2. Appropriate Level of Deference. The lack of a clearly defined standard of judicial review for science policy and trans-scientific issues has fueled the debate on the appropriate level of judicial deference to agency findings. Some courts have undertaken a very stringent, critical review of agency risk assessments,[36] while others have adopted a much more deferential approach.[37] In the 1983 *Baltimore Gas* decision, the Supreme Court instructed reviewing courts to be at its "most deferential" when reviewing risk assessment findings at the frontiers of scientific knowledge.[38] Since this decision, the lower courts have generally responded with a "super deferential" standard of review.[39]

There are strong arguments for judicial deference when reviewing agency risk assessments. First, it is the agencies, and not the courts, which have the necessary expertise and resources to make decisions on highly technical risk assessment issues. Second, since the massive records usually needed to support risk assessments will always contain some flaws, courts will have the opportunity to substitute their policy judgment for that of the agency whenever it chooses under a less deferential review standard. Third, active participation by the courts in making the controversial policy judgments involved in risk assessment may improperly politicize the courts.[40] Fourth and finally, while there is only a single EPA or OSHA, there are many different federal courts and thus the danger of inconsistent decisions is much greater.

While the arguments for judicial deference are persuasive, there are equally strong arguments for judicial scrutiny. To begin with, Congress did not intend to delegate unlimited discretion to agencies, since it provided for judicial review under regulatory statutes and the Administrative Procedure Act. Furthermore, the high stakes involved in health and environmental regulation—including protection of human life, possibly irreversible environmental damage, and billions of dollars in compliance costs by industry—support heightened judicial scrutiny. Some agency findings have been described as "an elaborate evidentiary house of cards"[41] or as "a blind stab through a curtain of ignorance."[42] In the absence of meaningful judicial review, the prevalence of poor quality risk assessments using substandard data or unjustified assumptions would likely increase. Thorough judicial review would also minimize the danger of "agency capture." Furthermore, judicial scrutiny provides a useful "second look" that occasionally detects serious errors in the agency's record.[43] Finally, creating a more relaxed standard for judicial review of technical issues will provide an incentive for agencies to attempt to disguise policy judgments as scientific matters in order to elude judicial scrutiny.[44]

In summary, courts face a dilemma in determining the appropriate level of deference when reviewing technical risk assessments. "[A] court must reconcile its more limited capacity with a greater need for close review."[45] This tension will only be resolved by developing a set of clearly articulated principles for ensuring reasoned decision making that can be easily and consistently applied by the courts, but which recognize the limitations of the technical competency of judges and the institutional role of courts.

Five Principles for Reasoned Decision Making

Given the shortcomings of judicial review of technical risk assessment issues described above, the goal of judicial review should not be to ensure that an agency makes the "right" or "best" decision. Rather, the goal should be to require agency findings to meet a minimal level of rationality, and to ensure that the key choices and assumptions made by the agency are exposed to the political process. Five principles that can be used by the courts to evaluate the reasonableness of agency risk assessments are suggested below.

1. *Best Available Evidence.* Since risk assessments are no better than the data on which they are based, courts should require agencies to use the most up-to-date and reliable data available. Several courts have remanded agency rulemakings that were not based on the best available evidence.
2. *Disclosure of Uncertainties.* Many agency risk assessments currently do not disclose the uncertainties in their risk estimates,[47] perhaps in part to minimize vulnerability to political second-guessing. By requiring full disclosure and explanation of all uncertainties and assumptions in risk assessments, the courts can ensure that there is an opportunity for the political process to evaluate the agency's policy judgments.

While some court opinions have been criticized for their insensitivity to requiring disclosure of uncertainties,[48] other courts have held that it is "incumbent" on the agency to "estimate the possible degree of error" in its findings.[49] Courts are generally more deferential when an agency openly acknowledges the uncertainties and weaknesses in its analysis.[50]

3. *Explanation for Departure from Past Practice.* Any significant deviation from past agency practices creates a suspicion that the agency may be acting in a capricious or biased manner. Therefore, departures from past practices should only be upheld if supported by a reasoned explanation of why such a change is necessary or strongly desirable. The Supreme Court's recent *State Farm* decision holds that an agency must provide a "reasoned analysis" for a change from a settled course of behavior.[51]

4. *Scientific Peer Review.* Under some regulatory statutes, agencies are required to submit their findings and proposed standards to scientific advisory panels for comment. Whether required by statute or not, scientific peer review can strengthen the technical soundness of agency rulemakings. Given the holding of *Vermont Yankee* proscribing courts from requiring additional procedures by agencies, the courts clearly cannot mandate agencies to use peer review when not required by statute. Nonetheless, the courts can give greater deference to findings supported by peer review, and less weight to evidence that could have been reviewed by a scientific panel, but was not.[52] In practice, courts have often given greater deference to agency findings because they were supported by peer review.[53] Unfortunately, the courts have not always been consistent in giving greater deference to peer-reviewed findings.[54]

5. *Generic Risk Assessment Guidelines.* The use of uniform risk assessment guidelines by agencies should help reduce the inconsistency and arbitrariness of agency findings. Accordingly, agency risk assessments employing generic guidelines should be given greater deference by the courts. As the D.C. Circuit explained in upholding the EPA's use of risk assessment guidelines, the "specific enunciation of [EPA's] underlying analytical principles, derived from its experience in the area, yields meaningful notice and dialogue, enhances the administrative process and furthers reasoned agency decision making."[55] In another recent case, the court treated the guidelines themselves as substantial evidence to support an agency's finding.[56]

CONCLUSION

The problem with the reasonableness standard for judicial review of agency risk assessments is the lack of clear criteria for judging the rationality of agency findings. Courts can best achieve the appropriate balance between deference and close scrutiny by using the five principles for reasoned decision making suggested here. Namely, courts should insist that agencies use the best available data, fully disclose uncertainties and assumptions, and provide a reasoned explanation for any departure form past practice. The courts should also encourage agencies (through the promise of greater deference) to utilize scientific peer review and generic risk assessment guidelines.

Although the courts have been sporadic in applying the five principles for reasoned decision making identified here, they do frequently and increasingly use these principles in determining whether an agency risk assessment is sufficient and adequate to support a proposed rulemaking (see Table 2). Agencies that do not follow these principles risk a much higher likelihood that their proposed regulation will be overturned or remanded by the courts. Accordingly, risk practitioners, risk managers, and policy makers in federal agencies should incorporate these five principles at all levels of their risk assessment process. Taken together, these five principles of reasoned decision making can be applied

Table 2. Case Law Supporting Five Principles

	COURT APPLIED PRINCIPLE . . .		COURT CONTRADICTED PRINCIPLE
	To Support Agency	To Overturn Agency	
BEST AVAILABLE EVIDENCE	Public Citizen v. Tyson	API v. OSHA EDF v. Costle National Lime Ass'n v. EPA	
DISCLOSURE OF UNCERTAINTIES	Public Citizen v. Tyson Building & Constr. Trades v. Brock API v. Costle	Int'l. Harvester Portland Cement NRDC v. NRC (overturned)	Baltimore Gas v. NRDC ???????
EXPLAIN DEPARTURE FROM PAST PRACTICE	Asarco v. OSHA	Motor Vehicle Manufacturers v. State Farm Mutual	
SCIENTIFIC PEER REVIEW	Lead Industries v. EPA Foundation on Economic Trends v. Thomas Friends of Endangered Species	Asbestos Info. Ass'n	API v. Costle Gulf South
GENERIC RISK ASSESSMENT GUIDELINES	NRDC v. EPA EDF v. EPA		Industrial Union Dept. v. API ???????

predictably and consistently, will ensure a minimum standard of reasonability, and will expose agency choices and assumptions to the political process for ultimate judgment.

REFERENCES

1. National Research Council, *Risk Assessment in the Federal Government Managing the Process*, National Academy Press, Washington, DC (1983).
2. United States General Accounting Office, *Health Risk Analysis—Technical Adequacy in Three Selected Cases*, Report to the Chairman, Committee on Science, Space, and Technology, House of Representatives, General Accounting Office, Washington, DC (1987).
3. U.S. Congress, Office of Technology Assessment, *Identifying and Regulating Carcinogens*, OTA-BP-H-42, U.S. Government Printing Office, Washington, DC (1987).
4. Technical adequacy criteria for the practice of "required carcinogenicity testing," accepted scientific study design and toxicity experiment techniques, issues of dosing regimen, pathology techniques, personnel qualifications, have not been included in this category. For a good review of these issues, see OTA, 1987.
5. T. O. McGarity, Substantive and Procedural Discretion in Administrative Resolution of Science Policy Questions: Regulating Carcinogens in EPA and OSHA, *Georgetown Law J.* **67**:729-810 (1979).
6. A. Weinberg, Science and Trans-Science, *Minerva* **10**:209 (1972).
7. Environmental Protection Agency, Guidelines for Carcinogenic Risk Assessment, *Federal Register* **51(185)**:33992-34003 (September 24, 1986).

8. Food and Drug Administration, Sponsored Compounds in Food-Producing Animals; Criteria and Procedures for Evaluating the Safety of Carcinogenic Residues, *Federal Register* **50(211)**:45530-45556 (October 31, 1985).
9. Occupational Safety and Health Administration, Identification, Classification, and Regulation of Potential Carcinogens, *Federal Register* **45(15)**:5002-5296 (January 22, 1980).
10. Office of Science, Technology and Policy, Chemical Carcinogens—A Review of the Science and Its Associated Principles, *Federal Register* **50(50)**:10372-10442 (March 14, 1985).
11. J. V. Rodricks, Personal Communication.
12. Environmental Protection Agency, A Cancer Risk-Specific Dose Estimate for 2,3,7,8-TCDD, Review Draft (1987).
13. A. M. Findel, Dioxin: Are We Safer Now Than Before? *Risk Analysis* **8(2)**:161-166 (1988).
14. F. Perera, EPA Cancer Risk Assessments, Letters to the Editor, *Science*, p. 1227 (March 11, 1988).
15. M. Gough, Science Policy Choices and the Estimation of Cancer Risk Associated with Exposure to TCDD, *Risk Analysis* **8(3)**:337-342 (1988).
16. E. Silbergeld, Risk Assessment, Letters to the Editor, *Science*, p. 1399 (September 18, 1987).
17. E. Silbergeld, The Uses and Abuses of Scientific Uncertainty in Risk Assessment, *Natural Resources Environ.* **2**:17-20,57-59 (1986).
18. *Vermont Yankee Nuclear Power Corp. v. Natural Resources Defense Council, Inc.*, 435 U.S. 519 (1978).
19. *Texas Independent Ginners Assoc. v. Marshall*, 630 F.2d 398, 405 (5th Cir. 1980).
20. E.g., *American Petroleum Institute v. Costle*, 665 F.2d 1176, 1186 (D.C. Cir. 1981); *Ethyl Corp. v. EPA*, 541 F.2d 1, 40 (D.C. Cir. 1976).
21. E.g., *Industrial Union Dep't. v. American Petroleum Inst.*, 448 U.S. 607, 656 (1980); *Lead Industries Assoc. v. EPA*, 647 F.2d 1130, 1162 (D.C. Cir. 1980).
22. D. Sive, Environmental Decision Making: Judicial and Political Review, *Case Western L. Rev.* **28**:827 (1978).
23. *Chevron, U.S.A., Inc. v. Natural Resources Defense Council, Inc.*, 467 U.S. 837 (1984).
24. J. T. O'Reilly, *Administrative Rulemaking*, pp. 119-123, McGraw-Hill, Colorado Springs (1983).
25. A. Oleinick, L. D. Disney, and K. S. East, Institutional Mechanisms for Converting Sporadic Agency Decisions into Systematic Risk Management Strategies, in *Risk Evaluation and Management*, pp. 381-411, V. Covello, J. Menkes, and J. Mumpower, eds., Plenum Press, New York (1986).
26. *Industrial Union Department v. American Petroleum Institute*, 448 U.S. at 653 (1980).
27. *Natural Resources Defense Council v. EPA*, 824 F.2d 1211, 1217 (D.C. Cir. 1987); *Environmental Defense Fund v. EPA*, 598 F.2d 62, 85 (D.C. Cir. 1978); *Environmental Defense Fund v. EOA*, 548 F.2d 998, 1003 (D.C. Cir. 1976).
28. Compare *International Harvester Co. v. Ruckelshaus*, 478 F.2d 615, 648 (D.C. Cir. 1973) ("Administrator must sustain the burden of adducing a reasoned presentation supporting the reliability of EPA's methodology") with *Dry Color Mnfrs. Assoc. Inc. v. Dept. of Labor*, 486 F.2d 98, 109 (3rd Cir. 1973) ("Obviously the petitioner must bear the burden of proof").
29. *Gulf South Insulation v. U.S. CPSC*, 701 F.2d 1137, 1147 n.19 (5th Cir. 1983).
30. *Public Citizen Health Research Group v. Tyson*, 796 F.2d 1479, 1501 (D.C. Cir. 1986); *Asarco, Inc. v. OSHA*, 746 F.2d 483, 493 (9th Cir. 1984).
31. *Natural Resources Defense Council v. EPA*, 812 F.2d 712, 725 (D.C. Cir. 1987); *Texas Independent Ginners*, 630 F.2d at 407-09 (1980).
32. *Building & Construction Trades Dept., AFL-CIO v. Brock*, 838 F.2d 1258, 1266 (D.C. Cir. 1988); *EDF v. EPA*, 598 F. 2d at 87 (1978).

33. *Asbestos Information Assoc. v. OSHA*, 727 F.2d 415, 425 (5th Cir. 1984).
34. *Public Citizens v. Tyson*, 796 F.2d at 1503 (1986).
35. D. L. Davis, The "Shotgun Wedding" of Science and Law: Risk Assessment and Judicial Review, *Col. J. Envtl. L.* **10**:67 (1985); W. H. Rodgers, Judicial Review of Risk Assessments: The Role of Decision Theory in Unscrambling the Benzene Decision, *Envtl. L.* **11**:301 (1981).
36. E.g., *Gulf South*, 746 F.2d at 1137 (1983); *L.U.D. v. A.P.I.*, 448 U.s. at 607 (1980).
37. *Asarco*, 746 F.2d at 483 (1984); *Ethyl Corp.*, 541 F.2d at 1 (1976).
38. *Baltimore Gas & Electric Co. v. Natural Resources Defense Council, Inc.*, 462 U.S. 87, 103 (1983).
39. A. D. Siegal, The Aftermath of *Baltimore Gas & Electric Co. v. NRDC*: A Broader Notion of Judicial Deference to Agency Expertise), *Harv. Envtl. L. Rev.* **11**:331 (1987).
40. T. O. McGarity, Judicial Review of Scientific Rulemaking, *Science, Technology & Human Values*, pp. 97-106 (Winter 1984).
41. *EDF v. EPA*, 598 F.2d at 79 (1978).
42. *Ethyl Corp.*, 541 F.2d at 111 (1976).
43. *Asbestos Info. Assoc.*, 727 F.2d at 419 n.8 (1984).
44. J. Yellin, Science, Technology, and Administrative Government: Institutional Designs for Environmental Decision Making, *Yale L. J.* **92**:1300 (1983).
45. D. L. Bazelon, Science and Uncertainty: A Jurist's View, *Jurimetrics J.* **22**:372 (1982).
46. *American Petroleum Institute v. OSHA*, 581 F.2d 493, 507 (5th Cir. 1978) (remanding agency finding on cancer risk from dermal contact with benzene because a much more reliable experimental methodology had become available); *Environmental Defense Fund v. Costle*, 578 F.2d 337 (D.C. Cir. 1978) (remanding proposed regulation in light of new sources of available data); *National Lime Assoc. v. EPA*, 627 F.2d 416, 454 (D.C. Cir. 1980) (requiring agency to consider real-life test data when available).
47. D. Scroggins, EPA Health Risk Policy Will have Broad Impact, *Legal Times*, July 15, 1985 at 19.
48. See, e.g., Yellin, *supra* (criticizing the Supreme Court's *Baltimore Gas* decision).
49. *International Harvester*, 478 F.2d at 647 (1973); *Portland Cement Assoc. vs. Ruckelshaus*, 486 F.2d 375, 396 (D.C. Cir. 1973).
50. See, e.g., *Public Citizen v. Tyson*, 796 F.2d at 1479 (1986); *A.P.I. v. Costle*, 665 F.2d at 1185 (1981).
51. *Motor Vehicle Manufacturers Association of the United States, Inc. v. State Farm Mutual Automobile Insurance Company*, 463 U.S. 29 (1983).
52. T. S. Burack, Of Reliable Science: Scientific Peer Review, Federal Regulatory Agencies, and the Courts, *Va. J. Natural Resources L.* **7**:27 (1987).
53. *Asbestos Info. Assoc.*, 727 F.2d at 421, n. 15 (1984); *Lead Industries Assoc.*, 647 F.2d at 1157 (1980); *Friends of Endangered Species v. Jantzen*, 596 F.Supp. 518, 523 (N.D.Cal. 1984); *Foundation on Economic Trends v. Thomas*, 637 F. Supp. 25, 27 (D.D.C. 1986).
54. E.g., see *A.P.I. v. Costle*, 665 F.2d at 1189 (1981) (upholding standard that was required to be peer reviewed but was not); *Gulf South*, 701 F.2d at 1137 (1983) (vacating proposed rule that had been supported by a highly qualified review panel).
55. *EDF v. EPA*, 548 F.2d at 1007 (1976).
56. *NRDC v. EPA*, 824 F.2d at 1217 (1987).

Risk Assessment of the Army's Chemical Stockpile Disposal Program

Willard Fraize, Robert Cutler, William Duff, John Perry, and Brian Price
The MITRE Corporation
McLean, VA

Thomas Kartachak
U.S. Army
Aberdeen Proving Ground, MD

Michael Stamatelatos
General Atomics
San Diego, CA

ABSTRACT

The Army's Chemical Stockpile Disposal Program is intended to destroy the nation's stockpile of unitary chemical weapons. The stockpile, consisting of three basic chemical agent types in both explosive and bulk storage configurations, is stored at eight Army sites across the conterminous United States. This paper describes the probabilistic risk assessment that was carried out to assist the Army in determining which of five proposed disposal program alternatives, all large scale efforts involving multiple activities at multiple sites, pose the least risk to public safety for the population groups living near the sites or along the proposed transportation corridors. The risk analysis rests on a foundation of approximately 3000 hypothesized accidents—a mix of modeled and historic data. Consequences for each accident are expressed as potential fatalities and the extent (length and area) of the resulting agent dispersion plume; probability is expressed as the chance that the accident will happen during the stockpile disposal program. Results are expressed in terms of five different risk measures. Uncertainty in the risk assessment results was estimated. The results showed that the "on-site disposal" option is expected to pose the least programmatic risk.

KEYWORDS: Risk assessment, chemical weapons, programmatic risk, individual risk, atmospheric dispersion

INTRODUCTION

The U.S. Army was directed by Congress (Public Law 99-145) to destroy the nation's stockpile of lethal, unitary chemical agents and munitions in a manner which provides for maximum protection to the public. This paper describes the analytical

Risk Analysis, Edited by C. Zervos
Plenum Press, New York, 1991

approach used in the comparative assessment of risk for the several alternatives within the Army's Chemical Stockpile Disposal Program (CSDP).

The Chemical Stockpile Disposal Program

The Chemical Stockpile consists of a wide range of munitions and bulk agent storage containers. Three chemical agent types are included: the persistent nerve agent, VX; the non-persistent nerve agent, GB; and the persistent blister agents known as mustards and designated by the symbols H, HT, and HD. The stockpile is currently stored in eight locations throughout the conterminous U.S. (CONUS): Anniston Army Depot (ANAD), Alabama; Aberdeen Proving Ground (APG), Maryland; Lexington Blue-Grass Army Depot (LBAD), Kentucky; Newport Army Ammunition Plant (NAAP), Indiana; Pine Bluff Arsenal (PBA), Arkansas; Pueblo Depot Activity (PUDA), Colorado; Tooele Army Depot (TEAD), Utah; and Umatilla Depot Activity (UMDA), Oregon.

The method selected for disposal consists of mechanical disassembly of the munitions, separation into material classes (dunnage, metal parts, energetics, and agent), and incineration.

Five disposal alternatives were evaluated: (1) continued storage of the stockpile in its present locations (the "no-action" alternative required by the National Environmental Policy Act); (2) on-site destruction of the stockpile at its present storage locations; (3) movement of the CONUS stocks to two regional disposal centers (at ANAD and TEAD); (4) movement of the CONUS stocks to one national disposal center (at TEAD); (5) movement of the stocks from two sites (APG and LBAD) by air to the national disposal site (TEAD) with the remainder of the stockpile destroyed on-site. The disposal alternatives and the activities involved in each are illustrated by Fig. 1.

Purpose and Context of the Risk Analysis

The purpose of the analysis was to provide a consistent and quantitative basis for comparing the risks to the public for each of the disposal alternatives. Risk was defined as the potential impact on public safety of a set of possible accidents that could result from the storage, handling, transporting, and physical destruction of the munitions in the stockpile. Risk was measured by both the probability of occurrence of a lethal event and the number of fatalities that would result if the event took place. The results of the analysis were used to support the selection of the environmentally preferred disposal alternative in the Final Programmatic Environmental Impact Statement (FPEIS).[1] They were also used as one of several factors considered by the Army in arriving at the decision to proceed with the on-site disposal alternative (Record of Decision of February 23, 1988, U.S. Army).

Participants and Roles in the Risk Analysis

The risk analysis of the CSDP involved several organizations.

General Atomics (formerly GA Technologies) was responsible for identifying the accident scenarios and characterizing each in terms of agent release and probability of occurrence. Subcontractors supporting General Atomics included H&R Technical Associates, JBF Associates, and Battelle Columbus Division.

The U.S. Army defined the disposal alternatives and disposal technology and provided access to the Army-developed agent dispersion model (D2PC).

Oak Ridge National Laboratory (ORNL) provided demographic data, meteorological assumptions, and generic fatality estimates (number of potential fatalities for a chemical accident of a given size category). ORNL was also responsible for preparation of the FPEIS

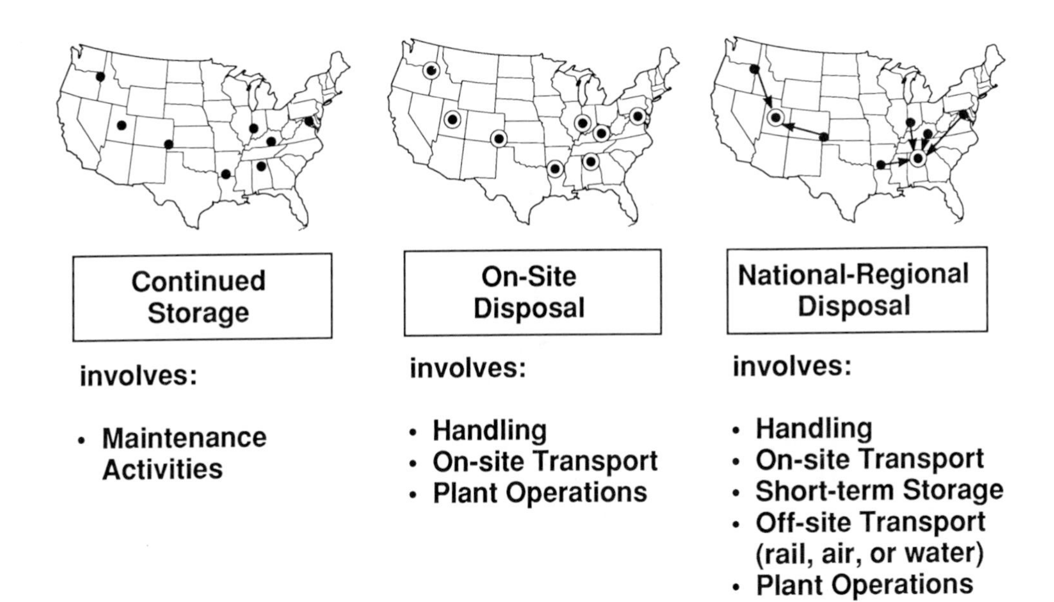

Fig. 1. Chemical stockpile disposal program alternatives.

and the use of the risk analysis results in the determination of the environmentally-preferred alternative.

Finally, the MITRE Corporation was responsible for developing and implementing the risk analysis methodology which integrated the data provided by the other participants and provided useful quantitative estimates of several selected risk measures in a variety of formats.

RISK ELEMENTS OF THE CHEMICAL STOCKPILE DISPOSAL PROGRAM

The analysis of risk associated with the CSDP took the following factors into account: (1) the nature and the severity of the hazards to individuals posed by exposure to a chemical agent; (2) the munitions and bulk containers in which the agents are contained; (3) the activities within the CSDP that could lead to accidental release of agent; (4) the accident initiators appropriate for each activity class and munition type; (5) the disposal alternatives which specify the activities and the location at which they take place; and (6) the population groups that could be affected by an accidental agent release.

Hazards of Chemical Agents

The chemical agents are, by design, highly lethal; relatively small exposures via inhalation (measured as the product of atmospheric concentration and exposure time, i.e., mg-min./m^3) or via skin contact (measured in mg/kg of body weight) can be lethal. For inhalation of dispersed agents lethality is given by the exposures listed in Table 1.

The Munitions and Bulk Containers

The chemical agents are stored in both munitions and bulk storage configurations. Munitions include cartridges, mortars, projectiles, rockets, mines, bombs, and spray tanks; most are explosively configured to provide for rapid dispersion of the agent and, in the case of rockets, for propulsion toward the target area. The bulk storage containers hold up to 1700 pounds of liquid agent and do not contain explosives. The explosively-configured

Table 1. Lethality of Chemical Agents

Agent Type	Exposure [mg-min./m^3] for 50% Lethalities[6]
GB	70
VX	30
HD	1500

munitions have agent fills in the 1 to 15 lb. range. A 10 lb. release of either agents GB or VX can lead to lethal exposures at distances of 1 km from the release site under average meteorological conditions.

CSDP Activity Categories

The major activity categories associated with the disposal program alternatives include storage, handling, on-site transport, off-site transport, and plant operations. The sequencing and the location of these potentially risky activities for the several disposal alternatives is illustrated in Fig. 2.

Accident Initiators

The accident initiators considered in the risk analysis are appropriate to the activity categories described above. Causes of an accidental release of an agent include "external" events (e.g., tornados, earthquakes, meteor strikes, and airplane crashes), transportation accidents (truck, rail, or aircraft while carrying chemical agent), handling accidents (dropping of a munition or puncturing it with a forklift tine), and accidents associated with plant operations (human error, control system failure, mechanical equipment breakdown, fire). A list of the accident initiators considered, by activity category, is presented in Table 2.

Disposal Alternatives

The disposal alternatives define which of the disposal activities take place where. The alternatives are illustrated in Fig. 1.

For the continued storage alternative, risk is due to the storage and storage-related handling activities at the current storage locations.

For on-site disposal, risk arises from the (short-term) storage of the stockpile awaiting disposal, from handling and on-site transport activities as the munitions are moved to the disposal facility, and from the plant operations themselves — all occurring at the current eight storage locations.

The risk associated with the regional/national disposal and partial relocation alternatives (the so-called collocation alternatives) is distributed between the originating sites, the transportation corridors, and the destination/disposal sites. At the originating sites, risk results from handling, on-site transport, and short-term storage activities. The originating sites (APG and LBAD) also bear the risk of take-off aircraft accidents for the partial relocation alternative. The transportation corridors are exposed to the en-route transport risks. The destination sites experience the risks due to handling, on-site transport,

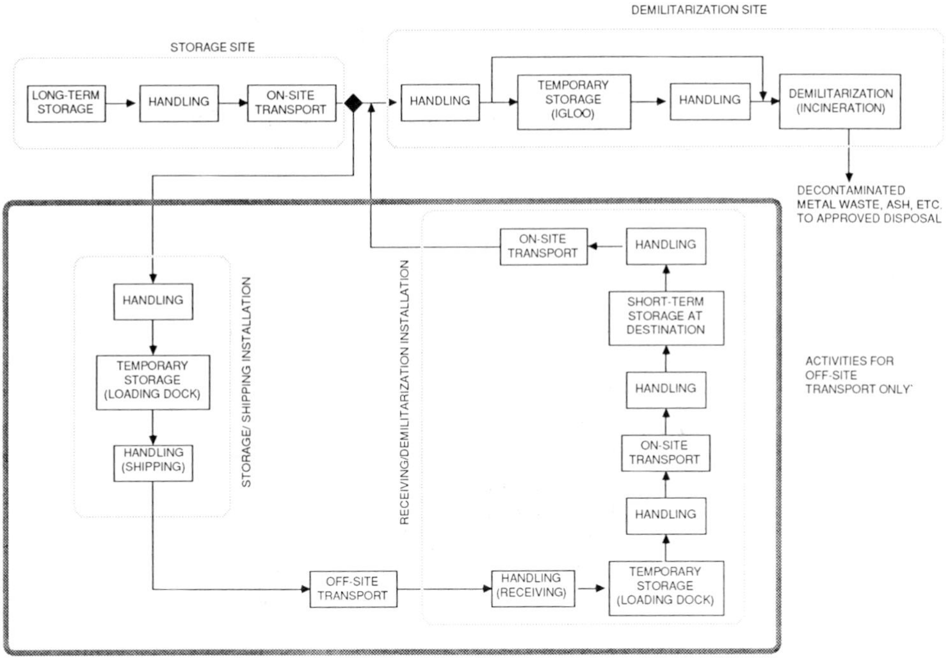

Fig. 2. CSDP disposal activities by locale and disposal alternative.

and short-term storage of the imported munitions as well as all the risks associated with disposing of the resident and collocated stockpiles.

Affected Population Groups

Any population groups living or working within the maximum hazard distance ("no-deaths" distance for most severe accident) of a potential accident site are at some risk due to the CSDP. Hence, the risk analysis had to consider the risk to the population groups surrounding the eight current stockpile sites plus those along the several transportation corridors.

DATA SOURCES

Accident Scenarios

Accident scenario data were developed by General Atomics.[2-4] The accident scenarios are described by the following: (1) a ten-character identification code, described in Fig. 3, which uniquely defines operational activity (handling, plant operations, etc.); munition type, agent type, and release mode; (2) a brief textual description of each scenario, as defined by activity code and scenario number (a representative sampling of scenarios for the plant operations activity category is given in Table 3); and (3) agent release and probability data.

Agent release data includes agent type, release mode, release time (where relevant), surface character for evaporative releases (i.e., porous or non-porous), and location of evaporative releases (indoor, outdoor).

Table 2. Accident Initiators, by CSDP Activity Category

Activity Category	Accident Initiators
Storage	Spontaneous munition leak Puncture by forklift tine Spontaneous rocket motor ignition Small or Large aircraft crash into storage area Tornado-generated missiles Tornado-induced building collapse Severe earthquake Meteorite strike Lightning strike Munition(s) dropped during handling Fire from internal or external sources
Handling	Munition(s) dropped Forklift collision Puncture by forklift tine Undetected leak
On-site Transport	Munition vehicle collides/overturns Aircraft crash onto/near munitions vehicle Severe earthquake causing vehicle accident Tornado-generated missile Tornado-induced vehicle overturn
Rail Transport	Train accident (various severity levels) Aircraft crash onto munitions railcar Severe earthquake causing rail accident Tornado-generated missile Tornado-induced rail accident
Air Transport	Aircraft crash on takeoff, while in flight, or on landing On-board fire
Plant Operations	Tornado-generated missile Meteorite strike Aircraft crash (various severity levels) Earthquake (various severity levels) Excess agent feed to liquid incinerator Furnace explosion due to failure of fuel shut-off Furnace explosion due to feed of unpunched bulk container Fire due to spill of bulk container contents Munition detonation Burstered munition fed to the dunnage incinerator

General Form: XXYZWQnnnS

where: XX = Activity code
Y = Munition code
Z = Agent code
W = Release mode code
Q = Special code defining storage configuration
nnn = Scenario number
S = Site code

Example: POKVC 029N meaning:

"Earthquake damages the MDB (munition demilitarization building); munitions are intact; fire occurs; fire suppression system fails" [plant operations scenario PO 029]. The accident occurs at Newport [N] and involves bulk (ton) containers [K] of agent VX [V] in a complex release model [C].

Fig. 3. Accident scenario ID code.

Table 3. Representative Scenario Descriptions — Plant Operations Only

Scenario ID Code*	Scenario Description
PO___ 001	Tornado-generated missile punctures munitions in the munitions holding igloo (MHI).
PO___ 004	Tornado-generated missile detonates munitions in the unpack area (UPA).
PO___ 006	Meteorite strikes the UPA.
PO___ 010	Direct large aircraft crash onto the MHI results in a fire which is not contained in 0.5 hours.
PO___ 014	Direct large aircraft crash damages the munitions demilitarization building (MDB), causing a fire which is contained in 0.5 hours.
PO___ 023	Earthquake causes munitions in the MHI to fall and be punctured.
PO___ 024	Earthquake causes munitions in the MHI to fall and detonate.
PO___ 026	Earthquake damages the MDB structure, munitions fall and are punctured; a fire is initiated and the fire suppression system fails.
PO___ 041	Failure to stop agent feed to the liquid incinerator overloads the ventilation system.
PO___ 042	Explosion in the metal parts furnace due to failure to stop fuel flow after a shutdown.
PO___ 045	Ton container spills and the building structure fails due to a subsequent fire.
PO___ 048	Munition detonation occurs in the explosion containment vestibule; fire occurs and propagates.
PO___ 049	Munition detonation occurs in the explosion containment room, causing structural and ventilation system damage.
PO___ 051	Ton container spills in processing bay with a fire causing structural failure.
PO___ 052	Burstered munition is fed to the dunnage furnace and detonates.

*Scenarios are defined by the activity code (first two characters of ID code) and the scenario number; individual accidents are the munition and agent-specific variations on the scenario.

Event probability data are based on the site-specific expectation that an event will occur per unit time, per mile, per operation, or per storage unit-year (e.g., per igloo year), as appropriate to the activity type. Converting this unit probability data to a per-munition-stockpile basis for a given site is discussed below.

Dispersion Model

The Army's chemical agent dispersion model, D2PC, is a Gaussian diffusion model.[5] It is available as a compiled FORTRAN code, suitable for use on IBM/PC-compatible computers. It accepts a wide range of input, including munition type, agent type, amount of agent released, release mode, location, meteorological conditions. Its principal output are distances to downwind locations where a specified fatality rate or lethal "dose" can be expected.

Demographic Fatality Data

The Oak Ridge National Laboratory (ORNL) has access to an extensive national demographics data base based on 1980 census. Demographic data combined with predictions for plume contours (constant dose lines) for given meteorological conditions, lead to potential fatalities for a given location, accident size, and meteorological condition. A portion of the fatality data file is displayed in Table 4.

RISK ASSESSMENT APPROACH & METHODOLOGY

The means for combining the hazard data for individual accidents into an assessment of overall risk, as indicated by several risk measures, is outlined next. An overview of the approach is depicted in Fig. 4. The ovals represent the four major data inputs to the risk analysis. These four major data sets are integrated in ways that represent the disposal alternatives defined by the Army to yield the two principal categories of risk (shown on the right side of Fig. 4): Individual risk, describing the probability of an individual at a given distance from a potential accident site receiving a lethal exposure to released agent; and societal risk, describing the probability of there being an accident of given consequence as measured by potential fatalities.

The societal risk, whose consequence is expressed in terms of potential fatalities, is a measure that can be aggregated over the disposal sites and transportation routes as necessary in order to compare the programmatic impact of each alternative.

Risk to the individual is strictly site-specific and is dependent on the aggregate effect of the particular set of accidents that could happen at a given site for a specified disposal alternative.

Some of the key steps and assumptions in the assessment, including the estimation of agent plume size, the assumptions regarding meteorology, the estimation of potential fatalities, and the treatment of accident probability data, are outlined below.

Lethal Plume Size

Lethal plume size was estimated for each event using the results of the Army's D2PC model. Results were presented in a parametric form from which plume sizes could be obtained for the full spectrum of accident scenarios. The dispersion model was used to predict downwind distances to, and arc widths of, the 'no-deaths,' 'one-percent-deaths,' and 'fifty-percent-deaths' dosage boundaries for given meteorological conditions as a function of the following scenario-specific factors: agent type, quantity released, release mode, event duration (based on the emergency response capability at the accident site for a given event),

Table 4. Representative Potential Fatality Data — Selected Fixed Sites

No-Deaths Hazard Distance	Weather and Population Density*	Potential Fatalities at Stockpile Sites			
		ANAD	APG	LBAD	TEAD
1	Extreme	0.2	44	0.2	0
2		0.4	83	0.6	0
5		3	276	19	0.2
10		57	835	469	0.4
20		1439	2294	1801	2
50		4986	42007	6570	1072
100		10731	120185	18640	19812
1	Average	0	2	0	0
2		0.2	6	0.1	0
5		2	54	7	0.2
10		53	219	112	0.6
20		508	909	335	2
50		2393	10186	1901	116
100		7483	38715	5350	4722

*Average = Most-likely weather and azimuthally-averaged population
Extreme = Worst-case weather and wind direction over actual population distribution.

Data Source: ORNL (U.S. Army, 1988).

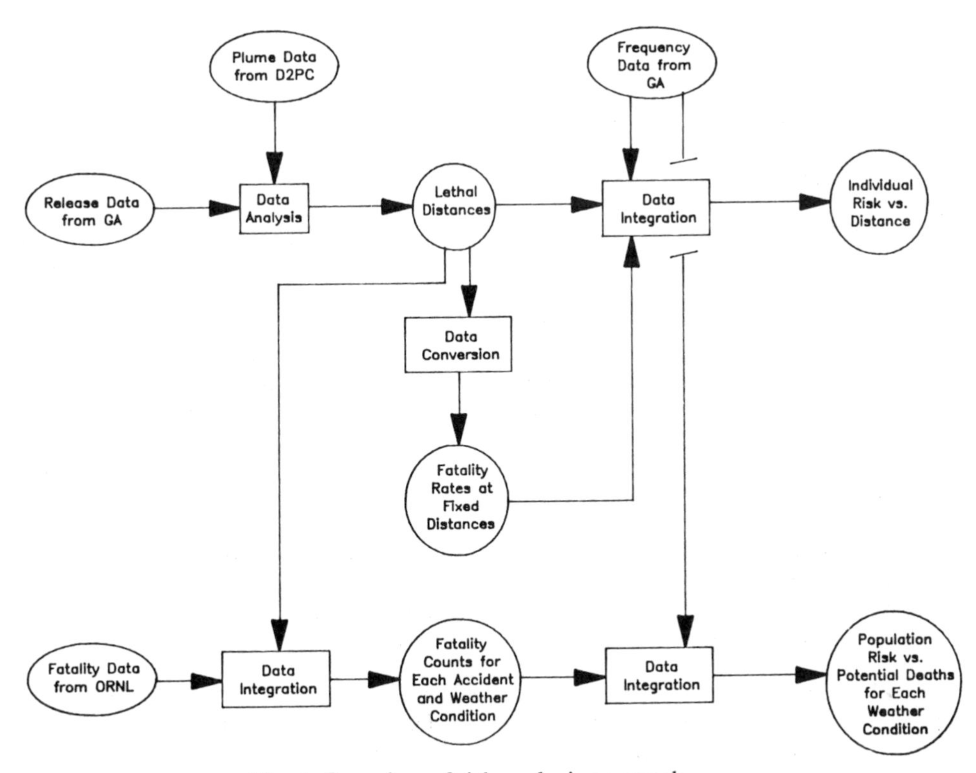

Fig. 4. Overview of risk analysis approach.

surface type (gravel or non-porous), and spill area, if special conditions pertain to limit puddle size for spill releases.

More details on the determination of plume size and representative lethal plume data are presented in the description of the D2PC model[5] and in the report of the CSDP risk analysis.[6]

Meteorological Conditions

Specific meteorological conditions were assumed for the agent dispersion calculations. The critical meteorological parameters are presented in Table 5. Most-likely meteorological conditions represent non-site-specific averages which account for the full ranges of actual conditions and, hence, are appropriate for obtaining best estimates of the expected public health impacts of accidental agent releases. Worst-case meteorological conditions were selected for use in obtaining upper bound estimates of public health impacts. A stability class of E (a stable or inversion condition) was employed, since the extreme stability class of F was judged to be characterized by light meandering breezes such that the resulting downwind agent exposures would be only intermittent. A very low worst-case wind speed of one m/sec was selected, as was a high worst-case temperature of 30°C.

Potential Fatality Estimates

The use of the term "potential" refers to the lack of quantification of the preservation of lives that would result from preplanned emergency response measures that would be implemented by the U.S. Army and cooperating agencies. For example, no credit was taken for evacuation, or even for the protection afforded by remaining indoors. Thus, actual fatalities are likely to be less than the calculated potential fatalities for most cases.

Potential fatality counts were computed by Oak Ridge National Laboratory as functions of accident location (any of the eight agent storage sites in the CONUS, and locations along the proposed 11 rail routes and two air routes), lethal downwind distance (to the 0 percent fatality, or 'no-deaths' dose), and meteorological conditions. Data were generated for a set of uniform 'no-deaths' distance values: 0.1, 0.2, 0.5, 1, 2, 5, 10, 20, 50, 100, 200, 500, 1000 km. The 'no-deaths' distances obtained using the D2PC model were used to determine which of the ORNL fatality counts was applicable for a given accident at a specified location. When 'no-deaths' distances were intermediate between the uniform distance values defined above, we used the next higher uniform distance in order to select a fatality count. Since some of these 'no-deaths' distances were expected to exceed 100 km, the standard distances were extended to include 200, 500 and 1,000 km. However, although the releases resulting in these longer distances resulted in higher fatality rates within 100 kilometers, no fatalities occurring beyond 100 km were counted by ORNL. Furthermore, in no case was a fatality count used that would correspond to a 'no-deaths' distance exceeding 1,000 km. The data in Table 4 illustrate the results of this computation.

The ORNL fatality counts based on most-likely meteorological conditions and average population density (within any given ring for which the inner and outer radii are defined by adjacent uniform downwind distance values) about an accident site were used to develop probabilities of fatal accidents, expected fatality values, and risk curves.

The ORNL fatality counts based on worst-case meteorological conditions, actual population distribution, and worst-case (highest fatality count) wind direction were used only to estimate the upper limits of numbers of fatalities (i.e., maximum fatalities).

Table 5. Major Meteorological Assumptions

Meteorological Parameters	Worst-Case Weather (WC)	Most-Likely Weather (ML)
Atmospheric Stability Class	E	D
Wind Speed [m/s]	1	3
Temperature [deg. C]	30	20
Mixing Layer Height [m]	750	750

Probability Analysis

The frequency or probability data, expressed in units appropriate to the particular activity type (e.g., events per train-mile or events per year of processing) need conversion in order that they relate to the entire munition stockpile at a specific site. The computational algorithms for combining the unit probability data with other global and site-specific data to yield stockpile probability data are illustrated in Fig. 5. The probability estimates, as provided by General Atomics, represented median values for a presumed log-normal distribution. The width of the distribution was given by a range factor assigned to each probability value; the range factor is the ratio of the 95 percentile value to the mean value. Range factors were used in the estimation of uncertainty, as discussed below.

The Computation of Risk

If the set of accident scenarios which contribute to the risk for a given disposal alternative at a given location or site are sorted in decreasing order of consequence, and the probability values for each accident are added cumulatively beginning with the highest consequence accident, then the resulting vectors, potential fatalities and cumulative probability, will define the societal or community complementary cumulative risk curve (hereafter referred to as, simply, "risk curve") for the alternative and location. If the accident scenarios applicable to all locations are combined into one data set, then the resulting risk curve is the programmatic risk curve for the alternative. A representative risk curve is shown in Fig. 6.

For the estimation of individual risk, a different approach is required. For each applicable accident scenario, the probability of an individual's death at a given distance from the site of the agent release is estimated as the product of three terms: (1) the probability of the event occurring; (2) the probability of an individual being within the plume, given a uniform wind-rose (equal to the ratio of plume width to the perimeter of the circle designating the individual's given distance from the release site); and (3) the fatality rate associated with the centerline dosage within the plume at a given distance from the release site. This product, determined for the fixed distance increments of 0.1, 0.2, 0.5, 1.0, 2.0, etc. out to 100 km, is then summed for each distance value for all applicable potential accidents. The result is an individual risk curve, defining the probability of an individuals' death as a function of distance from the site. A representative individual risk curve is also shown in Fig. 6. For individuals living along a transportation corridor, a separate approach, illustrated in Fig. 7, had to be used.

Several aggregate measures of public risk, each providing a different perspective on overall program risk, were estimated; each is illustrated in Fig. 6 and defined in the text following.

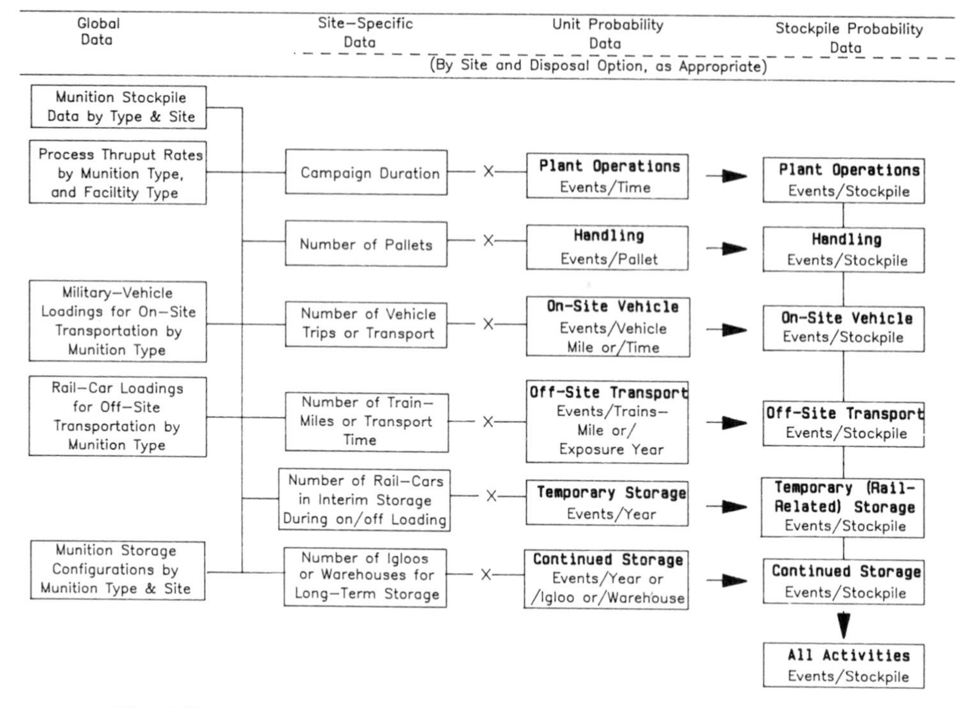

Fig. 5. Procedure for estimating accident probability (events/stockpile).

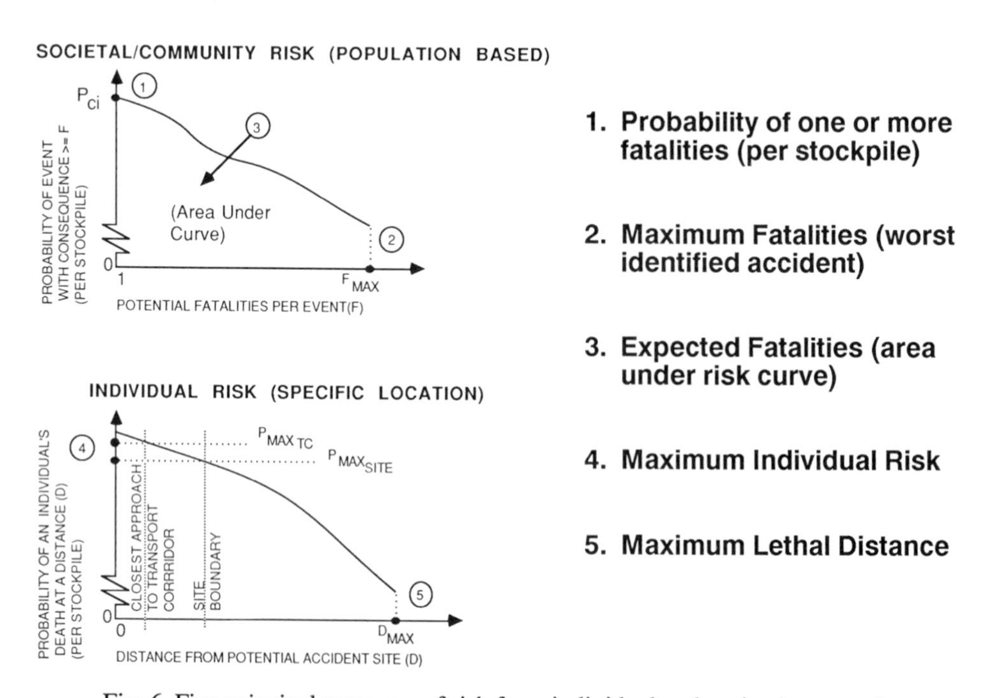

Fig. 6. Five principal measures of risk from individual and societal perspectives.

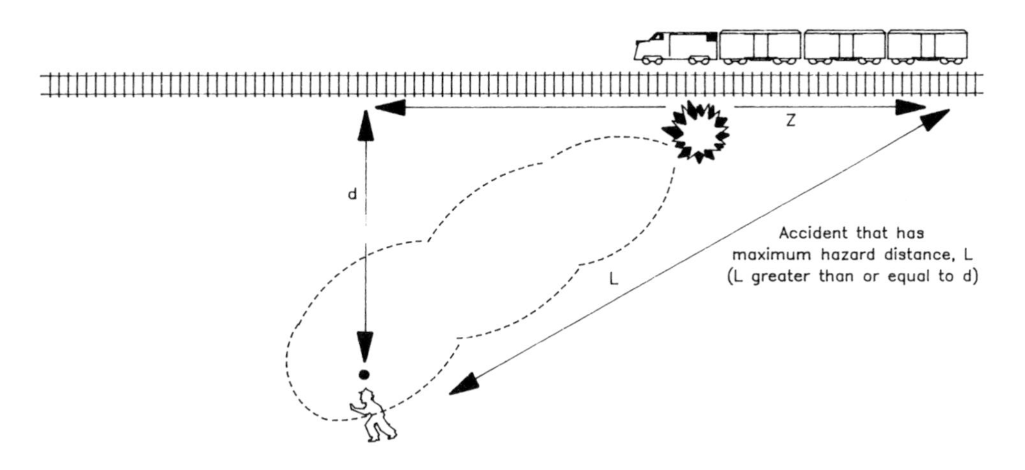

- Estimation of risk due to that accident takes into account the occurrence anywhere within track length, 2 x Z
- Total individual risk is the sum of risks due to all accidents that can result in hazard distances greater than individual's distance from track

Fig. 7. Estimation of individual risk along a transportation corridor.

Probability of one or more fatalities is a public risk indicator equal to the chance that there will be at least one fatality at a given site or for the nation as a whole during the CSDP. This measure is calculated by summing the probabilities of all accidents that could cause one or more fatalities. Included in this sum are all accidents for which the potential fatality estimate, based on assuming uniform population densities, is less than unity. (This means that that accident is expected to cause a fatality for only a fraction of the times it occurs; for the remaining fraction of occurrences, that event would not cause a fatality. For such accidents, the probability of occurrence is reduced so that only the fraction of events expected to cause a fatality are counted).

Maximum number of fatalities is equal to the maximum consequence of all accidents at a site or for the nation. This risk measure is based on worst-case weather conditions, actual population densities, and worst possible wind direction (i.e., plume striking the highest number of people without any allowance for preventive/emergency response measures).

Expected fatalities is equal to the sum of the risk contribution of all accidents at a site or for the nation, where risk for each accident is the potential fatality count (if the accident were to occur) multiplied by the probability of the accident occurring. At the programmatic level, the expected fatalities value is the sum of the expected fatality contribution of several hundreds of potential events and might lie somewhere around 0.001. This typical value can be interpreted in the following way: The program can be expected to cause, on average, one fatality every 1000 times the program is executed. Since the program consists of many events which could cause multiple fatalities, a more typical interpretation would be made up of several parts, such as one fatality every 10,000 programs (expected fatality contribution of 1/10,000 = 0.0001) plus a 10-fatality event every 25,000 programs (contribution of 10/25,000 = 0.0004) plus a 100-fatality event every 200,000 programs (contributing 100/200,000 = 0.0005), for a total expected fatality value of 0.001.

Maximum individual risk is equal to the probability of a fatal exposure at the site boundary (assumed to be 0.5 km from the on-site disposal/storage operations) or as close as

0.1 km to the centerline of a transportation corridor. This indicator is equal to the vertical intercept of the individual risk curve at the appropriate distance value (0.5 or 0.1 km); it is dependent only on the mix of potential accidents that could happen at the individual's location and, since it applies only to an individual, is independent of population density.

Maximum lethal distance is equal to the maximum downwind length (given by the 'no-deaths' dose) of the plume from the worst of all identified potential accidents under worst-case weather conditions at a specific location. Conversely, it is also the minimum distance an individual could be from a given site or transportation corridor and have no risk of lethal exposure during the disposal program. It is equal to the horizontal intercept of the individual risk curve at some minimum accepted level of credibility — say, 1×10^{-10} per stockpile.

In addition, two time-dependent risk measures were defined.

Maximum total time at risk represents the maximum length of time an individual could be at risk at a fixed location near a site or along a transportation corridor. For those living within a radius equal to or less than the maximum lethal hazard distance, the time at risk is the total time during which stockpile disposal activities will take place at that site, regardless of where the individual is located. For those individuals along the transportation corridors, the time depends on the distance from the rail line or air corridor; the maximum time is assumed to occur if the individual is located at a 0.1 km distance from the rail track or centerline of the air corridor. These persons are exposed to a hazard only when a train or aircraft is in the vicinity (defined as the maximum lethal hazard distance in either direction) of them. This time is summed for each agent-bearing train or aircraft that would pass by in each alternative. Since maximum lethal hazard distance is used in this determination, the worst-case meteorological conditions apply. The probabilistic measures of individual risk are preferred over this time-based measure because the former contains more information, accounting for relative magnitude and probability of occurrence of all contributing accidents. However, maximum time-at-risk is the only risk measure appropriate to the question in the mind of that potentially affected individual who asks: "For how long must I and my family be away from home if we will accept no additional risk at all from the program?"

Person-years-at-risk is equal to the population living within all zones that could experience potentially lethal agent exposure multiplied by the time period over which that worst-case event could take place (typically, the duration of disposal operations at fixed sites or the time during which transport vehicles might be within lethal plume reach of population groups along the corridors). This measure does not account for the fact that individuals within the affected population groups who are farther from the potential accident site are at lower risk of suffering ill effects of exposure; all affected individuals are counted if they have any risk at all.

Uncertainty Analysis

Uncertainties in risk estimation arise due to many causes, including the inadequacy of data, inaccuracies in modeling, and the incomplete identification and understanding of accident phenomena. The risk analysis methodology provides for the treatment of uncertainty in the basic hazard data that goes into the analysis. Uncertainty arises in the estimation of both probability and consequences. The uncertainty analysis discussed herein considers probability uncertainty only. The contribution to risk uncertainty of consequence estimation (i.e., estimation of fatalities as a result of an agent release) is represented separately (though incompletely) by considering most-likely and worst-case meteorological conditions.

RISK ANALYSIS RESULTS

Risk Portrayal Options

Risk is portrayed in this analysis using the following:

- Risk curves, which portray, for the full set of applicable accident scenarios, the probability of exceeding a given number of potential fatalities per event (vertical axis), against the potential fatalities per event (horizontal axis);
- Risk pictograms, which provide a pictorial indication (the darkness of the shading) of the relative magnitude of each of the measures of risk along with a key to the numerical range represented by each of the four shading categories; and
- Expected fatalities plots, showing mean estimated values of expected fatalities, with uncertainty bands.

Representative Results

Below are representative samples of the results of the risk analyses that were performed in support of the FPEIS.

Figure 8 is a pictogram of the comparative risk for the five major CSDP alternatives at a programmatic level — i.e., all locations combined. Risk is displayed in terms of four major health risk measures and the expected value of the plume area which is an ecological risk indicator. Higher risk is connoted by darker shading. The shading assigned to any entry in the pictograms is defined by the mean value of the risk measure relative to the numerical boundaries of the ranges. Differences in shading should not be interpreted as defining a statistically significant difference in risk.

Risk curves for three CSDP alternatives — continued storage, on-site disposal, and regional disposal — are compared in Fig. 9. The risk curves indicate the probability that an accident having a consequence equal to or greater than the number of fatalities given by the horizontal scale will occur during the course of the disposal program.

Uncertainty bounds are not shown, because the purpose of the figure is to illustrate the difference in character and shape of the risk curves for these three representative disposal alternatives.

In Fig. 10, the five disposal alternatives are compared on the basis of risk, as measured by expected fatalities (equivalent to the area under a linear plot of the respective risk curves). For each alternative, the upper and lower bounds on the mean values for expected fatalities are also shown to demonstrate graphically the importance of uncertainty considerations in making risk comparisons.

Risk Data Ranges for Major Risk Measures

Although not evident in the graphical displays presented above, quantitative data on each of the risk measures for each CSDP alternative and for each location involved in the program (storage/disposal sites and transportation corridors) are available as an output of the risk analysis method.

Analysis of the actual quantitative risk data leads to the following summaries for each of the major risk parameters.

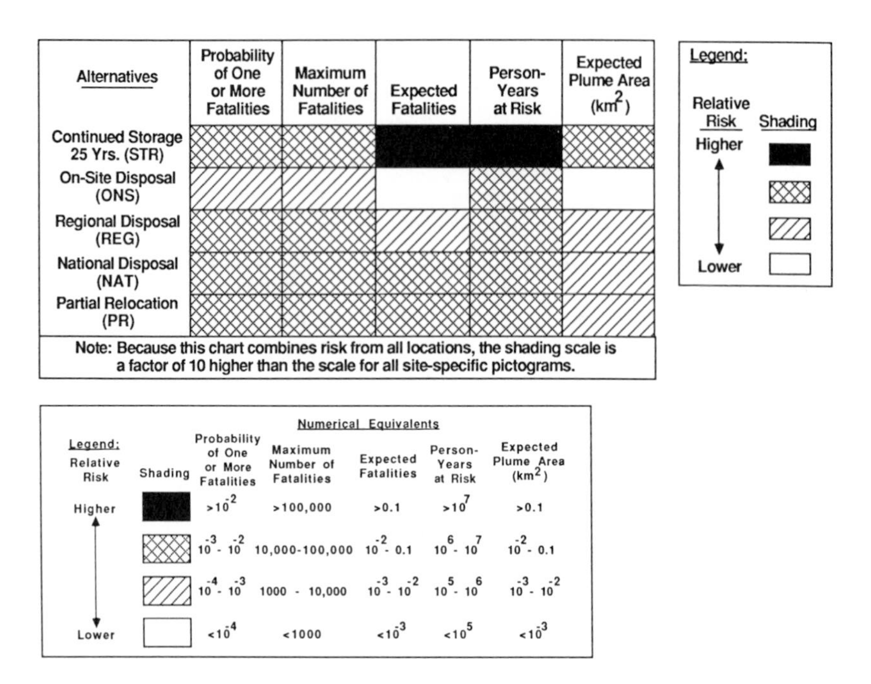

Numerical Equivalents

Legend: Relative Risk	Shading	Probability of One or More Fatalities	Maximum Number of Fatalities	Expected Fatalities	Person-Years at Risk	Expected Plume Area (km^2)
Higher		$>10^{-2}$	>100,000	>0.1	$>10^{7}$	>0.1
		10^{-3} - 10^{-2}	10,000-100,000	10^{-2} - 0.1	10^{6} - 10^{7}	10^{-2} - 0.1
		10^{-4} - 10^{-3}	1000 - 10,000	10^{-3} - 10^{-2}	10^{5} - 10^{6}	10^{-3} - 10^{-2}
Lower		$<10^{-4}$	<1000	$<10^{-3}$	$<10^{5}$	$<10^{-3}$

Fig. 8. Pictogram portrayal of five risk measures for all programmatic alternatives.

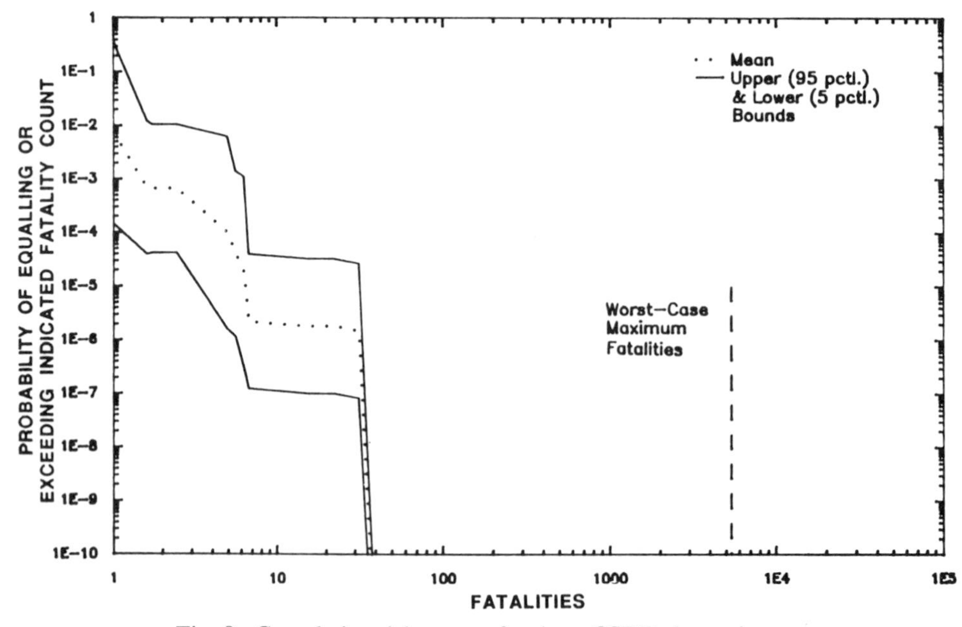

Fig. 9. Cumulative risk curves for three CSDP alternatives.

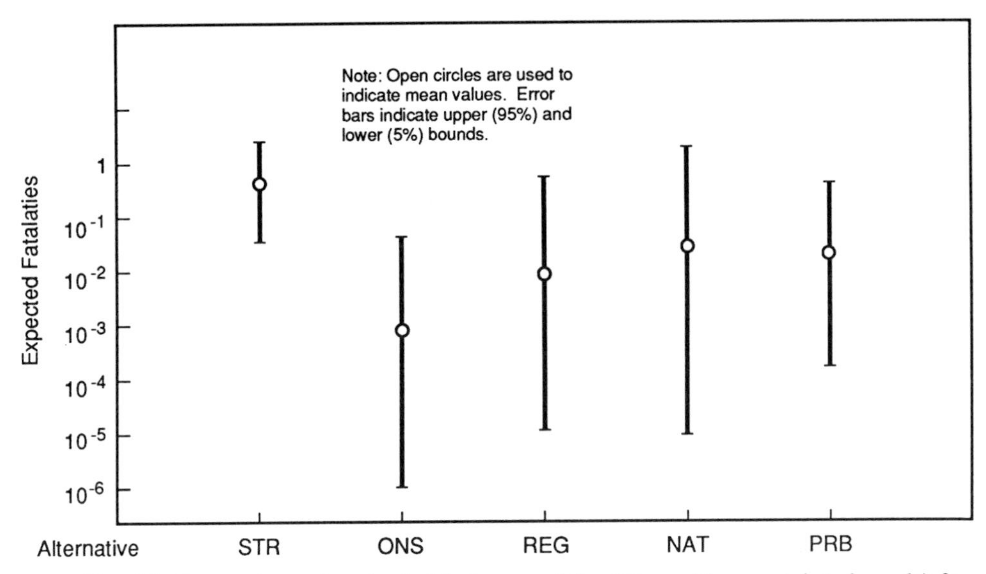

Fig. 10. Comparison of societal risk (expected fatalities, with uncertainty bounds) for five programmatic alternatives.

The probability of one or more fatalities falls within a narrow range — 0.0003 to 0.003 — for all alternatives, with on-site disposal having the lowest value. This means there is a chance of about 1-in-1000 that the CSDP will result in at least one fatality.

The maximum number of fatalities of the five FPEIS alternatives ranges between approximately 5,000 and 90,000, with continued storage having the greatest number and on-site disposal having the least.

Expected fatalities ranges from a low of less than 0.001 for on-site disposal to nearly 0.5 for 25 years of continued storage.

OBSERVATIONS AND RECOMMENDATIONS

The presentation of risk to a general audience is not an easy matter. What may be obvious to the risk analyst is by no means so to an audience not conditioned to think in terms of probabilistic descriptions of reality. Risk analysis, by its very nature must deal with the unknown; analysts are usually faced with the task of making predictions of future relative safety of complex systems on the basis of extrapolations of limited and, often, non-existing data. Risk is often dominated by very severe consequence but highly improbable events. Risk analysis must, therefore, be carried out with due respect for the inherent uncertainty in the base of relevant data and associated predictive models. Similarly, the risk analyst must be conscious of the difficulty the general public will have in accepting and/or interpreting the predictions of risk where the potential consequences are well beyond anyone's experience and the probabilities are too low to be easily comprehended.

By way of guidelines that may be of value to others faced with the need to carry out and present the results of a risk assessment, the following are offered:

1. *Know your audience.* Be sure that the level of detail in both the execution and the presentation of the risk analysis matches the needs of the audience. The risk manager will want a risk-ranked detailed listing of individual potential events. The

community leaders will want to know the societal impact on their locality and how it compares with risk imposed elsewhere, and may be best satisfied with credible graphical presentations such as the use of the pictogram. The risk analyst will appreciate best the cumulative risk curves and the presentation of uncertainty data. The program director who may have to chose between alternatives on the basis of relative risk may be most responsive to the risk curve and to the other risk measures that display expected values of risk according to the areas of interest (e.g., by site).

2. *Display the uncertainty.* A risk analysis which does not clearly indicate the level of uncertainty inherent in the process, whether due to data inadequacy, level of completeness, or methodology limitations, will lack for credibility and, more importantly, may be taken for more than it really is: a quantitative approximation of the public safety impact of a program or other set of activities. Deterministic comparisons of program alternatives without consideration of uncertainty can lead to the mistaken belief that one alternative is definitely less risky than another.

3. *Where public safety is involved, use expected fatalities as the preferred measure of risk.* Expected fatalities, while it may have an ominous label, is the most useful measure of societal risk because it best accounts for the consequences as experienced by the local affected population and because it reflects the estimated probability of occurrence of lethal events. Other measures, such as maximum hazard distance, may be used to supplement the portrayal and interpretation of risk, but they should not become the principal measure of risk.

4. *Avoid comparisons between voluntary and involuntary risk.* Although the risk analyst might be tempted to calibrate the magnitude of risk of an imposed program (representing an involuntary exposure to risk) by comparing the risk with the levels of risk the public might routinely accept (voluntary exposure to risk) in return for the benefits offered, the comparison should be avoided. The general public usually perceives involuntary risk as being in a completely different category, and not an appropriate basis for comparison with the risk of a government program over which the individual has no control.

5. *Include consideration of individual risk.* Some members of the public in the vicinity of a facility or transportation corridor are going to insist on knowing what impact the potentially risky program could have on their personal risk, no matter how many other members of the public might be affected or how severely. Individual risk computations will enable officials to answer such inquiries. Individual risk estimation will also enable the program manager to determine whether or not an acceptable level of societal/community risk arises at the expense of high risk borne by a relatively few people. Risk management/mitigation efforts which lead to reductions in societal risk by reducing the number of individuals affected could entail higher risk (e.g., through higher accident probability) for individuals closer to the site boundary or transportation corridor.

REFERENCES

1. U.S. Army Program Executive Office — Program Manager for Chemical Demilitarization, Chemical Stockpile Disposal Program, Final Programmatic Environmental Impact Statement, January 1988.
2. GA Technologies Inc., Risk Analysis of the Onsite Disposal of Chemical Munitions, GA-C18562, prepared for the U.S. Army, Office of the Program Executive Officer — Program Manager for Chemical Demilitarization, SAPEO-CDE-IS-87010, August 1987.

3. GA Technologies Inc., Risk Analysis of the Disposal of Chemical Munitions at National or Regional Sites, GA-C18563, prepared for the U.S. Army, Office of the Program Executive Officer — Program Manager for Chemical Demilitarization, SAPEO-CDE-IS-87008, August 1987.
4. GA Technologies Inc., Risk Analysis of the Continued Storage of Chemical Munitions, GA-C18564, prepared for the U.S. Army, Office of the Program Executive Officer — Program Manager for Chemical Demilitarization, SAPEO-CDE-IS-87009, August 1987.
5. C. G. Whitacre *et al.*, Personal Computer Program for Chemical Hazard Prediction, CRDEC-TR-87021, Aberdeen Proving Ground, MD: Chemical Research, Development & Engineering Center (1987).
6. U.S. Army Program Executive Office — Program Manager for Chemical Demilitarization, Risk Analysis in Support of the Chemical Stockpile Disposal Program, MTR87W00230, The MITRE Corporation, SAPEO-CDE-IS-87014, December 1987.

Municipal Solid Waste Management: Evaluating the Alternatives

Michael Marchlik
Ebasco Services, Inc.
New York, NY

Steven Anderson
Roy F. Weston, Inc.
West Chester, PA

ABSTRACT

The potential health risks from municipal solid waste (MSW) incineration have been the subject of an ongoing debate over MSW management strategies in the face of diminishing landfill space. Local citizen groups have successfully lobbied against proposed MSW incinerators by focusing on the uncertain health impacts from these facilities. This paper presents a more structured approach for evaluating waste management options by examining the currently available MSW management alternatives such as landfilling, recycling, and incineration, and exploring the impacts these technologies have on the community. These impacts include human health risks, ecosystem risks, economic considerations, and land use issues. The authors examine the generic application of multiattribute decision analysis techniques for the selection of an effective MSW management strategy, and the obstacles to employing such an approach to community decision making in an uncertain environment.

KEYWORDS: Municipal solid waste (MSW), multiattribute utility (MAU) analysis, incineration, landfills, public participation

INTRODUCTION

In 1985 it was estimated that Americans disposed of 250 million tons of garbage with that rate projected to increase at an annual rate of two to three percent.[1] Currently 95 percent of this refuse is landfilled. With landfill sites being filled to capacity, or closed because they violate environmental regulations, the need to address the solid waste crisis is apparent. This is further complicated when one considers that well-designed and engineered sanitary landfills will continue to remain the principal means of municipal waste disposal for the foreseeable future, despite an increasingly limited number of viable sites.

In view of the known or anticipated hazards to the environment and public health from landfilling municipal solid waste, along with the pending shortage of permitted landfills and escalating costs of operating landfills, other disposal options are being considered. Source separation, recycling, combustion, and beneficial use of ash residues are

Risk Analysis, Edited by C. Zervos
Plenum Press, New York, 1991

being evaluated and implemented as important components of municipal solid waste management plans. However, in order to select/implement from these various solid waste disposal options, the solid waste management authority, the regulatory agencies, and the public must be assured that the alternatives to landfilling are environmentally acceptable.

MANAGING THE CRISIS

This paper presents a decision framework for municipal solid waste management that relies on advanced planning to enumerate and evaluates multiple strategies, and which incorporates public participation throughout the evaluation process. There has been considerable opposition in a number of communities to the construction and operation of incinerators. Regardless of the technical merits of the arguments against these projects, this opposition has revealed considerable weaknesses in the traditional approach to managing municipal solid waste.

This traditional approach has been characterized by the selection and siting of landfills and incinerators by a local officials without any significant effort to involve the public in the decision making. In many cases involving mass burn incineration, local officials have been perceived as conspiring with the firm constructing the plant. Given a heightened public concern about the risk from hazardous materials and a populist bias against large, technically complicated projects, this perception has served to fuel public opposition to such projects.

Organized opposition to mass burn incineration has focused on the uncertain health risks of these facilities and the problem of disposing of potentially hazardous ash. Local officials do not gain respect when they brush off these concerns or reject suggested alternatives without giving them due consideration. There are a number of sociological and psychological factors contributing to this situation, and an explanation of this phenomenon is beyond the scope of this paper. What is obvious, however, is the need for a closer working relationship between the officials in charge of the problem and the community which they represent.

This paper presents an analytic decision framework that addresses this problem. It calls for a working group of officials and citizens that will enumerate and evaluate all potential municipal solid waste management strategies to arrive at an optimal waste management solution. This framework, outlined in Fig. 1, proceeds logically from a definition of the waste management needs through an evaluation of feasible alternatives to the selection of an optimal strategy. Each step in this process is discussed in the following sections.

PUBLIC PARTICIPATION

Participation of the public in managing solid waste can occur in one of two ways. The government agency responsible for making waste management decisions can solicit public involvement through public meetings or citizen advisory groups prior to making a final decision, or the agency can wait to solicit public input at formal hearings, possibly after the decision has been made. The second route to public participation is too often practiced, and it has resulted in establishing a combative atmosphere which can lead to long delays in the permitting and construction of needed projects.

The management framework set forth in this paper relies on active public participation throughout the entire decision making process. A number of authors have presented successful models for public participation in the waste management process. Our

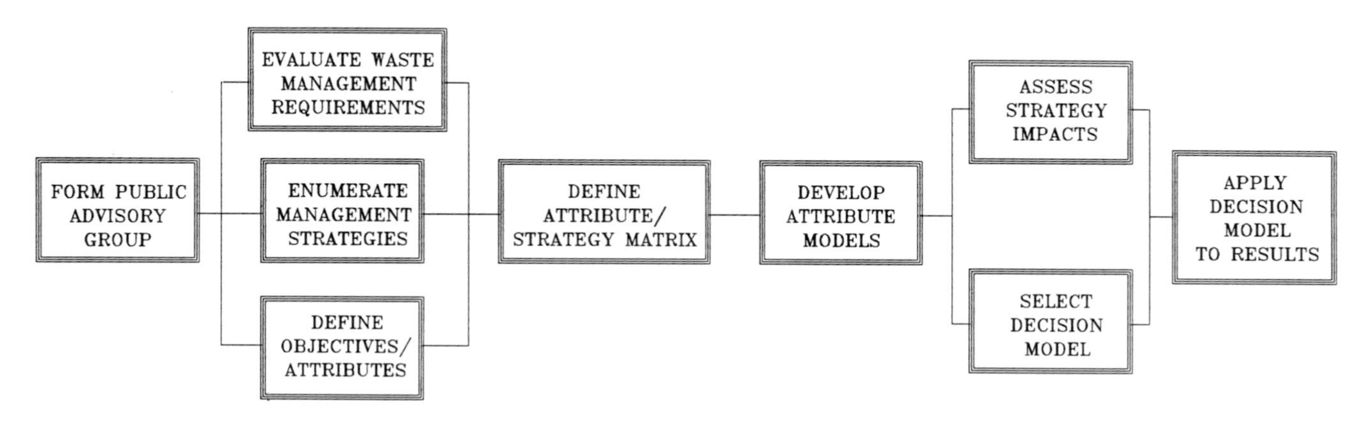

Fig. 1. Decision framework for managing municipal solid waste.

purpose in this paper is to present a more structured process by which a team of public officials, citizens, and consultants can evaluate and select the waste management strategy.

WASTE MANAGEMENT NEEDS

Planning for future waste management involves demographic projections and land use plans to evaluate the volume and composition of municipal solid waste. The techniques used for this evaluation are not addressed in this paper except to suggest improvements that are useful in the evaluation of waste management strategies. In commissioning these studies and presenting the results, it is desirable to identify key assumptions about the growth projections underlying the estimated waste disposal requirements.

In addition to identifying these assumptions, it is useful to examine alternative growth projections. When considering measures such as source separation or a ban on certain types of containers, it is helpful to be able to calculate the impact these alternatives have on waste generation by going back to the initial analysis of the waste management needs. The analysis, assumptions, and results should be presented in a manner that is readily understood.

ENUMERATION OF TECHNOLOGIES

The decision regarding final disposal/management of municipal solid waste is no longer just a decision of where to landfill. There are a multitude of alternative methods of disposal. Possible disposal alternatives include, but are not limited to landfilling, recycling, waste reduction, incineration (mass burn; RDF), ocean dumping, and composting. Many of these alternative methods can be combined into an integrated system for municipal solid waste management. New legislative mandates, such as recycling laws in Florida and New Jersey, are shaping the future direction of municipal solid waste management. There appears to be interest in composting, but at present the ultimate viability of this alternative is not clear. Resource recovery after incineration is still viable; however, the ash disposal issue is receiving ever increasing attention. A more detailed discussion of resource recovery is presented in the following subsection.

What does seem reasonable to expect in the future is a definite need to have an overall management strategy for municipal solid waste management. The ever changing regulatory environment will not allow anything else.

Resource Recovery

Concerns for the environment are not limited to detrimental effects of pollution, they also include recovery and utilization of resources recognized as finite, namely energy and fuels. Resource recovery possibilities have become apparent when one considers the economics associated with hauling off wastes for disposal. Resource recovery promise a

- contribution to energy supplies, and
- mitigation of adverse environmental effects associated with waste disposal.

Historically, industrial application of incineration technology involving energy recovery has concentrated on hazardous material and waste destruction. More recently, incineration technology has incorporated high heat recovery efficiency for cogeneration of steam to supply process needs or generate electricity. Various technologies considered applicable for energy recovery from municipal refuse were reported by Cheremisinoff.[2] These are presented in Table 1.

Table 1. Municipal Refuse Energy Recovery Technologies

Direct Combustion of MSW

- Modular incinerator
- Waterwall moving-grate boiler
- Waterwall rotary combustor-boiler

Refuse Derived Fuel (RDF) Preparation and Combustion

- Semisuspension-fired waterwall boiler
- Fluidized bed combustion
- Cofiring with coal in a utility boiler

Gasification/Pyrolysis

- Fixed bed
- Fluidized bed

Anaerobic

- Landfill gas recovery
- Anaerobic digestion
- Enzymatic hydrolysis

Pyrolysis and Gasification

Biological Processing

Adapted from Cheremisinoff.[2]

Kidder, Peabody, and Company[1] reported that there were 74 resource recovery units operating in the U.S. with a processing capacity of 34,744 tons per day (T/D). They identified 34 units (23,744 T/D) under construction, plans for 61 plants with capacity of 65,400 T/D and plans for 50 additional plants without a definite capacity rating. The companies surveyed by Kidder, Peabody, and Company expressed "universal frustration with the permitting processes which precede ground breaking for a plant." This "dead" time of an uncertain duration was viewed as an impediment to pricing contracts and as a factor in the riskiness of a resource recovery venture.

IMPACTS ANALYSIS

Statement of Objectives

As a list of feasible strategies are being enumerated to address the solid waste disposal requirements, a similar effort should be directed towards identifying the impacts that each technology has on the community. This list should be developed by the waste management committee and should start with a statement of objectives. The objective of a waste management strategy should be to ensure adequate disposal of current and future municipal solid waste streams in a manner that minimizes impacts on the health and well being of the community.

Attribute Selection

In order to measure how well a strategy meets this goal, it is necessary to define a number of attributes. These attributes will become the cornerstone of the decision process and should be selected with care. A well defined set of attributes is one which is "comprehensive" and "measurable." Comprehensive attributes are those which clearly identify the extent to which an objective has been met. Attributes are measurable if the alternatives can be assigned a value or range of values over the possible levels of the attributes and if preferences can be assigned for various levels of the attribute.

When an objective is nebulously described as minimizing the impacts on the "well being" of a community, it is often useful to reword the descriptive to be more specific. "Well being" could be replaced with a list of related objectives such as minimizing degradation of the environment, minimizing interference with existing and future land use patterns, minimizing traffic congestion, and other related objectives. When objectives are more focused, it easier to develop a list of corresponding attributes.

Table 2 contains a sample list of objectives and corresponding attributes. Once such a list is compiled, units of measure should be assigned to each attribute.

Define Attribute/Strategy Matrix

Once lists of attributes and strategies have been developed, it is informative to organize these lists in a matrix format to identify the attributes impacted by each strategy. Since a single strategy may involve several options, the cross matrix should reflect the impacts from each element of a strategy. This step is not necessary, but it results in a more organized analysis that can be referred to for a quick overview of what went into the decision process.

Estimating Impacts

Once the problem is defined, a thorough investigation should be made of each option and its impact on the appropriate attributes. This is begun with a definition of models relating each option to a measurable attribute. For some attributes such as cancer risk, this may entail the application of detailed environmental transport and dose response models.

Two concerns should be addressed in this stage of the analysis. First, the task of model development often requires that assumptions be made to simplify the analysis or to deal with a lack of adequate data. This process is acceptable as long as these assumptions are made known to the decision makers and their input is obtained in making these assumptions. In some cases, it is advisable to run the model with alternative assumptions to measure the change in the model output.

Similarly, some data such as dioxin emission rates are uncertain and are often at the center of controversies surrounding the health risk analysis. For these instances, the good alternative is to perform a sensitivity analysis using ranges of input data in order to generate a distribution of outputs. In any case, whenever the analyst makes decisions regarding the selection of input values to a model, these decisions should be brought to the attention of the decision maker.

A second concern in estimating attribute impacts is consistency between the models. Economic models of the various alternatives may be very different, and to compare the impacts of the alternatives requires that comparable accounting methods and parameters such as inflation rates and interest rates be used between the models. This consistency between models is required to insure that attribute impacts are comparable.

Table 2. Sample List of Objectives and Attributes

Objective:	Minimize risk to public health
Attributes:	Number of excess cancers; number of acute illnesses; number of accidental deaths or injuries
Objective:	Minimize effects on the environment
Attributes:	Amount of contaminants released to the air; amount of contaminants released to surface water; drinking water quality; degradation of wilderness/wildlife areas; decreased visibility; occurrence of noxious odors
Objectives:	Minimize financial costs
Attribute:	Cost per ton of refuse disposed; change in local tax revenues; change in the number of local jobs

Since the waste management strategies being examined may consist of mixed technologies, the component of each strategy should be analyzed and the results summed by strategy. For example, one strategy might be continued landfilling while another strategy combines source separation, incineration of the nonrecyclable waste and landfilling of the ash. For the first option, only the impacts of landfilling the entire volume of waste would be examined. In the second strategy, the impacts of all three technologies would need to be estimated and summed.

DECISION MAKING

Once each strategy has been adequately evaluated with respect to each attribute, it is possible to begin the process of selecting an optimal waste management strategy. Techniques such as benefit cost analysis, multiattribute utility (MAU) analysis, and analytical hierarchy process have been applied to select from alternatives in public policy settings. This section will discuss some of the advantages and disadvantages to each method and will discuss some of the generic problems associated with the application of decision analysis techniques in a group setting involving public participation.

With benefit cost analysis, each attribute is categorized as a cost or benefit. Valuation factors are then derived to convert all costs and benefits into dollars. Derivation of these valuation factors can be difficult and may limit the application of benefit cost analysis if there is disagreement over the values assigned to such attributes as affects on human health. Such monetary conversion factors can be controversial, especially in a diverse group setting.

The application of benefit cost analysis also assumes that the decision makers' preferences over the range in attribute values is a simple linear function. Another limiting assumption of benefit cost analysis is that the decision maker assesses his or her preferences one attribute at a time without considering trade-offs between the values of the other attributes. These trade-offs are captured entirely by valuation factors. These theoretical concerns may seem trivial, but in fact they are important in the ability to develop a decision model that yields sensible results. An advantage of benefit cost analysis is that it is possible to combine multiple attribute scores into a single measure that can be rank ordered, simplifying the task of picking the optimal strategy. Once the valuation factors are selected by the group; the results are easily obtained and can be easily presented to others for review.

MAU analysis is a decision analysis technique developed for situations involving a number of attributes with conflicting objectives. The application of this technique relies on explicitly assessing the decision makers' preferences and risk attitudes in a quantitative manner. This process can be quite complex and difficult to apply, especially in a group environment, however, it will allow decision makers to define a fairly complex decision model not afforded by other techniques.

MAU requires that utility preference curves be derived for each attribute over the range of values for each. This permits the decision makers to express their relative preferences, either linear of nonlinear, over a range of attribute impacts, a significant refinement over benefit cost analysis. MAU also permits the decision makers to exhibit nonlinear preferences between attributes; though to do so is an complicated process. One of the greatest problems with the use of MAU is that there are few analysts with the skill to apply this technique in the proper manner. Often the technique is reduced to the simple application of weighting factors assigned to each attribute, multiplied by the attribute value for a strategy and summed across all attributes. Such simplifications ignore the body of research regarding the elicitation of preferences and trade-offs.

The analytical hierarchy process (AHP) is a variation on MAU which does not explicitly evaluate and quantify the preferences of the decision makers. In practice, therefore, it is much easier to apply than MAU and yields comparable results. The selection of an optimal strategy is accomplished by asking the decision makers to make pairwise comparison of each strategy across each attribute. Weights between attributes are derived in the same manner, and a single score for each strategy is derived. AHP may require that a large number of pairwise comparisons be made, especially if there are many attributes or strategies.

All three of these approaches have been successfully applied to similar public policy problems, and there is no "best" technique. Selection of the appropriate decision analysis technique should be made in the context of the problem. The decision model should be carefully developed to yield results that make sense to the decision makers. If the rating of strategies does not make sense, then the effort will be perceived as a waste of time and resources.

CONCLUSION

This paper has addresses a need that became apparent from performing risk assessments on numerous proposed municipal solid waste incinerators for the state of California. The state permitting process provides for public involvement in town meetings on a regular basis, and it requires that all interactions between the licensing commission and the party submitting the application be held in public. This approach failed in that there was considerable public opposition to several of the projects; enough to defeat some projects being planned after considerable resources were expended by the state and private parties.

Much of the debate centered on the health risks from incinerators. It became obvious that a better model needed to include public involvement at the beginning of developing a waste management strategy and should be organized to include a more comprehensive analysis of options and impacts. While better models for public participation exist, there did not seem to be any models for organizing the development of a waste management strategy.

This paper addresses this need. While the approach has not been tested through practical experience, we believed it was necessary to present this idea before the professionals practicing risk assessment, risk management, and public participation. The authors welcome comments and criticisms and hope to pursue this concept further.

REFERENCES

1. Kidder, Peabody, and Company, Engineering-Construction Resource-Recovery Outlook, the Research Department, Industrial Analysis, March 5, 1986.
2. Paul N. Cheremisinoff, Resource Recovery: A Special Report, *Pollution Engineering* **14(11)**:52:59 (1987).

Toxic Air Pollutants and Noncancer Health Risks

Ila L. Cote, Larry T. Cupitt, and Beth M. Hassett
U.S. Environmental Protection Agency
Research Triangle Park, NC

ABSTRACT

In a recent agency-wide comparison of environmental risks, noncancer risks associated with exposure to toxic air pollutants were among the agency's highest concerns. To better understand these potential risks, a study was conducted comparing reported health effects of 132 pollutants to monitored or modeled concentrations in more than 700 geographic locations in the United States. The study assessed (1) individual chemicals, (2) mixtures of chemicals reported to effect the same organ systems, and (3) the impact of the combined emissions of multiple facilities on ambient air concentrations of toxics. The study concluded that data to adequately assess air toxics in the United States is very limited. Available data, however, suggests that (1) increased but ill-defined risks are associated with exposure to toxic air pollutants, (2) exposure to multiple chemicals are of concern in many geographic areas studied, and (3) the combined emissions of multiple facilities may add to levels of concern.

KEYWORDS: Risk assessment, air pollution, toxics, health

INTRODUCTION

Over the past two decades, there has been growing concern about the numbers and quantities of toxic air pollutants to which the public may be exposed. Of great importance are possible adverse effects to public health and the environment resulting from exposure to these pollutants. Previous assessments conducted by the Environmental Protection Agency (EPA) have most often been concerned with cancer. Less attention has been given to assessing other types of health effects that may be associated with exposure to toxic air pollutants. Thus, the EPA's Office of Air Quality Planning and Standards (OAQPS) has initiated a project which begins to evaluate the potential for noncancer public health risks as a result of short-term and long-term exposure to toxic air pollutants.

Noncancer health effects may range from subtle biochemical, physiological or pathological effects to gross effects, including death. Some broad categories may be used to describe these noncancer effects including respiratory toxicity, developmental and reproductive toxicity, central nervous system effects, and other systemic effects such as liver and kidney toxicity, cardiovascular toxicity, and immunotoxicity. The effects of greatest concern are the ones that are irreversible and/or impair the normal functioning of the exposed individual.

The main focus of this study is an evaluation of risk from exposure to toxic air pollutants that are routinely emitted from industrial or commercial sources. Excluded from detailed consideration in this analysis are occupational exposures, indoor air pollutants, criteria air pollutants, (carbon monoxide, ozone, nitrogen oxides, sulfur dioxide, particulates, and lead), secondary atmospheric reaction products and accidental releases. These are excluded because they are the subject of other efforts and are outside this office's current air toxics regulatory efforts.

STUDY OBJECTIVES

The specific goals of this project are (1) to develop various hypotheses for broadly assessing noncancer public health risks associated with short-term and long-term exposure to releases of toxic air pollutants; (2) to determine the availability of relevant information; (3) to conduct any analyses of data which appear reasonable and feasible within the time and resource constraints of this project; and (4) to make recommendations for future actions such as the conduct of additional studies.

Any analysis of air pollutant impacts on public health must consider and account for multiple factors such as exposure to multiple air pollutants, exposure via other media, smoking habits, etc. Issues associated with the assessment of the effects of air pollution have been previously discussed.[1,2] The establishment of causal relationships between public health risk on the one hand and exposure to routine releases of toxic air pollutants on the other is outside the scope of this project. It is hoped, however, that the groundwork for more detailed analyses can be laid.

AVAILABLE DATA AND PROTOCOLS

At this time, there is no comprehensive data base suitable for assessing noncancer public health risks associated with exposure to toxic air pollutants. The data sets that are available were originally collected for a variety of reasons using different protocols. As a consequence, these data sets are not completely comparable or well suited for the assessment of health risks. By analyzing these disparate sets of information, however, it is hoped that some insight into the overall problem can be gained.

The following types of approaches were considered: (1) analysis of ambient monitoring and exposure modeling data available to EPA; (2) review of existing epidemiologic literature and data bases; (3) descriptions of regional toxic air pollution problems, including health, source and exposure information provided by EPA Regional offices, state and local air pollution control agencies, state health departments, and regional representatives of the Agency for Toxic Substances and Disease Registry; and (4) new exposure modeling of small sources emitting toxicants into the atmosphere in a midwestern urban county and a comparison of resulting air concentrations to estimated health effect levels. These analyses are independent; that is, data from one analysis do not serve as input for another analysis. It is thought that the uncertainties associated with each data set are such that to use the results of one analysis as a component of a second analysis would be inappropriate. Rather, it is hoped that the results from each analysis may provide information on a different aspect of potential noncancer health impacts resulting from exposure to toxic air pollutants. The work that has been completed thus far, a broad screening study of readily available health and exposure data, will be the topic of this paper.

COMPARISON OF MONITORING AND EXPOSURE MODELING DATA TO HEALTH DATA

Analysis of Existing Data

This portion of the project involved a comparison of exposure levels from monitoring and modeling data to health effects levels determined from the literature. The results of this analysis must be considered in the context of the limitations of the supporting data base. These limitations and accompanying uncertainties are discussed in the risk characterization section of this paper.

Exposure

1. Monitoring. Information on exposure was obtained from existing ambient monitoring data (annual, 24-hour median concentrations, and 1-hour averages) that were tabulated for 319 volatile organic chemicals from approximately 123,000 samples collected in 310 U.S. cities.[3] The 24-hour median concentration underestimates peak exposures of 24 hours and less. Based upon EPA analysis of two data sets from Louisiana and Virginia containing unique, extensive, hourly monitoring data, maximum short-term concentrations (less than 24-hour exposure) may be underestimated by a factor of 25 to 100.[4,5] Data sets from a variety of special EPA projects such as the Total Exposure Assessment Methodology Studies and Geographic Studied Project were included in the data base.
2. Modeling. Existing exposure modeling data (annual and short-term, less than 24-hour, averages) have been tabulated for approximately 40 chemicals emitted from approximately 3600 facilities.[6] This information was developed for regulatory assessment of specific chemicals under the Clean Air Act. Input parameters (e.g., source and emissions information) for the exposure models were either estimated by EPA or were provided by industry. To our knowledge, these modeling data and the monitoring data described above represent the most comprehensive collection of quantitative exposure data for toxic air pollutants available.

Health. Existing inhalation reference dose (RfD)[a] values and acceptable daily intake (ADI[a]) levels for chronic exposures were used when available. Oral RfDs/ADIs were converted to inhalation values when better data was not available, using the same conversion factors as used by the RfD Working Group.[7,8] Additional health reference levels, for annual and 24-hour averaging times were developed by identifying lowest observed effect levels (LOELS)[b] reported in EPA peer-reviewed health documents or in the Registry of Toxic Effects of Chemical Substances (RTECS) and dividing by uncertainty factors (UF) of 10 to 1000 (10 for the use of a LOEL rather than a no-observed-effect level (NOEL), 10 for variability in the human population, and 10 for the use of animal data rather than human data, when appropriate). A disadvantage of the RTECS data base is that acute lethality is often the only acute health endpoint reported. No additional uncertainty factor was incorporated when lethality was the basis of the health reference level thus, underestimating possible deaths. Health endpoints associated with adverse reproductive or developmental effects of deaths were considered in the determination of short-term health

---

a. The RfD or ADI is an estimate of the exposure dose that is likely to be without deleterious effect even with continued exposure. They are developed by dividing the estimated lowest concentration at which an effect occurs (see footnote *b*, next page) by uncertainty or "safety factors." Often RfD or ADI refers to chronic exposure situations. In this study, ADIs were also calculated based on short-term exposures to enable evaluation of 24-hour exposure data. The term RfD denotes an ADI which has received EPA-wide review and approval.

b. Lowest observed effect levels (LOELS) are the lowest exposure concentrations associated with some health effect or response.

effect levels because of the potential for these effects to result from brief exposure periods. It is recognized that this may overestimate reproductive or developmental effects which depend on more prolonged exposures.

If health data were not available from any of the sources described above, original data referenced by the American Conference of Industrial and Governmental Hygienists were used in place of LOELs. Health reference levels were determined by dividing by uncertainty factors as described above.

In total, 88 chronic LOELs and RfDs or ADIs were identified or developed. One hundred nine LOELs and ADIs were identified and developed for 24-hour exposure periods. For chronic health effects, data from agency reviewed documents were used for 61 percent of the LOELs. For acute health effects (≤24-hour exposure) data from agency-reviewed documents was available for 6 percent of the LOELs.

Chronic RfDs or ADIs were always based on LOELs from subchronic of chronic studies. Acute (24 hour) ADIs were always based on LOELs from short-term exposure studies (24 hours or less). Acute exposures differing from 24 hours were converted to units of 24 hours arithmetically. Disregarding dose-rate effects in such fashion can obviously lead to serious errors in estimation of LOELs.

The approach described above was judged to be a reasonable first step in conducting screening analyses of air concentration data. Uncertainty factors of 100 of 1000 were most common. Chemicals that appeared to be a problem after the screening step received additional review. Some of the more serious limitations in the data are noted later in this paper. A complete discussion of the limitations of the uncertainty factor approach and the use of RTECS data are discussed elsewhere.[7,9,10]

Risk Characterization. The air concentration data from both monitoring and modeling were compared to the LOELs and the RfDs or ADIs to identify potential chemicals of concern. In assessing exposure to individual pollutants potentially resulting in noncancer health effects, the lowest LOELs, RfDs, or ADIs identified were compared to average annual and maximum short-term 24-hour modeled concentrations as well as median 24-hour and less than 24 hours maximum acute monitored concentrations. This analysis, illustrated in Figs. 1-4, indicates exceedances of 42 and 59 percent of chronic and acute RfDs or ADIs, respectively, for the chemicals assessed. The chronic and acute LOELs were exceeded for 1 percent and 12 percent, respectively, of the chemicals assessed. When a LOEL, RfD or ADI was exceeded, the extent of the exceedances, the anticipated health effects, and the geographic areas in which they occur were identified. For the chronic exposure modeling data, additional analyses were under taken to assess the exposure concentrations between the RfD or ADI and the LOEL. Figure 5 illustrates for a representative chemical, chloroform, the range of annual modeled concentrations compared to the ADI, the ADI × 10, and the LOEL. As one would anticipate, concentrations around many more facilities exceed the ADI than the LOEL. Few facilities included in this analysis are estimated to be below the ADI. Concentrations above the ADI indicate that additional analysis may be warranted.

A specific concern for evaluating environmental exposures to toxic air pollutants relates to the analyses of multipollutant exposures. If data are not available on an identical or reasonably similar mixture, a risk assessment may be based on the toxic properties of the components in the mixture.[11] Although substantial uncertainties exist, it was thought that some attempt to evaluate the extent of multipollutant exposure was warranted. The method of evaluation used, based on the toxicity of the components of the mixtures, is described below. Exposure to a single pollutant often results in elicitation of several different health endpoints. Where possible, LOELs for each different health endpoint (e.g., neurotoxicity, developmental/reproductive effects) were identified for each specific chemical (e.g.,

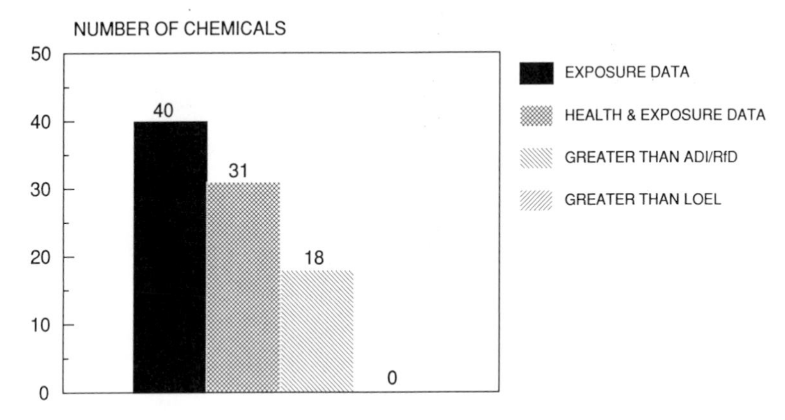

Fig. 1. Chronic modeling data — nonadditivity (maximum concentration).

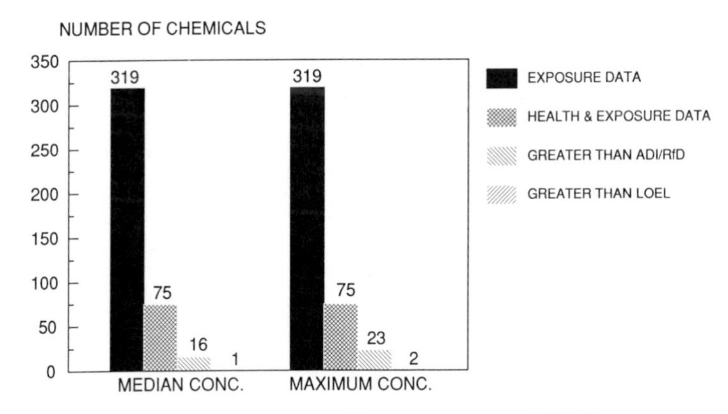

Fig. 2. Chronic modeling data — nonadditivity.

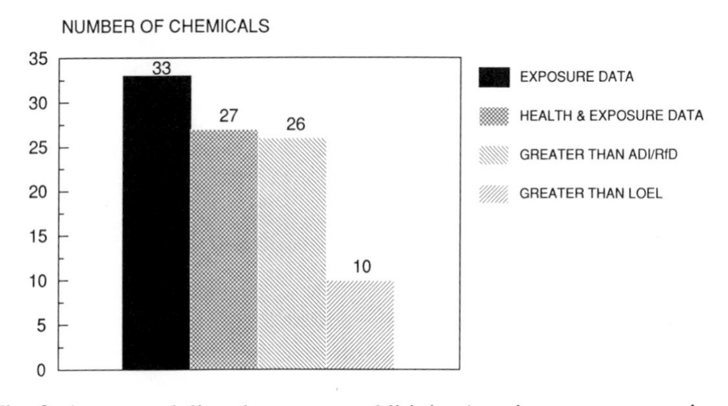

Fig. 3. Acute modeling data — nonadditivity (maximum concentrations).

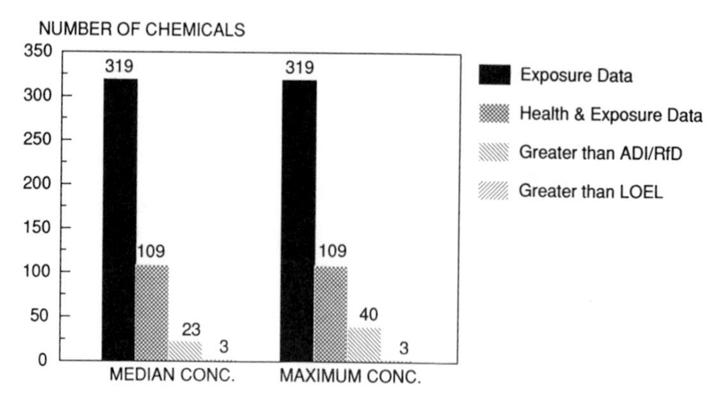

Fig. 4. Acute monitoring data — nonadditivity.

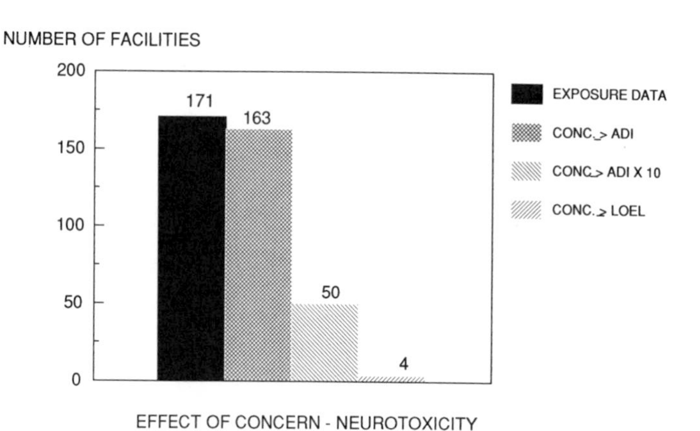

Fig. 5. Nonadditivity analysis — chloroform chronic — maximum modeling data.

chloroform). General descriptions of health endpoints (e.g., neurotoxicity) rather than very specific descriptions (e.g., distal axonopathy resulting from reduction in enzyme activity) were used. This approach resulted in some information loss. When assessing the additivity of similar effects of different pollutants, these general descriptions may group together what are, in reality, dissimilar health endpoints. No attempt to identify synergistic or antagonistic interactions was made.

A hazard index (HI) of a mixture for each health endpoint of concern, assuming dose addition, was developed as follows:

$$HI = \underline{E}_1/AL_1 + \underline{E}_2/AL_1 + \underline{E}_2/AL_2 \ldots + \underline{E}_2/AL_2 \tag{1}$$

where

E_i = exposure level of the *i*th toxicant
AL_i = maximum acceptable level for the *i*th toxicant.

The evaluation of potential additive noncancer health effects using the HI approach as described above indicated many locations where the HI was equal to or greater than one using the ADI for AL in Eq. 1 and several locations where the HI was equal to or greater

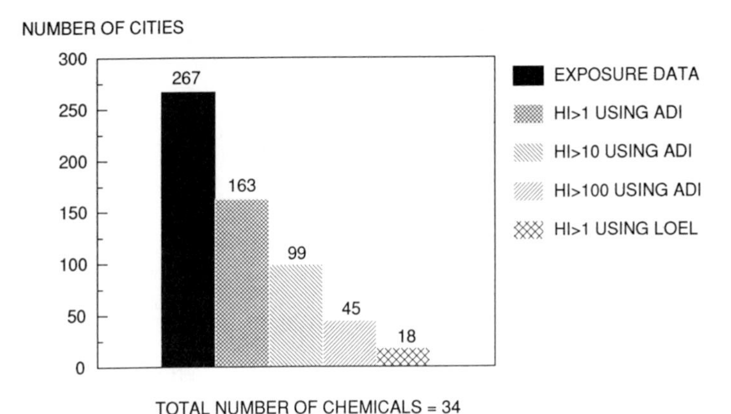

Fig. 6. Additivity analysis — repro/developmental acute — maximum monitoring data.

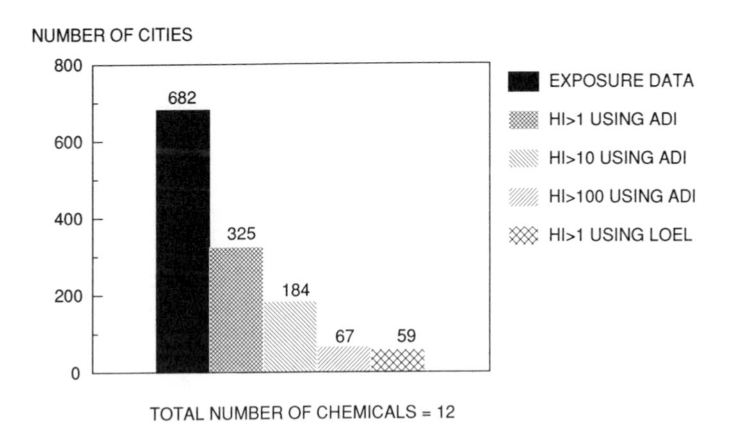

Fig. 7. Additivity analysis — neurotoxicity chronic — average modeling data.

than one using the LOEL for AL in equation (see examples Figs. 6 and 7). Endpoints of particular concern were neurotoxicity, reproductive/developmental toxicity, respiratory toxicity, blood related toxicity and death.

LIMITATIONS

When evaluating these data, one must recognize the many limitations associated with them. These limitations include:

1. Health and exposure data were available for only approximately 10 percent of the chemicals that have been monitored in ambient air.
2. Inhalation health data were available for only 5 percent of the 132 chemicals for which health and exposure data were available.
3. "True" LOELs may be lower or higher than the values used in the analyses.
4. The additivity analyses crudely groups health data and may add together health endpoints that may not truly be associated with one another; on the other hand, this

analysis did not take into account the interaction of chemicals affecting different target organs (e.g., the effect of a liver toxicant on the metabolism of a neurotoxicant).

5. The health data from other than agency documents have received very limited review.
6. The monitoring data were collected using a variety of sampling and analytical methodologies and locations.
7. The ability to model short-term exposure events ($\leq$24 hours) is at this time crude. These data, however, were not inconsistent with the monitoring data, especially when the hourly monitoring data was considered.
8. The RfD/ADI approach produces no quantitative estimate or risk in term of incidence.

SUMMARY

The noncancer risk project is being conducted (a) to collect available data on noncancer public health risks associated with exposure to toxic air pollutants, (b) to propose different approaches for analyzing the data, and (c) to identify data gaps for future efforts that could be undertaken. The work completed thus far involved the gathering and analysis of available exposure data (e.g., monitoring and modeling data) compared to chemical-specific health effect data.

The extent of exposure, the health effects of concern and the significance of multipollutant exposure were evaluated for approximately 132 chemicals. This is less than 10 percent of the chemicals that have been detected in ambient air.[12] Due to the limitations in the data, it is difficult at this time to determine the magnitude and nature of noncancer public health risks associated with exposure to nonaccidental releases of toxic air pollutants. The data evaluated to date, however, suggest a possible association between noncancer health effects and exposure to single chemicals as well as multiple chemicals affecting the same target organ. For approximately 50 percent of the situations studied, exceedances of ADIs were observed. For 16 percent of these chemicals, the health level of concern was exceeded at more than 25 percent of the sites where the chemical was modeled or monitored. Approximately 10 percent of the chemicals studied showed exceedances of exposure concentrations which have been reported in the literature to produce health effects. For the additivity analysis, the hazard indices based on both ADIs and LOELs were exceeded in many locations for most of the health effects observed.

In conclusion, while the preliminary results of this study must be interpreted in light of substantial data limitations, exposure to air toxics may be of concern for noncancer health effects. This tentative association is strengthened when exposures to multiple pollutants from numerous sources are considered. The results to date support the need for completing the comparison analyses described above that are now underway.

REFERENCES

1. National Research Council, *Epidemiology and Air Pollution*, National Academy Press, Washington, DC (1985).
2. Task Force on Environmental Cancer and Heart and Lung Disease, Environmental Cancer and Heart and Lung Disease, Sixth Annual Report to Congress (1983).
3. U.S. Environmental Protection Agency, National Ambient Volatile Organic Compounds/VOCs Data Base Update, prepared for Larry T. Cupitt, U.S. EPA,

Atmospheric Science Research Laboratory by Nero and Associates, Inc., EPA Contract No. 68-02-4190 (1988).

4. U.S. Environmental Protection Agency, Statistical Properties of Hourly Concentrations of Volatile Organic Compounds at Baton Rouge, Louisiana, prepared for Neil Frank, U.S. EPA, Office of Air Quality Planning and Standards by Systems Applications, Inc., September 30, 1987.
5. William A. McClenny, Karen D. Oliver, and Joachin D. Pleil, A Field Strategy for Sorting Volatile Organics into Source Related Groups, Environmental Science and Technology (submitted, 1988).
6. T. J. Mohin, Air Toxics Exposure and Risk Information System, Draft Report (1988).
7. U.S. Environmental Protection Agency, Integrated Risk Information System-Supportive Documentation Volume I, EPA/600/8-86/032a, March 1987.
8. U.S. Environmental Protection Agency, Identification of Health Data, prepared for Dr. Ila Cote, U.S. EPA, Office of Air Quality Planning and Standards by RADIAN Corporation, Research Triangle Park, N.C., EPA Contract No.68-02-4330, Work Assignment No. 33, January 20, 1988.
9. I. L. Cote, B. M. Hassett, F. W. Hauchman, T. J. Mohin, H. M. Richmond, B. L. Riddle, and L. Zaragoza, Noncancer Risk Assessment — Review of Issues and Methodologies, Draft Report, U.S. EPA, Office of Air Quality Planning and Standards, March 1987.
10. National Research Council, *Drinking Water and Health*, Vol. 3, National Academy Press, Washington, DC (1980).
11. U.S. Environmental Protection Agency, Guidelines for the Health Risk Assessment of Chemical Mixtures, 51 FR 34014, September 24, 1986.
12. T. E. Graedle, D. T. Hawkins, and L. S. Claxton, *Atmospheric Chemical Compounds: Sources, Occurrences, and Bioassay*, Academic Press, Orlando, Florida (1986)

Quantitative Risk Assessment of Commercial Hazardous Waste Facilities: A TSDF Rating Method for Generators

Kevin D. Grant
Kemron Environmental Services
Jupiter, FL

ABSTRACT

Waste generators often audit waste disposal facilities as a due diligence function: these audits are conducted by the generator's staff and hired consultants. These audits are traditionally compliance driven and convey little if any information about the potential liability exposure of sending waste to a site. A method of commercial waste risk assessment was developed to quantitatively assess risk. The method functions on a relative risk basis with the intention of supporting the generator's decision process in the selection of commercial waste facilities.

KEYWORDS: Risk assessment, TSDF liability, hazardous waste, audits, CERCLA

BACKGROUND

Generators of hazardous waste face the liability of cleaning up environmental contamination and providing environmental restoration where ever their wastes have been transported or managed. This liability stems from CERCLA aka the Superfund Act of 1980. In 1976, the Federal government enacted RCRA (the Resource Conservation and Recovery Act). RCRA establishes government enforced standards for the transportation and disposal of hazardous wastes. Though RCRA regulates disposal, many generators are realizing the current RCRA system of hazardous waste management does not protect them from CERCLA liability. Moreover, exemptions in RCRA rules allow hazardous waste to be sent to unregulated facilities for recycling or otherwise provide for exemptions that allow hazardous waste to escape the purview of government rules and inspectors.

This paper discusses a method to quantitatively assess the risk of commercial waste management facilities. The assessment method utilized goes beyond the criteria of a generator due diligence audit and also covers criteria which is not covered in government agency inspections of waste facilities. In quantitatively assessing waste facility risk, financial, regulatory, design/operation and site/location criteria were considered. Models were developed to evaluate each of these criteria to produce a risk score. The risk score is then used by the generator in the decision process of selecting least risk disposal sites.

Risk Analysis, Edited by C. Zervos
Plenum Press, New York, 1991

INTRODUCTION

A method to evaluate the potential risk of commercial hazardous transportation, storage, disposal facilities (TSDFs) was developed by the writer for generator due diligence assessments. The basic approach employed was initially developed for a risk assessment project involving five TSDFs for a client generator. The project budget allowed five man days for the development of assessment criteria, assessment methodology and assessment protocols. From this effort, a risk assessment method was designed to compare the relative risk of TSDFs employing both quantitative and qualitative risk scores.

The risk criteria selected included: regulatory and legal issues, site design and operation factors, site contamination, facility location and siting factors and the financial strength of the TSDF owner/operator. The methods used to evaluate risk and limitations associated with the assessment method (and other methods evaluated) and data interpretation are discussed. In addition, the results of nine TSDF assessments conducted utilizing this method are presented.

Several methods currently employed to audit or assess risks of TSDFs were reviewed for this presentation. Also considered for TSDF risk assessment were applications of engineering/hazard assessments of operations and site evaluation criteria for uncontrolled hazardous waste sites. Information covering audit approaches for hazardous waste TSDFs was found in EPA's Annotated Bibliography on Environmental Auditing.[1] Methods of hazard assessments and references were found in the Chemical Manufacturers "Process Safety Management".[2] Methods to assess hazardous waste sites were found in the CERCLA National Contingency Plan, 40 CFR 300[3] and in the Council on Economic Priorities publication on Hazardous Waste Management. Methods to assess the cost of remedial site actions can be found in various primers, RCRA/CERCLA documents and technical papers including the CH2M-Hill REM/FIT Cost Estimating Guide.

TSDF RISK ASSESSMENT METHODS

Environmental Audit Approaches

Auditing is the most common method employed by third parties to evaluate regulatory compliance. Generators, trade associations, government agencies and consulting firms conduct audits of TSDFs for due diligence functions. Most of the audits and audit protocols observed are based on regulatory compliance checklists available through EPA and environmental consulting firms. The EPA National Enforcement Investigation Center (NEIC) checklists are often utilized and the audits are conducted to review the TSDF compliance.

Audits are fine, as far as these are designed to go, but the audit protocols reviewed provide just a regulatory compliance model. The audit protocols provided no technique for quantitative or comparative evaluation of audits. Since this assessment project was intended to provide a quantitative assessment of risk having comparison value, it was determined that a typical audit wouldn't provide the required data for this project. An auditing protocol would need to designed to produce the desired information.

Hazard Assessment Approaches

Hazard identification techniques, engineering hazard assessment methods and hazard indexes have useful applications in qualitative and quantitative evaluations of process operations and designs. The available budget and time limitations project would not allow a full blown hazard assessment of TSDFs, nor would this method be a practical approach for generators to perform at a third party site. Hazard indexes were reviewed, these provide fire and explosion hazard data to rate facility risk. Indexing was considered to be an ideal approach, however, no data base was found for this application. Using hazard assessment techniques, an index was developed to rate types of treatment, storage and disposal units. Model TSDF units were conceptualized as reference units to which a TSDFs design and operation would be compared to produce a quantitative risk score.

Site Release Assessment Methods

The Hazard Ranking System (MITRE Model) or HRS used by the EPA to list sites on the National Priority List (NPL) has been widely used and adopted for quantitatively scoring risk from abandoned or uncontrolled waste sites. While the HRS has been the standard for qualifying Superfund sites, it has received significant criticism and is currently being revised (52 FR 11513, 4/9/87). While the HRS identifies some suitable risk criteria, it is not necessarily a suitable method for evaluating risk for TSDFs. The HRS risk criteria were modified to consider actual risk from an active, controlled operation. The writer's own experience and methods developed for evaluating industrial facilities and property for potential sale and acquisition were also incorporated into the assessment method.

TSDF RISK ASSESSMENT DESIGN

The risk assessment process involved several steps and tasks which are illustrated in Table 1. In referring to Table 1, Task 1 lists the generator concerns upon which the assessment was structured. The objective of this process was to identify risks which can result in financial liability to the generator or result in non-compliance for the generator. A matrix of potential risk criteria was developed, then reduced to the five criteria listed in Task II. A key factor in selecting criteria was the availability of information to evaluate risk since new information could not be produced. Reverse design was also used to establish criteria, knowing what data and information would be available for review.

RISK CRITERIA (Task II)

Five risk criteria were selected for the assessment; these are listed under Task II in Table 1. The risk criteria were then broken down into categories for risk scoring. Individual categories within the criteria had evaluation protocols developed for data collection.

TSDF Financial Strength

With generators facing CERCLA liability should the TSDF operator become financially unable to meet its RCRA requirements, the financial capacity of the TSDF was a key criteria. The assessment analyzed financial strength as a measure of assets, liquidity and indebtedness versus RCRA closure/post closure liabilities. The EPA financial test at 40 CFR 264.143(f) was used as one measure of financial strength used in the financial risk model. Changes in earnings, revenues, financial position and the TSDF ability to provide the EPA corporate guarantee (for TSDF closure) were also measures of financial strength utilized. TSDF closure liabilities identified by the TSDF (this is a regulatory requirement) were reviewed and modified by the assessor for the evaluation. The assessor reviewed site contamination reports and observed site conditions to revise the TSDF's closure estimates. Table 3b (discussed later) lists the financial risk categories employed in the assessment, and the TSDFs annual report and form 10-K, together with available bond and credit ratings provided by financial analysts on corporations, served as the basis of financial data.

Table 1. Risk Assessment Design

Assessment Method Element	Risk Issues
Task I Identify Generator Concerns	Financial Liability Own Compliance Concern Third Party Liability Polluter Image
Task II Establish Risk Criteria	TSDF Financial Strength Site Contamination Status Unit Design Factors/Unit Operation Factors (D&O) Regulatory/Legal Issues Site/Location Issues
Task III Develop Risk Model	Financial Strength Measurement Contamination Risk Measurement D/O Risk Components Regulatory/Legal Risk Components Site/Location Risk Components
Task IV Develop Data Collection Needs and Instruments	Annual Report & 10K Financial Assurances Hydrological Investigations Permit & Regulatory Documents Insurance Risk Assessments Regulatory Questionnaire (TBD) Facility Audit Protocols (TBD)
Task V Visit Site	Complete Observations and Audit Protocols
Task VI Evaluate Data and Information	Quantitative Score Qualitative Score Interpret Data

Site Contamination Status

The presence of contamination at existing hazardous waste sites or the potential to have releases is a site liability and a direct measure of a TSDF risk. RCRA required regulatory documents concerning groundwater contamination, groundwater assessments, waste releases, site investigations, exposure assessments, permit applications and solid waste management units (SWMUs) were reviewed to assess this criterion. A review of site utilization history and on-site inspections was an integral part of the contamination evaluation. Rough estimates of site corrective action costs were taken from RCRA site characterization reports and from the assessor's site observations. Cost estimates were made using clean up references such the REM/FIT Cost Estimating Guide.[4] These costs were transferred to the liability column in the financial strength assessment.

Design and Operation (D/O)

Risk assessment of the TSDF focused upon environmental release protection and control of each waste unit. The TSDF RCRA Part B permit application, facility engineering reports and on-site observations were evaluated against regulatory requirements and EPA technical and guidance documents for 40 CFR 264 regulations as well as standards from NFPA, ASTM and guidelines on SPCC plans. General operations of the TSDF were reviewed, including health and safety, materials handling and materials hazards. Table 3a (discussed later) provides the D/O categories which were evaluated at each facility.

Selected D/O risk categories cover subject areas not specifically addressed by environmental regulations, therefore, these are not typically inspected by agency personnel. Such categories not covered or inspect frequently include transportation staging areas, container processing areas such as drum crushing and general housekeeping. Audit protocols were specifically designed to collect information concerning these categories.

Regulatory/Legal (R/L)

Risk categories selected to assess potential regulatory and legal issues were those identified which could result in the loss of a TSDF's RCRA (or other statute) authority or lead to an agency's denial of permits. The categories of regulatory risk included the TSDF's compliance and the assessor's assessment of TSDF regulatory risk (compliance management and other compliance issues). The legal issue category considered siting challenges, CERCLA/RCRA suits and third party suits against the TSDF as potential risk factors. Table 2 lists the categories of regulatory/legal risk and provides the category assessment factors and source of risk data.

Site and Location (S&L)

The risk categories selected for S&L assessment are similar to those proposed by EPA in the HRS (50 FR 5912-14). In the model, potential harm to the human population and environment from the TSDF is based upon the proximity of the TSDF to occupied areas and sensitive environments: actual risk is not computed. The TSDF's risk is more directly assessed by the D&O criteria and the site contamination criteria previously discussed. The S&L criteria assesses the exposure risk potential, should releases occur.

Categories selected for the S&L assessment include the following: TSDF proximity to population centers (area occupied by 100 or more people [e.g. residences, schools, etc.] within a specific area around the facility boundary); proximity to occupied structures (distance to nearest building [e.g. residence, school] from a hazardous waste unit); and proximity to sensitive environments.

METHOD OF RISK ASSESSMENT SCORING (Task III)

Risk criteria were broken down into risk categories which were evaluated and comparatively scored. Tables 3a - 3c provide the selected risk categories and their scores.

Risk was evaluated on a one (1) to five (5) point scales as follows:

	Risk Score
Low risk	1
Less than average risk	2
Average risk	3
Above average risk	4
High risk	5

Table 2. Regulatory/Legal Risk Categories

Category	Evaluation Factor	Source of Data
Permit Status	Issued/To Be Issued	Regulatory Agency
	Technical Deficiencies	Regulatory Agency
	Remediation Requirements	Regulatory Agency
Regulatory Compliance	NOV's, Fines	Regulatory Agency
	Consent Orders	Regulatory Agency
	Regulator's Perception	Agency Staff
	Pending Actions	Regulatory Agencies
Regulatory Oversite	No. of Inspections	Regulatory Agency
	Staff Interaction w/TSDF	Regulatory Agency
	Regulatory Enforcement (exercising of authority)	Assessor
	Regulatory Authority (ability to cite or fine)	State Regulations
Facility Compliance (Risk Management)	Compliance Management (Proactive/Reactive/Fire Fighting)	Assessor/Facility
	TSDF Knowledge of Requirements	Assessor
	Standard Operating Procedures/ Control Systems	TSDF
	D&O Release Controls	TSDF
	TSDF Attitude Towards Compliance	Assessor
Other Compliance	Assessor Identified Exceptions	Assessor Audit Protocol
	OSHA Compliance	Audit Protocol
	Health & Safety Issues	Audit Protocol
Legal Issues	Siting Challenges	Regulatory Agencies & Form 10-K
	Government Suits	Regulatory Agencies & Form 10-K
	Third Party Suits	Form 10-K

The method used to rate or score the risk for each category was based upon a model which is described in each criteria.

Financial Strength Method

The financial strength criteria of a TSDF operation considered three categories, these being: financial strength versus liabilities; the ability of the TSDF to meet RCRA specific financial assurances; and the TSDF's financial position. The evaluation considered a complete analyses of a facility's financial ability to operate when stringent permit requirements are implemented during the next five years.

Table 3a. Quantitative Assessment Summary of TSDF Risk

	Facility								
Risk Criteria	1	2	3	4	5	6	7	8	9
Regulatory/Legal Issues									
Permit Status/Issues	1	1	1	1	1	1	2	1	1
Regulatory Compliance	2(-)	3	2	1	4*	3	3	2	2
Regulatory Oversite	2(-)	3	3	3	2	3	4	3	3
Compliance (Risk) Mgmt.	1(-)	3	4	2	3*	3	4	4	3
Other Compliance Issues	3	1	5	5	3	2	2	1	5
Legal Issues	2	1	1	1	4	1	5	2	3
R/L Criteria Score	12/30	12/30	16/30	13/30	17/30	13/30	20/30	13/30	17/30
Average Risk Score	18/30	18/30	18/30	18/30	18/30	18/30	18/30	18/30	18/30
Design and Operation (D/O)									
Bulk Storage Facilities	3	1	1	1	1	3	2	3	3*
Container Storage #	2	-	2	1	3	-	-	-	1
Mat'ls Handling/Transfer	2	2	4	2	1	4	-	2	4
Current Land Disp Facil	1	-	-	-	4	-	5	3<	-
Surface Impoundments	4	-	-	-	4	-	-	3	4
Fire/Spill Prevention	3	3	4	2	1	4	3	3	4
Housekeeping	2	2	3	2	2	3	3	2	2
Decontamination Procedures	2	-	-	1	N/A	-	2	-	2
Health & Safety	1	3	5	3	2	3	2	2	3
Mat'l Hazard	5	2	3	4	5	2	4	3	4
Tank Process Area	2	1	2	2	1(-)	2	-	3	-
Container Process Area	2	-	4	2	2	-	-	-	2
Transportation Staging	3(-)	2	4	3	1	4	4	2	2
Incineration Facilities	-	-	-	2	1	-	-	-	2
Treatment Facils (Other) (Having Disch/Emiss)	3	-	-	-	3	3	-	-	-
D/O Criteria Score	35/65	16/40	33/50	25/60	31/70	28/45	24/40	26/50	33/60
Average Risk Score	42/70	24/40	30/50	36/60	42/70	27/45	24/40	27/50	36/60

Financial Strength vs. Liability Category

The TSDF's financial strength versus liability was scored considering the TSDF's ability to pass the EPA's closure/post closure financial test at 40 CFR 264.143(f) and 264.147. Passing this test is only required of TSDFs which chose the available corporate financial guarantee mechanism of supplying RCRA mandated financial assurances for closure/post closure (firms may also select letters of credit, surety bonds and insurance). The TSDF's latest available annual report was utilized to provide the firm's financial data for the test. In conducting the test, the assessor included the estimated cost of required facility improvements (required means set by existing rules, standards) and the costs of cleaning up the site (a future regulatory requirement) respectively in the liability column. In applying the financial test in this manner, the TSDF's ability to pass the test against more stringent future requirements was evaluated.

Table 3b. Quantitative Assessment Summary of TSDF Risk

Risk Criteria	Facility 1	2	3	4	5	6	7	8	9
Site Contamination/Pathway Analysis									
Groundwater Contamination (Monitoring Data)									
From Active Units (if monitored)	-	1	1	-	1	5	-	5	-
From SWMUs (if monitored)	-	N/A	-	5	5	-	-	5	-
Off-site Contamination (if monitored)	-	-	-	-	5	-	-	-	-
Monitoring Coverage	3	1	5	2	1	5	4	3	5
Groundwater Pathway Analysis (use only if no contamination detected)	2.5	3	3	-	-	3.5	-	-	3.5
Surface Water Pathway	1	2	5	3	3	3	1	4	3.5
Surface Contamination (observed)	4	2	4	2	1	4	3	2	2
Potential SWMU Risk	5	-	3	-	-	-	-	-	4
SC/P Criteria Score	16.5/30	9/25	20/25	13/25	20/30	15.5/20	13/20	14/20	18/25
Average Risk Score	18/30	15/25	15/25	15/25	18/30	12/20	12/20	12/20	12/25
Site and Location (S/L)									
Proximity to Population Center	1	2	2	1	3	3	1	2	4
Nearest Building	1	2	4	3	5	2	1	2	4
Sensitive Environment	3	1	4	3	3	2	1	3	1
S/L Criteria Score	5/15	6/15	10/15	7/15	11/15	7/15	3/15	7/15	9/15
Average Risk Score	9/15	9/15	9/15	9/15	9/15	9/15	9/15	9/15	9/15
Financial Strength (F/S)									
Strength vs. Liability	2	3	2	1	3	4	5	2	3
Availability Assurances	1	4	1	1	3	4	3	1	3
Financial Position	1.5	2	2	1	3	-	4.5	2	2
F/S Criteria Score	4.5/15	9/15	5/15	3/15	9/15	8/15	12.5/15	5/15	8/15
Average Risk Score	9/15	9/15	9/15	9/15	9/15	9/15	9/15	9/15	9/15

Table 3c. Quantitative Assessment Summary of TSDF Risk

	Facility								
	1	2	3	4	5	6	7	8	9
Total risk score	73/155	52/125	84/135	61/145	88/160	71.5/120	72.5/120	65/130	84/143
Standardized risk score	2.35	2.08	3.11	2.10	2.75	2.98	3.02	2.49	2.93
# of categories with risk >3	4/32	1/26	12/28	3/30	9/33	8/25	10/25	3/26	9/30
# of categories with risk <3	21/32	16/26	10/28	20/30	14/33	8/25	10/25	14/26	13/30
# of criteria which were higher than average risk	0	0	3	0	1	3	3	1	2

Criteria	Risk Score
The TSDF closure/post closure cost estimates have been reviewed and approved by EPA. EPA has determined that the TSDF has the required RCRA financial assurances.	2
The TSDF closure/post closure cost estimates have not been reviewed by EPA. The TSDF has documentation that the required financial assurance mechanisms are in place.	3
The TSDF in the assessor's opinion is not in compliance with RCRA financial assurances requirements.	5

The risk score taken from the matrix was adjusted by using the following criterion:

- Decrease the TSDF risk score by 1, if the TSDF can meet the RCRA financial test for closure/post closure;
- Increase the TSDF risk score by 1, if in the assessor's opinion, the TSDF closure cost estimate is substantially low or the TSDF would not pass the financial test using the assessor's estimate of liability and more stringent future test criteria.

RCRA Liability Assurance Category

TSDFs must have liability insurance for sudden releases of hazardous waste (all RCRA sites) and non-sudden releases (land disposal sites). The availability of these insurance coverages is limited and the insurance is very costly where available: non-sudden release coverage is practically non-available. The liability insurance can be provided by a corporate guarantee, if the TSDF (or parent) can pass the EPA RCRA financial test or meet specified financial criteria.

Using the regulatory criteria for required insurance coverage(s), risk for this category was scored as follows:

Criteria	Risk Score
TSDF has required sudden coverage, but is operating (with regulatory approval) without non-sudden coverage.	3
TSDF has all required sudden and non-sudden liability coverages. (Reduce the risk score to one, if the TSDF passes the financial test requirement.)	2
The TSDF has neither of the required coverages.	5

The risk score taken from the matrix was adjusted by using the following criterion.

Financial Position

A company's change in financial position over time is a good measure of future financial strength. Regulations, technology advances and legal decisions (involving the TSDF) could significantly impact the TSDF future revenues and earnings. The financial position risk score was computed by adjusting a risk score of 5 (starting point) accordingly for any conditions listed below which were applicable to the TSDF's current financial status.

Financial Status	Reduced Risk By
The annual reports show increases in assets, revenues and earnings over the last 3 years.	1
Hazardous waste business revenues are less than 25% of the corporate business revenues and other corporate businesses are less risky than hazardous waste management.	
The TSDF has made substantial improvements in equipment and technology for the treatment, destruction or recovery of hazardous waste.	1
Changes in regulations concerning hazardous waste disposal are likely to maintain or increase the TSDF's waste business.	1
	Increased Risk By
Changes in regulations are likely to decrease the TSDF's market potential.	1
Pending legal cases involving the TSDF have substantial liability which could have an adverse financial impact on the TSDF.	1

Design and Operations (D&O)

Design and operating risks were evaluated from an environmental release perspective. Assessment criteria for the D&O of waste units were taken from the permitted facility rules (40 CFR 264), proposed rules and supporting EPA Technical Guidance Documents. Detailed checklists developed for the assessment, were used to identify the D&O elements of the TSDF waste unit which prevented, controlled or monitored potential releases. Table 3a shows the categories that were scored for the D&O criterion. A conceptual model for each type of unit D&O was developed as a low risk reference (risk score of 1) to which the TSDF unit was comparatively scored.

REGULATORY/LEGAL ISSUES (R&L)

The R&L category assessment method was developed by the assessor and based on perceived risk. The method of risk scoring is shown in the R&L risk score matrix in Fig. 1.

Siting and Location (S&L)

The selected risk categories and the method of risk scoring utilized are analogous to the National Contingency Plan HRS procedure. Waste toxicity and fire and explosion hazard were factored into scores as indicated. Fire and explosion hazard data were taken from Sax[5] and converted to the five point rating method used herein. The risk categories and risk rating procedure are provided in Fig. 2.

DATA AND INFORMATION COLLECTION (TASKS IV & V)

Data and information collection protocols were designed to collect risk information. These protocols included a regulatory agency telephone questionnaire, a pre-audit questionnaire sent to the TSDF operator and a site specific audit checklist/questionnaire to be completed by the assessor.

In addition to conducting a TSDF visit and reviewing facility documents, all state, local and Federal agencies having jurisdiction over toxic/hazardous waste management, water discharges or air emissions were contacted by telephone or visited to complete the Agency Questionnaire Form. Where regulatory agency offices were located nearby the TSDF to be visited, arrangements were made to visit the office and review facility files (this was done for 3 of the 9 assessments presented). Information from agencies was also requested in writing under the Freedom of Information Act (FOIA) when it was not obtainable through other means.

The TSDF site visit and the collection/review of site documents were the most important and time consuming tasks in the assessment. To facilitate the process, a pre-audit survey was provided to the TSDF three weeks before to the site audit. Prior to the on-site audit, the pre-audit survey responses were reviewed and clarified with the TSDF. The pre-audit survey requested reports and information which were sometimes too numerous reproduce and forward; therefore, arrangements were made to review requested information during the on-site audit.

While at the TSDF, performance audits of the TSDFs waste tracking systems and management controls were conducted. Records previous wastes shipped to the site by the generator were tracked. The existence of management and control systems for the tracking of RCRA inspection findings, maintenance and repairs, and instrument monitoring and calibration were also reviewed.

Category	Risk Score 1	2	3	4	5
Permit Status	Have all permits	Permits to be issued	Minor permit	Major permit issues	Permit to be denied
Regulatory Compliance	No agency non-compliance	Trivial non-compliance	Minor non-compliance	1 major non-compliance issue	Repeated major non-compliance issues
Agency Oversite	Staff on-site strong enforcement	Frequent inspections	>1 insp. year	<1 insp. year weak agency enforcement	Minimal regulatory oversite
Other Compliance Issues	None	Minor issues id by assessor	Many minor issues id by assessor	Potential major issue id by assessor	Critical issue id by assessor
Compliance (Risk) Management	Assessor considers proactive	Assessor considers compliance orientated	Assessor considers reactive but responsive		Fire fighting approach
Legal Issues	None identified		Issues not likely to have sig. impact on financial status		Issues likely to significant financial impact

Fig. 1. R&L risk matrix.

RESULTS (TASK VI)

The risk assessment evaluated TSDF risk for five (5) risk criteria and 34 risk categories. Table 3c provides the risk criteria/category scores for the nine (9) TSDFs assessed by the described method. Category risk scores are summarized by a standardized risk score (SRS) (the raw score divided by the number of categories). SRS ranged from 2.08 to 3.11. Data were also summarized to show the number of categories for which a TSDF risk score was greater than or less than 3. The TSDF scores for the five (5) major criteria were also summarized to indicate the number of criteria for which the TSDF score was greater than 3 (above average risk). Table 4 provides a description of the TSDF operations assessed in Tables 3a through 3c.

The TSDF assessment data is presented as a summary of separate due diligence assessments projects. The method is suitable as a risk evaluation procedure for a single

Category	Risk Score 1	2	3	4	5
1. Proximity to Population Center a. Select the corresponding score from the listed area occupied by 100 or more persons. b. Take score from Step 1.1 and multiply it by the ration of waste hazard(s) (e.g. x/5). c. List the score on the Quantitative Assessment Summary (QAS). Add 1 point to any computed score (up to score of 5) if the area is primarily residential.	1 sq mi		<1/2 sq mi		<1/4 sq mi
2. Proximity to Occupied Structure a. Select risk score which corresponds to the distance of the nearest off-site occupied structure. b. Take score from Step 2.1, and multiply it by the waste hazard(s) (take the highest score from either the toxic or physical hazard score). c. Add 1 point to score for any occupied structure less than 300 ft. from active waste area, list the score on the QAS.	1/2 mi		<1/4 mi		<300 ft
3. Proximity to Sensitive Environments a. Select the risk score from the sub-categories listed below. Take the highest score selected and carry it to the QAS. If no sub category is applicable, the risk score is 1.					
• Flood prone area	-	-	-	-	5
• Distance to public surface water	-	-	<1/4 mi	<1,000 ft	<300 ft
• Earthquake zone	-	-	-	-	5
• Distance to livestock, agriculture	-	-	<1/4 mi	<1,000 ft	<300 ft
• Distance to critical habitat	-	-	<1/4 mi	<1,000 ft	<300 ft
• Site located above potable water aquifer serving 10,000 people (depth to aquifer)					

Fig. 2. Siting and location (S&L) risk matrix.

Table 4. Description of Facilities

	Facility								
	1	2	3	4	5	6	7	8	9
Operations									
Landfill	X				X		X		X
Land Placement*	X				X				
Incineration				X	X				X
Aqueous Treatment					X	X		X	
Solvent Recovery	X		X						
Deep Well Injection								X	
Tank/Storage	X	X	X	X	X	X	X	X	X
(Container/Storage)	X		X	X	X				X
Offsite Mgmt. of Waste		X	X	X		X	X	X	X
History									
Age of Current Operation (yrs)	10	2	13	2	16	10	17	18	16
Past Usage	Farm-land	Vacant	Farm-land	Mili-tary (1940s)	Petro-chem (1960s)	Vacant	RAD Waste (1960s)	Vacant	Petro-leum
Contamination Risk									
Current Oper.	Low	Low	Mod	Low	High	Mod	High	Low	Mod
Past Oper.	High (1978-1984)	Mod (Neigh-bor)	Low	Mod	High	Low	High	High	High
Location									
Industrial				X				X	X
Rural	X		X	X			X	X	X
Urban		X				X			
Residential						X			
Commercial		X							
Volume of Waste Disposal	10MM	--	Spills	Spills	2MM	Spills	550K	100K	20K

*Land placement includes surface impoundments, waste piles, and land treatment facilities.

TSDF, or it can be used to compare the relative risks of similar disposal operations. The TSDFs evaluated in this paper were conducted as single facility evaluations, then later compared.

The facility information in Table 4 indicates that the TSDFs assessed had differing waste management capabilities. These differences limit the direct comparison of the quantitative data summaries. The summary score is not intended to be an absolute measure of TSDF risk, and the SRS should not be used to compare risks of unlike TSDFs. For that reason, qualitative assessments were all prepared to identify the risk factors important to the TSDF risk assessment. High risk scores in individual risk categories for any assessment criterion were flagged in written reports. A high risk score on a key category was considered to be a significant indicator of potential risk.

REFERENCES

1. U.S. EPA, Office of Policy, Planning and Evaluation, Annotated Bibliography on Environmental Auditing, March 1988.
2. Chemical Manufacturers Association, Process Safety Management, 1985.
3. 40 CFR 300, Appendix A. Also see the Michigan Priority Ranking System, Michigan Environmental Response Act (Act 307); and, Benjamin Goldman, *Hazardous Waste Management*, Island Press, Washington, DC (1986).
4. CH2M Hill, REM/FIT Cost Estimating Guide, July 1985.
5. N. Irving Sax, *Dangerous Properties of Industrial Materials*, Van Nostrand Reinhold Co., Inc., New York (1984).

Effects of Analytical Data Gathering and Handling Techniques on Calculated Risk Levels at Superfund Sites

Steven T. Cragg
Radian Corp.
Washington, DC

Robert J. Caprara
Roy F. Weston, Inc.
West Chester, PA

ABSTRACT

Large amounts of analytical chemical data are generated during the course of Superfund site investigations. Often, insufficient thought is given to the final uses of these data as they relate to risk assessment. The manner in which these large volumes of analytical data are reduced may have a large impact on calculated risk levels. For example, it may be desirable to ignore "non-detects" in some instances, whereas in others, gross overestimation of risks may result if this is done. Regarding the effect of the type of data gathered, the following example is revealing. Fish ingestion may be a significant pathway of concern, yet no fish data are gathered. Bioconcentration factors (BCFs) must then be used to estimate fish tissue levels and, subsequently, human intakes and risk levels. Large overestimates in risk levels may result from using BCFs as opposed to actual tissue levels. Situations where alternative data-gathering and data-handling techniques may profoundly influence calculated risk levels are shown. In addition, an attempt is made to establish guidelines for the gathering and handling of analytical data used in risk assessments.

KEYWORDS: Risk assessment, data handling, data reduction, statistics, Superfund site

INTRODUCTION

When conducting risk assessments of chemically contaminated sites, the risk assessment team will often receive large amounts of analytical data after it has been collected. Those conducting the risk assessment have little control over what data have been collected or how. There may be no means of ascertaining the quality of the data, in terms of its extent and appropriateness of sampling location, which may have been collected by another laboratory or consulting firm. The data may be inappropriate because no initial systematic identification has been conducted of possible contaminant migration pathways, plausible contact points, or potentially exposed populations.

Risk Analysis, Edited by C. Zervos
Plenum Press, New York, 1991

Data handling techniques may also greatly impact calculated risk levels. Particularly critical is the problem of reducing the large volume of data into average values which realistically reflect a discrete area of contamination. Contrary to data collection problems, data handling is within the control of the risk assessment team.

Both areas may profoundly influence the noncarcinogenic and carcinogenic risk levels calculated for a contaminated site. The quantified health threats are based directly upon the environmental concentrations measured on the site.

Non-carcinogenic risk is quantified by comparing the estimated dose (directly reflected by the environmental concentrations) to the acceptable dose. This ratio is called the Hazard Index (HI) and the overall HI for a site is calculated by summing the specific HI for each contaminant of concern, assuming that non-carcinogenic hazards are additive. Excess lifetime cancer risk is calculated by multiplying the cancer potency slope by the dose. The latter calculation is permitted by the assumptions of low dose linearity and zero intercept.

The errors introduced from analytical data which is either incomplete or incorrectly reduced will be directly reflected in the dose estimates and the calculated risk levels.

DATA GATHERING

The influence of inappropriate data gathering on calculated risk levels can best be illustrated by an example. Table 1 shows the difference in pesticide levels in fish using concentrations measured in fish tissue versus those projected from water concentrations using chemical specific bioconcentration factors (BCFs). When fish tissue data are absent, the risk assessment team must "default" to BCFs in order to project tissue levels as a consequence. These data were collected at a site contaminated with chlordane and heptachlor and show how overly conservative estimates may be when appropriate data are not gathered.

Using BCFs as reported in the Superfund Manual,[1] it can be seen that concentrations exceed actual fish tissue levels by approximately two orders of magnitude for these chlorinated pesticides. It is noteworthy that the empirical BCFs (i.e. the ratio of measured fish tissue levels to ambient water concentrations) are so much lower than those reported in the open literature. This may result from the relative short-term nature of BCF experiments, while the empirical values represent long-term exposure conditions.

The large differences observed in BCF-projected as opposed to measured tissue concentrations are also reflected in the hazard index and excess cancer risk derived from the tissue levels. The algorithm used to convert fish tissue levels to human intakes (and attendant assumptions) are reported in Table 2.

Using this algorithm to convert BCF-estimated and measured fish tissue concentrations to estimated human intakes, the Hazard Index and excess cancer risks from fish consumption are shown in Tables 3 and 4, respectively.

As for the tissue levels, the non-carcinogenic and carcinogenic risk levels are approximately 2 orders of magnitude less when based upon actual fish tissue levels as opposed to BCF-estimated levels.

If fish tissue data are lacking, it is quite likely that water concentrations at the fishing location are also absent (such was the case in these examples). This further necessitates surface water modeling to predict concentrations in the water body where fishing occurs. Although the data are not shown here, this additional step results in even greater differences

Table 1. Fish Tissue Concentrations (mg/kg) Measured Versus BCF-Projected (from Ambient Water)

	SPHEM Projected Concentration	Measured Concentration	Empirical BCF	BCF*
Chlordane	1.40E+04	2.04E+01	1.00E-01	6.85E+01
Heptachlor	1.57E+04	2.36E+00	2.55E-02	1.70E+02

*Reported in the Superfund Public Health Evaluation Manual (SPHEM).[1]

Table 2. Algorithm for Estimating Contaminant Intake: Oral Ingestion of Contaminants from Fish

Algorithm:

$$FID = \frac{CWATER \times BCF \times FCR}{BW}$$

Variables:

FID = Fish ingestion dose (mg/kg/day)
CWATER = Surface water concentration (mg/l)
FCR = Fish consumption rate (kg/day)
BCF = Bioconcentration factor (see below)
BW = Body weight (kg)

Assumptions:

1. Fish consumption rate from recreational sources: adults = 4.4E-03 kg/day; children 2.2E-03 kg/day.
2. Body weight = 70 kg for adults and 42.2 kg for children (Anderson[2]).

Table 3. Comparison of Hazard Indices from BCF-Projected versus Measured Fish Tissue Levels (for Fish Consumers)

	Estimated BCF-Based (mg/kg/day)	Intakes Tissue-Based (mg/kg/day)	Acceptable Daily Intakes (mg/kg/day)	HI BCF-Based	HI Tissue-Based
Chlordane	1.07E-03	5.21E-06	5.00E-05	2.13E+01	1.04E-01
Heptachlor	1.23E-04	1.33E-06	5.00E-05	2.46E+00	2.66E-02
Total				2.38E+01	1.31E-01

Table 4. Estimated Excess Lifetime Cancer Risk from Fish Consumption: BCF-Projected versus Measured Fish Tissue Levels

	Estimated Intakes (mg/kg/day)		Oral Cancer Potency Value*	Cancer Risk	
	BCF-Based	Tissue-Based		BCF-Based	Tissue-Based
Chlordane	1.07E-03	5.21E-06	1.30E+00	1.39E-03	6.78E-06
Heptachlor	1.23E-04	1.33E-06	3.40E+00	4.17E-04	4.52E-06
Total				1.80E-03	1.13E-05

*From the Superfund Public Health Evaluation Manual.[1]

between risk levels based on projected concentrations as opposed to those based on actual fish tissue measurements. The additional step of modeling further increases uncertainty due to requisite assumptions which necessarily must err on the conservative side in order to protect health.

DATA HANDLING/REDUCTION

Data reduction for the purpose of assigning average chemical concentrations to the various environmental media at a site may also has a critical impact on the health risk levels ultimately based upon them. An example of the criticality of data reduction techniques is provided in a decision as basic as how to address non-detects (samples where a chemical is not detected).

Ignoring non-detects introduces a bias into the data. However, the bias is health conservative in the sense that it will usually overestimate the average concentration of a particular medium. This is shown in Table 5 for a data set of soil samples where non-detects are ignored in one column and one-half the detection limit is substituted for non-detects in the next. There is great incentive to ignore non-detects because it may be a labor intensive procedure to insert one half the detection limit for non-detects where significant numbers of non-detects exist. This is because the detection limit may vary for each sample since its dilution depends upon the concentration of the predominant chemical. Thus, each individual concentration must be evaluated for each chemical in each sample. Further complicating this procedure is the question of which value to insert for non-detects (this is a subject of debate among statisticians).

If non-detects are ignored, the bias may become extreme when the proportion of non-detects to detects is high, resulting in gross overestimation of the average media concentration.[3] This is equivalent to assigning the average concentration of a small "hot-spot" to an entire sampling grid which may exceed the surface area (or volume) of the hot spot by orders of magnitude. Consequently, exposure and risk calculations based upon such data will be similarly overestimated. The health impacts of ignoring or including non-detects are compared in Tables 6 through 8.

Table 5. Contaminant Concentrations in Soil and Water

	Plant Soil (μg/kg) non-detects		Creek Water (μg/l) non-detects	
	(ignored)	(not ignored)	(ignored)	(not ignored)
benzene	1.80E+05	1.47E+01	6.13E+01	2.50E+00
chlordane	2.62E+04	8.68E+02	1.64E+00	1.46E–01
chloroform	-	1.04E+01	5.00E+00	2.50E+00
DEHP*	3.39E+03	1.44E+02	1.47E+01	8.40E+00
heptachlor	1.75E+03	4.20E+01	-	1.50E–01
hex**	1.60E+03	3.61E+02	6.30E+00	5.00E+00
lead	5.82E+01	4.06E+01	2.68E+00	2.05E+00
phenol	-	2.97E+02	5.10E+01	5.90E+00
toluene	7.10E+05	2.12E+01	-	2.50E+00

*DEHP = Di- or bis(2-ethylhexyl)phthalate
**Hex = Hexachlorocyclopentadiene

Ignoring and not ignoring non-detects, Table 6 compares the estimated dosages and hazard indices (HI) for each oral, inhalation, and dermal exposure pathway. Table 7 reports overall HI for oral, inhalation/dermal, and combined exposures and Table 8 reports similar information for estimated lifetime cancer risks. These tables show that the very large artificial increases in the contaminant concentrations in soil and other media (resulting from ignoring non-detects) translate directly to quantitative overestimates of health impacts.

DISCUSSION

Data Gathering. The great differences in risk levels resulting from projected data as opposed to actual data, range far beyond the examples given in this paper. The same principle applies to any situation where modeling is applied to predict concentrations at a contact location removed from the initially contaminated source. While it is not always possible to measure concentrations at distant contact points (the contaminants may not have had time to reach the site), it is important at least to attempt to base risk assessments on actual analytical levels. The examples provided clearly illustrate the importance of this principle, showing differences of as much as 2 or more orders of magnitude when media concentrations must be estimated using factors (such as BCFs) or predictive models.

The problem of insufficient data may only be solved if those applying the data to perform a risk assessment are included early in the site investigation to help derive the sampling plan.

Data Handling. Ignoring or not ignoring non-detects will also influence exposure scenarios beyond those illustrated in this paper. For example, any soil contact scenario, such as pica soil ingestion by small children or incidental ingestion by workers or trespassers will be affected by assigning an overly conservative average concentration to the soil. The dermal soil-contact pathway is similarly affected. Rather than insert concentrations which are one half the detection limit to avoid overly conservative estimates, it is far easier to define the area of the hot spot within a sampling matrix or field where

Table 6. Estimated Contaminant Dosages (mg/kg/day) and Noncarcinogenic Hazard Indices Oral Exposure

Indicator Chemical	Incidental Oral Soil Ingestion non-detects (ignored)	(not ignored)	Fish Ingestion non-detects (ignored)	(not ignored)	Swimmer Oral Ingestion non-detects (ignored)	(not ignored)	Total Ingestion non-detects (ignored)	(not ignored)	Oral Acceptable Daily Intake (mg/kg/day)	Oral Hazard Index non-detects (ignored)	(not ignored)
benzene	6.1E-02	5.0E-06	1.9E-04	7.6E-06	3.1E-05	1.3E-06	6.1E-02	1.4E-05	7.4E-04	8.2E+01	1.9E-02
chlordane	8.8E-03	2.9E-04	1.3E-02	1.2E-03	8.4E-07	7.5E-08	2.2E-02	1.5E-03	5.0E-05	4.5E+02	3.0E+01
chloroform	-	3.5E-06	1.1E-05	5.5E-06	2.6E-06	1.3E-06	1.4E-05	1.0E-05	1.0E-02	1.4E-03	1.0E-03
DEHP	1.1E-03	4.9E-05	1.2E-01	6.9E-02	7.5E-06	4.3E-06	1.2E-01	6.9E-02	2.0E-02	6.1E+00	3.4E+00
heptachlor	5.9E-04	1.4E-05	-	1.4E-03	-	7.7E-08	5.9E-04	1.4E-03	5.0E-05	1.2E+01	2.8E+01
hex	5.4E-04	1.2E-04	1.6E-05	1.3E-05	3.2E-06	2.6E-06	5.6E-04	1.4E-04	7.0E-03	8.0E-02	2.0E-02
lead	2.0E-05	1.4E-05	7.7E-05	5.9E-05	1.4E-06	1.0E-06	9.8E-05	7.4E-05	1.4E-03	7.0E-02	5.3E-02
phenol	-	1.0E-04	4.2E-05	4.8E-06	2.6E-05	3.0E-06	6.8E-05	1.1E-04	4.0E-02	1.7E-03	2.7E-03
toluene	2.4E-01	7.2E-06	-	1.6E-05	-	1.3E-06	2.4E-01	2.4E-05	3.0E-01	8.0E-01	8.0E-05
									Total =	5.5E+02	6.1E+01

DERMAL AND INHALATION EXPOSURES

Indicator Chemical	Dermal Absorption From Soil Contact non-detects (ignored)	(not ignored)	Dermal Absorption From Swimming non-detects (ignored)	(not ignored)	Inhalation non-detects (ignored)	(not ignored)	Total Dermal & Inhalation non-detects (ignored)	(not ignored)	Inhalation Acceptable Daily Intake (mg/kg/day)	Dermal & Inhalation Hazard Index non-detects (ignored)	(not ignored)
benzene	1.9E-01	1.5E-05	6.0E-06	2.5E-07	1.3E-04	1.1E-08	1.9E-01	1.6E-05	7.4E-04	2.6E+02	2.1E-02
chlordane	2.7E-02	9.1E-04	1.6E-07	1.4E-08	1.9E-05	6.3E-07	2.7E-02	9.1E-04	5.0E-05	5.5E+02	1.8E+01
chloroform	-	1.1E-05	4.9E-07	2.5E-07	-	7.6E-09	4.9E-07	1.1E-05	1.0E-02	4.9E-05	1.1E-03
DEHP	3.6E-03	1.5E-04	1.4E-06	8.3E-07	2.5E-06	1.1E-07	3.6E-03	1.5E-04	2.0E-02	1.8E-01	7.6E-03
heptachlor	1.8E-03	4.4E-05	-	1.5E-08	1.3E-06	3.1E-08	1.8E-03	4.4E-05	5.0E-05	3.7E+01	8.8E-01
hex	1.7E-03	3.8E-04	6.2E-07	4.9E-07	1.2E-06	2.6E-07	1.7E-03	3.8E-04	6.6E-05	2.5E+01	5.7E+00
lead	6.1E-05	4.3E-05	2.6E-07	2.0E-07	4.3E-08	3.0E-08	6.1E-05	4.3E-05	4.3E-04	1.4E-01	1.0E-01
phenol	-	3.1E-04	5.0E-06	5.8E-07	-	2.2E-07	5.0E-06	3.1E-04	2.0E-02	2.5E-04	1.6E-02
toluene	7.4E-01	2.2E-05	-	2.5E-07	5.2E-04	1.6E-08	7.4E-01	2.2E-05	1.5E+00	5.0E-01	1.5E-05
									Total =	8.7E+02	2.5E+01

Table 7. Estimated Contaminant Dosages (mg/kg/day) and Noncarcinogenic Hazard Indices (All Exposure Routes Combined)

Indicator Chemical	Intake by all Pathways non-detects ignored	not-ignored	Total Hazard Index non-detects ignored	not-ignored
benzene	2.5E-01	3.0E-05	3.4E+02	4.0E-02
chlordane	5.0E-02	2.4E-03	1.0E+03	4.8E+01
chloroform	1.4E-05	2.1E-05	1.4E-03	2.1E-03
DEHP	1.3E-01	6.9E-02	6.3E+00	3.5E+00
heptachlor	2.4E-03	1.4E-03	4.9E+01	2.9E+01
hex	2.2E-03	5.2E-04	2.6E+01	5.8E+00
lead	1.6E-04	1.2E-04	2.1E-01	1.5E-01
phenol	7.3E-05	4.2E-04	1.9E-03	1.8E-02
toluene	9.8E-01	4.7E-05	1.3E+00	9.5E-05
Total			1.4E+03	8.6E+01

exposure might occur and adjust the intake algorithm by a factor equal to the ratio of the area of the hot spot to the sampling matrix or plausible exposure field. This may be thought of either in terms of probability of contact time (with the hot spot) or probability of visiting the hot spot location and practically applied using the adjustment factor referred to above in the intake algorithm.

Another area where risk assessments might be improved lies more in the realm of data application rather than handling. The inclusion of standard scenarios common for all sites and using the same algorithms would benefit the practice of risk assessment. The scenarios comprising such a "standard set" should be simple and commonly encountered. For example, assuming an hypothetical well on site using the simple algorithm of 2 liters per day for 70 kg adult provides a common benchmark by which to compare site to site, no matter which consultant has performed the assessment. Another exposure scenario might consist of soil ingestion (incidental as well as pica) or dermal contact with soils. These scenarios would not have to be "realistic" under current use conditions but should be otherwise plausible. This would strengthen risk assessments in their ability to measure relative risks, comparing site to site and pathway to pathway in order to prioritize sites and contaminant migration pathways for remediation. This would be possible only with the consistent use of more standardized algorithms and supporting assumptions. Such a practice would not have to impede the application of more sophisticated intake algorithms or modeling techniques which could also be included in the risk assessment.

In summary, data gathering and handling practices may profoundly influence health risk levels estimated for a contaminated site. An awareness of how various procedures impact risk levels is essential in order to have sufficient information when it is initially gathered and to avoid bias when reducing data.

Table 8. Excess Carcinogenic Risk from Lifetime Exposure to Contaminants Oral Exposure

Indicator Chemical	Soil Ingestion non-detects (ignored)	Soil Ingestion non-detects (not ignored)	Fish Ingestion non-detects (ignored)	Fish Ingestion non-detects (not ignored)	Swimmer Ingestion non-detects (ignored)	Swimmer Ingestion non-detects (not ignored)	Total Ingestion non-detects (ignored)	Total Ingestion non-detects (not ignored)
benzene	3.2E-03	2.6E-07	9.7E-06	4.0E-07	1.6E-06	6.6E-08	3.2E-03	7.2E-07
chlordane	1.1E-02	3.8E-04	1.7E-02	1.6E-03	1.1E-06	9.7E-08	2.9E-02	1.9E-03
chloroform	-	2.8E-07	8.9E-07	4.4E-07	2.1E-07	1.0E-07	1.1E-06	8.3E-07
DEHP	7.8E-07	3.3E-08	8.2E-05	4.7E-05	5.1E-09	2.9E-09	8.3E-05	4.7E-05
heptachlor	2.0E-03	4.8E-05	-	4.7E-03	-	2.6E-07	2.0E-03	4.7E-03
Totals	1.7E-02	4.3E-04	1.8E-02	6.3E-02	2.9E-06	5.3E-07	3.4E-02	6.7E-03

DERMAL AND INHALATION EXPOSURES

Indicator Chemical	Dermal Absorption From Soil Contact non-detects (ignored)	Dermal Absorption From Soil Contact non-detects (not ignored)	Dermal Absorption From Swimming non-detects (ignored)	Dermal Absorption From Swimming non-detects (not ignored)	Inhalation non-detects (ignored)	Inhalation non-detects (not ignored)	Total Dermal & Inhalation non-detects (ignored)	Total Dermal & Inhalation non-detects (not ignored)
benzene	4.9E-03	4.0E-07	1.6E-07	6.4E-09	3.4E-06	2.8E-10	4.9E-03	4.1E-07
chlordane	3.6E-02	1.2E-03	2.1E-07	1.9E-08	2.5E-05	8.3E-07	3.6E-02	1.2E-03
chloroform	-	8.8E-07	4.0E-08	2.0E-08	-	6.2E-10	4.0E-08	9.0E-07
DEHP	2.4E-06	1.0E-07	9.9E-10	5.6E-10	1.7E-09	7.2E-11	2.4E-06	1.0E-07
heptachlor	6.2E-03	1.5E-04	-	5.0E-08	4.4E-06	1.0E-07	6.2E-03	1.5E-04
Totals	4.7E-02	1.3E-03	4.1E-07	9.6E-08	3.3E-05	9.3E-07	4.7E-02	1.3E-03

ALL EXPOSURE ROUTES COMBINED

Indicator Chemical	Total Ingestion non-detects (ignored)	Total Ingestion non-detects (not ignored)	Total Dermal & Inhalation non-detects (ignored)	Total Dermal & Inhalation non-detects (not ignored)	Intake by all Paths Combined non-detects (ignored)	Intake by all Paths Combined non-detects (not ignored)
benzene	3.2E-03	7.2E-07	4.9E-03	4.1E-07	8.1E-03	1.1E-06
chlordane	2.9E-02	1.9E-03	3.6E-02	1.2E-03	6.5E-02	3.1E-03
chloroform	1.1E-06	8.3E-07	4.0E-08	9.0E-07	1.1E-06	1.7E-06
DEHP	8.3E-05	4.7E-05	2.4E-06	1.0E-07	8.6E-05	4.7E-05
heptachlor	2.0E-03	4.7E-03	6.2E-03	1.5E-04	8.3E-03	4.9E-03
Totals	3.4E-02	6.7E-03	4.7E-02	1.3E-03	8.1E-02	8.1E-03

REFERENCES

1. EPA (Environmental Protection Agency), *Superfund Public Health Evaluation Manual*, Office of Emergency and Remedial Response, EPA 540/1-86/060 (1986).
2. E. Anderson, S. Browne, S. Duletsky, J. Ramig, and T. Warn, Development of Statistical Distributions or Ranges of Standard Factors Used in Exposure Assessments, U.S. EPA, Office of Health and Environmental Assessment, OHEA-E-161 (1985).
3. R. O. Gilbert, *Statistical Methods for Environmental Pollution Monitoring,* Van Nostrand Reinhold Co., New York (1987).

Measurement Uncertainty in Epidemiological Studies of Two Cohorts Exhibiting Benzene-Induced Leukemia

Elizabeth T. Barfield
BEST Consulting
Apex, NC

H. Gruenwald
Long Island Hospital
Long Island, NY

Steven H. Lamm and Anthony Walters
Consultants in Epidemiology and Occupational Health
Washington, DC

Richard Wilson
Harvard University
Cambridge, MA

Daniel M. Byrd
Consulting Toxicologist
Falls Church, VA

ABSTRACT

This paper reviews several epidemiology papers by Vigliani and his coworkers about benzene-associated leukemia in the Milan and Pavia areas of Italy. Although the data have generally been thought not suitable for risk assessment, we find that the application of expert judgment and a previously developed combinatorial procedure successfully yields a description of the range of risk of benzene-associated leukemias in these studies. We also compare this risk distribution to that obtained with the same model and data from risk assessments of a study by Rinsky, Young and coworkers about benzene-exposed workers in Ohio. The leukemogenic risks of benzene differ between the two cohorts but are not inconsistent. Based on a probability distribution representing an aggregate of opinions, however, experts' uncertainty about risk in the Italian cohort exceeds the assessors' uncertainty about risk in the Ohio cohort.

KEYWORDS: Benzene, leukemia, Vigliani, epidemiology, uncertainty

INTRODUCTION

Our previous work led to development of a general combinatorial procedure for the application of an empirical degree-of-belief method to risk assessment. We applied this method to fourteen risk assessments that were based on a historical prospective cohort study of Ohio rubber hydrochloride workers described by Rinsky, Young and their coworkers.[1,2] The risk distributions in these papers described the aggregate belief of a group of risk assessors about measurement uncertainty in the epidemiology data.

The applications of the procedure gave equal weight to each unique, competing value in a data set for each parameter in a risk model. As such, these results could have been congruent with similar evaluations in which different experts gave values for each parameter of a risk model, but no differential weight was accorded the skills of each expert. If the experts were the same as the risk assessors, presumably the distributions would be identical.

Unlike the cohort described by Rinsky, Young and their coworkers, other epidemiology studies of benzene-exposed persons have not been subjected to extensive, multiple risk assessments.[3,4] To examine measurement uncertainty in one of the other cohorts, we modified our combinatorial procedure to utilize expert judgment. Several investigators were invited to describe their opinions about the data in Vigliani's epidemiology studies of benzene by estimating the value of each parameter in a risk model; that is, population size, exposure, and so forth.

Delore and Borgomano first reported benzene-associated leukemia in the literature in 1928.[5] By 1938, Vigliani and Penati prepared a critical survey of the literature and identified 10 cases of benzene leukemia, plus many cases that today would be classified as pre-leukemia.[6] In the mid-1970's Vigliani reported on the outcomes of an epidemic of chronic benzene poisoning that occurred in the Italian rotogravure printing industry between 1949 and 1965 and in the Italian shoe making industry from 1959 to 1963.[7,8,9] These epidemics of chronic benzene poisoning were traced back to the use of inks and glues which contained benzene as a solvent at concentrations up to nearly 100 percent. These epidemics were brought to a close with the prohibition by law of benzene as a solvent for inks and glues.

By 1945, another Italian worker, Saita, had accumulated 23 published cases.[10] Vigliani continued to observe cases of benzene-associated leukemia and, in 1964 with Saita, reported the experiences of the occupational medicine clinic in Milan.[11] This led to a series of papers that later additionally included the experience of Professors Pollini and Maugeri at the occupational medicine clinic in Pavia.[7]

The resulting literature, however, became confused, because some later papers refer in part to cases which were previously reported. Vigliani reported numerous cases of benzene leukemia and benzene hemopathy in his studies, and the total number of cases varied from report to report. In Pavia and outside of Milan, he found 13 reported cases of benzene leukemia (9 acute myelogenous leukemia, 1 chronic myelogenous leukemia, 2 acute erythemia, and 1 acute erythroid leukemia). In Milan, he found 47 reported benzene hemopathy cases between 1942 and 1963, of which 6 were leukemias. (See case descriptions below).

To some extent, the desirability of the current exercise arises from the limited descriptions of risk parameters in these papers. At the time of Vigliani's publications, the practice of quantitative risk assessment had not been invented, and his papers do not contain all of the data elements that modern risk assessors seek in publications. Probably for this reason, most investigators have rejected the use of these data in risk assessments. While

Vigliani's studies do not contain all of the information necessary to assess risk, the present authors find that use can be made of them.

METHODS

Cases

We extracted the original Milan cases from the multiple descriptions in the Italian reports.[6-8,10,12,13] For Pavia the cases have been reported.[9]

1. A 49 year old man started as a leather worker in 1933, became symptomatic with asthenia in 1934, and was diagnosed with acute myelogenous leukemia in 1942, 1.5 months before his death and after 9 years of exposure.

2. A 38 year old man started at rotagravure in 1940 with inks containing 40% benzene, was exposed to benzene air levels of 0.6 to 2.1 mg/liter for 5 years, developed asthenia and pallor in 1944, splenomegaly and petechiae in 1945, and died in May of 1945 with an autopsy diagnosis of myeloid metaplasia.

3. A 29 year old man with an 8 year history of spraying nitrocellular varnishes dissolved in a 60% benzene solvent first exhibited asthenia in 1956 and was diagnosed with acute myelogenous leukemia in 1958.

4. A 24 year old man who began in 1938 in the same rotagravure department as case 2, above, was well until 1961 except for a tendency to mild leukopenia, when he developed asthenia, was treated for acute myelogenous leukemia, and died. The reported benzene levels were 200 to 400 ppm with peak excursions to 1,500 ppm. Benzene use in his department terminated in 1949, and he continued in a quarterly examination program.

5. A 50 year old man who glued rubber ribbons to billiards with 100% benzene glue from 1943 to 1961 for 2-3 hours/day presented in November of 1961 with asthenia and was treated successfully for acute myelogenous leukemia with corticosteroids and transfusions into 1963, when he went home and was lost to follow up.

6. A 53 year old woman who used 25% benzene solvent to glue artificial flowers for 3 years was treated for acute myelogenous leukemia from June to October of 1963, when she died from undifferentiated stem cell leukemia.

7. A 36 year old woman, who worked as an electric cable finisher from 1942 to 1964 using benzene as a solvent, presented with severe anemia in September of 1964, aplastic anemia in December of 1965, and myeloid metaplasia in May of 1966. She died in April of 1967 with acute myelogenous leukemia superimposed on aplastic anemia.[13]

8. A 37 year old woman, who used a glue diluted with benzene on her finger to assemble beauty cases from 1959 to 1966, had a vaginal bleed in 1965, presented with acute erythroblastic leukemia in 1966, and died in 1967 with erythroid and myeloid infiltration of the liver and spleen.[14]

9. A 31 year old man, who worked as a shoemaker from 1959 to 1961, and who heated and shaped shoes softened with a 40% benzene solvent, presented with a pallor in the spring of 1962, anemia in October of 1962, erythroblastic marrow in May of 1963, myeloblastic leukemia in March of 1965, and died in May of 1965 of subacute benzene erythroleukemia.

10. A 66 year old woman, who glued artistic leatherware from 1954 to 1957 with a 75% benzene adhesive, presented with pancytopenia in 1957, 1965, and 1972, and with erythroblastic and myeloblastic marrow at death January of 1973, was diagnosed as having benzene erythroleukemia.

11. A 55 year old male shoemaker, who worked close to other shoemakers using benzene from 1958 to 1965, presented in 1961, 1964, and 1969 with hyporegenerative anemia and was admitted in 1970 with acute ethryremia superimposed on aplastic anemia.

Experts

We solicited estimates from four medical experts, each with some familiarity with epidemiology, industrial hygiene, and leukemia. They were promised anonymity. All expressed severe doubts about the value of the exercise, especially the prospect of forcing a cohort design onto essentially a record of case studies, with the unlikely assumption that no cases escaped the attention of the Italian physicians. While the effort involved was offhand, however, it was qualitatively of the same historical prospective nature as the studies of the Ohio cohort, in that reporting of several cases led to specification of a group with disputable numbers of cases, controversial exposures, and arguable outcomes.

In one case, where an expert did not state a value for a parameter, we inferred it by back calculation from the expert's guess of an overall risk value. Statements of boundary conditions (between x and y) were accepted as a pair of values, as if the distribution was square wave, and the two results were each given half weight.

Combinatorial Procedure

The combinatorial procedure operates according to a recursive formula,

$$a_i \cdot b_j \cdot c_k \cdot .... d_l = r_z,$$

where a_i, b_j, c_k, and d_l each represents one value taken from a set for each factor (or its reciprocal), taken in all possible combinations, and r_z represents the resulting set of risk estimates. Because the risk calculation is multiplicative in essence, the resulting distribution is log-normal distributed. The following formula, which assumes absence of a threshold, no latency, and Haber's rule, was used.

$$\mathrm{R} = \frac{[\mathrm{O} - (P \times M)]}{D \times P \times E}$$

where:

R = Risk of excess deaths
O = Observed leukemic deaths
P = Exposed population
M = Risk of leukemia in the control population
D = Duration of exposure (years)
E = Exposure concentration (ppm).

Calculations were carried out using *Clipper*, a compiled version of dBase III and checked occasionally and independently with APL68000. When compared, virtually identical results were obtained with both programs. The *Clipper* program is available on request from the authors. The program currently displays the results in both tabular and graphical form and gives geometric average and variance. Geometric mean and variance were calculated according to the formulas given by Aitchison and Brown.[15]

RESULTS

The Italian authors reported cases 1-6 (seen between 1942 and 1963) as examples of hematocytoblastic leukemia (with myeloid characteristics) and also reported never observing a case of chronic myeloid or lymphatic leukemia in workers poisoned with benzene.[11] For comparison, the authors reported that in 1959-61 the annual leukemia incidence rate in the general Milan population was 0.01% or 10^{-4} year^{-1}, with a distribution of 46% acute leukemias, 28% chronic myelogenous leukemia and 26% chronic lymphocytic leukemia. The annual acute leukemia rate was estimated at 0.46 × 0.01%, or 5×10^{-5} year^{-1} (1/20,000).

Vigliani and Saita state that fewer than 5,000 persons were occupationally exposed to benzene in Milan and Pavia together and that fewer than 3,000 of those were exposed to "dangerous" concentrations of benzene vapors.[11] During 1960-61, one leukemia death (Milan or Pavia) was registered as a blood dyscrasia due to chronic benzene poisoning with the National Institute for Insurance Against Accidents and Occupational Diseases, and 10 were registered for the 1962-63 period. The authors also cited an unpublished case of a 66 year old woman with benzene anemia in 1957 and normal blood counts, which proceeded her 1972 onset of an acute erythroleukemia that was fatal in five months.

Assuming that the exposed population was 5,000 persons, the leukemia rate for 1960-61 would be 5,000 persons × 2 years × 0.01% year^{-1} = 1 death and for acute leukemia would be half of this rate (5,000 × 2 × 0.01% × 0.46 = 0.5 death). For 1962-63, however, the leukemia rate was 10 times that expected (10 observed/1 expected) and for acute leukemia was approximately 20 times expected (10 observed/0.5 expected).

The Milan Clinic reported eleven cases of benzene-associated leukemic deaths between 1943 and 1974. Not all came from Milan or Pavia, not all were benefit cases, but all had acute hematocytoblastic leukemia (eight cases) or erythroleukemia (three cases). Additionally, one acute erythremia death and six aplastic anemia deaths occurred. The Pavia Clinic reported thirteen cases of death from acute leukemia and three aplastic anemia deaths between 1959 and 1974, all of which were acute hematocytoblastic in type. Nine leukemia cases were initially seen in the clinic and 4 were referred in from other hospitals in Pavia. Five of these 9 cases from the clinic had leukemia superimposed on aplastic anemia.

Another risk comparison that can be extracted from these statements is that the category of persons "exposed to dangerous concentrations of benzene vapors" had a risk estimate of about 33 (10 observed among 3,000 persons with 0.3 expected).

The Milan Clinic reported 66 benzene hemopathy cases and 11 benzene leukemia cases, who were first seen between 1942 and 1975, and who were reported by industry and gender. The benzene exposure at the rotagravure plant, from which cases 2 and 4 came, and exposure was later reported as 200 to 400 ppm with peaks to 1,500 ppm. The eleven cases would now be described as myeloblastic (7), erythremic (1), or erythroleukemic (3).

The Pavia Clinic reported cases from the shoe making industry, with air measurements in the range of 25-600 ppm benzene, but mostly at about 200-500 ppm from use of glues and solvents containing up to 100% benzene. For the 9 cases originally seen at the clinic (as opposed to the 4 cases referred to them, for whom data are lacking), ages at diagnosis ranged from 35 to 66 with a mean of 53.7 years and a median of 54 years and durations of exposure for two cases of 1-2 years, one of 8 years, and five of 38-46 years. All cases were acute myeloid (stem, hematocytoblast, myeloblast, paramyeloblast, or erythro) leukemia.

Between 1942 and 1975 the Milan clinic had a total of 10 or 11 acute leukemia cases and additional acute erythremia cases, not all from Milan.

We are told that the crude leukemia mortality rate for Milan is 0.01%/year with 46% of them being acute leukemias. The peak relative risk for acute leukemia among the benzene exposed population in Milan and Pavia together supposedly was about 20 fold for 1962-1963.

An alternative calculation might be that of 3,000 heavily exposed workers × (15 years in Pavia or 33 years in Milan, we assume an average of 24 years) × 0.01% × 0.46 = 3,000 persons × 24 years × 0.01% leukemia deaths $year^{-1}$ × 0.46 acute leukemia death/leukemia death = 3.3 cases expected. A total of 24 acute leukemia deaths were observed in the two clinics (though not all from the Milan and Pavia areas) for an overall relative risk of about 7.2 (24/3.3). Therefore, one estimate of the relative risk of acute leukemia is 7.2.

Besides the report of 200-400 ppm with peaks up to 1,500 ppm in one Milan rotagravure plant, levels of 25-600 ppm (with most measurements about 200-500 ppm) were noted in the shoe factories of Pavia. The Pavia data appear most closely related to the sites where most of the cases occurred. Therefore, an exposure estimate of 350 ppm could be used, with a range of 200-500 ppm covering perhaps 3/4 of these workers.

Among the Milan cases an exposure lasted between 3 to 22 years, with a mean of 12.3 and a mode of about 8 years. The duration of exposure for the non-cases was not given. Similarly, the range of latencies was 3 to 24 years, with a mode of about 7 years and mean of about 21 years. The Pavia cases have, as exposure durations, one person each at 1, 2, and 8 years, and five with a range of 32 to 46 years with both median and mode at 40 years. No latency information was given for the Pavia cases.

These estimates can be compared to the distribution of risk estimates parsed from aggregation the experts' values for the parameters for the Italian studies in the risk formula shown in Fig. 1. The comparable distribution for acute myelogenous leukemia cases in the 1987 NIOSH study is illustrated in Fig. 2.

DISCUSSION

We have proposed that risk assessors describe each parameter of a risk model as a probability distribution, instead of as a point value, to incorporate measurement uncertainty into the final result.[1,2] The outcome of this approach is a risk distribution, and, of necessity, it requires a procedure to integrate probability distributions and to estimate the distributions.

The primary purpose of this paper is to demonstrate that, given some wide-ranging assumptions and imaginative experts, it is possible to integrate fragmentary data to produce a risk distribution, albeit of a highly uncertain nature, through the use of a published error propagation techniques. From this perspective, the differences among historical prospective epidemiology studies are only quantitative in nature, differing in the nature of the probability distribution for each parameter, and therefore in uncertainty in risk. The current effort tends toward one extreme of the spectrum. Given this perspective, it also is noteworthy that the median risk in the distribution derived from the expert opinion about the studies by Vigliani and coworkers is similar in magnitude to that obtained from the risk assessors' valuations of Rinsky, Young and coworkers' study, as a comparison of Figs. 1 and 2 illustrates.

Based on the Italian studies, the aggregated risk distribution reflects, as expected, greater uncertainty among the experts, reflecting greater measurement uncertainty. The

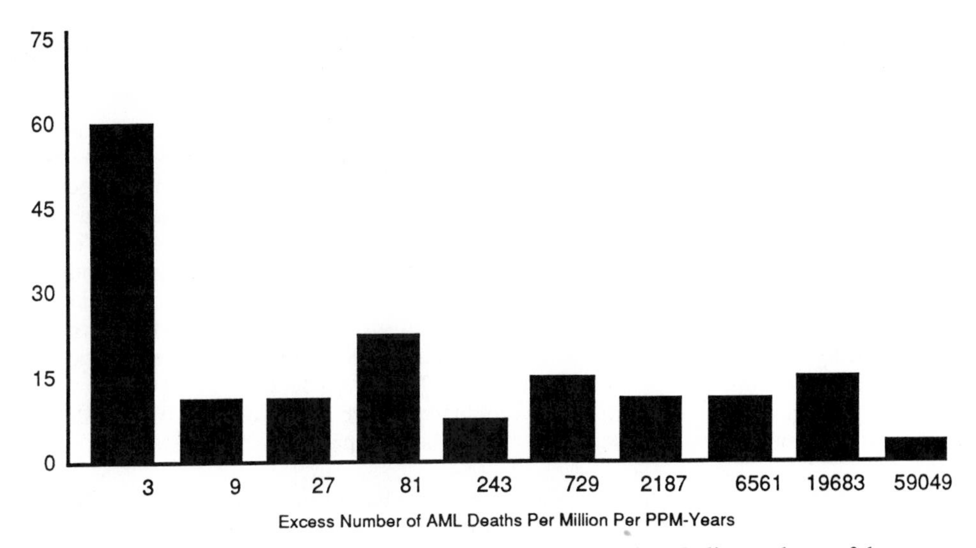

Fig. 1. Aggregate risk estimates of four experts using Italian cohort of benzene-exposed workers.

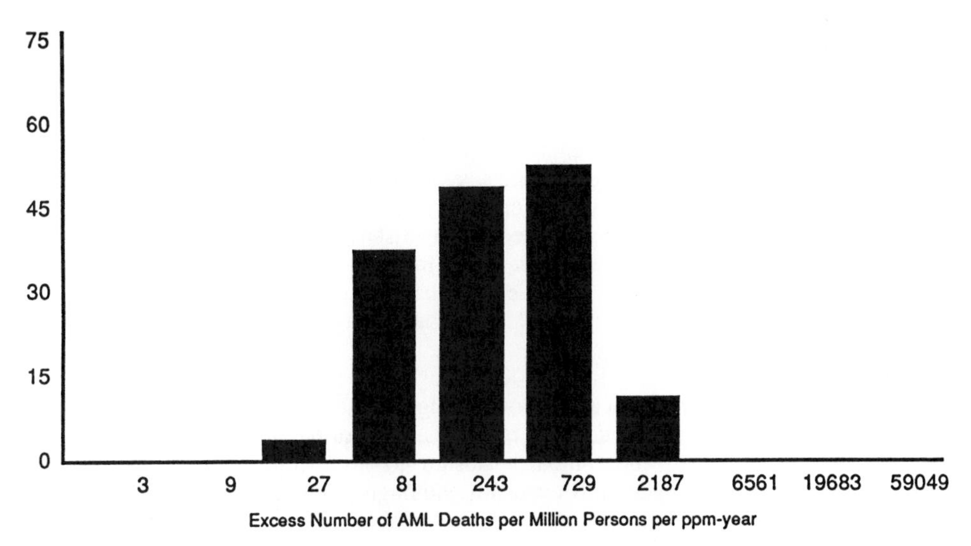

Fig. 2. Aggregate risk estimates from twelve risk assessors using Ohio cohort of benzene-exposed workers.

experts who agreed to provide us with their estimates of risk parameters experienced great difficulty and discomfort in producing these "as if" data.

This example also shows that the current approach is neither case control nor cohort in nature. A philosophical and statistical problem arises when cases noted initially are then used to construct exposure groups. This problem arises in both our use of Vigliani's studies and in the studies by Rinsky, Young and coworkers, but it is not intrinsic to all historical prospective studies. In essence, the assessor does not know whether to include or exclude the triggering cases in statistical analyses that led to conduct of the study and construction of the cohort. The groups have not been randomly defined, but the analytical procedures only apply to randomly constructed groups.

While the traditional admonition to describe all of the assumptions in a risk assessment does not necessarily address the sources of model uncertainty, most such assumptions relate to the structure of a proper risk model. Risk assessors tend to agonize over the question of model choice[16] but clinicians often do not. Vigliani's studies illustrate some consequences of this practice, because in places they omitted some relatively easily obtained parameters that are immediately necessary for any descriptive risk estimation (for example, the number of observed cases, population at risk, exposure levels, duration of exposure, latency of effect and/or appropriate control group for comparison). This paper suggests, however, that experts can reconstruct, if only crudely, these parameters. If we had used the same experts to review the study by Rinsky, Young and coworkers, then presumably the data sets could be directly compared, since the effect of having different experts produce the probability distributions would be eliminated.

The reader should not mistake that these procedures lead to accurate estimates of benzene potency or prove that the similarity of median risk estimates somehow proves that the model used is correct to describe the dose-response curve for benzene. In the present instance, the risk model almost certainly is wrong. Human erythroleukemic risk is not a linear function of benzene exposure.

Our procedure has flexibility with respect to risk models; almost any mathematical specification can be assumed. Because the procedure primarily elicits measurement uncertainty, the distributions simply are contingent on the assumptions in the risk model. In effect, the procedure integrates all differences of opinion about the values of parameters, instead of allowing, for example, compensating estimates of two different parameters to produce identical risk estimates, even if by coincidence. The procedure is not useful, however, in comparing two different models, as differences between risk distributions created by error propagation with two different models does not provide any information about which one best represents physical reality. A lesser problem can arise in estimating measurement uncertainty, when the assumed risk model omits an important variable (or includes an irrelevant one) about which the experts have opinions, because the specification of measurement uncertainty will be incomplete (or masked).

The mechanism of benzene-induced leukemogenesis is not well-understood. In this regard, our review of the Italian cases strongly suggests that direct dermal contact with liquid benzene often was an important risk factor, as many of the cases had such exposure. Similarly, in mouse studies intermittent exposure to high concentrations of benzene generates greater risk than continuous exposure, although the murine T-cell leukemias do not completely resemble the human acute erythroleukemias.[17]

REFERENCES

1. D. M. Byrd and E. T. Barfield, Empirical Degree-of-belief Methods for Risk Assessments Based on Epidemiology Data: Application of a Procedure for Combinatorial Analysis of Risk-related Components to a Series of Occupational Studies of Leukemia Incidence Associated with Benzene Exposure at Several Rubber Hydrochloride Plants in Ohio, in *Risk Assessment and Risk Management of Industrial and Environmental Chemicals*, pp. 209-223, R. Cothern and M. Mehlman, eds., Princeton Scientific, Princeton, NJ (1988).
2. D. M. Byrd and E. T. Barfield, Uncertainty in the Estimation of Benzene Risks: Application of an Uncertainty Taxonomy to Risk Assessments Based on an Epidemiology Study of Rubber Hydrochloride Workers, *Environ. Health Perspect.* **82**:283-287 (1989).

3. Occupational Safety and Health Administration, Occupational Exposure to Benzene: Final Rule, *Federal Register* **52**:34,460-34,578 (1987).
4. H. Austin, E. Delzell, and P. Cole, Benzene and Leukemia: A Review of the Literature and a Risk Assessment, *American J. Epidemiol.* **127**:419-139 (1988).
5. P. Delore and C. Borgomano, Leucemie sigue as couen [???] l'intoxication benzenique: sur l'origine toxique de certaines mies aiques et leurs relations avec les anemies graves, *J. Med. Lyon* **9**:227-233 (1928).
6. F. Penati and E. C. Vigliani, Sui problema delle mielopatie aplastiche, psuedoaplastiche e leucemiche da benzolo, *Rassegna Med. Indust.* **9**:345 (1938).
7. E. C. Vigliani, Leukemia: Occupational Chemical Factors, Proc. XI Internat. Congress Cancer, pp. 248-252, Florence, Italy (1974).
8. E. C. Vigliani and A. Forni, Benzene and Leukemia, *Environ. Res.* **11**:122-127 (1976).
9. E. C. Vigliani, Leukemia Associated with Benzene Exposure, *Ann. NY Acad. Sci.* pp. 143-151 (1976).
10. G. Saita, Mielosi aplastica e successiva mielosi leucemica leucopenica, provocate da benzolo, *Medicina De Lavoro* **36**:143 (1945)
11. E. C. Vigliani and G. Saita, Benzene and Leukemia, *New England J. Med.* **271**:872-876 (1964).
12. E. C. Vigliani and A. Forni, Benzene, Chromosome Changes and Leukemia, *J. Occup. Med.* **11**:148-149 (1969).
13. A. Forni and L. Moreo, Cytogenetic Studies in a Case of Benzene Poisoning, *Eur. J. Cancer* **3**:251-255 (1967).
14. A. Forni and L. Moreo, Chromosome Studies in a Case of Benzene-Induced Erythroleukemia, *Eur. J. Cancer* **5**:459-63 (1969).
15. J. Aitchison and J. A. C. Brown, *The Lognormal Distribution*, Cambridge University Press, Cambridge, MA (1973).
16. A. S. Whittemore, Quantitative Theories of Oncogenesis, *Advances in Cancer Research* **27**:55-88 (1978).
17. R. D. Irons, D. A. Neptun, and R. W. Pfeifer, Inhibition of Lymphocyte Transformation and Microtubule Assembly by Quinone Metabolites of Benzene: Evidence for a Common Mechanism, *J. Reticuloendothel. Soc.* **30**:359-371 (1981).

Organ Specificity of Rodent Tumor Induction: A Test of Statistical and Graphical Methods by Examination of Tumor Induction from Ingestion of Selected Substances

Daniel M. Byrd III
Consulting Toxicologist
Falls Church, VA

Edmund A. C. Crouch
Cambridge Environmental
Cambridge, MA

Richard Wilson
Harvard University
Cambridge, MA

ABSTRACT

With few exceptions current federal risk assessment policy regards the induction of tumors at one site as equivalent to the induction of tumors at any other site for purposes of risk assessment.[1] Sufficient bioassay data exist to test this policy with the closely related rodent species, mouse and rat.

We made estimates of organ-specific concordance between these two species for 102 organ sites, taking statistical variation into account and using the peer reviewed data of the National Toxicology Program and National Cancer Institute (NTP/NCI). We devised a graphical method to display the concordance results in two dimensions. We calculated the ratio of the number of substances that yield statistically positive results in both species to the number of substances the yield statistically positive results in a particular organ or site of one species. We plotted this ratio against a second ratio, the number of substances that do not yield statistically positive results in either species against the number of substances that do not yield statistically positive results at the same specific organ site and species.

Our approach leads to extensive results. Two of the more interesting, if expected, findings are that, (a) within the NTP/NCI data, concordance varies with the stringency of statistical criteria and with the kind of statistical test (for example, trend with dose instead of confidence that differences of tumor frequency exist between different dose groups), and (b) male and female mice have a greater concordance of tumor induction than do mice and rats.

Overall, our results support the present federal regulatory agency policy of estimating a general increase in cancer risk at *any* site for one species exposed to a substance, based on

Risk Analysis, Edited by C. Zervos
Plenum Press, New York, 1991

a statistically positive increase in tumors of a second species at a specific organ site after exposure to the same substance. However, our results also suggest a modification of current risk assessment practice in which the qualitative and quantitative implications of tumor induction at a specific organ site will vary, depending on which specific organ site is involved and the history of concordance of tumor induction between rodent species at the same site for all previously tested substances.

KEYWORDS: Rodent tumor induction, organ-specific concordance, animal carcinogens, risk assessment

INTRODUCTION

Whenever researchers think that some feature of carcinogenesis can simplify our thinking about the general phenomenon, further studies tend to develop complications. This tendency particularly applies to decision rules for the discovery and/or control of exposure to potential carcinogens.

Direct information on human carcinogenesis comes from accidental exposures, and these occur less and less frequently. Regulation of known human carcinogens to minimize risk seems obvious, so exposures trend lower. In addition, we can not ethically expose people to a substance to discover whether it causes cancer in man. Accidental exposures tend not to provide a reliable guide to potential toxicity, especially for carcinogens, which may pose risks at lower doses than apparent in small populations. The resulting information deficit forces a search for other methods of prediction.

This paper inquires about the relevance of cancer induction in laboratory animals to human carcinogenesis, but indirectly, by asking about the relevance of induction in one rodent species, the mouse, to another, the rat. With these two species better data exist.

Such an inquiry has considerable limitations, among which are the following:

1. Statistical relationships do not necessarily indicate causality or mechanism and may yield spurious results.
2. The National Toxicology Program and National Cancer Institute (NTP/NCI) did not choose the chemical substances to test in the bioassays at random or according to a prior, well-defined algorithm. It does not appear possible to state precisely what bias the nonrandom nature of the test substances will introduce into any results.
3. Mouse and rat have a close phylogenetic relationship. A concordance relationship between mouse and rat does not necessarily imply a similar relationship between either species and man.

Nevertheless, the methods described below, when applied to the best current data for cancer induction in rodents, will illuminate the limitations of our current decision rules for other species, such as rodent to man, for which the data are sparse and the methods, if stated at all, often lack precision.

DECISION RULES FOR HUMAN RISK ASSESSMENT

Thirty years ago, many persons hoped that only a few substances caused cancer. If that were true, it would be possible, with perhaps a few legislated exceptions, to ban the use of all human carcinogens. This idea, together with the idea that all animal carcinogens would prove carcinogenic in man, led to the Delaney amendment to the Federal Food, Drug and Cosmetic Act.[2-4] However, this decision rule now seems naive and impractical.[5]

The extent to which current methods of testing will yield a statistically positive result with a substance chosen at random from the chemical universe is a matter of controversy. Estimates range from 5 to 70%. Over 1,000 substances are known that can cause cancer in animals, and many of these substances are essential to commerce. A more sophisticated approach becomes necessary, in order not to destroy the industrial society that has afforded a high standard of living and long life expectancy.

Following the approach of the classical animal model, which has been used throughout biomedical science with many diseases, it seemed reasonable to look for cancer in the same organ where a substance caused acute toxicity. Organ specificity of toxicity might suggest specific metabolic activation and/or accumulation in the organ. If so, this second decision rule would suggest that an animal carcinogen with concordance of organ toxicity should be regulated as if it were a known human carcinogen. For example, when aflatoxin B1 was shown to cause liver toxicity in man, a search began for liver tumors caused by this substance in rats and mice. Indeed, aflatoxin B1 has been shown to cause liver tumors in rats quite readily. Moreover, early studies suggested that aflatoxin B1 also causes liver tumors in exposed human populations, although another association with hepatitis B virus infection now confounds this association.

A third decision rule derived from the same classical paradigm of the animal model for a human disease, namely that a substance which causes a particular cancer in one species might cause the same cancer at the same site in a different species. For example, vinyl chloride causes angiosarcoma in both men and rats. This decision rule suggests a particularly tissue sensitivity of the organ for the substance or its metabolites.

Tomatis and coworkers[6] proposed a fourth decision rule. They showed that animal bioassays for those substances which caused cancer in man usually cause tumors in animals, but at a variety of different sites, not always the same organ site seen in man. Tomatis[7] proposed that, in screening substances for possible human carcinogenic effects, all animal tumors should be considered as evidence for possible human carcinogenesis. As described, for example by EPA's Carcinogen Assessment Group,[8] Tomatis' proposal has been the basis of calls for regulation of each and every animal carcinogen *as if* it were known to cause cancer in man. This decision rule dominates current regulatory practice. It has the effect of treating tumor induction at any animal organ site as quantitatively equivalent to any other site with respect to human carcinogenic risk.

In order to study the validity of this decision rule, Crouch and Wilson[9] compared carcinogenic potency of a number of substances in rats and mice, and showed that potencies in the two species correlated better if the site was not specified. (On the average, the potency estimated from the induction of tumors by a substance at a specific organ site in the mouse agrees better with the potency estimated from the induction of tumors by the same substance at any organ site in the rat than does the potency estimated from the induction of tumors at the same site as that used for estimation with the mouse.) Using the same strategy of correlation between potencies of a substance at any organ site in two different species, Crouch[10,11] showed that few, if any, cases exist in which the carcinogenic potency in one rodent species differs by more than a factor of 100 from the potency in the other. Gaylor and Chen[12] confirmed the findings of Crouch and Wilson and also compared "estimated safe doses" derived from data in mice and rats. Both groups of investigators found a better correlation using body weight, not body surface area, as the basis for interspecies extrapolation of dose.

Perhaps the above correlations arose spuriously because the bioassays in both species used toxic doses. Regulators might, therefore, want to pay special attention to a substance which induces tumors at, for example, more than one site, a rarely observed site, or a site at which tissue toxicity does not occur. Such a substance might, for example, exhibit a linear dose response relationship at low doses and pose an otherwise undetected risk to large human populations. If so, better correlations of carcinogenic potency between the same organ site in two species should exist among animal carcinogens with these properties. Such a decision rule, differing from that of Tomatis and coworkers, would lead to risk assessments in which regulatory practice would vary with the biological characteristics of the animal tumor(s) induced by a substance.[13] EPA's Science Advisory Board has investigated several organ sites for possible variance from the usual risk assessment procedures.[14]

This paper initiates an investigation of what, if any, support exists for the latter decision rule by attempting to predict tumor induction by a chemical substance in one rodent species, given results in another species with the same substance.

CONCORDANCE

Concordance refers to the similarity between two objects in one or more characteristics. In the context of this paper it describes the agreement between two bioassays of the same substance in two different species, usually agreement on the statistical significance of tumor induction (see for example Ref. 15). With each organ site, we construct a 2 × 2 concordance table as follows:

		Columns	
		+	–
Rows	+	A	B
	–	C	D

Each of the columns and rows can indicate a combination of any desired characteristic of the bioassay, such as species or strains tested. They can include or exclude particular findings. The numbers A, B, C, D represent numbers of tested substances. Any desired statistical test of significance of the bioassay result can be applied, and the option exists of including weakly positive responses in either the (+) positive or (–) negative column or row.

"A" is the number of substances which are + at the chosen site(s) in the row selection and + at any chosen site(s) in the column selection.

"B" is the number of substances which are + at the chosen site(s) in the row selection and – at any chosen site(s) in the column selection.

"C" is the number of substances which are – at the chosen site(s) in the row selection and + at any chosen site(s) in the column selection.

"D" is the number of substances which are – at the chosen site(s) in the row selection and – at any chosen site(s) in the column selection.

If $B = C = 0$, the data are completely concordant for the chosen site(s), meaning that finding a tumor at some site in the row selection always guarantees a tumor at some site in the column selection. Not finding a tumor at the chosen site in the row selection guarantees not finding a tumor at any site in the column selection.

MATERIALS AND METHODS

A set of carcinogenesis bioassays performed with a relatively uniform protocol simplifies the statistical analysis of bioassay data. The NCI/NTP bioassay program has produced such data and made a summary of these data available through the Carcinogenesis Bioassay Database System (CBDS) computer tapes (Mike Rowley, personal communication). The CBDS tapes hold data on each individual animal tested in the carcinogenesis bioassays and have an additional advantage of undergoing peer review. These tapes contain a complete list of all lesions, benign and cancerous, and their sites. To obtain some measures of concordance between tumor occurrence in different tissue types and in different strains of animals, requires extensive computation. We staged these calculations, starting from the data in the CBDS tapes. At each stage of the computation, various decisions have to be made on methods of analysis, as described in the following subsections.

Tumor Site

For each animal, CBDS codes the type of neoplasia (and other lesions) found at necropsy and/or histopathological examination, according to a standard classification. The coding has considerable detail; over 4400 different classifications exist for primary neoplasia. Excessive detail would obviate the desired comparisons because the resulting small numbers would create a high variance in the results.

In the usual analyses of such bioassays pathologists combine many of the standard neoplasia classifications (for example, tumors of the same types at nearby sites or different types at the same site). Our less detailed system classified 36 organ sites as benign primary neoplasia and 66 as malignant primary neoplasia. These 102 classifications contained all the original (more detailed) classifications. This classification ignores metastatic lesions (or lesions classified as undecidable as to primary or metastatic). Nothing in this procedure prevents our returning to more interesting associations and analyzing the "fine structure" by not combining the standard classifications. Table 1 summarizes the 102 tumor classifications used in this paper.

Data Base

The CBDS data tape does not include NTP/NCI bioassays of several substances which Gulf South Research Institute conducted but which do not meet current standards of quality control. A total of 489 combinations of substances plus route of administration have some data. Most of these bioassays have data for both male and female sexes and for rat and mouse species, classified as MR, FR, MM, and FM, respectively. The data base subsumes bioassays on 18 strains of mice, hamsters and rats [7 of mice (B6C3F1, C57Bl/6Cr, Swiss Albino, Swiss CD-1, Swiss ICR, Swiss NIH, Swiss Webster), 10 of rats (ACI, August 28807, Charles River CD, F344, Long Evans, Marshall, Osborne Mendel, Sherman, Sprague Dawley, and Wistar), and 1 of hamsters (Syrian Golden)] and 7 routes of administration [intramuscular (IM), skin painting (SD), intraperitoneal (IP5), food (PO1), water (PO2), gavage (PO4) and inhalation (RE2)].

All of the CBDS experiments that met certain criteria were analyzed for the 102 tumor classifications. Each experiment consisted of groups of animals of the same strain and sex, with every group in the experiment exposed to a single substance (or a well-defined mixture of substances assigned a unique name) at a different dose. Each route of exposure counts as a separate experiment. There were 1968 such experiments potentially available for analysis. To be included in our concordance studies, an experiment also had to meet the following criteria:

a. Each experiment had to have at least one control (i.e. undosed) group, and there had to be data available on some animals in each group. Of the 1968 original experiments, 121 lacked either a control group or information on any dosed group. For some experiments, there were more than one control group and/or there were both gavage and untreated control group(s). For gavage experiments,

Table 1. Tumor Classification and Numbering

1 skin, breast papilloma, +
2 respiratory, oral + papilloma, +
3 GI papilloma, +
4 urinary, reproductive papilloma +
5 skin, breast adenoma, +
6 respiratory, oral adenoma,
7 liver adenoma, +
8 GI adenoma, +
9 urinary, reproductive adenoma, +
10 pituitary adenoma, +
11 endrocrine + adenoma, +
12 skin, urinary + adenomas
13 reproductive, endocrine + adenomas
14 tubular-cell adenoma +
15 follicular, C cell adenomas
16 cortical adenoma
17 skin, breast, liver and cystadenomas
18 GI, urinary, reproductive cystadenomas
19 endocrine cystadenomas
20 acinar cell adenoma
21 keratoacanthoma +
22 tubular adenoma +
23 interstitial cell tumor
24 pheochromocytoma +
25 skin, breast fibroma
26 blood, bone fibroma
27 fibroma, other sites
28 lipoma +
29 leiomyoma +
30 endometrial stromal polyp, +
31 fibroadenoma +
32 hemangioma +
33 osteoma +
34 hamartoma +
35 ganglioneuroma +
36 chromophobe adenoma
37 skin, breast carcinoma
38 blood, bone carcinoma
39 lung carcinoma
40 oral, GI carcinoma
41 urinary carcinoma
42 reproductive carcinoma
43 pituitary carcinoma
44 endrocrine carcinoma
45 brain carcinoma
46 skin, breast papillar carcinoma
47 lung papillary carcinoma
48 GI, urinary papillary carcinoma
49 uterus, ovary papillary carcinoma
50 thyroid papillary carcinoma
51 skin + squamous carcinoma
52 lung squamous carcinoma
53 oral, GI squamous carcinoma
54 urinary, reproductive squamouse carcinoma
55 skin, GI basal cell carcinoma
56 urinary transitional cell carcinoma
57 skin, breast adenocarcinoma
58 lung adenocarcinoma +
59 oral, GI adenocarcinoma
60 urinary, reproductive adenocarcinoma
61 endocrine, brain adenocarcinoma
62 islet cell carcinoma
63 bile duct carcinoma
64 hepatocellular carcinoma
65 alveolar, broncheolar carcinoma
66 chromaphobe carcinoma
67 tubular-cell adenocarcinoma
68 thyroid follicular cell carcinoma
69 cortical carcinoma
70 C-cell carcinoma
71 adnexal, sebaceous, + carcinoma
72 thymoma
73 granulosa-cell carcinoma
74 interstitial cell carcinoma
75 pheochromocytoma +
76 skin sarcoma +
77 other sites sarcoma +
78 blood, bone sarcoma +
79 liposarcoma
80 leimyosarcoma +
81 endometrial stromal sarcoma, +
82 carcinosarcoma +
83 mesothelioma, osteosarc, +
84 teratoma +
85 hemagiosarcoma +
86 granular cell tumor +
87 glioma
88 oligodendroglioma +
89 astrocytoma
90 olfactory neuroblastoma
91 neurofibrosarcoma
92 lymphoma
93 lymphocytic lymphoma
94 histocytic lymphoma 95 mixed lymphoma
96 malignant reticulosis
97 leukemia
98 myelomonocytic leukemia
99 lymphocytic leukemia
100 plasmactic leukemia +
101 granulocytic leukemia
102 monocytic leukemia

untreated control groups were ignored, if there was a control group subjected to sham gavage. All remaining control groups for a single experiment were combined and treated as a single control group.

b. The CBDS tapes record the details of dosing. For purposes of this analysis, relative magnitudes of the first dose administered to the different dose groups were taken as representative. However, we were not able to decipher the meaning of the data available for some of the combinations of dose route and dosing information. Other experiments (137 in all) were excluded for this reason.

c. The experiment had to continue for a sufficient period for tumor induction to occur. This analysis required that the longest lifetime recorded for any animal in the experiment exceed 70 weeks. Since control groups typically were sacrificed as soon as all dosed animals died (or sooner, if the experimental protocol demanded it), this criterion ensured that only long-term experiments were included. Seventeen of the 1968 experiments were excluded by this criterion.

Overall, applying these three criteria reduced the available number of experiments to 1693.

Statistical Methods

We first calculated statistical significance within each experiment, taking one species and sex pair at a time for each of the 102 combinations of organ site, and asking for the statistical significance separately. The results of the statistical analysis can be tabulated for any tumor site out of the 102. The most powerful use of such results is to prepare correlations directly from the results within a computer program and print the graphs. (Instead of printing intermediate results and rekeying them for further analysis.) The analysis applied to each experiment resulted in standardized measures of significance of the results and the background rate of tumor occurrence. The same procedure was followed for each of the 102 classifications of neoplasia in the 1693 experiments — a total of 172,686 analyses.

For each dosed group two measures of significance were obtained with the Fisher exact test. The first ("unadjusted") test took no account of early deaths in the experiment, while the second ("adjusted") test made some adjustment for early deaths. In addition, a mortality adjusted measure of the occurrence of a dose response relationship was computed. The exact procedure followed was as follows:

a. The total number of tumors (of the classification under analysis) in the experiment (i.e. in all groups, including the control group) was counted. If this was less than 4 no further analysis was performed, because even if all the tumors occurred in a single dose group, no measure of significance would reach a critical value. If the organ site combinations of tumors included in the classification were not examined, due to this exclusion, no further analysis was performed.

b. The tumors in each dose group were counted, and a one-sided Fisher exact significance value was computed to compare the incidence in each group with the incidence in the control group. The numbers of tumors were those at the end of the experiment. The numbers of animals at risk were taken to be either the initial numbers of animals in any given dose group (for the unadjusted analysis), or the number of animals in the given dose group at the time the first animal in any dose group was found to have a tumor of the classification under analysis (for the adjusted analysis).

c. A mortality-adjusted trend analysis was performed to obtain a measure of significance of the dose-response relationship of tumors at the organ site.[16]

d. If any of the significance values obtained by steps b or c above, was less than 0.1, all values were recorded. If all significance values exceeded 0.1, then no data on significance were recorded. Of the 172,686 products of experiments and classifications, 161,219 had fewer than 4 tumors in any dosed group, 8385 had all significance values greater than 0.1, and full data on significance values were recorded for 3082.

e. In addition to the computations performed on individual experiments, a record was kept of the background incidence of tumors in the control groups. Each experiment was classified according to its combination of species, strain, sex and route of administration of the test material to the dosed groups. For each combination, a grand total was obtained of the number of tumors of each classification seen, the total number of control animals placed on test, and the total "adjusted" number of animals as described in 2 above.

   Since there were a few experiments that shared control groups, the procedure described in the last paragraph may double count some control groups. However, since only an approximate background incidence was required at this stage, no attempt was made to correct for this. The "adjusted" numbers of animals were chosen at different times for different classifications and experiments, so that they are not truly comparable. At this stage, however, these values have not been used. The background rate of tumors are estimated by dividing the total observed number of tumors by the total (unadjusted) animals placed on test.

f. With the results of the analyses described so far, summary results were obtained for all the distinct combinations of substance, species, strain, sex and route of administration occurring in the 1693 experiments that met the inclusion criteria. For each of the 1693 experiments analyzed, a summary response classification was obtained for each of the 102 tumor classifications.

   For this analysis we defined a test as positive (+) if, at the end of the experiment, a difference of any dosed group from the control was significant at the level of $P < 0.025$ by a Fisher exact test (either adjusted or unadjusted), or two dosed groups both exhibited a significant difference from control at a level of $P < 0.05$ with the same test. We defined evidence as weak (w), if a slope test, carried out by the procedures recommended by IARC, gave a significant result at $P < 0.025$, but other results, as defined above, were not positive. Otherwise the response was labelled negative (–), provided this tumor classification had been examined in the experiment, or blank (" ") if it had not been examined. If the CBDS tapes listed more than one experiment for a given substance, both results were listed.

g. Any duplications of combinations of substance, species, strain, sex and route of administration occurring in the 1693 experiments were combined together by assigning the order + > w > – > " " to the responses, and choosing the largest response among duplicates, for each of the 102 classifications.

h. With the procedures described, each substance has an associated file of species/strain/route/sex combination, each of which has 102 associated results (+, w, –, or " "). Any list entry with entirely blank (" ") results was eliminated, since it contained no information. In addition, the summation of control animal results gave information on the background tumor rates for all species/strain/route/sex combinations. These files represent the basic data from which concordance information can be obtained.

Graphical Display

Our concordance plots graphically summarize the information contained in the files developed according to the procedures described in the previous section. The plots illustrate the concordances of tumor induction over the set of tested substances and between different species/strain/route/sex combinations. To achieve this result, we define the desired combinations and write 2 × 2 tables of numbers of chemicals classified as + or – in various groups of organ sites specified in the columns and rows of the table, as defined earlier.

		Columns		Totals
		+	–	
Rows	+	A	B	A + B
	–	C	D	C + D

From each such 2 × 2 table, we define the following coordinates for rows:

$$X = A/(A + B)$$

$$Y = D/(C + D)$$

and plot the corresponding points as X,Y coordinates in a two dimensional graph. In the figures, X = Y = 1 for complete concordance, and X = Y = 0 for a complete lack of concordance. For the trivial result of X = 1 and Y = 0, the row and column species/strain/route/sex/organ site combinations would give statistically positive results for all substances tested, whereas for X = 0 and Y = 1 the row and column species/strain/route/sex/organ site combinations would give negative results with all tested substances.

We plotted only sites where A + B > 5 and C + D > 5, omitting rare sites, unless these sites were the object of specific inquiry. Weak tumor responses (w) can be counted as either positive (+) or negative (–) in these plots. Generally, both possibilities were tested.

Confidence limits for each point were obtained by treating A/(A + B) or D/(C + D) as binomial samples from an infinite population of substances. Where shown, points for each tumor site with a specific species/strain/route/sex combinations have associated error bars representing a confidence interval corresponding to a 68%, one-sided binomial distribution (approximately one standard deviation).

The values of X = A/(A + B) and Y = D/(D + C) are respectively the positive and negative predictive values of the results defined by the rows for the results defined by the columns. Alternatively, they are respectively the sensitivity and specificity of the results defined by the columns for the results defined by the rows. We will use them in the former sense and abbreviate them as PPV and NPV (for positive and negative predictive values) because prediction is the object of our inquiry. (Thus X = PPV and Y = NPV.)

We can "amplify" visual discrimination by expanding the scale of X and/or Y and printing only a part of the coordinate system. This has been done in several of the figures in this paper, so the reader should note the coordinates of each figure before making comparisons between them.

An example may make our graphical display system clearer. We could specify the rows for mouse results with strain B6C3F1, any oral route of administration, and both sexes. We may then define the mouse organ sites to be included. The column entries could be selected from experiments using any rat strain, all oral routes, and both sexes. "All" rat organ sites could be included. (In this context the meaning of "all" is that all sites are searched and if any yields a statistically positive increase, we include it.)

Such definitions yield two 2 × 2 tables describing the appropriate results for all such tested substances. Tables 2 and 3 illustrate this example for the NTP/NCI data base. Each table compares mouse against rat by any of 3 oral routes of administration, for either sex.

Mouse		Rat
any tumor	v	any tumor

For each set of row definitions, any substance that has an associated experiment matching the row criteria, and an associated experiment matching the column criteria will contribute to one of the entries in the corresponding 2 × 2 table. In some cases our graphical procedures display the results of these tabulations as several points in one graph corresponding to different tumors to facilitate comparisons.

RESULTS

For purposes of comparison in this paper we selected all routes of ingestion for both species: gavage, diet (food), and water. This step involves selecting the options "PO1, PO2, and PO4," as noted in the legends to the accompanying figures. Unless otherwise noted we did not differentiate between strains but selected all the mouse strains listed above for the row selection and all rat strains for the column selection. Similarly, unless otherwise noted we did not differentiate the sexes but selected any male or female result. Except where noted, we display experiments with only weak (w) evidence of tumor induction as positive. (Weak responses have a statistically positive dose-response trend but no statistically significant group comparisons.)

Table 2 shows the concordance plot for all results in both species, when an experiment with weak significance is included as a negative result. Of the 145 substances found to give a statistically positive result (+) at one or more organ sites in mice, 92 (63.4%) were positive (+) at one or more sites in rats. Figure 1 shows the computer generated concordance plot of the same data. It has one point and the error bars indicate one standard deviation. The legend below the graph lists the options selected. The row options (strains, routes sexes and groups of tumors) are on the left, whereas the column options are on the right.

Table 3 and Fig. 2 show the same data when weak significance is included as a positive result. Note the change in the coordinate system. PPV improves. Now 137/187 or (73.3%) of substances which are positive in mice are also positive (+) in rats. NPV decreases. Of the substances negative (–) in mice, only 39/103 (37.9%) are also negative (–) in rats.

The remainder of the results of this paper are presented only in figures. The strains, sexes, and groups are varied as marked on the figures.

Figure 3 shows the results for many mouse organ sites, each in comparison to the induction of tumors at any rat organ site. Each mouse site was chosen separately, and a smear of points numbered in accordance with the sites listed in Table 1 results, each with approximately the same PPV but differing widely in NPV. The two points lying above this horizontal plane (7,64) represent mouse liver adenomas and carcinomas respectively as listed in Table 1. The value of the Y coordinate is greater than for other tumors or groupings. A separate paper discussed this finding in detail.[17]

As another example, we may also choose only one species of mouse — the B3C3F1 hybrid. Figure 4 repeats Fig. 1 with the variation that results refer only to the B6C3F1

Table 2. Concordance of Rat Tumor Induction with Mouse Tumor Induction
[Weak (w) significance included as (–)]

	ANY RAT TUMOR			
		+	-	totals
ANY MOUSE TUMOR	+	92	53	145
	-	60	85	145
	totals	152	138	290

Table 3. Concordance of Rat Tumor Induction with Mouse Tumor Induction
[Weak (w) significance included as (+)]

	ANY RAT TUMOR			
		+	-	totals
ANY MOUSE TUMOR	+	137	50	187
	-	64	39	103
	totals	201	89	290

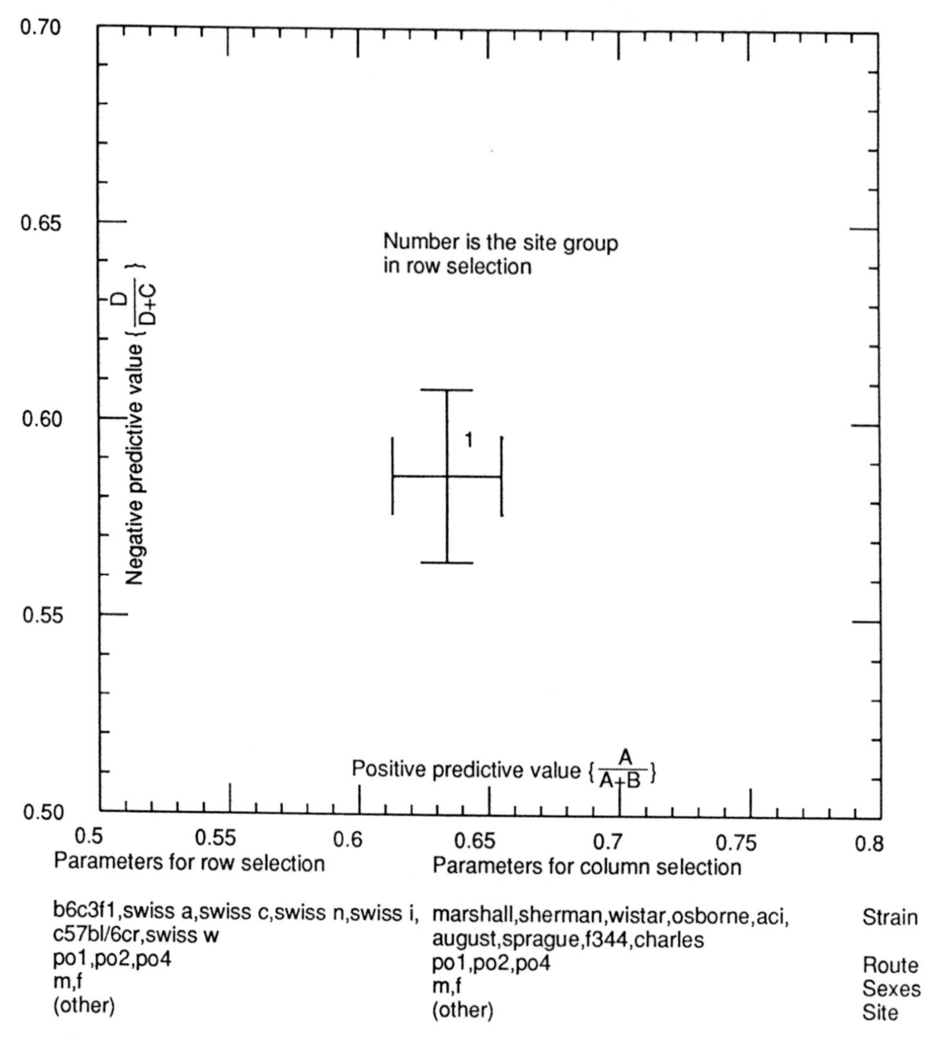

Fig. 1. A computer generated concordance plot for all results in both species when an experiment with weak significance is included as a negative result.

mouse. There is little difference because the NCI/NTP database mainly consists of experiments with B6C3F1 mice.

Figure 5 displays concordance of results between male and female B6C3F1 mice. The concordance between male and female mice is better than the concordance (Fig. 4) between rats of both sexes and mice of both sexes. Figure 6 illustrates concordance between the B6C3F1 mouse and itself. It can be regarded as a systematic check on our methods, and it yields the desired results of high concordance (unity) when rare tumors predict rare tumors but low concordance when liver tumors (either adenomas or sarcomas) (7,64) predict rare tumors in the same animal.

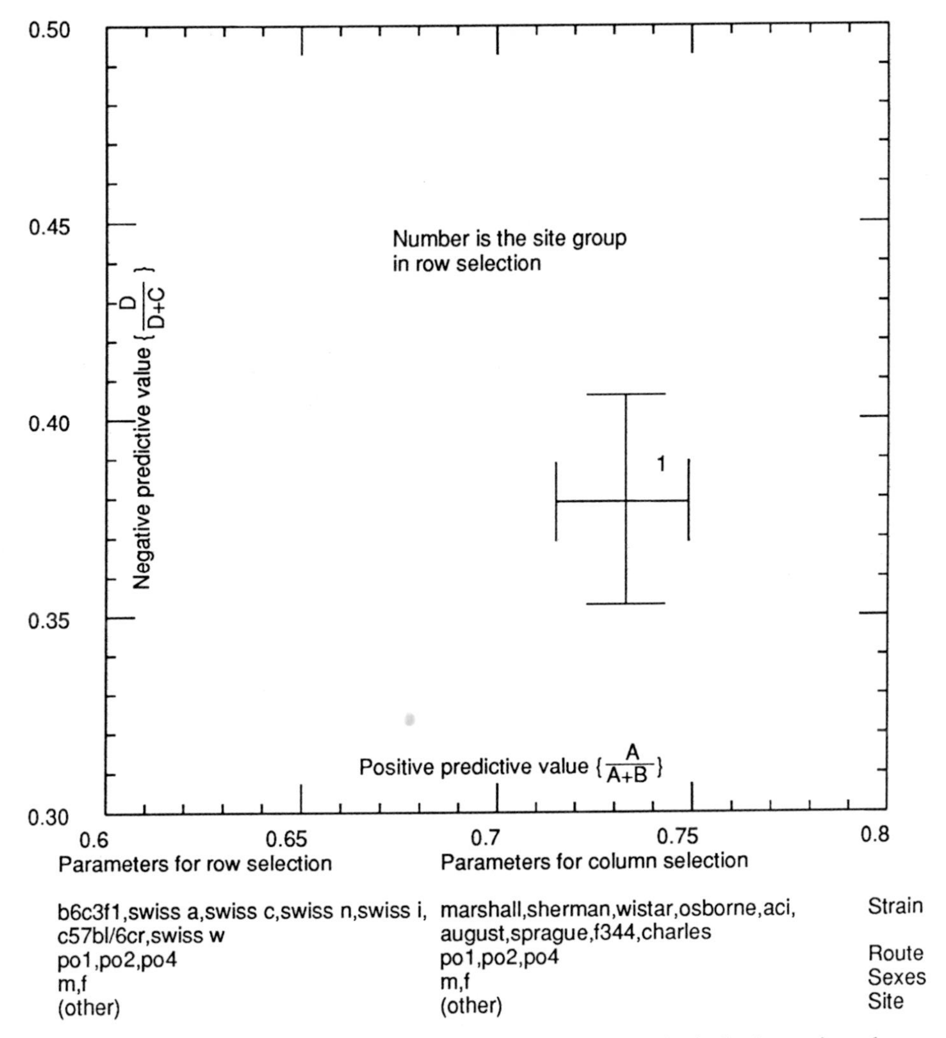

Fig. 2. A computer generated concordance plot for all results in both species when an experiment with weak significance is included as a positive result.

DISCUSSION

This paper demonstrates of some methods we devised to explore the issue of organ site concordance or tumor induction. The numerous variables within the data will require further, detailed investigation. How different choices for confidence limits will alter the amplitude of the trends, or change rankings of tumor sites, also remains for future work. Here, we limited our current analysis to only one route of administration but will compare others eventually.

Over 102 × 102 variations on these plots can be prepared with little effort. We hope that close examination of these analyses will provide leads for those studying biological mechanisms. For example the plots presented above describe all of the substances in the

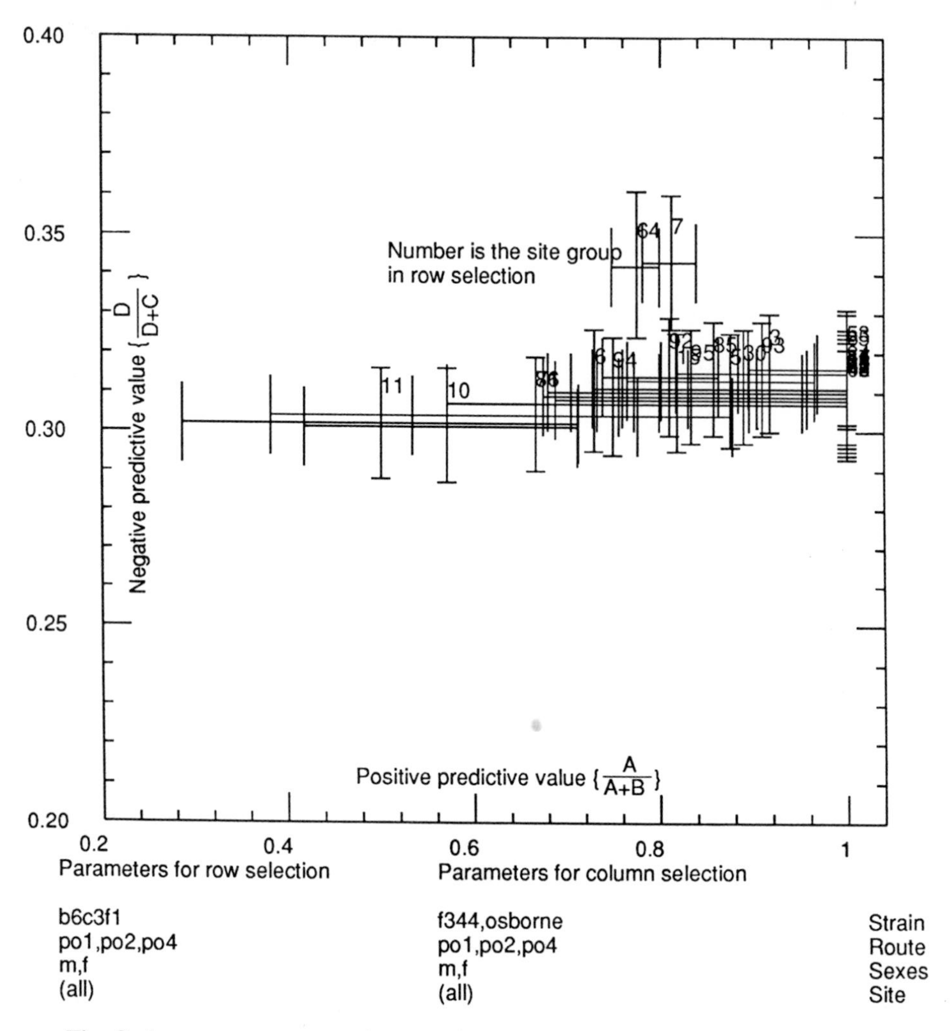

Fig. 3. A computer generated concordance plot of the results for many mouse organ sites, each in comparison to the induction of tumors at any rat organ site with weak significance counted as a positive result.

NCI/NTP computer tape. It is possible to select classes of substances from the substances in the tape and repeat the correlations. We could compare substances that are positive or negative in the Salmonella and structural analysis tests of Ashby and Tennant.[18] We could review only substances that are pesticides, only substances that are chlorinated hydrocarbons and so forth.

Concordance usually is far from complete ($X < 1$ and $Y < 1$), except in trivial situations, such as shown by point 1 in Fig. 6. In other words, if a substance yields statistically positive tumor induction at one organ site in mice, it does not always yield positive results, even for any site in rats. Moreover, a negative result for any mouse site is not particularly predictive of a negative response in rats ($Y < 0.5$).

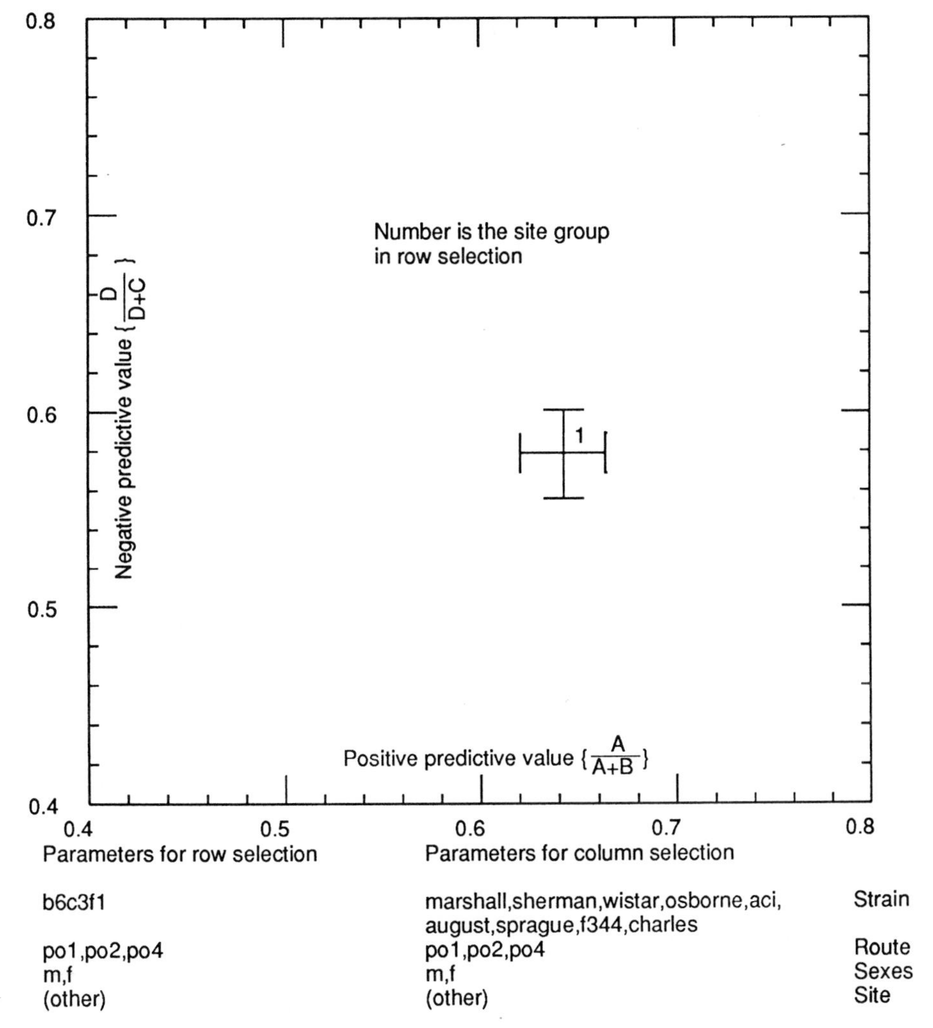

Fig. 4. A computer generated concordance plot for all results in the B6C3F1 mouse with weak significance counted as negative.

Our results (Fig. 3) show that tumors induced by a substance at a particular organ site in the mouse are not generally equivalent to tumors at other mouse organ sites in predicting the results likely to occur in another rodent species, the rat. Across all organ sites and the substances tested, the differences in prediction of a positive result in the rat, given a positive result in the mouse, varies more than the prediction of a negative result in the rat, given a negative result in the mouse (i.e., PPV varies more than NPV), although NPV was fairly low.

Different organ sites of the mouse could be quantitatively ranked according to their general utility in predicting results in the rat. The implication of this finding is that induction of tumors at the mouse organ sites with greater concordance for rat are likely to have greater capability for prediction of induction in other, nonrodent species. Conversely, we also expect that on the average those mouse tumor sites with poor concordance for rat

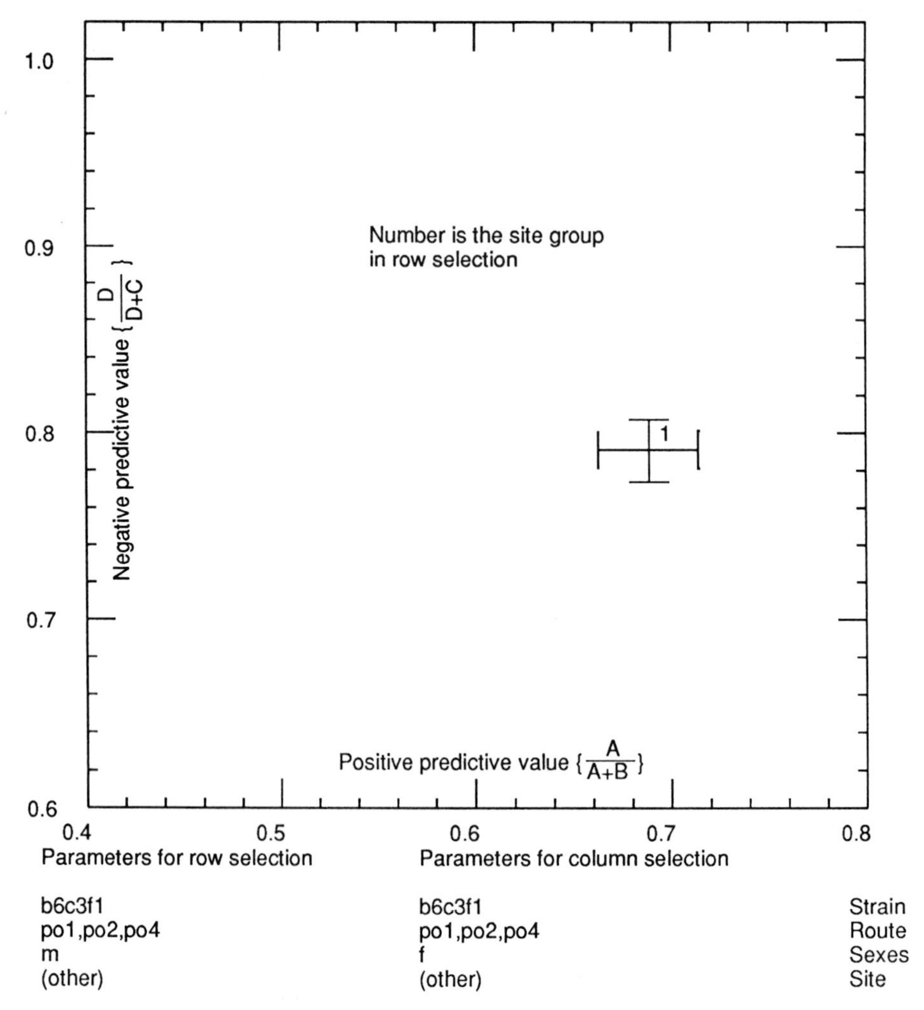

Fig. 5. A computer generated concordance plot of results between male and female B6C3F1 mice with weak significance counted as negative.

tumor induction will tend not predict the presence or absence of tumor induction in species other than the rat.

If true, the suggestion of organ specificity in extrapolation of rodent tumor induction between species will modify the current practice of both qualitative and quantitative risk assessment. When a substance induces tumors at a particular organ site, assessors could apply a relative prediction factor (possibly a quantitative factors stated as a probability) in evaluating the weight-of-the-evidence regarding the possibility of carcinogenesis in another species. When evaluating the potential potency of the substance in another species based on induction of tumors at a particular organ site, assessors also would utilize the relative prediction factor for that organ site in their quantitative model. This procedure agrees with a decision rule in which regulatory practice would vary with the biological characteristics of the animal tumor(s) induced by a substance.

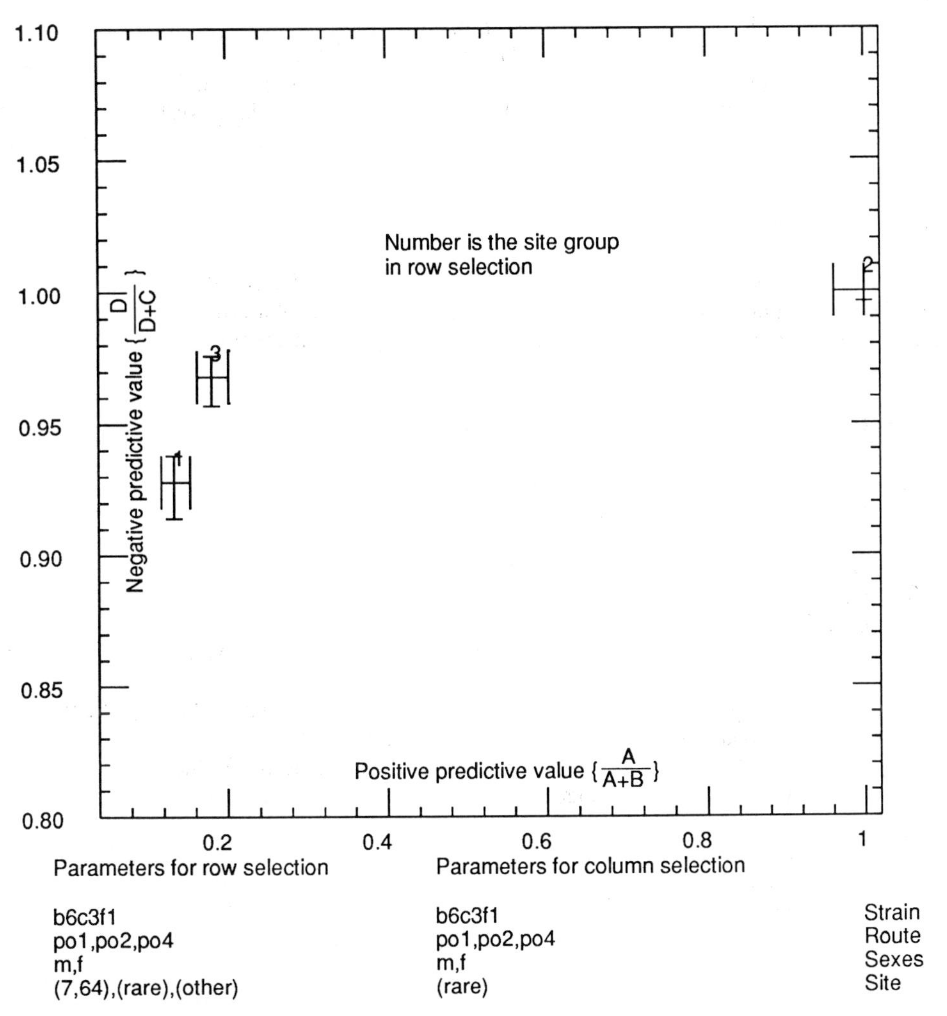

Fig. 6. A computer generated concordance plot between the B6C3F1 mouse and itself with weak significance counted as positive.

CONCLUSIONS

A graphical method has been devised to display concordance results in two dimensions. These plots facilitate the discernment of patterns in the data. Data from the NTP/NCI bioassay data base have been compiled and applied to demonstrate the method. As one example, the method demonstrates a greater concordance of tumor induction between two sexes of the same species, such as male and female mice, than between two different species, mice and rats.

Our results support the current practice of assessing carcinogenic risk at an unspecified site in one species, based on the induction of tumors at a specific organ site in a different species. However, our results also show that the magnitude of either a qualitative or quantitative risk assessment varies, when the species are rats and mice, depending on the organ site involved. Based on the assumption that induction of tumors at mouse organ sites having a greater concordance for rat sites better predicts the relevance of induction for other species. This suggests that predictions of human risk, based on tumor induction at a specific rodent site, could well vary in relation to the history of the concordance of tumor induction between rats and mice for all previously tested substances.

ACKNOWLEDGEMENTS

We thank Mike Rowley for the CBDS tapes, Bob MacDonald for assistance in modifying and running programs, and Donna Speigelman and John Bailar, who participated in the development of the 102 categories while working on a different project.

REFERENCES

1. Environmental Protection Agency, Guidelines for Carcinogen Risk Assessment, *Federal Register* **51**:33991-34003 (1986).
2. U.S. Code, Food Drug and Cosmetic Act: Food Additive Amendments of 1958, USC 21: Section 348(c)(3)(A) (1958).
3. U.S. Code, Food Drug and Cosmetic Act: Color Additive Amendments of 1960, USC 21: Section 376(b)(5)(B) (1960).
4. U.S. Code, Food Drug and Cosmetic Act: New Animal Drug Amendments of 1968, USC 21: Section 360(d)(1)(H) (1968).
5. M. R. Taylor, The *de minimis* Interpretation of the Delaney Clause: Legal and Policy Rationale, *J. Amer. Col. Toxicol.* **7**:529-537 (1988).
6. L. Tomatis, C. Partensky, and R. Montesano, The Predictive Value of Mouse Liver Tumor Induction in Carcinogenicity Testing — A Literature Survey, *Int. J. Cancer* **12**:1-20 (1973).
7. L. Tomatis, The Contribution of Epidemiological and Experimental Data to the Control of Environmental Carcinogens, *Cancer Lett.* **26**:5-16 (1985).
8. E. L. Anderson and the Carcinogen Assessment Group of the U.S. Environmental Protection Agency, Quantitative Approaches in Use to Assess Cancer Risk, *Risk Analysis* **3**:277-295 (1983).
9. E. A. C. Crouch and R. Wilson, Interspecies Comparisons of Carcinogenic Potency," *J. Tox. Environ. Health* **5**:1095-1118 (1979).
10. E. A. C. Crouch, Carcinogenic Risk Assessment: The Consequences of Believing Models, in *Organ and Species Specificity in Chemical Carcinogenesis*, pp. 653-665, R. Langenback, S. Nesnow and J. M. Rice, eds., Plenum Press, New York (1982).
11. E. A. C. Crouch, Uncertainties in Interspecies Extrapolations of Carcinogenicity, *Environ. Health Perspect.* **50**:321-327 (1983).
12. D. W. Gaylor and J. J. Chen, Relative Potency of Chemical Carcinogens in Rodents, *Risk Analysis* **6**:283-290 (1986).
13. D. M. Byrd, New Statistical Approaches to the Qualitative Interpretation of Toxicology Data, *J. Amer. Coll. Toxicol.* **7**:559-563 (1988).
14. C. R. Cothern, Summary of a Workshop on Mouse Liver Tumors and Rat Kidney Tumors, Environmental Health Committee, pp. 1-12, Science Advisory Board, U.S. EPA, Washington, DC (1987).
15. J. K. Haseman and J. E. Huff, Species Correlation in Long-Term Carcinogenicity Studies, *Cancer Lett.* **37**:125-132 (1987).
16. R. Peto, M. C. Pike, N. E. Day, R. G. Gray, P. N. Lee, S. Parish, J. Peto, S. Richards, and J. Wahrendorf, Guidelines for Simple, Sensitive Significance Tests for Carcinogenic Effects in Long-Term Animal Experiments, in *Long-Term and Short-Term Screening Assays for Carcinogenesis: A Critical Appraisal*, IARC Monographs on the Evaluation of the Carcinogenic Risk of Chemicals to Humans, Supplement 2, Lyon France (1980).

17. D. M. Byrd, E. A. C. Crouch, and R. Wilson, Do Mouse Liver Tumors Predict Rat Tumors? A Study of Concordance Between Tumors Induced at Different Sites in Rats and Mice, in *Mouse Liver Carcinogenesis: Mechanisms and Species Comparisons*, pp. 19-41, Alan R. Liss, Inc. (1990).
18. J. Ashby and R. W. Tennant, Chemical Structure, Salmonella Mutagenicity and Extent of Carcinogenicity as Indicators of Genotoxic Carcinogenesis Among 222 Chemicals Tested in Rodents by the US NCI/NTP, *Mutation Research* **204**:17-115 (1988).

Author Index

Subject Index

A

B

C

S

T

U

V

W